pharmacy review

The National Medical Series for Independent Study

pharmacy review

EDITOR

Leon Shargel, Ph.D., R.Ph.

ASSOCIATE EDITORS

Alan H. Mutnick, Pharm.D., R.Ph.
Paul F. Souney, M.S., R.Ph.
David C. Kosegarten, Ph.D., R.Ph.
Sunil Jambhekar, Ph.D.
Edward F. LaSala, Ph.D., R.Ph.
Robert L. McCarthy, M.S., R.Ph., F.A.C.A.
Anthony V. Rozzi, M.S., R.Ph.

A WILEY MEDICAL PUBLICATION
JOHN WILEY & SONS
New York • Chichester • Brisbane • Toronto • Singapore

Harwal Publishing Company, Media, Pennsylvania

The authors and publisher have made a conscientious effort to ensure that the drug information and recommended dosages in this book are accurate and in accord with accepted standards at the time of publication. However, pharmacology is a rapidly changing science, so readers are advised, before administering any drug, to check the package insert provided by the manufacturer for the recommended dose, for contraindications for administration, and for added warnings and precautions. This recommendation is especially important for new, infrequently used, or highly toxic drugs.

Senior editor: Jane Velker
Project editors: Susan Kelly, Keith LaSala, Gloria Hamilton
Editorial assistant: Judy Johnson
Illustrator and layout artist: Adriana Kulczycky
Compositors: June Sangiorgio Mash, Richard Doyle

Library of Congress Cataloging-in-Publication Data

Pharmacy review/editors, Leon Shargel . . . [et al.].
p. cm.—(A Wiley medical publication)
Includes index.
ISBN 0-471-85700-9 (pbk.)
1. Pharmacy—Examinations, questions, etc. I. Shargel, Leon, 1941– . II. Series.
[DNLM: 1. Pharmacy—examination questions. QV 18 P53751]
RS97.P49 1988
615'.1'076—dc19
DNLM/DLC
for Library of Congress 88-39083
CIP

10 9 8 7 6 5 4 3 2

Dedication

To Deborah Ptak, R. Ph., Brigham and Women's Hospital, catalyst for this book, with gratitude and love.

Contents

Contributors

Lyndon D. Braun, Pharm.D., M.B.A., R.Ph.
Staff Pharmacist
Brigham and Women's Hospital
Boston, Massachusetts

Robert J. Cersosimo, Pharm.D., R.Ph.
Associate Professor of Clinical Pharmacy
Northeastern University College of Pharmacy and Allied Health Professions
Boston, Massachusetts

Louise Glassner Cohen, Pharm.D., R.Ph.
Associate Professor of Clinical Pharmacy
Massachusetts College of Pharmacy and Allied Health Sciences
Clinical Pharmacist, Infectious Diseases and Pharmacokinetics
Brigham and Women's Hospital
Boston, Massachusetts

Helen L. Figge, Pharm.D., R.Ph.
Clinical Research Fellow
Brigham and Women's Hospital
Boston, Massachusetts

Kathryn A. Huntley, B.S., M.B.A., R.Ph.
Health Physicist
Health Physics Services, Inc.
Rockville, Maryland

Sunil Jambhekar, Ph.D.
Associate Professor of Pharmaceutics and Industrial Pharmacy
Massachusetts College of Pharmacy and Allied Health Sciences
Boston, Massachusetts

John E. Janosik, Pharm.D., R.Ph.
Manager, Drug Information
Kaiser Foundation Health Plan of Ohio
Cleveland, Ohio

David C. Kosegarten, Ph.D., R.Ph.
Associate Professor of Pharmacology and Toxicology
Massachusetts College of Pharmacy and Allied Health Sciences
Boston, Massachusetts

Susan A. Krikorian, M.S., R.Ph.
Assistant Professor of Clinical Pharmacy
Massachusetts College of Pharmacy and Allied Health Sciences
Boston, Massachusetts

E. Paul Larrat, M.B.A., R.Ph.
Coordinator, Ambulatory Care Programs
University of Rhode Island
Kingston, Rhode Island

Edward F. LaSala, Ph.D., R.Ph.
Professor of Chemistry
Massachusetts College of Pharmacy and Allied Health Sciences
Boston, Massachusetts

S. James Matthews, Pharm.D., R.Ph.
Associate Professor of Clinical Pharmacy
Northeastern University College of Pharmacy and Allied Health Professions
Boston, Massachusetts

Robert L. McCarthy, M.S., R.Ph., F.A.C.A.
Assistant Professor of Pharmacy
Massachusetts College of Pharmacy and Allied Health Sciences
Boston, Massachusetts

Glenda Meneilly, Pharm.D., R.Ph.
formerly Assistant Professor of Clinical Pharmacy
Massachusetts College of Pharmacy and Allied Health Sciences
Boston, Massachusetts

Alan H. Mutnick, Pharm.D., R.Ph.
Associate Director, Clinical Support Services
Memorial Medical Center
Springfield, Illinois

Joseph F. Palumbo, M.S., R.Ph.
Clinical Assistant Professor of Pharmacy (retired)
Northeastern University College of Pharmacy and Allied Health Professions
Boston, Massachusetts

Barbara Schlienz Prosser, B.S.
Pharmacy Supervisor
New England Health Resources
Boston, Massachusetts

Gurvinder Singh Rekhi, M.S.
Formulation Scientist
Barr Laboratories, Inc.
Pomona, New York

Anthony V. Rozzi, M.S., R.Ph.
formerly Assistant Professor of Pharmacy Practice
Massachusetts College of Pharmacy and Allied Health Sciences
Boston, Massachusetts

Leon Shargel, Ph.D., R.Ph.
Associate Professor of Pharmacy and Pharmacology
Massachusetts College of Pharmacy and Allied Health Sciences
Boston, Massachusetts

Robert A. Smaglia, M.S., R.Ph.
Director of Pharmacy Services
New England Health Resources
Boston, Massachusetts

Paul F. Souney, M.S., R.Ph.
Assistant Director of Pharmacy for Research Education and Drug Information
Brigham and Women's Hospital
Assistant Clinical Professor
Northeastern University College of Pharmacy and Allied Health Professions
Adjunct Professor of Clinical Pharmacy
Massachusetts College of Pharmacy and Allied Health Sciences
Boston, Massachusetts

Cheryl A. Stoukides, Pharm.D., R.Ph.
Drug Information Fellow
Brigham and Women's Hospital
Boston, Massachusetts

Larry N. Swanson, Pharm.D., R.Ph.
Associate Professor of Clinical Pharmacy
Northeastern University College of Pharmacy and Allied Health Professions
Boston, Massachusetts

Barbara Szymusiak-Mutnick, M.H.P., R.Ph.
Staff Pharmacist
Memorial Medical Center
Springfield, Illinois

Nelson S. Yee, B.S., R.Ph.
Medical Student
Cornell University Medical College
New York, New York

Preface

Our initial plan for *Pharmacy Review* was modest enough—to produce a comprehensive study guide for pharmacy students who are preparing for the NABPLEX®. Accordingly, we set out to develop outlines and practice questions for the subjects in the pharmacy school curriculum. These, along with the separate booklet of simulated NABPLEX® exams that supplements this review, would provide both guidance and test practice for NABPLEX® candidates.

What actually materialized is something more ambitious. While the principal market for *Pharmacy Review* remains NABPLEX® candidates, the book is also intended for a broader audience of pharmacy undergraduates and professionals who seek detailed summaries of pharmacy subjects. Encompassed by the review is a range of topics central to the study of pharmacy—chemistry, pharmaceutics, pharmacology, pharmacy practice, clinical pharmacy—organized to parallel the pharmacy curriculum and presented in outline form for easy use. It can therefore be used as a quick review (or preview) of essential topics by a diverse group of readers, including:

- Matriculating pharmacy students. The organization and topical coverage of *Pharmacy Review* is such that many pharmacy students will want to purchase it in their freshman year and use it throughout their undergraduate training in preparing for course examinations.
- Instructors and preceptors. *Pharmacy Review* also functions as a generic instructor's manual and a reference for teachers and tutors in pharmacy schools. Chapter outlines can be used to organize courses and to plan specific lectures.
- Professional pharmacists. *Pharmacy Review* offers practitioners a convenient handbook of pharmacy facts. It can be used as a course refresher and as a source of recent information on pharmacy practice. The appendices include prescription dispensing information, common prescription drugs, and general pharmacy references.

This volume represents the contributions of nearly 2 dozen specialists, each delivering a state-of-the-art summary of his or her field to a review guide that is not only accurate and up-to-date, but also comprehensible to students, teachers, and practitioners alike. If you have any suggestions on how we might improve *Pharmacy Review*, please write us at Harwal Publishing Company, P.O. Box 96, Media, PA 19063.

Introduction to the NABPLEX®

The profession of pharmacy has changed significantly during the last 3 decades. Pharmacy has evolved from the practice of preparing, preserving, compounding, and dispensing drugs to a patient-oriented practice, in which the pharmacist not only must understand the biologic and chemical nature of drugs but also must be a knowledgeable health professional. The formal education of the pharmacist has reflected these changes by an increase in the required years of education and by an increase in the emphasis on both behavioral and clinical sciences.

After graduating from an accredited pharmacy program, the prospective pharmacist must demonstrate that he or she has the competency to practice pharmacy. Currently, every state and the District of Columbia require that the graduate pass an examination for licensure to practice pharmacy. Most states use the National Association of Boards of Pharmacy Licensure Examination (NABPLEX®), which is administered three times a year (January, June, and September) by the National Association of Boards of Pharmacy (NABP®).

The standards of competence for the practice of pharmacy are set by each state board. The NABPLEX® is not a competitive examination; however, it is the principal instrument used by the state boards of pharmacy to assess the knowledge and proficiency necessary for a candidate to practice pharmacy. All NABPLEX® questions are based upon competency statements, which are reviewed and revised periodically. The competency statements summarize the knowledge that the candidate is expected to have acquired and to be able to demonstrate.

The NABPLEX® was introduced to state boards in 1976 and was composed of five subtests: pharmacy, mathematics, chemistry, pharmacology, and pharmacy practice. These tests examined basic skills and knowledge without regard to geographic or practice setting. Because of the evolution of pharmacy practice, the current NABPLEX® has a new integrated format, focusing on patient profiles and practice situations. According to NABP®, the intent of the test is to approximate practice conditions as closely as possible and to examine the basic skills and knowledge a pharmacist needs.

Competency Statements

The following Competency Statements are those in effect for the 1989–1990 NABPLEX® testing cycle. Please consult the latest edition of *NABPLEX: A Condidate's Review Guide*, published by NABP®, for a current listing of competency statements.

1.00.00 Interpreting and Dispensing Prescriptions/Medication Orders

(25% of total test)

1.01.00 Given a prescription or medication order, or relevant information about the patient's disease state, the candidate shall demonstrate the ability to gather, accurately interpret and evaluate the information, and to make a professional judgment whether or not the prescription/medication order should be filled.

- 1.01.01 Given medication orders, the candidate shall exhibit an understanding of these orders as they relate to a patient's condition and therapy.
- 1.01.02 Given physicians' orders other than those for medications (eg, radiological procedures, respiratory therapy, diet), the candidate shall be able to interpret them and to identify their relationship to drug therapy.
- 1.01.03 Given relevant information about a patient, the candidate shall be able to identify the disease, symptoms, or medical disorder.
- 1.01.04 Given relevant information about a patient, the candidate shall be able to identify agents or tests used in diagnosis and parameters useful to monitor response to treatment.
- 1.01.05 Given a medical or scientific term, the candidate shall be able to define and exhibit knowledge of such terminology.

1.02.00 The candidate shall be able to identify a drug or product ingredient in a prescription/medication order by its generic, trade, and/or common name, to identify the therapeutic use or pharmacological rationale for use of the drug(s), and to identify the known or postulated site and/or mechanism of action, and shall be able to:

- 1.02.01 identify the pharmacologically active ingredients of a combination product and the rationale for their presence.

Reprinted by permission from *NABPLEX®: A Candidate's Review Guide*, copyright 1989, NABP®.

1.03.00 Given the name of a drug, its pharmacological or chemical class, or the name of a drug and its chemical formula/structure, the candidate shall be able to:

1.03.01 identify the functional group (eg, alcohol, amide, ester) and/or major class (eg, alkaloid, glycoside, thiazide) to which it belongs, and shall be able to identify:

- those physical/chemical factors that can lead to deterioration of the drug and to recognize the signs of such deterioration;
- those physical/chemical properties that affect solubility;

1.03.02 predict its metabolic transformations (eg, conjugation, hydrolysis, oxidation) and those of chemically related substances;

1.03.03 define and interpret commonly used terms associated with chemical and physical phenomena (eg, pKa, pH, adsorption, complexation, ionization, radiation, titration) that are relevant to the drug.

1.04.00 The candidate shall be able to determine the rationale of the dosage regimen, and shall be able to:

1.04.01 determine if the dose or dosage regimen prescribed is nontoxic or falls within the usual range for the patient and the condition being treated to achieve the desired therapeutic response;

1.04.02 determine whether it is practical to measure and administer the prescribed dose;

1.04.03 calculate the dose and/or rate of administration of a drug when given appropriate data;

1.04.04 determine whether the desired dose or drug strength is commercially available;

1.04.05 identify and/or evaluate the appropriate route of administration (eg, oral, parenteral, rectal, inhalation, percutaneous, ophthalmic); and shall be able to:

- apply pertinent physical and chemical characteristics of drugs to evaluate the suitability of the route of administration;
- describe the pharmacokinetic characteristics of the route of administration;
- determine the method of delivery for the route of administration (eg, enteral/parenteral nutritional administration, IV administration sets, infusion pumps, hyperalimentation techniques, retention enema procedures);

1.04.06 evaluate the suitability of the dosage form to best accommodate patient compliance; to describe/compare characteristics of dosage forms (eg, parenteral, solid versus liquid, suppository versus enema); and to define/explain:

- terminology related to dosage forms and delivery systems (e.g., film coating, enteric coating);
- release mechanisms, performance characteristics and manufacturing processes for dosage forms and delivery systems (eg, osmotic pumps).

1.05.00 The candidate shall demonstrate the ability to dispense a prescription/medication order by using proper techniques for measuring, counting, or transferring the medication, and shall be able to:

1.05.01 select the appropriate product and dosage form, identify the characteristic physical appearance of commercially available drugs, and identify the quantities required to be dispensed and/or the prepackaged unit-of-use;

1.05.02 recognize the purpose(s) for the inclusion of pharmaceutical ingredients (eg, excipients, preservatives, lubricants) in the formulation of a commercial dosage form;

1.05.03 select the packaging and container most appropriate for the quantity of the dosage form to ensure stability to light, temperature, and/or moisture, and to provide patient convenience, including:

- selection of a container to encourage patient compliance;
- recommendation of any appropriate additional apparatus necessary for drug administration.

1.05.04 identify the appropriate storage and/or handling conditions for the prescription/medication order.

1.06.00 Given a prescription/medication order, the candidate shall be able to select the proper labeling, including auxiliary/cautionary labeling, and to demonstrate knowledge of why such labeling is appropriate.

2.00.00
Assessing Prescriptions/Medication Orders and the Drugs Used in Dispensing Them
(10% of total test)

2.01.00 The candidate shall be able to identify patient and pharmacokinetic factors that affect either the efficacy or safety of individual drug therapy, including:

2.01.01 the influence of patient factors on drug therapy (eg, age, weight, sex, occupation, compliance, exercise, stress, placebo effect);

2.01.02 biopharmaceutical principles and pharmacokinetic factors (eg, absorption, distribution, metabolism, excretion) as they relate to dosage regimen design and evaluation of experimental and patient data, including the:

- definition and explanation of biopharmaceutical terminology;
- recognition of the effects of patient health status and concurrent drug therapy on bioavailability;
- determination of pharmacokinetic parameters and dosing regimens (eg, loading dose estimations, maintenance dose calculation, elimination half-life, determinations of clearance and volume of distribution);
- recognition of biosocial factors that affect pharmacokinetic parameters (eg, smoking, alcohol consumption, work environment).

2.02.00 The candidate shall be able to assess the physical/chemical equivalency of multisource drugs, and shall be able to:

- 2.02.01 demonstrate knowledge of how quality assurance data (eg, tests for assay, contamination level, identity, purity, content uniformity, disintegration, dissolution, and sterility) are used to determine equivalency among manufactured drug products;
- 2.02.02 demonstrate familiarity with the procedures used to analyze drugs and/or their metabolites in dosage forms and in body fluids, and shall be able to:
  - define physicochemical terminology and evaluate those properties that can affect product formulation;
  - predict formulation stability by evaluating drug molecular structure;
  - interpret stability data.

2.03.00 Given appropriate information and/or data regarding bioavailability, the candidate shall demonstrate the ability to:

- 2.03.01 interpret and utilize in vitro dissolution test results used to predict bioequivalence and distinguish these from in vivo tests;
- 2.03.02 define, interpret, and distinguish between relative and absolute bioavailability;
- 2.03.03 interpret the area under the curve for plasma concentration versus time as an assessment of bioavailability;
- 2.03.04 explain the effects of rate of absorption on peak concentrations and time of peak concentrations after oral administration;
- 2.03.05 predict the possible effect of excipients and formulation factors on the rate and extent of drug absorption;
- 2.03.06 identify drugs that are suitable for bioavailability testing by urinary excretion rate, including the application of urinary excretion rate data, when feasible;
- 2.03.07 identify the drugs for which documented evidence of bioinequivalence exists and to suggest how their use might lead to serious adverse drug effects.

2.04.00 The candidate shall demonstrate the ability to locate information necessary to provide clarification or answers to prescription, medication order, or health care questions and demonstrate the ability to evaluate that information, to:

- 2.04.01 select appropriate books and references concerning bioequivalence, drugs for emergency situations, physical and chemical stability, incompatibility, etc;
- 2.04.02 evaluate the appropriateness, accuracy, and reliability of information from literature sources (eg, pharmacokinetic characteristics, adverse effects, therapeutic efficacy);
- 2.04.03 distinguish between adequate and inadequate experimental design;
- 2.04.04 apply statistical principles to the interpretation of drug literature (eg, P-value, null hypothesis, test for significance);
- 2.04.05 analyze and interpret data presented in tabular or graphic form;

2.04.06 apply information appropriately when given an excerpt from scientific literature, recognized reference texts, professional papers/articles, or manufacturer's labeling/promotional material.

3.00.00 Compounding and Calculation Involved in the Extemporaneous Preparation of Prescriptions/Medication Orders

(15% of total test)

3.01.00 Given a prescription/medication order, the candidate shall demonstrate competent professional judgment and proper technique in compounding and dispensing, such as:

- 3.01.01 knowledge of the special procedures, ingredients, appropriate equipment, possible problems, and correct techniques needed to compound extemporaneous prescriptions; knowledge of the correct strength and concentration of active ingredients, and appropriate labeling; and the ability to perform the required tasks for the preparation of dosage forms such as capsules, creams, lotions, ointments, suppositories, urethral and vaginal inserts, powders, emulsions, suspensions, and nonsterile solutions;
- 3.01.02 recognition of the techniques needed to combine ingredients into an appropriate dosage form by using the most effective method based on the properties of the ingredients and the product to be compounded in the practice environment;
- 3.01.03 selection of proper labeling including auxiliary/precautionary labeling.

3.02.00 Given one or more prescriptions/medication orders, the candidate shall be able to determine if the formulation(s) should be altered, to identify the course of action/suitable remedy for physical and/or chemical incompatibilities, and to demonstrate knowledge of:

- 3.02.01 the condition of the ingredient(s) by recognizing the physical and chemical signs of degradation;
- 3.02.02 physical and/or chemical incompatibilities (eg, acid-base, precipitation, oxidation, color change, hydrolysis) and terminology (eg, activation energy, decomposition constant);
- 3.02.03 methods of stabilization, including data interpretation (eg, complexation, micellization, selection of buffers and/or vehicles).

3.03.00 Given a prescription or medication order, the candidate shall be able to make necessary basic calculations required to compound and dispense, including the ability to:

- 3.03.01 reduce or enlarge a given quantity expressed in usual units or proportional parts;

3.03.02 interpret the meaning of molarity, normality, weight in weight, volume in volume, or weight in volume percentage or ratio strength preparations, and to calculate the quantity of active ingredient(s) or diluent needed to make the proper amount of the preparation.

3.04.00 The candidate shall demonstrate the ability to select proper ingredients used to compound and dispense extemporaneous preparations and shall identify:

3.04.01 appropriate ingredients by various chemical or common names;

3.04.02 physicochemical properties of an ingredient (eg, acid-base characteristics, solubility, particle size).

3.05.00 The candidate shall demonstrate the ability to perform specialized pharmaceutical calculations.

3.05.01 Given a prescription/medication order, the candidate shall be able to calculate the amount of agent needed to render a solution isotonic with body fluids.

3.05.02 Given a prescription/medication order, the candidate shall demonstrate knowledge of the relationship of pH and pK_a to ionization and solubility.

3.05.03 Given the appropriate data, the candidate shall be able to convert the concentrations of solutions expressed in usual units to milliequivalents, millimoles, and milliosmoles per unit volume of solution.

3.05.04 Given a nutritional order, the candidate shall be able to convert concentration units for each source to calories, and vice versa, and to determine nutritional content in appropriate units.

3.06.00 The candidate shall demonstrate knowledge of proper aseptic technique and the ability to prepare sterile products. The candidate shall demonstrate knowledge of the methods used to:

3.06.01 extemporaneously prepare small and large volume preparations for immediate use (eg, IV admixtures, parenteral nutrition, cancer chemotherapy; IM, SC, and intradermal preparations; ophthalmic preparations; and bladder irrigations);

3.06.02 sterilize products (eg, filtration, gas, dry heat, moist heat).

3.07.00 The candidate shall demonstrate knowledge of proper storage of compounded preparations in accordance with temperature, light, and moisture conditions, and shall be able to:

3.07.01 evaluate vulnerability of compounded medications to oxygen, pH, solvent, light, temperature, and moisture; and identify proper storage conditions (eg, evaluate published stability data);

3.07.02 evaluate stability in various containers and administration devices (eg, glass, plastic, catheters, sets, infusion pumps, unit dose).

4.00.00
Monitoring Drug Therapy
(25% of total test)

4.01.00 Given a medical history, medication record, drug therapy history, or a set of prescriptions/medication orders, the candidate shall be able to monitor the patient's therapy as assessed by the ability to:

- 4.01.01 recognize appropriate drug therapy, including the drug of choice and other therapeutic measures to treat the condition;
- 4.01.02 recognize therapeutic endpoints (eg, appropriate length of therapy, desired response versus observed response, specific maximum and/or minimum drug serum levels);
- 4.01.03 identify, collect, and evaluate patient information (eg, pharmacokinetic parameters, lab test results, sensitivities, and clinical observations);
- 4.01.04 recognize and remedy therapeutic problems such as:
  - inappropriate prescribing, duplicate prescribing;
  - iatrogenic and/or drug-induced illness;
  - noncompliance;
  - signs of drug misuse and abuse.

4.02.00 The candidate shall recognize and recommend appropriate action regarding interactions or contraindications that involve prescription/OTC products in conjunction with:

- 4.02.01 other drugs being taken;
- 4.02.02 disease states;
- 4.02.03 diagnostic tests and procedures;
- 4.02.04 personal habits, sensitivities, allergies, genetic, and environmental factors;
- 4.02.05 diet.

4.03.00 The candidate shall demonstrate the ability to recognize major precautions, warnings, adverse/side effects, and toxicity associated with a drug in a patient's regimen, and shall be able to:

- 4.03.01 identify the mechanism(s) responsible for an adverse effect;
- 4.03.02 determine if a drug in the patient's regimen is causing an adverse/side effect or toxicity;
- 4.03.03 identify major symptoms of drug toxicity;
- 4.03.04 identify appropriate action to remedy or prevent an adverse/side effect or toxicity.

5.00.00
Counseling Patients and Health Professionals
(25% of total test)

5.01.00 The candidate shall demonstrate the ability to counsel a patient or health professional on the indications, benefits, administration, storage, and adverse effects of prescription medications, and shall be able to:

- 5.01.01 explain the proper procedure to take or administer the drug (eg, dosage, time of day, method and time of administration—before or after meals, duration of use), and to provide auxiliary instructions about the medication;
- 5.01.02 describe the principal untoward effects of drug use, and be able to demonstrate knowledge of how to minimize the chance of significant side effects;
- 5.01.03 explain cautions regarding food and/or drugs to avoid while taking the medication;
- 5.01.04 explain cautions for use by special populations (eg, geriatrics, racial groups) and for use in special conditions (eg, diabetes, cystic fibrosis);
- 5.01.05 explain the proper storage conditions for a given medication.

5.02.00 Given a patient's profile or medication record, the candidate shall be able to provide specific information about the patient's disease state or medical condition.

5.03.00 The candidate shall be able to describe activities for emergency patient care, and shall be able to:

- 5.03.01 recognize the manifestations of poisoning from prescription and OTC drugs and from other toxic substances;
- 5.03.02 identify the recommended corrective treatment and/or referral for ingestion of toxic doses of drugs and for substance abuse;
- 5.03.03 select the main indications, when given a common antidote or antidotal procedure; to describe the suspected or identified mechanism of antagonism; to identify the major side effects and drawbacks; and to suggest additional supportive antidotal measures;
- 5.03.04 identify emergency procedures for burns, wounds, eye/ear problems, etc.

5.04.00 The candidate shall be able to identify the name, correct therapeutic classification, pharmacological action, and/or ingredients of OTC drugs, and shall be able to:

- 5.04.01 determine whether a given drug is for prescription only or is also available OTC;
- 5.04.02 evaluate OTC drugs based on available literature and product information.

5.05.00 The candidate shall be able to advise consumers on the selection, proper use, effects, precautions, and contraindications of OTC drugs, and to:

- 5.05.01 determine whether the patient's condition requires medical supervision or self-medication;
- 5.05.02 explain the drug's action in terms that the consumer can understand;
- 5.05.03 explain the correct way to take the drug (eg, dosage, time of day, before or after meals);

5.05.04 explain auxiliary instructions about the medication;

5.05.05 communicate the recommended duration of use for the medication;

5.05.06 identify and explain the effects and potential interactions of the OTC drug;

5.05.07 communicate cautions to special populations, if appropriate (eg, diabetic, asthmatic, hypertensive, and geriatric/pediatric patients);

5.05.08 explain the implications of product stability and describe the proper storage conditions for the medication;

5.05.09 recommend seeking professional advice if the medication causes an untoward effect or lacks therapeutic effect.

5.06.00 The candidate shall demonstrate an understanding of the use of medical/surgical appliances and devices, durable medical equipment, and prescription accessories and shall demonstrate the ability to counsel properly concerning their selection, use, and storage (eg, thermometers; ostomy appliances; contraceptives; catheters; needles, syringes, and diabetic supplies; diagnostics; and contact lens preparations).

5.07.00 The candidate shall demonstrate knowledge of contemporary public health issues and the principles of nutrition in relation to the disease and treatment of a patient, and shall be able to:

5.07.01 recognize and describe nutrient needs and identify:

- interactions of vitamins, minerals, and other food components with medications;
- common disease conditions and symptoms caused by vitamin and mineral deficiencies or overutilization;
- natural sources of vitamins and minerals;
- nonessential substances found in nutritional supplements;

5.07.02 apply knowledge of biochemistry to nutrition and drug treatment that relate to:

- prenatal/postnatal care;
- pediatric nutritional requirements (formulas);
- adult care;
- enteral alimentation and hyperalimentation;

5.07.03 recognize procedures appropriate to prevent and/or minimize the progression of a disease (eg, herpes, AIDS, cancer, chemical dependency, cardiovascular disease).

Part I
Pharmaceutics and Biopharmaceutics

Sunil Jambhekar
Leon Shargel

1
Pharmaceutical Calculations

Sunil Jambhekar

I. FUNDAMENTALS OF MEASUREMENT AND CALCULATION

A. Numbers and numerals

1. A **number** is a total quantity or amount of units.
2. A **numeral** is a word, sign, or group of words and signs representing a number. For example, the numeral 2 represents the number that is two times the unit 1.

B. Arabic numerals

1. Arabic numerals—a zero and nine digits—are a form of notation based on a **decimal system**, in which values assigned to digits depend on the place they occupy in a row.
2. The value of a digit **increases tenfold** each time it moves one place to the **left** of the decimal point; the value **decreases tenfold** each time it moves one place to the **right**.
3. A **zero** marks any place not occupied by a digit.
4. The **total value** of any number expressed by Arabic numerals is the sum of the values of its digits as determined by their position.

C. Roman numerals

1. **Roman numerals**, in contrast to Arabic numerals, express numbers by use of a few letters of the alphabet. They **are customarily used to designate quantities on prescriptions** when ingredients are measured by the apothecaries' system.
2. The **position** of a Roman numeral **indicates whether to add or subtract the numeral from a succession of bases** ranging from values of 1 to 1000. These eight fixed values (bases) are used:
   a. **ss** = ½
   b. **I** (or **i**) = 1
   c. **V** (or **v**) = 5
   d. **X** (or **x**) = 10
   e. **L** (or **l**) = 50
   f. **C** (or **c**) = 100
   g. **D** (or **d**) = 500
   h. **M** (or **m**) = 1000
3. Other quantities are expressed by **combining these letters** (Table 1-1).

II. CONVERSIONS

A. Necessity. Conversions—translations of measurements made in one system into equivalent values in another system—are **frequently required in pharmacy.**

B. Practical equivalents

1. The **metric**, **avoirdupois** (weight), **U.S. liquid measure** (volume), and **apothecaries'** (volume and weight) systems all differ and require conversion when quantities must be compared. That is, **all quantities must be converted to a single system** (Table 1-2).
2. The accuracy of conversion factors for pharmacy has not been satisfactorily established. The United States Pharmacopeia (USP) permits the pharmacist to dispense **prepared dosage forms** (such as tablets and capsules) in approximate equivalents; that is, for a prepared drug

Table 1-1. Guidelines for the Use of Roman Numeral Designations of Pharmaceutical Quantities

Rule

Two or more letters express a quantity that is the **sum of their values** if they are **successively equal or smaller in value.**

Examples

ii = 2	xxii = 22	ci = 101	mx = 1010
iii = 3	li = 51	cl = 150	mc = 1100
vi = 6	lv = 55	cc = 200	md = 1500
xi = 11	lx = 60	dv = 505	mdclxvi = 1666
xv = 15	lxxvii = 77	dc = 600	mm = 2000
xx = 20			

Rule

Two or more letters express a quantity that is the **sum of the values remaining after the value of each smaller letter is subtracted from the value of a following greater letter.**

Examples

iv = 4	xxiv = 24	xcix = 99	cm = 900
ix = 9	xl = 40	cd = 400	cmxcix = 999
xiv = 14	xliv = 44	cdxl = 440	mcdxcii = 1492
xix = 19	xc = 90	cdxliv = 444	

prescribed in metric values, an approximate equivalent in apothecaries' values may be dispensed, and vice versa.

a. These **equivalent values** are listed in the USP Table of Metric–Apothecaries' Approximate Dose Equivalents. Table 1-3 provides conversions sufficient for all practical purposes.

b. The USP directs that **exact equivalents** must be used for conversion of specific quantities when converting formulas; exact equivalents rounded to three significant figures must be used for compounding prescriptions.

III. RATIOS, PROPORTIONS, AND PERCENTAGES

A. Ratios. A ratio is the **relation of two like quantities expressed as a common fraction** (e.g., 10/5 represents the ratio of 10 and 5). When a fraction is to be interpreted as a ratio, it is written **10:5** and always read as "10 to 5." The rules governing common fractions apply to ratios.

1. If the two terms of a ratio are **multiplied or divided by the same number**, the **value of the ratio is unchanged**. For example, the ratio of 15:3 (or 15/3) has a value of 5. If both terms are multiplied by 2, the ratio becomes 30:6 (or 30/6) and still has the value of 5.

Table 1-2. Common Conversion Equivalents

Length

1 meter (m) = 39.37 inches (in)
1 in = 2.54 centimeters (cm)

Volume

1 milliliter (ml) = 16.23 minims (♏)
1 ♏ = 0.06 ml
1 fluidram (*f* ʒ) = 3.696 ml
1 fluidounce (*f* ℥) = 29.573 ml
1 pint (pt) = 473 ml
1 gallon U.S. (gal) = 3785 ml

Weight

1 gram (g) = 15.432 grains (gr)
1 kilogram (kg) = 2.20 pounds avoirdupois (lb avoir.)
1 gr = 0.065 g [65 milligrams (mg)]
1 ounce avoirdupois (oz avoir.) = 28.35 g = 437.5 gr
1 ounce apothecaries' (℥) = 31.103 g = 480 gr
1 lb avoir. = 454 g
1 pound apothecaries' (lb apoth.) = 373.2 g

Table 1-3. Apothecaries' System and Metric Equivalents

Apothecaries' System	Metric Equivalent
Fluid measure	
1 minim (♍)	0.062 milliliters (ml)
60 ♍ = 1 fluidram (fluidrachm) [*f*ʒ]	3.696 ml
8 *f*ʒ, or 480 ♍ = 1 fluidounce (*f* ℥)	29.573 ml
16 *f* ℥ = 1 pint (pt or 0)	473 ml, or 0.473 liter (L)
2 pt, or 32 *f* ℥, = 1 quart (qt)	946 ml, or 0.946 L
4 qt, or 8 pt, = 1 gallon (gal or C)	3785 ml, or 3.785 L
Weight	
1 grain (gr)	0.065 gram (g)
20 gr = 1 scruple (℈)	1.295 g
3 ℈ , or 60 gr, = 1ʒ	3.887 g
8 ʒ , or 480 gr, = 1℥	31.103 g
12 ℥ , or 5760 gr, = 1 pound (lb apoth.)	373 g, or 0.373 kilogram (kg)

2. **Ratios having the same values are equivalent**. Their **cross products** are equal (the product of the numerator of one and the denominator of the other always equals the product of the denominator of one and the numerator of the other). Their **reciprocals** are also equal.

B. Proportions

1. A proportion **expresses the equality of two ratios**. These standard forms may all be used to express proportions:
   a. a:b = c:d
   b. a:b :: c:d
   c. a/b = c/d

2. The terms of a proportion are designated as the **extremes** (the outer members, or **a** and **d** in the examples above) and the **means** (the middle members, or **b** and **c** in the examples above).

3. In any proportion, the **product of the extremes equals the product of the means**, allowing determination of any missing term when the other three terms are known. For example, if a/b = c/d, then:
   a. a = bc/d
   b. b = ad/c
   c. c = ad/b
   d. d = bc/a

4. **Many pharmaceutical calculations can be solved directly by using proportions**. For example, suppose one has the information that 15 tablets contain 75 grains (gr) of aspirin, and one needs to know how many grains 4 tablets contain. Proportions provide the answer as follows:

$$\frac{15 \text{ tablets}}{4 \text{ tablets}} = \frac{75 \text{ gr}}{x \text{ gr}}$$

$$x = \frac{75 \times 4}{15}, \text{ or } 20 \text{ gr}$$

C. Percentages

1. Percentage indicates the **rate per hundred** expressed by a number and a percent sign (%). A percentage may also be expressed as a **ratio**, given as a common or decimal fraction. That is, 25% indicates 25 parts of 100 parts and may also be expressed as 25/100 or 0.25.

2. For **computational purposes**, percents are generally changed to **equivalent decimal fractions**, by dropping the percent sign and dividing the numerator by 100. Thus, 15% = 15/100, or 0.15; and 0.01% = 0.01/100, or 0.0001.

3. Percentages play an important role in **pharmaceutical calculations**. Often, they are used to express the **concentration of a solute in solution, the amount of active material in a drug or preparation**, or **the quantity of an active ingredient in a dosage form**.

4. **Percent concentrations** are expressed in a variety of ways.
   a. **Percent weight-in-volume** (% w/v) expresses the number of grams (g) of constituent in 1 decaliter (dl), which is 100 milliliters (ml), of solution or liquid preparation.

(1) In the **metric system**, the required number of milliliters are multiplied by the percentage strength (expressed as a decimal) to determine the number of grams of solute or constituent in the liquid preparation. (The volume in milliliters represents the weight in grams of the solution or liquid preparation as if it were pure water). For example, if one needs to know how many grams of dextrose are required to prepare 3000 ml of 4% solution, then this calculation is used:

$$3000 \text{ ml} = 3000 \text{ g of solution}$$
$$4\% = 4/100 = 0.04$$
$$3000 \text{ g} \times 0.04 = 120 \text{ g}$$

(2) In the **apothecaries' system**, the weight of a fluidounce (*f* ℥) of water (455 gr) must be multiplied by the required number of fluidounces of solution and by the percentage strength to determine the number of grains of solute in the liquid preparation. (Volume in fluidounces multiplied by 455 gr represents the weight in grains of the solution.) For example, if one needs to know how many grains of atropine sulfate are required to prepare ½ *f* ℥ of a 2.5% solution, then this calculation is used:

½ *f* ℥ × 455 gr/ *f* ℥ = 227.5 gr of solution
2.5% = 0.025
227.5 gr × 0.025 = 5.687 gr

b. Percent volume-in-volume (% v/v) expresses the number of milliliters of a constituent in 1 dl of solution or liquid preparation. For example, if one needs to find the % v/v of liquified phenol in 300 ml of a lotion containing 6 ml of liquified phenol, then the following calculation is used:

$$\frac{300 \text{ ml}}{6 \text{ ml}} = \frac{100\%}{x\%} \qquad x = 2\% \text{ v/v}$$

c. Percent weight-in-weight (% w/w) expresses the number of grams of a constituent in 100 gr of solution or mixture. Because liquids are not customarily measured by weight, weight-in-weight solutions or liquid preparations should be designated as such (e.g., 8% w/w).

(1) A specified volume of a solution or liquid preparation of given % w/w strength is often impossible to prepare because the volume displaced by the active component is unknown. However, if the **specific gravity of the solvent** is known, the weight of the active component may be calculated. For example, if one needs to know how to prepare 200 ml of a 3% w/w solution of a substance in a solvent having a specific gravity of 1.25, then this calculation is used:

$$200 \text{ ml} \times 1.25 \text{ specific gravity} = 250 \text{ g (weight of solvent)}$$
$$3\% \text{ w/w} = 3 \text{ g of drug} + 97 \text{ g of solvent in } 100 \text{ g of solution}$$
$$\frac{97 \text{ g solvent}}{250 \text{ g solvent}} = \frac{3\%}{x\%}$$
$$x\% = 7.73 \text{ g of drug to be dissolved in } 250 \text{ g (or } 200 \text{ ml) of solvent}$$

(2) If the **specific gravity of the solvent is not known**, other data, such as the weight of solvent and solute, or the volume and specific gravity of the finished solution, must be given to complete the computation. For example, if one needs to know the percentage strength (% w/w) of a solution of 10 g of boric acid dissolved in 1 dl of water, then this calculation is used:

$$100 \text{ ml of water} = 100 \text{ g of water}$$
$$100 \text{ g of water} + 10 \text{ g of boric acid} = 110 \text{ g of solution}$$
$$\frac{110 \text{ g}}{10 \text{ g}} = \frac{100\%}{x\%}$$
$$x\% = 9.09\% \text{ (w/w)}$$

5. In **pharmacy practice**, the percent sign (%) used without qualification has these meanings:
   a. For **mixtures of solids and semisolids**, % = % (w/w).
   b. For **solutions or suspensions of solids in liquids**, % = % (w/v). For example, a 2% solution is prepared by dissolving 2 g of solid, or 2 ml of liquid, in sufficient solvent to make 1 dl of solution.

6. **Additional terms** are sometimes used to express concentrations.
   a. **Milligrams percent** (mg %) expresses the number of milligrams of substance per 1 dl of liquid. It is used to express the concentration of a drug or natural substance in a biologic fluid, such as blood. The equivalent term **mg/dl** is preferred.
   b. For **very dilute solutions**, concentration may be expressed in **parts per million** (ppm). For example, 6 ppm corresponds to 0.0006%.

IV. CALCULATION OF MILLIEQUIVALENTS

A. Electrolytes

1. **Electrolyte ions in plasma** include the cations Na^+, K^+, Ca^{2+}, and Mg^{2+}; the anions Cl^-, HCO_3^-, and SO_4^{2-}; organic acid; and protein. They play an important role in the maintenance of acid–base balance, regulation of body metabolism, and control of body water volume.

2. **Electrolyte solutions** are liquid preparations used to treat electrolyte disturbances of body fluids. The concentrations of these solutions are almost always expressed in chemical units known as **milliequivalents** (mEq).
   a. A **milliequivalent unit** is related to the total number of **ionic charges** in solution and also takes into account the **valence** of the ions. Thus, it **measures the amount of chemical activity of an electrolyte**.
   b. Under normal circumstances, **plasma** contains 155 mEq of cations and 155 mEq of anions. The total concentration of cations always equals the total concentration of anions.

B. Calculating milliequivalents

1. A milliequivalent represents the **amount of solute** (in milligrams) equal to 1/1000 of its gram equivalent weight. For example:

   Molecular weight (Mol wt) of KCl = 74.5
   Equivalent weight of KCl = 74.5 g
   1 mEq KCl = 1/1000 × 74.5 g = 0.0745 g (74.5 mg)

2. The **equivalent weight** of a bivalent compound is obtained by dividing the molecular weight by the total valence of the positive or negative radical. For example:

   Mol wt of $CaCl_2 \cdot 2H_2O$ = 147
   Equivalent weight of $CaCl_2 \cdot 2H_2O$ = 147/2 = 73.5 g
   1 mEq $CaCl_2 \cdot 2H_2O$ = 1/1000 × 73.5 g = 0.0735 g (73.5 mg)

3. The mEq value for a **cation present in a solution** can be computed similarly. For example, for a solution containing 15 mg/dl of Ca^{2+}, the mEq/L value can be calculated as follows:

   Mol wt of Ca^{2+} = 40
   Equivalent weight of Ca^{2+} = 40/2 = 20 g
   1 mEq of Ca^{2+} = 1/1000 × 20 g = 0.02 g (20 mg)
   A solution containing 15 mg/dl of Ca^{2+} = 150 mg Ca^{2+}/L

$$\frac{150 \text{ mg/L}}{20 \text{ mg/mEq}} = 7.5 \text{ mEq/L}$$

4. For the **milliequivalent weights of some important ions**, see Table 1-4.

V. CALCULATION OF MILLIOSMOLES

A. Osmotic pressure. Electrolytes help **control body water volumes** by establishing **osmotic pressure**. This pressure is proportional to the total number of particles in solution and is expressed in units of **milliosmoles** (mOsmol).

B. Calculating milliosmoles

1. For **nonelectrolytes** (such as dextrose), 1 millimole (mmol) [1 formula weight in milligrams] represents 1 mOsmol.

2. For **electrolytes** this relationship does not hold, because the total number of particles in solution depends on the degree of dissociation of a substance. For example, 1 mmol of KCl (completely dissociated) represents 2 mOsmol of total particles ($K^+ + Cl^-$). Similarly, 1 mmol of $CaCl_2$ represents 3 mOsmol of total particles ($Ca^+ + Cl^- + Cl^-$).

Table 1-4. Valences, Atomic Weights, and Milliequivalent Weights of Selected Ions

Ion	Formula	Valence	Atomic or Formula Weight	Milliequivalent Weight (mg)
Ammonium	NH_4^+	1	18	18
Lithium	Li^+	1	7	7
Potassium	K^+	1	39	39
Sodium	Na^+	1	23	23
Calcium	Ca^{2+}	2	40	20
Magnesium	Mg^{2+}	2	24	12
Acetate	$C_2H_3O_2^-$	1	59	59
Bicarbonate	HCO_3^-	1	61	61
Chloride	Cl^-	1	35.5	35.5
Gluconate	$C_6H_{11}O_7^-$	1	195	195
Lactate	$C_3H_5O_3^-$	1	89	89
Carbonate	CO_3^{2-}	2	60	30
Phosphate	$H_2PO_4^-$	1	97	97
	HPO_4^{2-}	2	96	48
Sulfate	SO_4^{2-}	2	96	48
Citrate	$C_6H_5O_7^{3-}$	3	189	63

3. The **milliosmolar value of the separate ions of an electrolyte** may be obtained by dividing the concentration of the ions in milligrams per liter (mg/L) by the ions' atomic weight. The **milliosmolar value of the complete electrolyte in solution** equals the sum of the milliosmolar values of the separate ions. For example, to determine how many milliosmoles are represented in 2 L of 0.9% NaCl solution, this calculation is used:

   1 mmol NaCl = 2 mOsmol of total particles ($Na^+ + Cl^-$)
   Mol wt of NaCl = 58.5
   1 mmol of NaCl = 58.5 mg = 2 mOsmol
   2000 ml (2 L) × 0.009 g/ml (0.9% solution) = 18 g (18,000 mg) NaCl
   18,000 mg/58.5 mg = 307.69 mOsmol for each ion
   Total mOsmol = 307.69 × 2 ($Na^+ + Cl^-$) = 615 mOsmol

STUDY QUESTIONS

Directions: Each question below contains five suggested answers. Choose the **one best** response to each question.

1. A physician requests ½ kg of Bacitracin Ointment containing 250 units of Bacitracin per gram. How many grams of Bacitracin Ointment (500 units/g) must be used to make this ointment?

(A) 100
(B) 250
(C) 280
(D) 300
(E) 400

2. How many grains of benzocaine are needed to prepare the following prescription?

Rx

Benzocaine	1% w/w
Glycerin	2.5%
Hydrophilic ointment q.s. ii℥	
sig: Apply as needed	

(A) 1.2
(B) 6.0
(C) 9.6
(D) 10.0
(E) 10.5

3. How many 8-f℥ bottles can be packaged from a 2-gal bottle of cough syrup?

(A) 10
(B) 15
(C) 20
(D) 28
(E) 32

4. A solution contains 2.5 mEq of calcium per 50 ml. Express the solution strength of calcium in terms of mg per L. (The atomic weight of Ca^{2+} is 40.)

(A) 250
(B) 350
(C) 500
(D) 1000
(E) 1500

5. How many grams of potassium chloride are used in making 500 ml of a solution containing 3 mEq of potassium per teaspoonful? (The atomic weight of K^+ = 39 and Cl^- = 35.5.)

(A) 5
(B) 10
(C) 15
(D) 22.62
(E) 32.62

6. How many grams of water are needed to make 150 g of a 4% w/w solution of potassium acetate?

(A) 100
(B) 130
(C) 135
(D) 144
(E) 156

ANSWERS AND EXPLANATIONS

1. The answer is B. (*II B; Tables 1-2, 1-3*) ½ kg = 500 g

$$\frac{1\text{ g}}{500\text{ g}} = \frac{250\text{ units}}{x\text{ units}}$$

$$x = 125{,}000\text{ units}$$

$$\frac{500\text{ units}}{125{,}000\text{ units}} = \frac{1\text{ g}}{x\text{ g}}$$

$$x = 250\text{ g}$$

2. The answer is C. (*III C 4 c*) ij℥ = 960 gr

$$\frac{100\text{ gr}}{960\text{ gr}} = \frac{1\text{ gr}}{x\text{ gr}}$$

$$x = 9.6\text{ gr}$$

3. The answer is E. (*II B 1; Table 1-3*) 2 gal = 256 *f* ℥

$$\frac{8\ f℥}{256\ f℥} = \frac{1\text{ bottle}}{x\text{ bottles}}$$

$$x = 32\text{ bottles}$$

4. The answer is D. (*IV B; Table 1-4*) The valence of calcium is + 2; hence,

$$1\text{ mEq} = \frac{40\text{ mg}}{2} = 20\text{ mg}$$

1 mEq = 20 mg of calcium. Therefore, 2.5 mEq = 50 mg

$$\frac{50\text{ ml}}{1000\text{ ml}} = \frac{50\text{ mg}}{x\text{ mg}}$$

$$x = 1000\text{ mg}$$

5. The answer is D. (*IV B; Table 1-4*) The atomic weight and equivalent weight of KCl = 74.5 g; 1 mEq = 74.5 mg of KCl

$$\frac{1\text{ mEq}}{3\text{ mEq}} = \frac{74.5\text{ mg}}{x\text{ mg}}$$

$$x = 223.5\text{ mg}$$

1 tbls = 5 ml; hence,

$$\frac{5\text{ ml}}{500\text{ ml}} = \frac{223.5\text{ mg}}{x\text{ mg}}$$

$$x = 22{,}350\text{ mg} = 22.35\text{ g of KCl}$$

6. The answer is D. (*III C 4 c*) 4% w/w is 4 g of potassium acetate in 100 g of solution; therefore, 100 g − 4 g of potassium acetate = 96 g of water

$$\frac{100\text{ g}}{150\text{ g}} = \frac{96\text{ g}}{x\text{ g}}$$

$$x = 144\text{ g of water}$$

2
Drug Solution Chemistry

Sunil Jambhekar

I. INTRODUCTION

A. A **solution** may be defined as a homogeneous substance that has, within certain limits, a continuously variable composition. Its properties and composition are uniform at a non-molecular level. A great variety of drugs exist in this form, requiring an understanding of the basic properties of solutions.

B. Solutes. The **components** of a solution may be defined as the **solvent** (usually the component present in greatest quantity) and the **solutes** (other components dissolved in the solvent). Solutes may be nonelectrolytes or electrolytes.

1. **Nonelectrolytes** are substances that **do not form ions** when dissolved in water and thus do not conduct an electric current through the solution. Examples include sucrose, glucose, glycerin, and urea.

2. **Electrolytes** are substances that **do form ions** in solution and thus can conduct an electric current through the solution. Examples include sodium chloride (NaCl), hydrochloric acid (HCl), and ephedrine hydrochloride. Electrolytes include strong electrolytes and weak electrolytes.
   a. **Strong electrolytes** are **completely ionized** in water at all concentrations, as with HCl and NaCl.
   b. **Weak electrolytes** are **partially ionized** in water at most concentrations, as with aspirin and ephedrine hydrochloride.

II. CONCENTRATION EXPRESSIONS.

The concentration of a solution may be expressed in terms of the **quantity of solute in a definite volume of solution** or as the **quantity of solute in a definite mass of solvent or solution** (Table 2-1).

A. Molarity. The molarity **(M)** of a solution is the number of moles **(mol)** of solute in 1 liter **(L)** of solution.

1. **All solutions of the same molarity contain the same number of solute molecules** in a definite volume of solution.

2. When a solution contains **more than one solute**, it may have **different molarities for each solute**. For example, a solution may be 0.001 M for phenobarbital, and 0.1 M for NaCl. One liter of such a solution is prepared by adding 0.001 mol of phenobarbital (0.001 mol × 232.32 g/mol = 0.2323 g) [g = gram] and 0.1 mol of NaCl (0.1 mol × 48.45 g/mol = 4.845 g) to sufficient water to make one liter of solution.

3. A solution containing only **one solute** may have **different molarities for the various ionic components of the solute**. For example, a molar solution of NaCl is 1 M for both sodium and chloride ions, whereas a molar solution of sodium carbonate (Na_2CO_3) is 1 M for the carbonate ion and 2 M for the sodium ion (each mole of this salt contains 2 moles of sodium ions).

4. Molarity **changes value with temperature** because of the contraction and expansion of liquids. It should not be used when the properties of the solution are to be studied at various temperatures.

B. Normality. The normality **(N)** of a solution is the number of gram-equivalent weights of solute in 1 L of solution.

Table 2-1. Summary of Concentration Expressions

Expression	Symbol	Definition
Molarity	M	Moles (gram molecular weights) of solute in 1 L of solution
Normality	N	Gram equivalent weights of solute in 1 L of solution
Molality	m	Moles of solute in 1000 g of solvent
Mole fraction	x	Ratio of the moles of one component (e.g., the solute) of a solution to the total moles of all components (e.g., solute and solvent)
Mole percent	. . .	Moles of one component in 100 moles of the solution (obtained by multiplying the mole fraction by 100)
Percent weight-in-weight	% w/w	Grams of solute in 100 g of solution
Percent volume-in-volume	% v/v	Milliliters of solute in 1 dl (100 ml) of solution
Percent weight-in-volume	% w/v	Grams of solute in 1 dl (100 ml) of solution
Milligrams percent	mg % or mg/dl	Milligrams of solute in 1 dl (100 ml) of solution

1. The **equivalent weight** of any material is the weight that would react with, or be produced by, its reaction with 7.999 g of oxygen or 1.008 g of hydrogen (see section III for more details).
2. A molar solution of NaCl is also 1 N for both its ions. However, a molar solution of Na_2CO_3 is 2 N for both its ions.
3. Normality provides a convenient unit of measurement for certain quantitative analyses. However, like molarity, it **changes value with temperature.**

C. Molality. The molality **(m)** of a solution is the number of moles of solute in 1000 g of solvent.

1. Molality is used more frequently than molarity or normality, because molal solutions are **prepared in units of weight** and **do not change with temperature.**
2. Molal solutions are prepared by adding the proper weight of solvent to the carefully weighed amount of solute.
3. Molality may be **converted to molarity or normality** if the final volume of the solution is known or if the density is determined. In dilute aqueous solutions ($<$ 0.1 M), **molarity and molality may be assumed to be equivalent for practical purposes.**

D. Mole fraction. The mole fraction **(x)** provides a measure of the ratio of the moles of one component of a solution to the total moles of all components.

1. For a **two-component system** (solvent and solute), the mole fraction is expressed as:

$$x_1 = \frac{n_1}{n_1 + n_2} \qquad x_2 = \frac{n_2}{n_1 + n_2}$$

where x_1 is the mole fraction of component 1 (usually the solvent), x_2 is the mole fraction of component 2 (usually the solute), and n_1 and n_2 are the number of moles of components in the solution.

2. The **sum of the mole fractions for a solution** (x_1 and x_2 in the example above) **must be equal to 1.**
3. **Mole percent** (the number of moles in 100 mol of solution) is obtained by multiplying the mole fraction by 100.

E. Percent expressions. Percent expressions are commonly used to express the concentrations of pharmaceutical solutions. These include percent weight-in-weight **(% w/w)**, percent volume-in-volume **(% v/v)**, percent weight-in-volume **(% w/v)** and milligrams percent **(mg %, or mg/dl)**. For more details, see Table 2-1 and Chapter 1, section III C.

III. EQUIVALENT WEIGHTS

A. Gram atoms

1. As stated above, the **equivalent weight** of any material is the weight that would react with, or be produced by, its reaction with 7.999 g of oxygen or 1.008 of hydrogen.
2. A **gram atom of hydrogen** weighs 1.008 g and consists of 6×10^{23} (Avogadro's number) of hydrogen atoms. This amount of hydrogen combines with other atoms in proportions that depend on the **valence** of the atoms.
3. One gram atom of hydrogen (1.008 g) combines with 19 g of fluorine (atomic weight of 19); however, it combines with only 8 g of oxygen (atomic weight of 16). The **quantity of an element combining with 1.008 g of hydrogen** is referred to as the **equivalent weight** of the combining element.

B. Calculation of equivalent weight

1. One equivalent weight of fluorine (19 g) is identical to its atomic weight; however, one equivalent weight of oxygen (8 g) is half its atomic weight. This equation relates equivalent weight (g/Eq) and atomic weight:

$$\text{Equivalent weight} = \frac{\text{atomic weight}}{\text{number of equivalents/atomic weight (valence)}}$$

2. The **number of equivalents/atomic weight** (e.g., 1 for fluorine and 2 for oxygen) indicates the common valence of an element.
3. Equivalent weights may be calculated for **molecules** as well as atoms.
   a. For example, the **equivalent weight of NaCl** is identical to its molecular weight (58.5) and is the **sum of the equivalent weights of sodium (23 g/Eq) and chlorine (35.5 g/Eq)**. Both sodium and chlorine have a valence of 1.
   b. In contrast, the **equivalent weight of Na_2CO_3** is 53 g/Eq, or half its molecular weight of 106. Two atoms of sodium are present, each with an atomic weight of 23 ($2 \times 23 = 46$); these have a **total valence of 2** and an equivalent weight of 23 g/Eq. One carbonate group has a molecular weight of 60 and a **valence of 2**, for an equivalent weight of 30 (23 + 30 = 53 g/Eq). This equation shows the relation of equivalent weight to molecular weight:

$$\text{Equivalent weight} = \frac{\text{molecular weight (g/mol)}}{\text{equivalents/mol}}$$

4. In **hospital situations**, solutions containing various electrolytes may be administered to correct serious electrolyte imbalances. Concentrations of these solutions are usually expressed as **equivalents/liter** (Eq/L) or as **milliequivalents/liter** (mEq/L) [see Chapter 1, section IV]. For example, normal sodium ion concentration in human plasma is about 142 mEq/L. These equations are used to calculate the quantity of an electrolyte needed to prepare an electrolyte solution:

$$\text{Equivalent weight (g/Eq)} = \frac{\text{g/L}}{\text{Eq/L}}$$

$$\text{Equivalent weight (mg/Eq)} = \frac{\text{mg/L}}{\text{mEq/L}}$$

IV. COLLIGATIVE PROPERTIES.

The colligative properties of a solution are those properties that are **dependent on the number of particles of solute in the solution** and **independent of the chemical nature of the solute**.

A. Lowering of vapor pressure. A solute lowers the vapor pressure of a solution in an amount dependent on the mole fraction of the solute.

B. Elevation of boiling point. The boiling point is the temperature at which the vapor pressure of a liquid equals an external pressure of 760 mm Hg. The boiling point of a solution of a nonvolatile solute is higher than that of the pure solvent because the solute lowers the vapor pressure of the solvent. The amount of elevation of the boiling point depends on the mole fraction of the solute.

C. Depression of freezing point. The freezing point (or melting point) of a pure compound is the temperature at which the solid and liquid phases are in equilibrium under a pressure of 1 atmosphere (atm). The freezing point of a solution is the temperature at which the solid phase of the pure solvent and the liquid phase of the solution are in equilibrium under a pressure of 1 atm. The amount of depression of the freezing point depends on the molality of the solution.

D. Osmotic pressure

1. **Osmosis** is the process by which solvent molecules pass through a **semipermeable membrane** (a barrier through which only solvent molecules may pass) from a region of dilute solution to one of more concentrated solution.
2. The pressure that must be applied to the more concentrated solution to prevent the flow of pure solvent into the solution is known as the **osmotic pressure.**
3. Solvent molecules move from a region where their **escape tendency** is **high** to one where their escape tendency is **low.** The presence of dissolved solute lowers the escape tendency of the solvent in proportion to solute concentration.

V. ELECTROLYTE SOLUTIONS AND IONIC EQUILIBRIA

A. Acid–base equilibria

1. According to the original **Arrhenius ionic dissociation theory,** an **acid** is a substance that liberates hydrogen ions in aqueous solution and a **base** is a substance that liberates hydroxyl ions in aqueous solution. This definition applies only under aqueous conditions, however.
2. The **Lowry-Bronsted theory** is a more powerful concept that applies in both aqueous and nonaqueous systems.
   - **a.** According to this definition, an **acid** is a substance (charged or uncharged) capable of **donating a proton** and a **base** is a substance (charged or uncharged) capable of **accepting a proton from an acid.**
   - **b.** The **dissociation of an acid** (HA) always produces a base (A^-) according to this formula:

$$HA \rightleftharpoons H^+ + A^-$$

   - **c.** HA and A^- are referred to as a **conjugate acid–base pair** (an acid and a base that differ in their structure by a proton and exist in equilibrium). The proton of an acid does not exist free in solution but combines with the solvent. (In water, this hydrated proton is known as a **hydronium ion.**)
   - **d.** The **relative strengths** of acids and bases are determined by their ability to donate or accept protons.
     - **(1)** For example, in water, HCl donates a proton more readily than does acetic acid. Thus, it is a stronger acid.
     - **(2)** Acid strength is also determined by the **affinity of the solvent for protons.** For example, HCl may dissociate completely in liquid ammonia but only very slightly in glacial acetic acid. Thus, HCl is a strong acid in liquid ammonia and a weak acid in glacial acetic acid.
3. The **Lewis theory** extends the acid–base concept to reactions in which protons are not involved. It defines an **acid** as **a molecule or ion that accepts an electron pair** from some other atom and a **base** as a **substance that donates an electron pair** to be shared with an atom.
4. The **Lowry-Bronsted theory is most commonly used** for pharmaceutical and biologic systems because these are primarily aqueous systems.

B. Hydrogen ion concentration

1. Hydrogen ion concentration values are very small and are thus expressed in **exponential notation** as **pH.**

2. The pH is defined as the **logarithm of the reciprocal of the hydrogen ion concentration,** or:

$$pH = \log \frac{1}{[H^+]}$$

where $[H^+]$ indicates the molar concentration of hydrogen.

3. Since the logarithm of a reciprocal equals the **negative logarithm** of the number, this equation may be rewritten as:

$$pH = -\log [H^+]$$

or

$$[H^+] = 10^{-pH}$$

4. The pH value may thus be defined as the **negative logarithm of the hydrogen ion value.**
   a. For example, if the hydrogen ion concentration $[H^+]$ of a solution is 5×10^{-6}, the pH value may be calculated as follows:

$$pH = -\log[5 \times 10^{-6}]$$

$$\log 5 = 0.6990 \qquad \log 10^{-6} = -6.0$$

$$\begin{aligned} pH &= -[-6 + 0.7] \\ &= -[-5.3] \\ &= 5.3 \end{aligned}$$

   b. **As pH decreases, hydrogen ion concentration increases exponentially.**
      (1) When the pH decreases from 6 to 5, the hydrogen ion concentration increases from 10^{-6} to 10^{-5}, or 10 times its original value.
      (2) When the pH falls from 5 to 4.7, the hydrogen ion concentration increases from 1×10^{-5} to 2×10^{-5}, doubling its initial value.

C. Dissociation constants

1. **Ionization** refers to the complete separation of the ions in a crystal lattice when the salt is dissolved.
2. **Dissociation** refers to the separation of ions in solution when the ions are associated by interionic attraction.
3. The dissociation of **weak electrolytes** is a reversible process. The equilibrium of this process may be expressed by the **law of mass action**, which states that the rate of the chemical reaction is proportional to the product of the concentration of the reacting substances, each raised to a power equal to the number of moles of the substance in solution.
4. For **weak acids**, dissociation in water is expressed as:

$$HA \rightleftharpoons H^+ + A^-$$

   a. The **dynamic equilibrium** between the simultaneous forward and reverse reactions is indicated by the arrows. By the law of mass action:

$$\text{Rate of forward reaction} = K_1[HA]$$

$$\text{Rate of reverse reaction} = K_2[H^+][A^-]$$

   b. At equilibrium, the **rates are equal**. Therefore,

$$K_1[HA] = K_2[H^+][A^-]$$

   c. Thus, the **equilibrium expression for the dissociation of a weak acid** may be written as:

$$K_a = \frac{K_1}{K_2} = \frac{[H^+][A^-]}{[HA]}$$

   where K_a represents the acid dissociation constant.

   d. For a weak acid, the **acid dissociation constant** is conventionally expressed as **pK_a**, as follows:

$$pK_a = -\log[K_a]$$

e. For example, the K_a of acetic acid at 25°C is 1.75×10^{-5}. The pK_a may be calculated as follows:

$$pK_a = -\log[1.75 \times 10^{-5}]$$

$$\log 1.75 = 0.2430 \qquad \log 10^{-5} = -5$$

$$pK_a = -[0.2430 - 5]$$

$$= -[4.75]$$

$$= -4.75$$

5. For **weak bases**, dissociation may be expressed using the K_a expression for the **conjugate acid of the base** (the acid formed when a proton reacts with the base). For a base that does not contain a hydroxyl group,

$$BH^+ \rightleftharpoons H^+ + B$$

a. The **dissociation constant** for this reaction can be expressed as:

$$K_a = \frac{[H^+][B]}{[BH^+]}$$

b. However, a **base dissociation constant** has traditionally been defined for the reaction of a weak base, using this expression:

$$B + H_2O \rightleftharpoons OH^- + BH$$

$$K_b = \frac{[OH^-][BH^+]}{[B]}$$

where K_b represents the dissociation constant of a weak base.

c. This **dissociation constant** can be expressed as pK_b, as follows:

$$pK_b = -\log[K_b]$$

6. Certain compounds (acids or bases) may accept or donate more than one proton and consequently have **more than one dissociation constant.**

D. Henderson-Hasselbalch equations

1. The Henderson-Hasselbalch equations describe the relationship between ionized and non-ionized species.

2. For **weak acids**, the equation is obtained from the equation in section V C 4 c as follows:

$$\frac{1}{[H^+]} = \frac{1}{K_a} \cdot \frac{[A^-]}{[HA]}$$

a. The **logarithm** of this equation is:

$$-\log[H^+] = -\log[K_a] + \log\frac{[A^-]}{[HA]}$$

b. Since $-\log[H^+] = pH$, and $-\log[K_a] = pK_a$, this equation may be expressed as:

$$pH = pK_a + \log\frac{[base]}{[acid]}$$

c. For practical purposes, the anion $[A^-]$ is assumed to be coming from the highly dissociated salt. Thus, the **Henderson-Hasselbalch equation for a weak acid** can be written as:

$$pH = pK_a + \log\frac{[salt]}{[acid]}$$

3. For **weak bases**, the Henderson-Hasselbalch equation is obtained from the equation in section V C 5 a as follows:

$$\frac{1}{[H^+]} = \frac{1}{K_a} \cdot \frac{[B]}{[BH]}$$

a. The **logarithm** of this equation is:

$$-\log[H^+] = -\log[K_a] + \log\frac{[B]}{[BH]}$$

b. Since $-\log[H^+] = pH$, and $-\log [K_a] = pK_a$, this equation may be expressed as:

$$pH = pK_a + \log \frac{[B]}{[BH]}$$

c. For practical purposes, the conjugate acid [BH] is assumed to be coming from the highly dissociated salt. Thus, the **Henderson-Hasselbalch equation for a weak base** can be written as:

$$pH = pK_a + \log \frac{[\text{base}]}{[\text{salt}]}$$

E. Degree of ionization

1. The degree of ionization (α) is the fraction of a weak electrolyte ionized in solution. Because gastrointestinal membranes act like a lipoid barrier, the **nonionized form** of an acidic or basic drug is **preferentially absorbed** by passive routes. Thus, the **greater the fraction of drug in the nonionized form at an absorption site, the faster the absorption.**

2. The value of α **increases** the more the drug is ionized. For a **weak electrolyte,** α can be calculated as follows:

$$\alpha = \frac{I}{T}$$

where I represents the ionized species and T represents the total species, or ionized (I) plus un-ionized (U).

a. The equation above can thus be represented as:

$$\alpha = \frac{I}{I + U}$$

or

$$\frac{1}{\alpha} = \frac{I + U}{I} = 1 + \frac{U}{I}$$

or

$$\frac{1}{\alpha} - 1 = \frac{U}{I}$$

b. Therefore,

$$\frac{1 - \alpha}{\alpha} = \frac{U}{I}$$

or

$$\frac{I}{U} = \frac{\alpha}{1 - \alpha} = \frac{[\text{ionized}]}{[\text{un-ionized}]}$$

3. For a **weak acid,** the **Henderson-Hasselbalch equation** is:

$$pH = pK_a + \log \frac{[\text{ionized}]}{[\text{un-ionized}]}$$

a. By substituting the equation in section V E 2 b into the Henderson-Hasselbalch equatic this equation is obtained:

$$pH = pK_a + \log \frac{[\alpha]}{[1 - \alpha]}$$

b. It is apparent from this that the ratio of ionized to un-ionized species dep upon pH and pK_a. For a **weak acid,** the **degree of ionization increases as p** For example, when the pH of a weakly acid drug is equal to the pK_a, 50 is ionized. When pH is one unit higher than pK_a, approximately 90% ionized. When pH is two units higher than pK_a, approximately 99% of th

4. For a **weak base,** the equation expressing the degree of ionization is

$$pH = pK_a + \log \frac{[1 - \alpha]}{[\alpha]}$$

a. For a **weak base**, the **degree of ionization decreases as pH increases.**

b. When the pH of a weakly basic drug is equal to the pK_a, 50% of the drug is ionized, as with a weak acid. However, when pH is one unit higher than pK_a, approximately 90% of the drug remains in the un-ionized form; when pH is two units higher than pK_a, approximately 99% of the drug remains in the un-ionized form.

F. Solubility

1. The **solubility of a weak acid or base** varies considerably as a function of pH. As a result, the dissolution rate of the drugs differs in various regions of the gastrointestinal tract.

2. For a **weak acid**, the total solubility (C_s) is given by this expression:

$$C_s = [HA] + [A^-]$$

where [HA] is the intrinsic solubility of the nonionized acid (denoted as C_0) and $[A^-]$ is the concentration of its anion.

a. The **anion concentration** can be expressed in terms of the dissociation constant (K_a) and C_0, giving this equation:

$$C_s = C_0 + \frac{K_a C_0}{[H^+]}$$

b. This equation indicates that the **solubility of a weak acid increases with increasing pH** (i.e., with decreasing H^+ concentration). Solubility is optimal at higher pH.

3. For a **weak base**, the total solubility is given by this expression, which indicates that the **solubility of a weak base decreases with increasing pH** (i.e., is optimal at lower pH):

$$C_s = C_0 + \frac{C_0[H^+]}{K_a}$$

G. Buffers and buffer capacity

1. A buffer is a **compound or mixture of compounds that, by its presence in solution, resists changes in pH upon addition of small quantities of acid or base.**

2. The resistance to a change in pH is known as **buffer action.**

3. A buffer may be a **combination of a weak acid and its conjugate base** or a **combination of a weak base and its conjugate acid**. However, buffer solutions are **more commonly prepared from weak acids and their salts.** They are not ordinarily prepared from weak bases and their salts, because of the instability and volatility of weak bases and because their pH depends on the dissociation constant of water (pK_w), which is affected by temperature changes.

a. For a **weak acid and its salt,** this buffer equation is satisfactory for calculations within the pH range of 4 to 10 and is important in the preparation of buffered pharmaceutical solutions:

$$pH = pK_a + \log \frac{[salt]}{[acid]}$$

b. For a **weak base and its salt,** the buffer equation is similar but also depends on the dissociation constant of water (pK_w). The equation becomes:

$$pH = pK_w - pK_b + \log \frac{[base]}{[salt]}$$

4. **Buffer capacity** is the ability of a buffer solution to resist changes in pH. The **smaller the pH change** caused by addition of a given amount of acid or base, the **greater the buffer capacity** of the solution.

a. Buffer capacity may be defined as the **number of gram equivalents of an acid or base that changes the pH of a liter of buffer solution by one unit.**

b. Buffer capacity is **influenced by the concentration of the buffer constituents** because a higher concentration of these provides a greater acid or base reserve. Buffer capacity (β) is related to the total concentration (C) as follows:

$$\beta = 2.3\,C\,\frac{K_a[H^+]}{[K_a + (H^+)]^2}$$

where C represents the molar concentrations of the acid and the salt.

c. Thus, **buffer capacity depends on the value of the ratio of the salt to the acid form.** It increases as the ratio approaches unity; maximum buffer capacity occurs when pH = pK_a and is represented by $\beta = 0.576$ C.

VI. CHEMICAL KINETICS AND DRUG STABILITY

A. Introduction

1. The **stability of a drug's active component** is a major criterion in the rational design and evaluation of dosage forms for a drug.
2. **Stability problems** may determine the acceptance or rejection of a given formulation.
   a. Extensive chemical degradation of the active ingredient may cause **substantial loss of active ingredient from the dosage form.**
   b. Chemical degradation may produce a **toxic product with undesirable side effects.**
   c. Instability of the drug product may result in **decreased bioavailability**, which can lead to a substantial reduction in the therapeutic efficacy of the dosage form.

B. Rates and orders of reactions

1. The **rate of a reaction** is the velocity with which it occurs, expressed as dC/dt (the change in concentration, or C, within a given time interval, or dt).
   a. Reaction rates depend on such conditions as **reactant concentration, temperature, pH,** and **presence of solvents or additives.** Radiation and catalytic agents such as polyvalent cations also have an effect.
   b. The effective study of reaction rates requires application of **pharmacokinetic principles** (discussed in detail in Chapter 4, section V A).
2. The **order of a reaction** refers to the way in which the concentration of the drug or reactant in a chemical reaction influences the rate. The study of reaction orders also requires application of pharmacokinetic principles (see Chapter 4, section V). For the most part, **pharmaceutical degradation** can be treated as a **zero-order** or a **first-order reaction**, as summarized below.
   a. A **zero-order reaction** is one in which the **rate is independent of the concentration of the reactants** (see Chapter 4, section V A 1 b for more details). Other factors, such as absorption of light in certain photochemical reactions, determine the rate.
      (1) A **zero-order reaction** can be expressed as:

$$C = -k_0 t + C_0$$

where C is the drug concentration, k_0 is the zero-order rate constant in units of concentration/time, t is the time, and C_0 is the initial concentration.

      (2) When this equation is plotted with C on the vertical axis (ordinate) against t on the horizontal axis (abcissa), the **slope of the line is equal to $-k_0$** (Fig. 2-1). The negative sign indicates that the slope is decreasing.
   b. A **first-order reaction** is one in which the **rate depends on the first power of the concentration of a single reactant** (see Chapter 3, section V A 1 c for more details).
      (1) The **reaction rate** is directly proportional to the concentration of the reacting substance, according to this equation:

$$C = C_0 e^{-kt}$$

where C is the concentration of the reacting material, C_0 is the initial concentration, k is the first-order rate constant in units of reciprocal time, and t is time.

      (2) In a first-order reaction, **concentration decreases exponentially with time**. A plot of the logarithm of concentration against time produces a straight line with a slope of $-k/2.303$ (Fig. 2-2).
      (3) The **half-life** of a reaction is the period of time required for the concentration of a drug to decrease by one-half ($t_{1/2}$). For a first-order reaction, this is expressed by:

$$t_{1/2} = \frac{0.693}{k}$$

      (4) The **time required for 10% of a drug to degrade** ($t_{10\%}$) is also important, as it represents a reasonable limit of degradation for the active ingredients. The $t_{10\%}$ can be calculated as:

$$t_{10\%} = \frac{2.303}{k} \log \frac{100}{90} = \frac{0.104}{k}$$

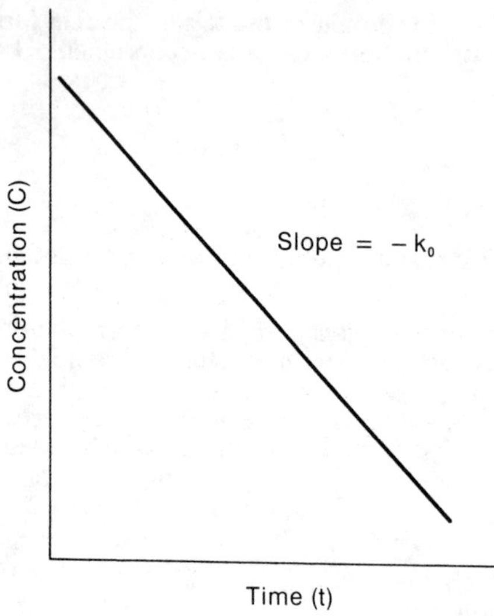

Figure 2-1. Linear plot of concentration (C) versus time (*t*) for a zero-order reaction. The slope of the line is equal to the zero-order rate constant, $-k_o$.

since $$k = \frac{0.693}{t_{1/2}}$$

then $$t_{10\%} = \frac{0.104}{0.693/t_{1/2}} = 0.152t_{1/2}$$

(5) Both $t_{1/2}$ and $t_{10\%}$ are **concentration-independent**; that is, it takes the same amount of time to reduce the concentration of the drug from 100% to 50% as it does from 50% to 25%.

C. Factors affecting reaction rates. Factors other than concentration may affect a drug's reaction rate and stability. Among these are temperature, the presence of a solvent, pH, and the presence of additives.

1. **Temperature.** An **increase in temperature** causes an increase in reaction rate, as expressed in the equation first suggested by Arrhenius:

$$k = Ae^{-Ea/RT}$$

or

$$\log k = \log A - \frac{Ea}{2.303} \times \frac{1}{RT}$$

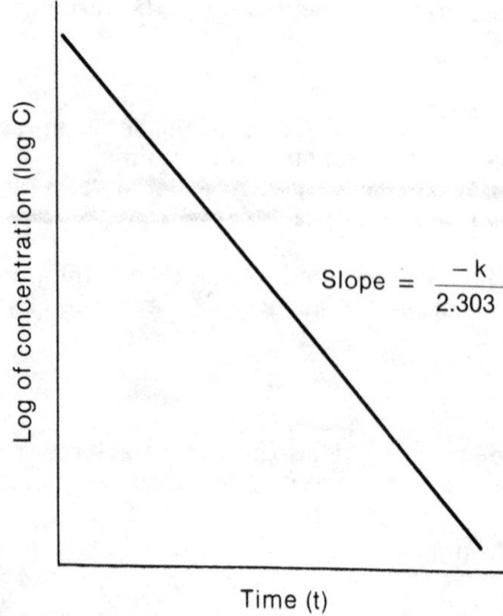

Figure 2-2. Linear plot of the logarithm of concentration (*log C*) versus time (*t*) for a first-order reaction. The slope of the line is equal to $-k/2.303$.

where k is the specific reaction rate constant, A is a constant known as the frequency factor, Ea is the energy of activation, R is the gas constant (0.987 cal/degree × mole), and T is the absolute temperature.

a. The **constants A and Ea** may be obtained by determining k at several temperatures and then plotting log k against 1/T. The slope of the resulting line equals –Ea/2.303R, and the intercept on the vertical axis equals log A.

b. The activation energy (Ea) is the amount of energy required to put the molecules in an **activated state**—molecules must be activated in order to react. As **temperature increases,** more molecules are activated and the **reaction rate increases.**

2. Presence of solvent. Many dosage forms require the incorporation of a water-miscible solvent [low molecular-weight alcohols, such as the polyethylene glycols (PEGs)] to stabilize the drug.

a. In addition to **altering the activity coefficients** of the reactant molecules and the transition state, a change in the solvent system may bring about simultaneous changes in such physicochemical parameters as pK_a, surface tension, and viscosity, **indirectly affecting the reaction rate.**

b. In some cases, **additional reaction pathways** may also be generated. For example, with an increasing concentration of ethanol in the solvent, aspirin degrades by means of an extra route, forming the ethyl ester of acetylsalicylic acid. However, a **change in solvent may also stabilize the drug.**

3. Change in pH. The magnitude of the rate of a hydrolytic reaction catalyzed by hydrogen and hydroxyl ions can vary considerably with pH.

a. Hydrogen ion catalysis predominates at **lower pH,** whereas **hydroxyl ion catalysis** operates at **higher pH.** At **intermediate pH,** the rate may be **pH-independent** or it may be catalyzed by **both hydrogen and hydroxyl ions.** (Rate constants in the intermediate pH range are generally less than those at higher or lower pH values, however.)

b. To determine the **influence of pH on degradation kinetics,** decomposition is measured at several hydrogen ion concentrations. The **pH of optimum stability** can be determined by plotting the logarithm of the rate constant (k) versus pH (Fig. 2-3). The **point of inflection** of such a plot represents the pH of optimum stability, useful in the development of a stable dosage formulation.

4. Presence of additives

a. Buffer salts must be added to many drug solutions to maintain the formulation at optimum pH. These salts **may affect the rate of degradation,** primarily from salt effect results of the increasing ionic strength.

(1) Increasing salt concentrations (particularly from polyelectrolytes such as citrate and phosphate) can **substantially affect the magnitude of pK_a,** causing a change in the rate constant.

(2) Buffer salts can also **promote drug degradation** through general acid or base catalysis.

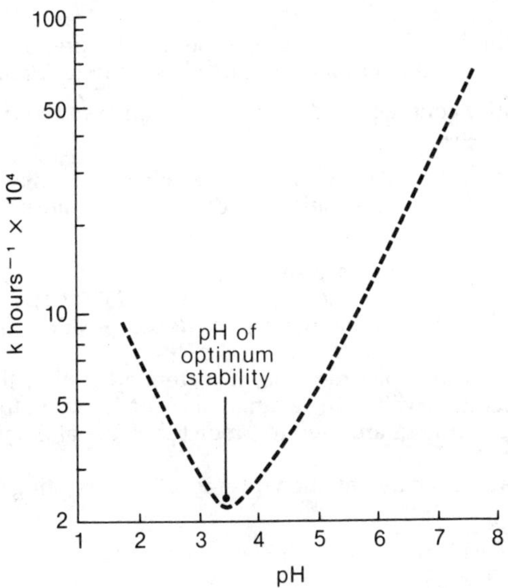

Figure 2-3. A plot of the logarithm of the rate constant (*k*) versus *pH*, used to determine the pH of optimum stability.

b. **Addition of surfactant agents** may accelerate or decelerate drug degradation.
   (1) **Acceleration of degradation** is frequently observed because micellar catalysis may provide a model for enzyme reactions.
   (2) **Stabilization of a drug** through addition of a surfactant is less frequently observed.

c. **Complexing agents** may improve drug stability. Aromatic esters such as benzocaine, procaine, hydrochloride, and tetracaine **increase in half-life** in the presence of caffeine. This increased stability appears to result from the formation of a less reactive complex between the aromatic ester and caffeine.

D. **Modes of pharmaceutical degradation**. The decomposition of active ingredients in a dosage form can occur through several pathways (e.g., hydrolysis, oxidation, and photolysis). (For further details, see Chapter 7, section II A.)

1. **Hydrolysis** is the most frequent type of degradation because many medicinal compounds are esters, amides, or lactams.
   a. **Hydrogen and hydroxyl ions** are the most common catalysts of hydrolytic degradation in solution.
   b. **Esters** most frequently undergo hydrolytic reactions that result in drug instability. Because esters are rapidly degraded in aqueous solution, formulators are reluctant to incorporate drugs having ester functional groups into liquid dosage forms.

2. **Oxidation** is usually mediated through reaction with atmospheric oxygen under ambient conditions (auto-oxidation).
   a. Medicinal compounds that undergo auto-oxidation at room temperature are affected by **oxygen dissolved in the solvent and in the void space of their packages**. These compounds should be packed under an **inert atmosphere** (e.g., nitrogen and carbon dioxide) to exclude air from their containers.
   b. Most oxidation reactions involve a **free-radical mechanism** and a **chain reaction**. (Free radicals tend to take electrons from other compounds.)
      (1) **Antioxidants** in the formulation react with the free radicals by providing electrons and easily available hydrogen atoms, thus preventing the propagation of chain reactions.
      (2) **Commonly used antioxidants** include ascorbic acid, butylated hydroxyanisole (BHA), butylated hydroxytoluene (BHT), propyl gallate, sodium bisulfite, sodium sulfite, and the tocopherols.

3. **Photolysis** is the degradation of drug molecules by normal sunlight or room light.
   a. Molecules may absorb the proper wavelength of light and **acquire sufficient energy to undergo reaction**. Generally, photolytic degradation occurs upon exposure to light of wavelengths less than 40 μm.
   b. An **amber glass bottle** or an **opaque container** acts as a barrier to this light, preventing or retarding photolysis. For example, sodium nitroprusside in aqueous solution has a shelf life of only 4 hours if exposed to normal room light. When protected from light, the solution is stable for at least 1 year.

E. **Determination of shelf life**

1. The **shelf life** of a drug preparation is the length of storage time before the preparation becomes unfit for use, either through chemical decomposition or physical deterioration.

2. **Storage temperature** affects shelf life and is generally understood to be ambient temperature unless special storage conditions are given.

3. In general, a preparation is considered fit for use if it **varies from the nominal concentration or dose by no more than** $\pm$ **5%**, provided the decomposition products are not more toxic than the original material.

4. **Shelf testing** aids in determining a formulation's standard shelf life.
   a. Samples are stored at about 3° to 5°C and at room temperature (20° to 25°C). They are then analyzed at various time intervals to determine the **rate of decomposition**, from which shelf life may be calculated.
   b. Because storage time at these temperatures may result in an extended testing time, **accelerated testing** is generally conducted as well, using a range of higher temperatures. The **rate constants** obtained from these samples are used to predict shelf life at ambient or refrigeration temperatures.
   c. **Prediction of stability at room temperature** can be obtained from accelerated testing data by the Arrhenius equation:

$$\log \frac{k_2}{k_1} = \frac{Ea(T_2 - T_1)}{2.303\ RT_2T_1}$$

where k_2 and k_1 are the rate constants at the absolute temperatures T_2 and T_1, respectively, R is the gas constant, and Ea is the energy of activation.

d. As an **alternate method**, an expression of concentration can be plotted as a linear function of time. Rate constants (k) for degradation at several temperatures are obtained; the logarithm of the rate constant (log k) is then plotted against the reciprocal of absolute temperature (1/T) to obtain, by extrapolation, the rate constant for degradation at room temperature (Fig. 2-4).

e. The **length of time the drug will maintain its required potency** can also be predicted by calculation of the drug's $T_{10\%}$ [see section VI B 2 b (4)]. This method applies to chemical reactions with activation energies in the range of 10 to 30 kcal/mol, which is the magnitude of the activation energy for many pharmaceutical degradations occurring in solution.

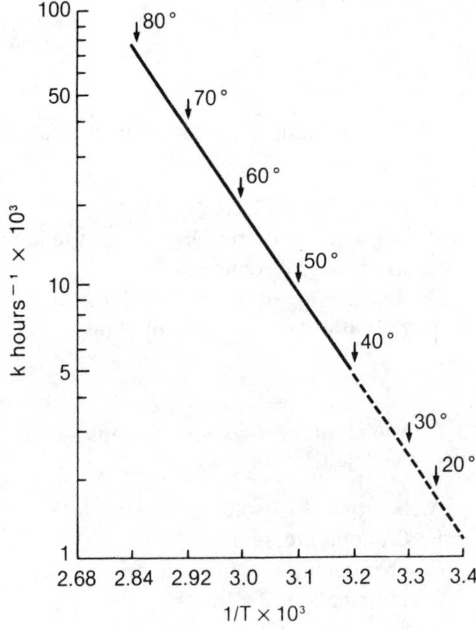

Figure 2-4. A plot of the logarithm of the rate constant (*k*) versus the reciprocal of absolute temperature (*1/T*), showing the temperature dependency of degradation rates.

STUDY QUESTIONS

Directions: Each question below contains five suggested answers. Choose the **one best** response to each question.

1. All of the following statements concerning chemical degradation are true EXCEPT

A. as temperature increases, degradation decreases
B. most drugs degrade by a first-order process
C. chemical degradation may produce a toxic product
D. chemical degradation may result in a loss of active ingredients
E. chemical degradation may affect the therapeutic activity of a drug

2. Molarity is defined as

A. gram molecular weight of solute in 1 L of solution
B. gram equivalent weight of solute in 1 L of solution
C. saturated solution of a solute in 1 L of solution
D. ml of solvent required to dissolve 10 g of solute
E. supersaturated solution of a solute

3. All of the following statements concerning zero-order degradation are true EXCEPT

A. its rate is independent of the concentration
B. a plot of concentration versus time yields a straight line on rectilinear paper
C. its half-life is a changing parameter
D. its concentration remains unchanged with respect to time
E. the slope of a plot of concentration versus time yields a rate constant

4. All of the following statements concerning first-order degradation are true EXCEPT

A. its rate is dependent on the concentration
B. its half-life is a changing parameter
C. a plot of the logarithm of concentration versus time yields a straight line
D. its $t_{10\%}$ is independent of the concentration
E. a plot of the logarithm of concentration versus time allows determination of the rate constant

5. Which of the following substances is classified as a weak electrolyte?

A. Glucose
B. Urea
C. Ephedrine hydrochloride
D. Sodium chloride
E. Sucrose

6. The pH value is calculated mathematically as the

A. log of the OH^- concentration
B. negative log of the OH^- concentration
C. log of the H^+ concentration
D. negative log of the H^+ concentration
E. ratio of H^+/OH^- concentration

7. Which of the following properties is classified as a colligative property?

A. Solubility of a solute
B. Osmotic pressure
C. Hydrogen ion concentration
D. Dissociation of a solute
E. Miscibility of the liquids

8. The colligative properties of a solution are related to the

A. pH of the solution
B. number of ions in the solution
C. total number of solute particles in the solution
D. number of un-ionized molecules in the solution
E. pK_a of the solution

9. The pH of a buffer system can be calculated by using the

A. Noyes-Whitney equation
B. Henderson-Hasselbalch equation
C. Michaelis-Menten equation
D. Yong equation
E. Stokes equation

10. Which of the following mechanisms is most frequently responsible for chemical degradation?

A. Racemization
B. Photolysis
C. Hydrolysis
D. Decarboxylation
E. Oxidation

11. Which of the following equations is used to predict the stability of a drug product at room temperature from experiments at accelerated temperatures?

A. Stokes equation
B. Yong equation
C. Arrhenius equation
D. Michaelis-Menten equation
E. Hixson-Crowell equation

12. Based on the relationship between the degree of ionization and the solubility of a weak acid, the drug aspirin (pK_a 3.49) will be most soluble at

A. pH 1.0
B. pH 2.0
C. pH 3.0
D. pH 4.0
E. pH 6.0

ANSWERS AND EXPLANATIONS

1. The answer is A. (*VI B 1, 2, C Figures 2-1, 2-2*) A number of factors may affect the reaction velocity, or degradation rate, of a pharmaceutical product. Among these are temperature, solvents, and light. The degradation increases two to three times with each 10° increase in temperature. The effect of temperature on reaction rate is given by the Arrhenius equation:

$$k = Ae^{-Ea/RT}$$

where k is the reaction rate constant, A is the frequency factor, Ea is the energy of activation, R is the gas constant, and T is the absolute temperature.

2. The answer is A. (*II A; Table 2-1*) Molarity is the number of moles (gram molecular weights) of solute in 1 L of solution. Molarity is the expression of concentration commonly used in analytical work. All solutions of the same molarity contain the same number of solute molecules in a definite volume of solution. When a solution contains more than one solute, it may have different molar concentrations with respect to the various solutes.

3. The answer is D. (*VI B 2 a; Figure 2-1*) In zero-order degradation, the concentration of a drug decreases over time; it is the *change* of concentration with respect to time that is unchanged. In the equation:

$$\frac{-dC}{dt} = k$$

the fact that dC/dt is negative signifies that the concentration is decreasing; however, the *velocity* of concentration change is seen to be constant.

4. The answer is B. (*VI B 2 b; Figure 2-2*) The half-life ($t_{1/2}$) is the time required for the concentration of a drug to decrease by one-half. For a first-order degradation,

$$t_{1/2} = \frac{0.693}{k}$$

both k and 0.693 are constants. Hence, $t_{1/2}$ is a constant.

5. The answer is C. (*I B 2 b*) Glucose, urea, and sucrose are nonelectrolytes, while sodium chloride is an example of a strong electrolyte. Electrolytes are substances that form ions when dissolved in water and thus can conduct an electric current through the solution. Ions are particles that bear electrical charges: Cations are positively charged ions, and anions are negatively charged. Strong electrolytes are completely ionized in water at all concentrations; weak electrolytes are only partially ionized at most concentrations. Nonelectrolytes do not form ions when in solution, and thus are nonconductors.

6. The answer is D. (*V B*) The pH is a measure of the acidity or alkalinity of an aqueous solution. The pH is the logarithm of the reciprocal of the H^+ ion concentration expressed in moles per liter. Since the logarithm of a reciprocal equals the negative logarithm of the number, the pH is the negative logarithm of the H^+ concentration. A pH of 7.0 indicates neutrality; as the pH decreases, the acidity increases. The pH of arterial blood is 7.35 to 7.45; of urine, 5 to 8; of gastric juice, about 1.4; of cerebrospinal fluid, 7.35 to 7.40. The concept of pH was introduced by Sörensen in the early 1900s.

7. The answer is B. (*IV*) Colligative properties depend upon the number of solute particles and are independent of the chemical nature of the solute. Osmotic pressure is an example of a colligative property. The osmotic pressure is the amount of pressure needed to stop osmosis across a semipermeable membrane between a solution and pure solvent. Other colligative properties of solutes are the reduction in vapor pressure of a solution, elevation of its boiling point, and depression of its freezing point.

8. The answer is C. (*IV*) The colligative properties of a solution are related to the total number of solute particles in a solution. Examples of colligative properties are osmotic pressure, lowering of vapor pressure, elevation of the boiling point, and depression of the freezing (or melting) point.

9. The answer is B. (*V D*) The Henderson-Hasselbalch equation for a weak acid and its salt is represented as:

$$pH = pK_a + \log\frac{[salt]}{[acid]}$$

where pK_a is the negative log of the dissociation constant of a weak acid, and [salt]/[acid] is the ratio of the molar concentration of salt and acid used to prepare a buffer.

10. The answer is C. (*VI D*) Although it is true that all of the mechanisms listed in the question can be responsible, the chemical degradation of medicinal compounds is most frequently due to hydrolysis. This is especially true of esters in liquid formulations, and drugs having ester functional groups are therefore formulated in dry form whenever possible. Oxidation, another common mode of degradation, is minimized by including antioxidants such as ascorbic acid in drug formulations. Photolysis is reduced by packaging susceptible products in amber or opaque containers. Decarboxylation, the removal of COOH groups, affects carboxylic acid compounds. Racemization neutralizes the effects of an optically active compound by converting half its molecules into the mirror-image configuration, so that the dextro- and levorotatory forms cancel one another out. This form of degradation affects only drugs characterized by optical isomerism.

11. The answer is C. (*VI E 4; Figure 2-4*) Testing of a drug formulation to determine its shelf life can be accelerated by applying the Arrhenius equation to data obtained at higher temperatures. The method involves the determination of rate constant (k) values for the degradation of a drug at various elevated temperatures. The log of k is then plotted against the reciprocal of the absolute temperature, and the k value for degradation at room temperature is obtained by extrapolation.

12. The answer is E. (*V E 3 b, F*) The solubility of a weak acid varies as a function of pH. Since pH and pK_a (the dissociation constant) are related, solubility is also related to the degree of ionization. The drug aspirin is a weak acid and will be completely ionized at pH that is 2 units above its pK_a. Therefore, it will be most soluble at pH 6.0.

3
Pharmaceutical Drug Forms

Sunil Jambhekar
Gurvinder Singh Rekhi

I. SOLUTIONS

A. Introduction

1. Drugs in **solution form** are more homogeneous and easier to swallow than drugs in solid dosage forms. For a drug with a slow dissolution rate, onset of action and bioavailability are also improved. However, drugs in solution are bulkier and more liable to degradation and interactions between constituents than those in solid dosage forms.

2. **Water**, the physiologic fluid of the human body, is the most commonly used vehicle for drug solutions. The United States Pharmacopeia (USP) recognizes four standards of water for the preparation of dosage forms.
   a. **Purified water USP** is water obtained by distillation or by ion exchange treatment. It may contain not more than 10 parts per million (ppm) of total solids and should have a pH between 5 and 7. Purified water is used in prescriptions and in finished manufactured products, except for parenteral and ophthalmic products.
   b. **Water for injection USP** conforms to the standards of purified water but is also free of pyrogens. It is used as a solvent for the preparation of parenteral solutions.
   c. **Sterile water for injection USP** is water for injection that has been sterilized and packaged in single-dose containers of type I or type II glass that do not exceed a capacity of 1 L. The limitations for total solids depend on the container size.
   d. **Bacteriostatic water for injection USP** is sterile water for injection that contains one or more suitable bacteriostatic agents. It is packaged in single-dose or multiple-dose containers of type I or type II glass that do not exceed a capacity of 30 ml.

B. Aromatic waters

1. Aromatic waters are **saturated aqueous solutions of volatile oils or of other aromatic or volatile substances**.

2. An aromatic water may be used as a pleasantly flavored **vehicle for a water-soluble drug** or as the **aqueous phase in an emulsion or suspension.**
   a. If a large amount of water-soluble drug is added to an aromatic water, an **insoluble layer may form at the top**.
   b. This **salting-out** is a competitive process in which the molecules of water-soluble drug have more attraction for the solvent molecules of water than do the volatile oil molecules. The associated water molecules are pulled away from the volatile oil molecules, which are no longer held in solution.

3. Aromatic waters should be **stored in tight, light-resistant bottles** to reduce volatilization and degradation from sunlight.

4. Aromatic waters may be **prepared by any of three methods**.
   a. **Distillation** is a universal method, but it is neither practical nor economical for most products. However, it is the only way to prepare stronger rose water NF and orange flower water NF.
   b. For the **solution method**, 2 ml or 2 g of the volatile substance is agitated for 15 minutes with sufficient water to make 1000 ml of solution. The solution is set aside for 12 hours and then filtered through wetted filter paper to prevent passage of excess oil into the filtrate and to eliminate adsorption of the dissolved aromatics.
   c. The **alternate solution method** is the most expedient way to produce aromatic waters.
      (1) The volatile substance is thoroughly mixed with an **inert adsorptive agent** (e.g., talc or purified siliceous earth). Then, 1 L of purified water is added and agitated for 10 minutes. The solution is filtered until a clear filtrate is obtained.

(2) The volatile substance is **adsorbed on the inert agent**, increasing the total area of volatile substance exposed to water and facilitating formation of a saturated solution. The inert agent also acts as a **clarifier**, as the undissolved material remains adsorbed and does not pass through the filter.

C. Syrups

1. A syrup is a **concentrated or nearly saturated aqueous solution of sugar. Syrup NF** contains 850 g of sucrose and sufficient purified water (about 450 ml) to make 1 L of syrup but is not yet saturated; it is an 85% weight-in-volume (w/v) or an approximately 65% weight-in-weight (w/w) solution with a specific gravity of 1.30. The high sugar content gives syrups a moderately high viscosity and a high specific gravity.

2. The **sweet taste** of syrups makes them useful vehicles for orally administered drugs.
   a. Syrups containing no medicinal agent are known as **flavoring syrups** (e.g., cherry syrup, cocoa syrup, and tolu balsam syrup).
   b. The choice of a syrup as a masking and flavoring vehicle must be determined by a taste panel. Traditionally, **aromatic eriodictyon syrup** or **glycyrrhiza syrup** are thought to **mask the bitter taste** of alkaloids; **cherry syrup** or **raspberry syrup**, the **saline taste** of certain other drugs.
   c. Syrups containing therapeutically active compounds are known as **medicinal syrups** (e.g., chlorpheniramine maleate syrup and ephedrine sulfate syrup).

3. Syrups may be **prepared by any of three methods**.
   a. **Agitation** of sucrose and water produces an odorless, colorless syrup. As the sugar dissolves and saturation is approached, the dissolution rate and the concentration gradient decrease. Thus, agitation may be a slow process.
   b. **Agitation with heat** often produces a syrup with a pale yellow color. A sucrose solution undergoes hydrolysis to dextrose and fructose in the presence of heat; with excessive heat the sweet taste is destroyed and a dark brown liquid results. This method cannot be used to prepare a syrup containing a thermolabile or a volatile ingredient.
   c. **Percolation** is an extraction process in which the desired constituents are dissolved from a granulated or powdered drug by the controlled descent of a suitable solvent through a column of the drug.
      (1) **A percolator** is a cylindrical or tapered vessel with a lower outlet from which the flow may be controlled.
      (2) **Powdered drug** is packed into the percolator, which has a layer of loosely packed cotton over the lower outlet. Purified water or a suitable solvent is then added.

4. Syrups have a **low solvent capacity for water-soluble drugs** because the hydrogen bonding between sucrose and water is very strong. It may be difficult or impossible to dissolve a drug in a syrup; often, the drug is best dissolved in a small quantity of water to which the flavoring syrup is then added.

5. A syrup's **sucrose concentration** plays a critical role in control of microorganism growth.
   a. **Dilute sucrose solutions** are excellent media for microorganisms.
   b. As the concentration of sucrose approaches saturation, the syrup becomes **self-preserved**. However, a saturated solution is undesirable because **temperature fluctuations may cause crystallization**.
   c. **Syrup USP** is self-preserved but has only a minimal chance of crystallization.

D. Solutions. As a pharmaceutical class, solutions are **liquid preparations that contain one or more solutes but are not, by their method of preparation or ingredients, classified within another category**. Nasal, ophthalmic, and parenteral solutions are physically solutions; however, they are classified separately because of their specific uses and methods of preparation.

1. **Mouthwashes** are solutions used for cleansing the mouth or treating diseases of the oral mucous membrane. They frequently contain alcohol or glycerin to aid in dissolving the volatile ingredients and are most often used cosmetically rather than therapeutically.

2. **Astringent solutions** are locally applied solutions that precipitate protein, reducing cell permeability without injury.
   a. Astringents can cause **constriction**, with wrinkling and blanching of the skin.
   b. Because astringents **reduce secretions**, they may be used as antiperspirants.
   c. **Aluminum acetate solution** and **aluminum subacetate solution** are used as wet dressings for contact dermatitis. Precipitation of these solutions is minimized by addition of **boric acid**.
   d. **Calcium hydroxide solution** is a mild astringent employed in lotions as a reactant and an alkalizer.

3. **Antibacterial topical solutions** are solutions that kill bacteria when applied to the skin or mucous membranes in the proper strength and under appropriate conditions. Examples include benzalkonium chloride solution, strong iodine solution, and methylrosaniline chloride solution.

E. Elixirs

1. Elixirs are pleasantly flavored **hydroalcoholic solutions intended for oral use**. The presence of sugar and alcohol distinguishes them from other categories.
2. The **alcohol content** of elixirs varies from 5% to 40%—sufficient alcohol is added to maintain the drug in solution. Most elixirs become turbid when moderately diluted by aqueous liquids.
3. Elixirs are prepared by **dissolving the ingredients in the appropriate solvent**. Usually, the alcohol-soluble substances are dissolved in alcohol and the water-soluble substances in water; the aqueous solution is then added to the alcoholic solution and stirred.
4. An **iso-alcoholic elixir** is a vehicle for various drugs that require solvents of different alcoholic concentration. It consists of a **low-alcoholic elixir** (8% to 10% alcohol) and a **high-alcoholic elixir** (75% to 78% alcohol). By mixing appropriate volumes of the two elixirs, an alcoholic content sufficient to dissolve the drugs can be obtained.
5. Elixirs containing therapeutically active compounds are known as **medicinal elixirs** (e.g., phenobarbital elixir).
6. Elixirs are **not the preferred vehicle for salts**, as alcohol accentuates a saline taste. Salts also have limited solubility in alcohol, so the alcoholic content of a salt-containing elixir must be low.

F. Spirits

1. Spirits (also called **essences**) are **alcoholic or hydroalcoholic solutions of volatile substances**, containing 50% to 90% alcohol.
2. This **high alcoholic content** maintains water-insoluble oils in solution. If water is added to a spirit, the oils separate.
3. Some spirits are **medicinal spirits** (e.g., aromatic ammonia spirit). Many spirits (e.g., compound orange spirit and compound cardamom spirit) are used as **flavoring agents**.
4. Spirits should be **stored in tight containers** to reduce loss by evaporation.

G. Tinctures

1. Tinctures are **alcoholic or hydroalcoholic solutions of chemicals or soluble constituents of crude drugs**. Although tinctures vary in drug concentration (up to 50%), those prepared for potent drugs are usually 10% in strength (i.e., 100 ml of tincture has the activity of 10 g of the drug).
2. Most tinctures are **prepared by an extraction process of maceration or percolation**. The selection of a solvent (also known as a **menstruum**) is based on the solubility of the active and inert constituents of the crude drug.
   a. Ideally, the **solvent should extract only the active ingredient**.
   b. **Unwanted material** is frequently extracted as well; if this excess material is detrimental, it can be removed by additional processes.
3. Tinctures may **precipitate inactive constituents upon aging. Glycerin** may be added to the hydroalcoholic solvent (as with aromatic rhubarb tincture) to increase solubility of the active constituent and reduce precipitation upon storage.
4. Generally, tinctures are **stable preparations**. The alcohol content of official tinctures varies from 17% to 21% with opium tincture USP, to 77% to 83% with tolu balsam tincture NF (National Formulary).
5. Tinctures must be **tightly stoppered and kept from excessive temperatures**. Because many of the constituents found in tinctures undergo photochemical changes when exposed to light, they must be **stored in light-resistant containers**.

H. Fluid extracts

1. Fluid extracts are **liquid extracts of vegetable drugs containing alcohol as a solvent, a preservative, or both**. They are prepared by percolation, so that each milliliter contains the therapeutic constituents of 1 g of the standard drug involved.

2. Because of their high alcohol content, fluid extracts are sometimes referred to as **100% tinctures**. Fluid extracts of potent drugs are usually **ten times as concentrated** (or potent) **as the corresponding tincture** (e.g., the usual dose of belladonna tincture is 0.6 ml; the equivalent dose of the fluid extract is 0.06 ml).

3. Many fluid extracts are considered **too potent for self-administration**, and so they are almost never prescribed. In addition, many are simply **too bitter** to be acceptable to patients. Today, most fluid extracts are modified by the addition of flavoring or sweetening agents.

II. SUSPENSIONS

A. Introduction

1. A suspension is a **two-phase system composed of a solid material dispersed in a liquid**. The particle size of the dispersed solid is usually greater than 0.5 μm; the liquid can be oily or aqueous. However, most suspensions of pharmaceutical interest are aqueous.

2. **Lotions, magmas** (suspensions of finely divided material in a small amount of water), and **mixtures** are all considered to be suspensions. For the most part, these are preparations that have had official formulas for some time (e.g., calamine lotion USP and kaolin mixture with pectin NF). Official formulas are given in the USP and the NF.
   a. A **complete formula** and a **detailed method of preparation** are available for some official suspensions.
   b. For other official suspensions, **only the concentration of active ingredients is given**, allowing the manufacturer considerable latitude in formulation.
   c. Some drugs are provided in a package in a **dry form** to circumvent the instability of aqueous dispersions. Water is added at the time of dispensing to complete the suspension.

B. Purposes of suspension

1. Suspensions have a **sustaining effect**. For a sustained-release preparation, suspension introduces a dissolution or diffusion step as the drug goes from solid form to solution form to final absorption.

2. Suspensions can **overcome stability problems**. Drug degradation in suspension or solid dosage forms occurs much more slowly than degradation in solution form.

3. Suspensions can **overcome taste problems**. A bad-tasting material can be converted into an insoluble form and then prepared as a suspension, obviating the taste problem.

4. Suspensions can **overcome basic solubility problems**. When suitable solvents are not available, the suspension provides an alternative. For example, only water can be used as a solvent for ophthalmic preparations because of the possibility of corneal damage. Ophthalmic suspensions provide an alternative.

C. Suspension parameters

1. An **ideal suspension** has these properties.
   a. **Uniform particle size**—all particles behave alike and produce consistent behavior for the suspension as a whole.
   b. **No particle-particle interaction**—each particle remains discrete, with no aggregation or clumping (such a suspension is known as a **monodispersed suspension**).
   c. **No sedimentation**—drug particles are either stationary or move randomly throughout the dispersion medium, so the drug is always uniformly distributed.

2. These ideal properties are not usually realized. However, they can be approximated by **controlling some of the fundamental parameters of the suspension**.
   a. **Particle size** should be as **small as possible**. A small particle size favors a slower sedimentation rate, according to Stoke's law:

$$\text{sedimentation rate} = \frac{d^2(\varrho - \varrho_0)g}{18\eta}$$

   where d is the particle diameter, ϱ is the density of the solid, ϱ_0 is the density of the sedimentation medium, g is the acceleration due to gravity, and η is the viscosity of the dispersion medium.
   b. A **high concentration of solid** increases the possibility of particle–particle collisions and thus promotes particle–particle interactions. However, the concentration of solid is usually fixed in a given formula, so this parameter can seldom be changed.

c. Ideally, **particle–particle interactions** should be avoided. With aggregation, the resulting clumps will behave like larger particles and will settle at a faster rate.

(1) Aggregations can be **prevented** if the **particles have a similar electrical charge**. A solid dispersed in an aqueous system will always have some charge, resulting from ionization of chemical groups on the solid surface, absorption of surfactant molecules on the solid surface, or absorption of electrolytes from solution.

(2) The **sign of the charge can usually be predicted** if it results from **absorption of an ionic surfactant**. For example, sodium lauryl sulfate used as a dispersing agent yields a negative charge to solid particles. In contrast, the **sign of the charge can rarely be predicted** if it results from **absorption of an electrolyte**.

(3) The **magnitude of the charge** is the difference in electrical potential between the charged solid surface and the bulk of the liquid. Most important is the **zeta potential**, determined from the fixed layers of ions on the particle surface (Fig. 3-1). This layer of ions is tightly bound and is considered part of the particle for practical purposes.

(4) To maintain a **monodispersed system**, the zeta potential must be great enough for particles to repel each other (**critical zeta potential**). This value is specific for each given suspension.

d. **Density** and **viscosity** can be manipulated to reduce sedimentation.

(1) According to Stoke's law, the **sedimentation rate equals zero when the densities of the solid and the dispersion medium are equal**. However, it is difficult to prepare aqueous solutions with a density sufficient to match that of the solids commonly used in suspensions. In addition, solution density also changes with temperature.

(2) Stoke's law also indicates that the **sedimentation rate is inversely proportional to the viscosity of the dispersion medium**. However, an increase in viscosity only slows the sedimentation rate and cannot stop it completely.

D. Suspending agents. Common suspending agents include hydrophilic colloids, clays, and a few other agents. Some of these are also used as **emulsifying agents** (see section III).

1. **Hydrophilic colloids** increase the viscosity of water by binding water molecules, thus limiting their mobility or fluidity. Viscosity is proportional to the concentration of the colloid. These agents **support the growth of microorganisms** and require a preservative. They are **anionic** (with the exception of methylcellulose) and thus incompatible with quaternary antibacterial agents and other positively charged drugs. Most are **insoluble in alcoholic solutions**.

a. **Acacia** is usually used as the mucilage (35% dispersion in water). Viscosity is greatest between pH 5 and pH 9. It is susceptible to microbial decomposition.

b. **Tragacanth** is usually used as a 6% dispersion in water (mucilage) and has an advantage over acacia in that less is needed. Also, tragacanth **does not contain the oxidase present in acacia**, which catalyzes the decomposition of organic chemicals. Its viscosity is greatest at pH 5.

c. **Methylcellulose** is a polymer that is **nonionic** and **stable to heat and light**. It is available in several viscosity grades. Because it is soluble in cold water but not in hot water, dispersions

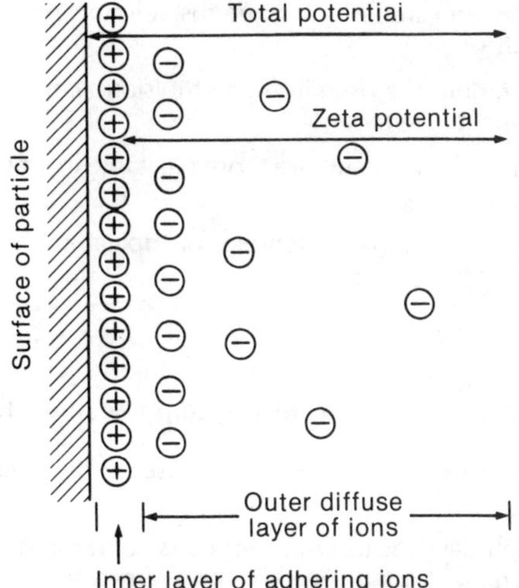

Figure 3-1. Schematic representation of the zeta potential of a particle in a suspension. The zeta potential is determined from the difference in the charge between the fixed layer of ions adhering to the particle surface and the bulk of the liquid.

are prepared by adding the material to boiling water and then cooling the preparation until the material dissolves.

d. **Carboxymethylcellulose** is an **anionic** material that is **soluble in water** and available in three viscosity grades. Prolonged exposure to heat causes loss of viscosity.

2. **Clays** (e.g., bentonite and Veegum) are silicates that are anionic in aqueous dispersions. Strongly hydrated, they exhibit **thixotropy** (the property of forming a gel-like structure on standing and becoming fluid on agitation).
   a. **Bentonite's** official form is as the 5% magma.
   b. **Veegum** is hydrated to a greater degree than bentonite and thus is more viscous at the same concentration.

3. **Other agents** include agar, chondrus (carrageenan), gelatin, pectin, and gelatinized starch. The use of all of these is limited by their susceptibility to bacterial attack, their incompatibilities, and their cost.

E. Methods of preparation

1. Initially, the **solid is wetted** to separate each individual particle and coat it with a layer of dispersion medium. Wetting may be accomplished by **levigation** (addition of a suitable nonsolvent, or **levigating agent**, to the solid material, followed by blending to form a paste), using a glass mortar and pestle; or a **surfactant** may be employed.

2. The **suspending agent** may then be added as a dry powder along with the active ingredient. For best results, however, the suspending agent should be added in the form of its **aqueous dispersion**.
   a. This dispersion may be added to the solid (or the levigated solid) by way of **geometric dilution** to ensure proper dispersion.
   b. The preparation is then **brought to the desired volume** by stirring in the appropriate vehicle.

III. EMULSIONS

A. Introduction

1. An emulsion is a **heterogeneous system consisting of at least one immiscible liquid intimately dispersed in another in the form of droplets** (droplet diameter usually exceeds 0.1 μm).

2. An emulsion is **inherently unstable** because the droplets of the dispersed liquid tend to coalesce to form larger droplets until all the dispersed material has coalesced.

3. An **emulsifying agent** (the third component of the system) must be employed to prepare a usable emulsion. Its purpose is to **prevent coalescence** and **maintain the integrity of the individual droplets of the dispersed liquid**.

B. Purposes of emulsion

1. Emulsions can **increase solubility**. Many drugs have limited solubility but have maximum activity in solution form. The **oil phase** of an emulsion allows the drug to be in solution form.

2. Emulsions can **increase stability**. Many drugs are unstable in aqueous solution but much more stable when incorporated into an emulsion.

3. Emulsions can **prolong drug action**. Incorporation of a drug into an emulsion alters its bioavailability, as with certain intramuscular injection preparations.

4. Emulsions can **improve taste**. Objectionable medicinal agents are more palatable in emulsion form and thus more conveniently administered.

5. Emulsions can **improve appearance**. Oleaginous materials intended for topical application are more appealing in an emulsified form.

C. Emulsion types

1. Emulsions are generally considered as **two-phase systems**.
   a. The liquid or phase in the **form of droplets** is known as the **dispersed phase**, the **internal phase**, or the **discontinuous phase**.
   b. The **other liquid** is known as the **dispersion medium**, the **external phase**, or the **continuous phase**.

2. In pharmaceutical applications, one of the phases is usually an **aqueous solution** and the other is **lipid or oily** in nature. The lipid can range from a vegetable or hydrocarbon oil to a semisolid hydrocarbon or a wax.

3. Conventionally, emulsions are described in terms of **water and oil** (oil represents the lipid, or nonaqueous, phase, regardless of its composition).
   a. If water is the **internal phase**, the emulsion is classified as **water-in-oil** (w/o).
   b. If water is the **external phase**, the emulsion is classified as **oil-in-water** (o/w).

4. The **type of emulsion** formed is primarily determined by two factors—the relative phase volumes and the emulsifying agent used.
   a. For an **ideal emulsion**, the maximum concentration of the internal phase is 74% (i.e., an o/w emulsion can theoretically be prepared containing up to but not more than 74% oil). This ideal factor usually holds true in practice.
   b. Choice of an **emulsifying agent** is perhaps more important in determining the final emulsion type. Most agents preferentially form one type of emulsion if the phase volumes permit.

D. Factors affecting emulsification

1. The **internal phase** (oil or water) must be **reduced to small droplets—**only possible if energy in the form of work is applied.
   a. The amount of work needed depends on the **interfacial tension** (the tension between the two phases of the system).
   b. Addition of an **emulsifying agent** reduces interfacial tension, reducing the amount of energy needed to produce an emulsion.

2. Energy, or work, can also be interpreted as the **surface free energy** or **excess potential energy** that makes an emulsion unstable.
   a. The surface free energy, however small, **promotes coalescence and emulsion instability**.
   b. **Emulsifying agents** provide a mechanical barrier to coalescence that counterbalances surface free energy. Three mechanisms appear to be involved.
      (1) Some emulsifying agents appear to function by forming strong, pliable **interfacial films** around the dispersed droplets.
      (2) **Charge repulsion** can cause droplets to repel each other and prevent coalescence. For example, oil droplets in an aqueous phase usually possess an electrical charge, developed either from the nature of the emulsifying agent or by absorption of ions from solution.
      (3) **Steric repulsion** occurs when the long hydrocarbon chains of the surfactant or the emulsifying agent prevent water droplets in an oily phase from contacting each other. Thus, a **more hydrophilic** emulsifying agent tends to produce an **o/w emulsion**, whereas a **more hydrophobic** agent tends to produce a **w/o emulsion**.

E. Emulsifying agents. Any compound that lowers interfacial tension and forms a film at an interface can function as an emulsifying agent. The effectiveness of an agent depends on its chemical structure, concentration, solubility, pH, physical properties, and electrostatic effects.

1. **True emulsifying agents** (primary agents) are capable of forming and stabilizing emulsions by themselves.

2. **Stabilizers** (auxiliary agents) do not form acceptable emulsions when used alone but do assist the primary agent in stabilizing the product. For example, they may increase viscosity.

3. Emulsifying agents may be natural or synthetic. **Natural emulsifying agents** include the following:
   a. **Acacia** forms a stable emulsion of low viscosity that tends to cream easily, is acidic, and is stable at a pH range of 2 to 10. Like other gums, it is negatively charged, dehydrates easily, and generally requires a preservative. It is incompatible with Peruvian balsam, bismuth salts, and carbonates (see also section II D 1 a).
   b. **Tragacanth** forms a stable emulsion that is coarser than acacia emulsion. It is anionic, difficult to hydrate, and used mainly for its viscosity effects. Less than one-tenth the amount as would be used for acacia is needed (see also section II D 1 b).
   c. **Agar** is an anionic gum used primarily to increase viscosity. Its stability is affected by heating, dehydration, and destruction of charge; it is also susceptible to microbial degradation.
   d. **Pectin** is a quasi-emulsifier that is used in the same proportion as tragacanth is used as an emulsifier.
   e. **Gelatin** provides good emulsion stabilization in the concentration range of 0.5% to 1.0%. It may be anionic or cationic, depending on the isoelectric point. Type A gelatin (+) is used in acid media; type B (−) in basic media.
   f. **Methylcellulose** is nonionic and induces viscosity. It is used as a primary emulsifier with mineral oil or cod-liver oil and yields an o/w emulsion. It is usually used in 2% concentration and forms a continuous film (see also section II D 1 c).

g. **Carboxymethylcellulose** is anionic and usually used to induce viscosity. It tolerates alcohol concentrations up to 40%, forms a basic solution, and precipitates in the presence of free acids (see also section II D 1 d).

4. **Synthetic emulsifying agents** may be anionic, cationic, or nonionic.
   a. **Anionic synthetic agents** include **sulfuric acid esters** (e.g., sodium lauryl sulfate), **sulfonic acid derivatives** (e.g., dioctyl sodium sulfosuccinate), and **soaps**.
      (1) **Soaps** are for **external use only**. They have a high pH and are sensitive to addition of acids and electrolytes.
      (2) **Alkali soaps** are hydrophilic and form o/w emulsions; **metallic soaps** are water-insoluble and form w/o emulsions; **monovalent soaps** form o/w emulsions; and **polyvalent soaps** form w/o emulsions.
   b. **Cationic synthetic agents** (e.g., benzalkonium chloride) are used as surface-active agents in 1% concentration. They are incompatible with soaps.
   c. **Nonionic synthetic agents** are resistant to the addition of acids and electrolytes.
      (1) The **sorbitan esters** known as **spans** are hydrophobic and form **w/o emulsions**. They have low hydrophilic–lipophilic balance (HLB) values (1 to 9).
      (2) The polysorbates known as **tweens** are hydrophilic in nature and form **o/w emulsions**. They may form complexes with phenolic compounds. They have high HLB values (11 to 20) [see section III E 4 c (1)].

5. The **HLB system** provides a means to rate an emulsifying agent's **balance between hydrophilic and lipophilic solution tendencies**.
   a. As an emulsifying agent becomes **more hydrophilic**, its solubility in water increases, favoring formation of an **o/w emulsion**. Conversely, **more lipophilic** agents favor formation of **w/o emulsions**.
   b. These observed tendencies led to the concept that the **type of emulsion** formed is related to the **balance between the hydrophilic and lipophilic solution tendencies** of the surface-active emulsifying agent. (Surface-active agents, or surfactants, are amphiphiles, in which the molecules or ions contain both hydrophilic and lipophilic portions.)
   c. The **HLB scale** is a numerical scale extending from 1 to approximately 50, based on the balance between these two opposing tendencies.
      (1) **More hydrophilic** surfactants have **high HLB numbers** (>10).
      (2) **More lipophilic** surfactants have **low HLB numbers** (1 to 10).
      (3) HLB values help **determine a surfactant's application** (Tables 3-1 and 3-2).
      (4) **Tweens** and **spans**, with their widely different HLB values, are often used in combination to provide an effective emulsifying agent, usually in a total concentration of approximately 2% w/v.

F. **Methods of preparation.** Emulsions may be prepared by the wet gum method, the dry gum method, the bottle method, or the nascent soap method.

1. For the **wet gum method** (also called the English method), a primary emulsion of the fixed oil, water, and acacia (in a 4:2:1 ratio) is prepared as follows:
   a. Two parts of water are added all at once to one part of acacia, and the mixture is **triturated** (rubbed together with a mortar and pestle) until a smooth mucilage is formed.
   b. Oil is added in small increments (1 to 5 ml) with continuous trituration until a primary emulsion is formed.
   c. The mixture (an o/w emulsion) is triturated for another 5 minutes and then brought to volume by mixing in water.

Table 3-1. HLB Values Affecting Surfactant Application

HLB Value Range	Surfactant Application
0–3	Antifoaming agents
4–6	w/o Emulsifying agents
7–9	Wetting agents
8–18	o/w Emulsifying agents
13–15	Detergents
10–18	Solubilizing agents

w/o = Water-in-oil.
o/w = Oil-in-water.
HLB = Hydrophilic–lipophilic balance.

Table 3-2. Commonly Used Surfactants and Their HLB Values

Agent	HLB Value
Sorbitan trioleate (Span 85, Arlacel 85)	1.8
Sorbitan tristearate (Span 65)	2.1
Propylene glycol monostearate (pure)	3.4
Sorbitan sesquioleate (Arlacel C)	3.7
Sorbitan monooleate (Span 80y)	4.3
Sorbitan monostearate (Arlacel 60)	4.7
Glyceryl monostearate (Aldo 28, Tegin)	5.5
Sorbitan monopalmitate (Span 40, Arlacel 40)	6.7
Sorbitan monolaurate (Span 20, Arlacel 20)	8.6
Gelatin	9.8
Triethanolamine oleate (Trolamine)	12.0
Polyoxyethylene alkyl phenol (Igepal CA-630)	12.8
Tragacanth	13.2
Polyoxyethylene sorbitan monolaurate (Tween 21)	13.3
Polyoxyethylene castor oil (Atlas G-1794)	13.3
Polyoxyethylene sorbitan monooleate (Tween 80)	15.0
Polyoxyethylene sorbitan monopalmitate (Tween 40)	15.6
Polyoxyethylene sorbitan monolaurate (Tween 20)	16.7
Polyoxyethylene lauryl ether (Brij 35)	16.9
Polyoxyethylene monostearate (Myrj 52)	16.9
Sodium oleate	18.0
Sodium lauryl sulfate	40.0

HLB = Hydrophilic–lipophilic balance.

2. For the **dry gum method** (also called the continental method), a primary emulsion of the fixed oil, water, and acacia (in a 4:2:1 ratio) is prepared as follows:
   a. The oil is added to the acacia and the mixture is triturated until the powder is distributed uniformly throughout the oil; then the water is added all at once, followed by rapid trituration to form the primary emulsion.
   b. Any remaining water and other ingredients are added to finish the product.
      (1) **Electrolytes in high concentration** tend to crack an emulsion; they should be added last and in as dilute a form as possible.
      (2) **Alcoholic solutions**, which tend to dehydrate and precipitate hydrocolloids, should also be added in as dilute a form as possible.
3. For the **bottle method** (a variation of the dry gum method used for **volatile oils**), the oil is added to the acacia in a bottle. The ratio of oil, water, and acacia should be 3:2:1 or 2:1:1, as the low viscosity of the volatile oil requires a higher proportion of acacia.
4. For the **nascent soap method**, a soap is formed by mixing relatively equal volumes of an oil and an aqueous solution containing a sufficient amount of alkali. The soap thus formed acts as an **emulsifying agent**.
   a. This method can be used for forming an **o/w** or a **w/o emulsion**, depending on the soap formed. For example, olive oil (contains oleic acid) and lime water are mixed during the preparation of calamine lotion to form calcium oleate, an emulsifying agent.
   b. A **50:50 ratio of oil to water** ensures sufficient formation of an emulsifying agent, provided the oil contains a sufficient amount of **free fatty acid**. (Olive oil usually does; cottonseed oil, peanut oil, and some other vegetable oils are deficient.)
   c. **Addition of an acid** destroys the emulsifying soap, causing separation of the emulsion.

G. **Incorporation of medicinal agents.** Medicinal agents may be incorporated into an emulsion during formation of the emulsion or after the emulsion is formed.

1. Generally, a **drug is best incorporated into a vehicle during emulsion formation**, when it can be incorporated in molecular form. Soluble drugs should be dissolved in the appropriate phase (e.g., a drug soluble in the external phase of the emulsion should be added as a solution to the primary emulsion).
2. Addition of a drug to a **preformed emulsion** may present some difficulty, which can be overcome by keeping in mind the type of the emulsion and the nature of the emulsifier (Table 3-3).

Table 3-3. Selected Commercial Emulsion Bases: Emulsion Type and Emulsifier Used

Commercial Base	Emulsion Type	Emulsifier Used
Allercreme Skin Lotion	o/w	Triethanolamine stearate
Almay Emulsion Base	o/w	Fatty acid glycol esters
Cetaphil	o/w	Sodium lauryl sulfate
Dermovan	o/w	Fatty acid amides
Eucerin	w/o	Wool wax alcohols
HEB Base	o/w	Sodium lauryl sulfate
Keri Lotion	o/w	Nonionic emulsifiers
Lubriderm	o/w	Triethanolamine stearate
Neobase	o/w	Polyhydric alcohol esters
Neutrogena Lotion	o/w	Triethanolamine lactate
Nivea Cream	w/o	Wool wax alcohols
pHorsix	o/w	Polyoxyethylene emulsifiers
Polysorb Hydrate	w/o	Sorbitan sesquioleate
Velvachol	o/w	Sodium lauryl sulfate

w/o = Water-in-oil.
o/w = Oil-in-water.

a. Addition of **oleaginous materials** to an **o/w emulsion** may be difficult after emulsion formation.
   (1) Occasionally, a small amount of oil material may be added if **excess emulsifier** was used in the original formulation.
   (2) A small quantity of an **oil-soluble drug** may also be added, if it is dissolved in a very small quantity of oil using geometric dilution techniques.

b. Addition of **aqueous material** to an **o/w emulsion** usually presents no problems if the added material does not interact with the emulsifying agent. **Potential interactions should be expected with cationic compounds and salts of weak bases.**

c. Small quantities of **alcoholic solutions** can also be incorporated directly into an **o/w emulsion**, provided the solute is compatible with or dispersible in the aqueous phase of the solution. If acacia or another gum is used as the emulsifying agent, the alcoholic solution should be diluted with water before addition.

d. Addition of **oleaginous materials** to a **w/o emulsion** presents no problems because of the miscibility of the additive with the external phase.

e. **Crystalline drugs may be incorporated more easily into a w/o emulsion** if they are dissolved in a small quantity of oil before addition.

f. Addition of **water or aqueous materials** to a **w/o emulsion** is extremely difficult unless enough emulsifier has been incorporated into the emulsion.

H. Emulsion stability. Creaming and coalescence may affect emulsion stability.

1. **Creaming** occurs when suspended particles or droplets rise or sediment, a process that depends on the specific gravities of the phases.
   a. **Larger particles** cream much more rapidly than smaller particles. Thus, formation of larger aggregates by coalescence accelerates creaming.
   b. If creaming takes place **without any aggregation**, the emulsion can be reconstituted by mixing or shaking.

2. **Coalescence** is the process by which emulsified particles merge with each other to form larger particles.
   a. The **major factor preventing coalescence** is the mechanical strength of the interfacial barrier. This is particularly true for o/w systems containing nonionic surfactants and for w/o emulsions in which electrical effects are negligible.
   b. Formation of a **thick interfacial film** is essential for minimal coalescence.

IV. OINTMENTS

A. Introduction

1. Ointments are **semisolid preparations intended for external use**. They are easily spread; their **plastic viscosity** may be controlled by modifications of the formulation.

2. Ointments are typically used as:
   a. **Emollients**, which make the skin more pliable

b. **Protective barriers**, which prevent harmful substances from coming in contact with the skin
c. **Vehicles** in which to incorporate medications

B. Ointment bases

1. **Oleaginous bases** are anhydrous and water-insoluble; they cannot absorb or contain water and are not washable in water.
   a. **Petrolatum** is a good base for oil-insoluble ingredients. It forms an occlusive film on the skin, absorbs less than 5% water under normal conditions, and does not become rancid. Wax may be incorporated to stiffen the base.
   b. A number of **synthetic esters** are used as oleaginous base constituents, including glyceryl monostearate, isopropyl myristate, isopropyl palmitate, and butyl stearate. **Longer-chain alcohols**, such as cetyl alcohol, stearyl alcohol, and polyethylene glycol (PEG), may also be used.
   c. Several **lanolin derivatives** are commonly used in topical and cosmetic preparations. Examples include lanolin oil (Lantrol) and hydrogenated lanolin.

2. **Absorption bases** are anhydrous, water-insoluble, and not washable in water; however, they can absorb water. They permit the inclusion of water-soluble drugs through prior solution and uptake of the solution in the internal phase.
   a. **Wool fat** (anhydrous lanolin) contains a high percentage of cholesterol as well as esters and alcohol-containing fatty acids. It absorbs twice its weight in water and melts between 36° and 42°C.
   b. **Hydrophilic petrolatum** is a white petrolatum combined with 8% white beeswax, 3% stearyl alcohol, and 3% cholesterol, added to a w/o emulsifier.
      (1) Prepared forms include **Aquaphor**, which employs wood alcohol to render white petrolatum emulsifiable; **Polysorb**, which uses sorbitan sesquioleate (Arlacel 83) as the emulsifier; and **Kessolin**.
      (2) **Kessolin** appears to be superior to the USP base. **Aquaphor** is superior in its ability to absorb water.

3. **Emulsion bases** may be **w/o emulsions**, which are water-insoluble and not washable in water but can absorb water because of their aqueous internal phase; or **o/w emulsions**, which are water-insoluble but washable in water and able to absorb water in their aqueous external phase.
   a. **Hydrous wool fat** (lanolin) is a w/o emulsion containing about 25% water. It acts as an emollient and forms an occlusive film on the skin, effectively preventing epidermal water loss.
   b. **Cold cream** is a w/o emulsion prepared by melting white wax, spermaceti, and expressed almond oil together and then adding a hot aqueous solution of sodium borate and stirring until cool.
      (1) Use of **mineral oil** rather than almond oil makes a more stable cold cream; however, cold cream prepared with **almond oil** is a better emollient base.
      (2) This ointment base should be **freshly prepared**.
   c. **Hydrophilic ointment** is an o/w emulsion employing sodium lauryl sulfate as the emulsifying agent. It will absorb about 30% to 50% of its weight in water without losing its consistency. It is readily miscible with water and can thus be removed from the skin easily.
   d. **Vanishing cream** is an o/w emulsion containing a large percentage of water as well as a **humectant** (such as glycerin or propylene glycol), which retards surface evaporation of the product. An excess of stearic acid in the formula helps form a thin film when the water evaporates.
   e. **Other emulsion bases** include **Dermovan**, a hypoallergenic, greaseless emulsion base, and **Unibase**, a nongreasy emulsion base that absorbs about 30% of its weight in water and has a pH close to that of skin.

4. **Water-soluble bases** may be anhydrous or may contain some water. They are washable in water and absorb water to the point of solubility.
   a. **PEG** ointment consists of a blend of water-soluble polymeric glycols that form a semisolid base capable of solubilizing water-soluble drugs and some water-insoluble drugs. It is compatible with a wide range of medications.
      (1) This base contains 40% PEG 4000 and 60% PEG 400 and is prepared by the **fusion method**.
      (2) Only **small amounts of liquid** ($< 5\%$) can be incorporated into the base without loss of viscosity. The base can be made stiffer by increasing the amount of PEG 4000 up to 60%.
   b. **Propylene glycol and propylene glycol-ethanol** form a clear gel when mixed with 2% hydroxypropyl cellulose. This base has become popular as a dermatologic vehicle.

C. **Methods of preparation.** Substances may be incorporated into an ointment base by **levigation** or by the **fusion method**. Insoluble substances should first be reduced to the finest possible form and levigated before incorporation, by levigating either with a small amount of compatible levigating agent or with the base itself.

1. For **levigation**, the substance is incorporated into the ointment by levigation on an ointment slab [see section VI A 4 b (3)]. (A mortar and pestle is preferred when incorporating a relatively large amount of liquid.)
   a. A **stainless steel spatula** with a long, broad flexible blade should be used for levigation. If interaction with the metal spatula is possible (as when incorporating iodine or mercuric salts), a **hard rubber spatula** may be used.
   b. **Insoluble substances** should be finely powdered in a mortar and then mixed with an equal quantity of ointment base until a smooth, grit-free mixture results. The rest of the base is then added in small increments.
   c. **Levigation of powder into a small portion** of base may be facilitated by using the melted base or by using a small quantity of a compatible levigation aid, such as mineral oil or glycerin.
   d. **Water-soluble salts** may be incorporated by dissolving them in the smallest possible amount of water and then incorporating the aqueous solution directly into the base, if the base is compatible.
      (1) Usually, **organic solvents** such as ether, chloroform, and alcohol should not be used to dissolve the drug because the drug may crystallize out as the solvent evaporates.
      (2) Solvents should be used as levigating aids **only if the solid will become a fine powder** following evaporation of the solvent.

2. The **fusion method** may be used when the base contains solids with higher melting points, such as waxes, cetyl alcohol, or glyceryl monostearate. This method is also particularly useful for solid medications that are readily soluble in the melted base.
   a. The **oil phase** should be melted separately, starting with the material that has the **highest melting point**. All other oil-soluble ingredients are then added in decreasing order of melting point.
   b. The ingredients in the **water phase** are combined and heated separately to a temperature equal to, or several degrees above, that of the melted oil phase.
   c. The **two phases are then combined**. If a **w/o system** is desired, the hot aqueous phase is incorporated into the hot oil phase with agitation. If an **o/w system** is preferred, the hot oil phase is incorporated into the hot aqueous phase.
   d. **Volatile materials** (such as menthol, camphor, iodine, alcohol, and perfumes) should be added after the melted mixture has cooled to 40°C or less.

V. SUPPOSITORIES

A. Introduction

1. A suppository is a **solid or semisolid mass meant to be inserted into a body orifice** (e.g., the rectum, the vagina, or the urethra) to provide either a local or a systemic therapeutic effect.

2. Once inserted, the suppository either **melts at body temperature** or **dissolves** (or disintegrates) **into the cavity's aqueous secretions**.

3. Suppositories are frequently used for **local effects**, such as relief of hemorrhoids or infection in the rectum, the vagina, or the urethra.

4. Suppositories can also provide **systemic medication** when used rectally.
   a. **Absorption of a drug** from a suppository through the rectal mucosa involves release of the drug from the vehicle, followed by diffusion of the drug through the mucosa and transportation by way of veins or lymph vessels into the circulation.
   b. Because the rectal veins bypass the liver, **first-pass effects** are avoided (see Chapter 4, section V E 5 f).
   c. Rectal suppositories are useful when **oral administration is inappropriate**, as with infants, debilitated patients, comatose patients, and patients with nausea, vomiting, or gastrointestinal disturbances. Some drugs given in rectal suppositories may cause gastrointestinal irritation.

B. Suppository types

1. **Rectal suppositories** are usually cylindrical and tapered to a point, forming a bullet-like shape. Contractions of the rectum cause a suppository of this shape to move inward, rather than outward. An adult suppository weighs about 2 g; a suppository for an infant or a child is smaller.

2. **Vaginal suppositories** are oval in shape and typically weigh about 5 g. Drugs administered by this route are intended to have local effects, but systemic absorption can occur. Antiseptics, contraceptive agents, and drugs used to treat trichomonal, monilial, or bacterial infections are commonly formulated into suppositories.

3. **Urethral suppositories** are long and tapered (typically about 60 mm long with a diameter of 4 to 5 mm). Drugs administered by this route (usually anti-infectives) have local action only. The only urethral suppository in common use is the nitrofurazone (Furacin) urethral insert.

C. Suppository bases

1. A **satisfactory suppository base** should meet these criteria:
   - **a.** Remains firm at room temperature for insertion (preferably it should not soften below 30°C to avoid premature melting during storage)
   - **b.** Has a narrow (or sharp) **melting range**
   - **c.** Yields a clear melt just below body temperature (or dissolves or disintegrates rapidly in the cavity fluid)
   - **d.** Is inert and compatible with a wide range of drugs
   - **e.** Is nonirritating and nonsensitizing
   - **f.** Has wetting and emulsifying properties
   - **g.** If the base is **fatty**, should also have an **acid value** below 0.2, a **saponification value** in the range of 200 to 245, and an **iodine value** less than 7
2. When selecting a suppository base, its **lipid–water solubility** must be considered because of its relationship to the rate of drug release.
   - **a.** If an **oil-soluble drug** is incorporated into an **oily base**, the rate of absorption is somewhat less than that achieved with a **water-soluble base**. The drug tends to remain dissolved in the oily pool from the suppository and has less tendency to escape into the mucous secretions from which it is ultimately absorbed.
   - **b.** Conversely, a **water-soluble drug** tends to pass more rapidly from the oil phase to the aqueous phase. If a rapid onset of action is desired, the **water-soluble form** of the drug should be incorporated into an **oily base**.
3. **Bases that melt** include cocoa butter, other combinations of fats and waxes, the witepsol bases, and the wecobee bases (Table 3-4).
   - **a. Cocoa butter** (theobroma oil) is the most widely used suppository base. It is a firm solid up to 32°C, at which point it begins to soften; it melts at 34° to 35°C, producing a thin, bland, oily liquid.
     - **(1)** Cocoa butter is a good base for **rectal suppositories** but less than ideal for vaginal and urethral suppositories.
     - **(2)** A mixture of triglycerides, cocoa butter exhibits **polymorphism**. Depending on the fusion temperature, it may crystallize into any one of four crystal forms.
     - **(3)** The **major limitation** of cocoa butter is its **inability to absorb aqueous solutions**. Addition of nonionic surfactants ameliorates this to some extent; however, the resulting suppositories have poor stability and may turn rancid rapidly.
     - **(4)** Another disadvantage is the **lowering of the melting point produced by certain drugs** (e.g., chloral hydrate).
     - **(5)** Because of these limitations, **many combinations of fats and waxes** have been suggested as substitutes (see Table 3-4).

Table 3-4. Composition, Melting Range, and Congealing Range of Selected Bases That Melt

Base	Composition	Melting Range (°C)	Congealing Range (°C)
Cocoa butter	Mixed triglycerides of oleic, palmitic, and stearic acids	34–35	28 or less
Cotmar	Partially hydrogenated cottonseed oil	34–75	. . .
Dehydag	Hydrogenated fatty alcohols and esters		
Base I		33–36	32–33
Base II		37–39	36–37
Base III		9 ranges	9 ranges
Wecobee R	Glycerides of saturated fatty acids C_{12} to C_{18}	33–35	31–32
Wecobee SS	Triglycerides derived from coconut oil	40–43	33–35
Witepsol	Triglycerides of saturated fatty acids C_{12} to C_{18}, with varied portions of the corresponding partial glycerides		
H-12		32–33	29–31
H-15		33–35	32–34
H-85		42–44	36–38

b. The **witepsol bases** contain natural saturated fatty acid chains between C_{12} and C_{18}, with lauric acid the major component. All 12 bases of this series are colorless and almost odorless; witepsol 15 has drug-release characteristics similar to those of cocoa butter.

(1) Unlike cocoa butter, the witepsol bases **do not exhibit polymorphism** when heated and cooled.

(2) The **interval between softening and melting temperatures** is very small. Because witepsol bases solidify rapidly in the mold, lubrication of the mold is unnecessary.

c. The **wecobee bases** are derived from coconut oil and appear similar in action to the witepsol bases. Incorporation of glyceryl monostearate and propylene glycol monostearate makes these bases emulsifiable.

4. Bases that dissolve include the PEG polymers in the molecular weight range of 400 to 6000.

a. At **room temperature**, PEG 400 is a liquid, PEG 1000 a semisolid, PEG 1500 and PEG 1540 fairly firm semisolids, and PEG 4000 and 6000 firm, wax-like solids.

b. These bases are **water-soluble**; however, the dissolution process is very slow. In the rectum and the vagina, where the amount of fluid is small, they dissolve very slowly but do soften and spread.

c. Several drugs may complex with PEG, influencing release and absorption.

d. Mixtures of PEG polymers in varying proportions provide bases of different properties (Table 3-5).

D. Methods of preparation. Suppositories may be prepared by hand rolling, by compression, or by the fusion method.

1. Hand rolling involves molding of the suppository with the fingers after formation of a plastic mass.

a. Finely powdered drug is mixed with the **grated base** in a mortar and pestle, using levigation and geometric dilution. A small quantity of fixed oil may be added to facilitate preparation of the mass.

b. The uniformly mixed semiplastic mass is **kneaded** further and then **rolled into a cylinder**.

2. Compression is generally employed when cocoa butter is used as a base.

a. A **uniform mixture of drug and base** is prepared as for the hand-rolling method.

b. The mixture is then **placed in a chamber mold**, and the mold is cooled.

c. This procedure usually produces a **2-g suppository**; however, the volume of active ingredient may affect the amount of cocoa butter required for an individual formula, if the active ingredient is present in a relatively large amount.

(1) The **amount of cocoa butter needed** may be determined by calculating the total amount of active ingredient to be used, dividing this by the **cocoa butter density factor of the active ingredient** (Table 3-6), and subtracting the resulting number from the total amount of cocoa butter needed for the required number of suppositories.

(2) For example, suppose 12 suppositories, each containing 300 mg of aspirin, are required. The mold has a 2-g capacity. For 13 suppositories (calculated to provide one extra), 3.9 g of aspirin (13 × 0.3 g) is required. This is divided by the density factor of aspirin (1.1) [see Table 3-6]. Thus, 3.9 g of aspirin replaces 3.55 g of cocoa butter. The total amount of cocoa butter needed for 13 suppositories of 2 g each equals 26 g; with aspirin added, the amount of cocoa butter required is 26 g minus 3.55 g, or 22.45 g.

Table 3-5. Mixtures of PEG Bases Providing Satisfactory Room-Temperature Stability and Dissolution Characteristics

Base	Comments	Components	Proportion (%)
1	Provides a good general-purpose water-soluble suppository base	PEG 6000 PEG 1540 PEG 400	50 30 20
2	Provides a good general-purpose base that is slightly softer than base 1 and dissolves more readily	PEG 4000 PEG 1000 PEG 400	60 30 10
3	Has a higher melting point than the other bases, which is usually sufficient to compensate for the melting-point lowering effect of such drugs as chloral hydrate and camphor	PEG 6000 PEG 1540	30 70

PEG = polyethylene glycol.

Table 3-6. Cocoa Butter Density Factors of Drugs Commonly Used in Suppositories

Drug	Cocoa Butter Density Factor	Drug	Cocoa Butter Density Factor
Aloin	1.3	Dimenhydrinate	1.3
Aminophylline	1.1	Diphenhydramine hydrochloride	1.3
Aminopyrine	1.3	Gallic acid	2.0
Aspirin	1.1	Morphine hydrochloride	1.6
Barbital sodium	1.2	Pentobarbital	1.2
Belladonna extract	1.3	Phenobarbital sodium	1.2
Bismuth subgallate	2.7	Salicylic acid	1.3
Chloral hydrate	1.3	Secobarbital sodium	1.2
Codeine phosphate	1.1	Tannic acid	1.6
Digitalis leaf	1.6		

3. The **fusion method** is the principal way of making suppositories commercially and is primarily used when cocoa butter, PEG, and glycerin–gelatin bases are used. Molds made of aluminum, brass, or nickel–copper alloys are employed, which can make from 6 to 50 suppositories (see section IV C 2).
   a. The **capacity of the molds** is determined by melting a sufficient quantity of base over a steam bath, pouring it into the molds, and allowing it to congeal. The sample suppositories are then trimmed, removed, and weighed. Once the weight is known, the suppositories can be prepared.
      (1) To prepare suppositories, the **drug is reduced to a fine powder**, and a small amount of **grated cocoa butter is liquified** in a suitable container placed in a water bath or a steam bath at 33°C or less.
      (2) The finely powdered drug is **mixed** with the melted cocoa butter by continuous stirring.
      (3) The **remainder of the grated cocoa butter is added by stirring**, while maintaining the temperature at 33°C or below. The liquid should appear creamy rather than clear.
      (4) The creamy melt is **poured into the mold at room temperature**. The mold must be very lightly lubricated with mineral oil; the melt should be poured continuously to avoid layering.
      (5) The suppositories are **allowed to congeal** and then are placed in a refrigerator for 30 minutes to harden. Then they can be removed from the refrigerator, trimmed, and unmolded.
   b. The fusion process presents certain problems. It should be used carefully with **thermolabile drugs** and **insoluble powders**.
      (1) **Insoluble powders** in the liquid may settle during pouring, collecting at the top of the suppository and causing nonuniform drug distribution.
      (2) **Hard crystalline materials** (e.g., iodine and merbromin) can be incorporated by dissolving the crystals in a minimum volume of suitable solvent prior to incorporation into the base.
      (3) **Vegetable extracts** can be incorporated by moistening with a few drops of alcohol and levigating with a small amount of melted cocoa butter.

VI. POWDERS

A. Introduction

1. A pharmaceutical powder is a **mixture of finely divided drugs and/or chemicals in dry form**, meant for internal or external use.

2. The **advantages** of powders include:
   a. **Flexibility of compounding**
   b. **Good chemical stability**
   c. **Rapid dispersion of ingredients** (because of the small particle size)

3. **Disadvantages** include:
   a. **Time-consuming preparation**
   b. **Dose inaccuracy**
   c. **Unsuitability for many unpleasant-tasting, hygroscopic, or deliquescent drugs**

4. Substances to be incorporated in a powder are frequently **milled** to reduce particle size (Tables 3-7 and 3-8). After milling, the various substances are mixed as needed. Milling is the

Table 3-7. USP Standards for Powders of Animal and Vegetable Drugs

Type of Powder	Sieve Size All Particles Pass Through	Sieve Size Percentage of Particles Pass Through
Very coarse (#8)	#20 sieve	20% through a #60 sieve
Coarse (#20)	#20 sieve	40% through a #60 sieve
Moderately coarse (#40)	#40 sieve	40% through a #80 sieve
Fine (#60)	#60 sieve	40% through a #100 sieve
Very fine (#80)	#80 sieve	No limit

mechanical process of reducing the particle size of solids (**comminution**) before incorporation into a final product. The particle size of a given powder is related to the proportion of the powder that can pass through the openings of standard sieves of varying dimension in a specified time period. (**Micrometrics** is the study of particle size.)

a. Milling has both advantages and disadvantages.

(1) Advantages

(a) Increases surface area, which may increase dissolution rate and bioavailability (e.g., griseofulvin)

(b) Increases extraction or leaching from animal glands (such as the liver and pancreas) and from crude vegetable extracts

(c) Facilitates drying of wet masses by increasing surface area and reducing the distance moisture must travel to reach the outer surface; micronization and subsequent drying, in turn, increase stability as occluded solvent is removed

(d) Improves mixing or blending of several solid ingredients if they are reduced to approximately the same size; minimizes segregation and provides greater dose uniformity

(e) Permits uniform distribution of coloring agents in artificially colored solid pharmaceuticals

(f) Improves the function of lubricants used in compressed tablets and capsules to coat the surface of the granulation or powder

(g) Improves the texture, appearance, and physical stability of ointments, creams, and pastes

(2) Disadvantages

(a) May change the polymorphic form of the active ingredient, rendering it less active, inactive, or unstable

(b) May degrade the drug as a result of heat buildup during milling, oxidation, or adsorption of unwanted moisture (due to increased surface area)

(c) Decreases the bulk density of the active compound and excipients, possibly causing flow problems and segregation

(d) Decreases raw material particle size, possibly creating static charge problems that may cause particle aggregation and decreased dissolution rate

(e) Increases surface area, which may promote air adsorption that may inhibit wettability of the drug

b. On a large scale, various mills and pulverizers (e.g., the rotary cutter, the hammer, the roller, and the fluid energy mill) may be used during manufacturing. On a small scale, as in a community pharmacy, the pharmacist usually uses one of the following **comminution techniques**:

(1) Trituration. The substance is reduced to small particles by rubbing it in a mortar with a pestle. The term is also used to designate the process by which fine powders are intimately mixed in a mortar.

(2) Pulverization by intervention. The substance is reduced and subdivided with an additional material that can be removed easily after pulverization is complete. The tech-

Table 3-8. USP Standards for Powders of Chemicals

Type of Powder	Sieve Size All Particles Pass Through	Sieve Size Percentage of Particles Pass Through
Coarse (#20)	#20 sieve	60% through a #40 sieve
Moderately coarse (#40)	#40 sieve	60% through a #60 sieve
Fine (#80)	#80 sieve	No limit
Very fine (#120)	#120 sieve	No limit

nique is often used with substances that are gummy and tend to reagglomerate or tend to resist grinding. For example, camphor can be reduced readily after addition of a small amount of alcohol or other volatile solvent, which is then permitted to evaporate.

(3) **Levigation.** The substance is reduced in particle size by adding a suitable nonsolvent (levigating agent) to form a paste and then rubbing the paste in a mortar and pestle or using an ointment slab and a spatula. This method is often used to incorporate solids into dermatologic or ophthalmic ointments and suspensions, to prevent a gritty feel. Mineral oil is a common levigating agent.

B. Mixing of powders. Powders may be mixed (blended) by spatulation, trituration, geometric dilution, sifting, or tumbling.

1. For **spatulation**, small amounts of powders are blended by the movement of a spatula through the powders on a sheet of paper or a pill tile.
   a. This method is **not suitable for large quantities of powders** or for **powders containing one or more potent substances** because homogeneous blending may not occur.
   b. It is **particularly useful for solid substances that liquify or form eutectic mixtures** (mixtures that melt at lower temperatures than any of their ingredients) **when in close and prolonged contact with one another** since very little compression or compaction results.
      (1) **Such substances** include phenol, camphor, menthol, thymol, aspirin, phenylsalicylate, phenacetin, and other similar chemicals.
      (2) To **diminish contact**, powders prepared from these substances are commonly mixed in the presence of an **inert diluent**, such as light magnesium oxide, magnesium carbonate, kaolin, starch, or bentonite.
      (3) **Silicic acid** (about 20%) prevents eutexia with aspirin, phenylsalicylate, and other troublesome compounds.

2. **Trituration** is used both to comminute and to mix powders.
   a. If **comminution** is desired, a **porcelain or Wedgwood mortar** with a rough inner surface is preferred to a glass mortar with a smooth working surface.
   b. A **glass mortar** may be preferred for chemicals that may stain a porcelain or Wedgwood surface and for **simple mixture** of substances without special need for comminution. A glass mortar cleans more readily after use.

3. **Geometric dilution** is employed when potent substances are to be mixed with a large amount of diluent.
   a. The **potent drug** is placed upon an approximately equal volume of the diluent in a mortar, and the substances are **thoroughly mixed by trituration**.
   b. A second portion of diluent **equal in volume to the powder mixture in the mortar** is added, and trituration is repeated. The process is continued, adding diluent equal in volume to the mixture in the mortar at each step, until all the diluent is incorporated.

4. During **sifting**, powders are mixed by passing them through sifters similar to those used in the kitchen to sift flour. This process results in a light, fluffy product and is generally not acceptable for incorporation of potent drugs into a diluent base.

5. **Tumbling** is the process of mixing powders in a large container rotated by a motorized process. These **blenders** are widely employed in industry, as are **large-volume powder mixers**, which use motorized blades to blend powders contained in a large mixing vessel.

C. Use and packaging of powders. Depending on their intended use, powders are packaged and dispensed by pharmacists as bulk powders or divided powders.

1. **Bulk powders** are dispensed by the pharmacist in bulk containers: a **perforated or sifter can** for external dusting; an **aerosol container** for spraying onto the skin; or a **wide-mouthed glass or pasteboard jar** that permits easy removal of a spoonful of powder.
   a. Powders **commonly dispensed in bulk form** include:
      (1) **Antacid powders** and **laxative powders**, meant to be used by mixing the directed amount (usually a teaspoonful or so) in a portion of liquid, which is then drunk
      (2) **Douche powders**, meant to be dissolved in warm water and applied vaginally
      (3) **Medicated or nonmedicated powders for external use**, usually dispensed in a sifter can to aid convenient application to the skin
      (4) **Dentifrices or dental cleansing powders**, used for oral hygiene
      (5) **Insufflations** (powders meant to be blown into body cavities, such as the ear, nose, throat, tooth sockets, or vagina), administered by means of an **insufflator** (powder blower)
   b. Generally, only **nonpotent substances** are dispensed in bulk powder form. Those intended for **external use** should bear a label indicating this.

c. Powders that are **hygroscopic, deliquescent**, or have **volatile ingredients** should be packed in **glass jars** rather than pasteboard containers. **Amber** or **green glass** should be used if needed to prevent the light-sensitive components of the powder from decomposition. All powders should be stored in tightly closed containers.

2. **Divided powders** are dispensed in the form of individual doses, generally in properly folded papers (known as **chartulae**). However, they may also be dispensed in metal foil, small heat-sealed plastic bags, or other containers.
   a. After weighing, comminution, and mixing of the ingredients, the powder must be **divided into the prescribed number of doses.**
   b. Depending on the **potency of the drug**, the pharmacist decides whether to weigh each portion separately before packaging or to approximate portions by the block-and-divide method.
   c. The **powder papers** may be of any convenient size that fits the required dose. There are **four basic types** of powder papers:
   (1) **Vegetable parchment**, a thin, semiopaque, moisture-resistant paper
   (2) **White bond**, an opaque paper that is not moisture-resistant
   (3) **Glassine**, a glazed, transparent, moisture-resistant paper
   (4) **Waxed paper**, a translucent, waterproof paper
   d. **Hygroscopic drugs** and **volatile drugs** are best protected with **waxed paper**, double-wrapped with **white bond** to improve the final appearance. Parchment and glassine papers are of limited use for these drugs.

D. Special problems

1. **Volatile substances**, such as camphor, menthol, or essential oils, may be lost by **volatilization** after incorporation into a powder. This process is **prevented** or **retarded** by use of heat-sealed plastic bags or by double-wrapping with waxed or glassine paper inside white bond paper.

2. **Liquids** may be incorporated into divided powders in small amounts.
   a. **Magnesium carbonate**, **starch**, or **lactose** may be added to increase the absorbability of the powder by increasing surface area.
   b. When the liquid is a **solvent for a nonvolatile, heat-stable compound**, it may be evaporated gently in a water bath. Some fluid extracts and tinctures may be treated this way.

3. **Hygroscopic and deliquescent substances** that become moist because of an affinity for moisture in the air may be prepared as divided powders by adding **inert diluents**. **Double-wrapping** provides further protection.

4. **Eutectic mixtures.** For a complete discussion, see section VI B 1.

VII. CAPSULES

A. Introduction

1. Capsules are **solid dosage forms in which one or more medicinal and/or inert substances are enclosed within a small gelatin shell.**

2. Gelatin capsules may be **hard** or **soft**; the majority are intended to be **swallowed whole**. However, occasionally the contents may be removed from the shell and employed as a **premeasured medicinal powder** (e.g., Theo-Dur Sprinkle, an anhydrous theophylline preparation meant to be sprinkled on a small amount of soft food before ingestion).

B. Hard gelatin capsules

1. **Empty hard capsule shells** are manufactured from a mixture of gelatin, colorants, and sometimes an opacifying agent such as titanium dioxide; the USP also permits addition of 0.15% sulfur dioxide to prevent decomposition of gelatin during manufacture.
   a. **Gelatin USP** is obtained by the partial hydrolysis of collagen from animal skin, white connective tissues, and bones. Type A gelatin is obtained by acid processing; type B, by alkali processing.
   b. Capsule shells are **cast** by dipping cold metallic molds, or pins, into a gelatin solution maintained at a uniform temperature and an exact degree of fluidity.
   (1) **Variation in gelatin solution viscosity** increases or decreases capsule wall thickness.
   (2) Once the pins have been withdrawn from the gelatin solution, they are **rotated while being dried in a kiln** through which a strong blast of controlled-humidity filtered air is forced. Each capsule is then mechanically stripped, trimmed, and joined.

2. Hard capsules should be **stored in tightly closed glass containers**, protected from dust and from extremes of humidity and temperature.
   a. These capsules contain **12% to 16% water**, varying with storage conditions. When **humidity is low**, capsules become **brittle**; when **humidity is high**, capsules become **flaccid and shapeless**.
   b. Storage in **high-temperature areas** also affects the quality of hard capsules.

3. Hard capsules are available in a **variety of sizes**.
   a. Empty capsules are numbered from **000** (the largest size that can be swallowed) to **5** (the smallest size). Approximate capsule **capacity** ranges from **600 mg to 30 mg** for capsules from sizes 000 to 5. However, capacity varies because of varying densities of powdered drug materials and the degree of pressure used in filling the capsules.
   b. Larger sizes are available for **veterinary medicine**.

4. **Preparation of filled hard capsules** includes preparing the formulation, selecting the appropriate capsule, filling the capsule shells, and cleaning and polishing the filled shells.
   a. Generally, hard capsule shells are used to **encapsulate between 65 mg and 1 g of powdered material**, including the drug and any diluents needed.
      (1) If the drug dose for a single capsule is **inadequate** to fill the capsule, a **diluent**, such as lactose, **must be added**.
      (2) If the amount of drug representing a usual dose is **too large** to be placed in a single capsule, **two or more capsules may be required** to provide the particular dose.
      (3) **Lubricants** such as magnesium stearate (frequently less than 1%) are added to facilitate the flow of powder when an automatic capsule-filling machine is used.
      (4) **Wetting agents** such as lithium carbonate may be added to capsule formulations to enhance drug dissolution.
   b. **Capsule size** should be chosen carefully. A properly filled capsule has its body filled with drug mixture and its cap fully extended down the body. The cap is meant to enclose the powder, not to retain additional powder.
   c. Capsules are usually **filled by the punch method**.
      (1) The powder is placed on paper and flattened with a spatula so that the layer of powder is no more than about one-third the length of the capsule. The paper is held in the left hand, and the body of the capsule, held in the right hand, is pressed repeatedly into the powder until the body is filled. Then, the cap is replaced and the capsule weighed.
      (2) **Granular material** that does not lend itself to the punch method may be poured into each capsule from the powder paper on which it was weighed.
      (3) **Crystalline material** (especially material consisting of a mass of filament-like crystals, as with the quinine salts) will not fit into a capsule easily unless first powdered.
   d. **Hand-operated capsule machines** may be used when capsules are prepared regularly or in large quantities. These machines are available in capacities of 24, 96, 100, or 144 capsules.
      (1) When efficiently operated, they can produce from **about 2000 capsules/day** (for the smallest machine) to **about 2000 capsules/hr** (for the largest machines).
      (2) Machines for **industrial use** automatically remove the caps from empty capsules, fill the capsules, replace the caps, and clean the outside of the capsules, at a rate of up to 165,000 capsules/hr.
   e. Once filled, capsules must be **cleaned and polished**.
      (1) On a **small scale**, capsules may be cleaned individually or in small numbers by rubbing them with a clean gauze or cloth.
      (2) On a **large scale**, many capsule machines have a cleaning vacuum that removes extraneous material from the capsules as they leave the machine.

C. Soft gelatin capsules

1. Soft gelatin capsules are prepared from **gelatin shells to which glycerin or a polyhydric alcohol** (such as sorbitol) **has been added**, rendering the shells elastic or plastic-like.

2. These shells also contain **preservatives** (such as methyl- and propylparabens and sorbic acid) to prevent the growth of fungi.

3. Soft gelatin shells may be **oblong, elliptic**, or **spherical in shape** and may be used to contain **liquids, suspensions, pasty materials, dry powders**, or **pelletized materials**.
   a. Drugs **commercially prepared in soft capsules** include ethchlorvynol (Placidyl), demeclocycline hydrochloride (Declomycin), chlorotrianisene (TACE), chloral hydrate (Noctec), digoxin (Lanoxicaps), vitamin A, and vitamin E.
   b. Soft gelatin capsules are usually prepared by the **plate process**, using a rotary or reciprocating productive die.

D. Uniformity and disintegration

1. **Uniformity of dosage** can be demonstrated by either weight variation or content uniformity methods. The official compendia should be consulted for details of these procedures.

2. **Disintegration tests** are usually not required for capsules unless they have been **enteric-coated** (treated to resist solution in gastric fluid) [see section VIII C 1 d]. In this case, they must meet the requirements for disintegration of enteric-coated tablets.

VIII. TABLETS

A. Introduction

1. The **oral route** is the most important method of drug administration when systemic effects are desired.

2. Oral drugs may be given as **solids** or **liquids**.
   a. **Solid dosage forms** have these **advantages**:
      (1) Accurate dosage
      (2) Easy shipping and handling
      (3) Less shelf space needed per dose than for liquids
      (4) No preservation requirements
      (5) No taste-masking problems
      (6) Generally more stable than liquids, with longer expiration dates
   b. **Liquid dosage forms** have these **advantages**:
      (1) The drug may be more effective in liquid than in solid form (e.g., adsorbents, antacids).
      (2) They may be useful for patients who have trouble swallowing solid dosage forms (e.g., pediatric and geriatric patients).

3. **Tablets** are the **most commonly used** solid dosage form.
   a. Tablets have these **advantages**:
      (1) Unit dose has great dose precision and low content variability
      (2) Low manufacturing cost
      (3) Easy to package and ship
      (4) Simple to identify
      (5) Easy to swallow
      (6) Lend themselves to special-release forms
      (7) Best suited to large-scale production
      (8) Most stable of all oral forms
      (9) Essentially tamperproof
   b. However, tablets also have these **disadvantages**:
      (1) Some drugs resist compression into tablets
      (2) Some drugs (e.g., those with poor wetting, slow dissolution, optimum absorption high in the gastrointestinal tract, or a combination of these) cannot be formulated as tablets with adequate drug bioavailability
      (3) Some drugs (e.g., bitter-tasting drugs, those with an objectionable odor, or those sensitive to oxygen or atmospheric moisture) require encapsulation or entrapment prior to compression or coating after compression. A capsule form may be a better approach for these.

B. Tablet design and formulation

1. An **ideal tablet** should be **free of such defects** as cracks, chips, discoloration, and contamination; should have the **strength** to withstand the mechanical stresses of production; should be **chemically and physically stable** over time; and should **release the medicinal agent in a predictable and reproducible manner**.

2. Tablets may be **manufactured** by **wet granulation, dry granulation**, or **direct compression**.

3. Regardless of their manner of manufacture, tablets for oral ingestion usually contain **excipients**, components added to the active ingredients that have special functions (Table 3-9).
   a. **Diluents** are fillers designed to make up the required bulk of a tablet when the drug dosage amount is inadequate. Diluents may also improve cohesion, permit use of direct compression manufacturing, or promote flow.
      (1) **Common diluents** include kaolin, lactose, mannitol, starch, powdered sugar, and calcium phosphate.
      (2) **Selection** of a diluent is based on the manufacturer's experience as well as on diluent cost and compatibility with other tablet ingredients. For example, calcium salts cannot

Table 3-9. Common Tablet Excipients

Diluents	**Disintegrants**
Calcium phosphate dihydrate NF (dibasic)	Alginates
Calcium sulfate dihydrate NF	Cellulose
Cellulose NF (microcrystalline)	Cellulose derivatives
Cellulose derivatives	Clays
Dextrose	PVP (cross-linked)
Lactose USP	Starch
Lactose USP (anhydrous)	Starch derivatives
Lactose USP (spray-dried)	**Lubricants**
Mannitol USP	PEGs
Starches (directly compressible)	Stearic acid
Starches (hydrolyzed)	Stearic acid salts
Sorbitol	Stearic acid derivatives
Sucrose USP (powder)	Surfactants
Sucrose-based materials	Talc
	Waxes
Binders and adhesives	**Glidants**
Acacia	Cornstarch
Cellulose derivatives	Silica derivatives
Gelatin	Talc
Glucose	**Colors, flavors, and sweeteners**
PVP	FD&C and D&C dyes and lakes
Sodium alginate and alginate derivatives	Flavors are available in two forms: spray-dried and oils
Sorbitol	Artificial sweeteners
Starch (paste)	Natural sweeteners
Starch (pregelatinized)	
Tragacanth	

PVP = polyvinylpyrrolidone; more commonly called povidone.
PEG = polyethylene glycol.

be employed as fillers for tetracycline products because calcium interferes with tetracycline's absorption from the gastrointestinal tract.

b. **Binders and adhesives** are materials added in either dry or liquid form to promote granulation during the wet granulation process or to promote cohesive compacts during the direct compression process.
   (1) **Common binding agents** include a 10% to 20% aqueous preparation of cornstarch; a 25% to 50% solution of glucose; molasses; various natural gums, such as acacia; cellulose derivatives, such as methylcellulose, carboxymethylcellulose, and microcrystalline cellulose; gelatins; and povidone. The natural gums are variable in composition and usually contaminated with bacteria.
   (2) If the drug substance is adversely affected by an aqueous binder, a **nonaqueous binder** may be used, or the binder may be added **dry**.
   (3) Generally, **binding is more effective** when the binder is added in **liquid form**.
   (4) The **amount of binder or adhesive** used depends on the manufacturer's experience and on the other tablet ingredients. **Overwetting** causes granules that are too hard for proper tablet formation; **underwetting** causes formation of tablets that are too soft and that tend to crumble easily.

c. **Disintegrants** are added to tablet formulations to facilitate tablet disintegration when the tablet contacts water in the gastrointestinal tract. They appear to function by drawing water into the tablet, swelling, and causing the tablet to burst apart.
   (1) Disintegration is **critical to subsequent drug dissolution** and **satisfactory drug bioavailability**.
   (2) **Common disintegrants** include cornstarch and potato starch; starch derivatives, such as sodium starch glycolate; cellulose derivatives, such as sodium carboxymethylcellulose; clays, such as Veegum and bentonite; cation-exchange resins; and others.
   (3) The **total amount of disintegrant** is not always added to the drug–diluent mixture. A portion may be added (with the lubricant) to the prepared granulation of the drug, causing **double disintegration** of the tablet. The portion of disintegrant added last causes breakup of the tablet into small pieces or chunks; the portion added first breaks the pieces into fine particles.

d. **Lubricants, antiadherents, and glidants** have overlapping functions.
   (1) **Lubricants** act during tablet ejection to reduce friction between the walls of the tablet and the walls of the die cavity in which the tablet was formed. Talc, magnesium stearate, and calcium stearate are among those commonly used.
   (2) **Antiadherents** reduce sticking or adhesion of the tablet granulation or powder to the punch faces or the die walls.
   (3) **Glidants** promote the flow of the tablet granulation or powder materials by reducing friction among the particles.

e. **Colors and dyes** serve three purposes: to disguise off-color drugs, to provide product identification, and to produce a more elegant product. **FD&C dyes and D&C dyes** are applied as solutions; **lakes** (dyes that have been absorbed on a hydrous oxide) are usually employed as dry powders.

f. **Flavoring agents** are usually used only with chewable tablets or tablets intended to dissolve in the mouth.
   (1) Generally, water-soluble flavors have poor stability; thus, **flavor oils** or **dry powder flavors** are usually used.
   (2) **Flavor oils** may be added to tablet granulations in solvents, dispersed on clays or other absorbents, or emulsified in aqueous granulating agents. Usually, the maximum amount of oil that can be added without affecting tablet characteristics is 0.5% to 0.75%.

g. **Artificial sweeteners**, like flavors, are usually used only with chewable tablets or tablets intended to dissolve in the mouth.
   (1) Some sweetness may come from the **diluent** (e.g., mannitol or lactose); agents such as saccharin and aspartame may also be added.
   (2) **Saccharin** has an unpleasant aftertaste.
   (3) **Aspartame** is unstable in the presence of moisture.

h. **Adsorbents** (e.g., magnesium oxide, magnesium carbonate, bentonite, and silicon dioxide) are substances capable of holding quantities of fluid in an apparently dry state.

C. **Tablet types and classes**. Tablets are classified by their route of administration, drug delivery system, and form and method of manufacture (Table 3-10).

1. **Tablets for oral ingestion** are designed to be swallowed intact, with the exception of chewable tablets. They may be **coated** to mask the drug's taste, color, or odor; to control drug release; to protect the drug from the stomach's acid environment; to incorporate another drug, providing sequential release or avoiding incompatibilities; or to improve appearance.
   a. **Compressed tablets** are formed by compression and have no special coating. They are made from powdered, crystalline, or granular materials, alone or in combination with such excipients as binders, disintegrants, diluents, and colorants.
   b. **Multiple compressed tablets** may be layered or compression-coated.
      (1) **Layered tablets** are prepared by compressing an additional tablet granulation around a previously compressed granulation. The operation may be repeated to produce multiple layers.
      (2) **Compression-coated tablets** (also called **dry-coated tablets**) are prepared by feeding previously compressed tablets into a special tableting machine and compressing an outer shell around them. This process applies a thinner, more uniform coating than sugar-coating and can be used safely with drugs sensitive to moisture. It can be used to separate incompatible materials, to produce repeat-action or prolonged-action products, or to provide a multilayered appearance.

Table 3-10. Tablet Types and Classes

Tablets for oral ingestion	Tablets used in the oral cavity
Compressed tablets	Buccal tablets
Multiple compressed tablets	Sublingual tablets
Layered tablets	Troches, lozenges, and dental cones
Compression-coated tablets	
Repeat-action tablets	**Tablets used to prepare solutions**
Delayed-action and enteric-coated tablets	Effervescent tablets
Sugar- and chocolate-coated tablets	Dispensing tablets
Film-coated tablets	Hypodermic tablets
Air suspension-coated tablets	Tablet triturates
Chewable tablets	

c. **Repeat-action tablets** are layered or compression-coated tablets in which the outer layer or shell provides an initial drug dose, rapidly disintegrating in the stomach.
   (1) The **inner layer** (or inner tablet) is formulated of components that are insoluble in gastric media but soluble in intestinal media.
   (2) **Examples** include Repetabs (Schering) and Extentabs (Robins).

d. **Delayed-action** and **enteric-coated tablets** delay the release of a drug from a dosage form to prevent drug destruction by gastric juices, to prevent stomach lining irritation by the drug, or to promote absorption, which may be better in the intestine than in the stomach.
   (1) Tablets coated so as to remain intact in the stomach but yield their ingredients in the intestines are said to be **enteric-coated**. Enteric-coated tablets are a form of delayed-action tablet, but not all delayed-action tablets are enteric or intended to produce an enteric effect.
   (2) Among the **agents** used to enteric-coat tablets are fats, fatty acids, waxes, shellac, and cellulose acetate phthalate.
   (3) **Examples** of commercially prepared enteric-coated tablets include Enseals (Lilly) and Ecotrin (Smith Kline & French).

e. **Sugar-** and **chocolate-coated tablets** are compressed tablets coated to protect the drug from air and humidity, to provide a barrier to the drug's objectionable taste or smell, or to improve the tablet's appearance. Chocolate-coated tablets are rare today.
   (1) **Sugar-coated tablets** may be coated with a colored or an uncolored sugar. The process includes **seal coating** (waterproofing), **subcoating, syrup coating** (for smoothing and coloring), and **polishing**, all of which take place in a series of mechanically operated coating pans.
   (2) **Disadvantages** of sugar-coating include the time and expertise required for the process and the increase in tablet size and weight. Sugar-coated tablets may be 50% larger and heavier than the original tablets.

f. **Film-coated tablets** are compressed tablets coated with a thin layer of a water-insoluble or water-soluble polymer (e.g., hydroxypropyl methylcellulose, ethylcellulose, povidone, or PEG).
   (1) The film is generally colored, and it is **more durable, less bulky**, and **less time-consuming to apply** than sugar-coating. It typically increases tablet weight by only 2% to 3% and provides increased formulation efficiency, increased resistance to chipping, and increased output.
   (2) **Film-coating solutions** generally contain a film former, an alloying substance, a plasticizer, a surfactant, opacifiers, sweeteners, flavors, colors, glossants, and a volatile solvent.
   (3) The **volatile solvents** used in these solutions are expensive and potentially toxic when released into the atmosphere. Hence, manufacturers are exploring the development and use of **aqueous-based solutions**.

g. **Air suspension–coated tablets** are fed into a vertical cylinder and supported by a column of air that enters from the bottom of the cylinder. As the coating solution enters the system, it is rapidly applied to the suspended, rotating solids (the **Wurster process**). Rounding coats can be applied in less than 1 hour with the assistance of warm air blasts released in the chamber.

h. **Chewable tablets** disintegrate smoothly and rapidly when chewed or allowed to dissolve in the mouth, yielding a creamy base (from specially colored and flavored mannitol).
   (1) These tablets are especially useful in **formulations for children** and are commonly used for multivitamin tablets.
   (2) They are also used for some **antacids** and **antibiotics**.

2. **Tablets used in the oral cavity** are allowed to dissolve in the mouth.
   a. **Buccal tablets** and **sublingual tablets** are absorbed through the oral mucosa after dissolving in the buccal pouch (buccal tablets) or below the tongue (sublingual tablets).
      (1) These forms are useful for **drugs that are destroyed by gastric juice** or **poorly absorbed from the intestinal tract.**
      (2) **Examples** include sublingual nitroglycerin tablets, which dissolve very promptly to give rapid drug effects, and buccal progesterone tablets, which dissolve slowly.
   b. **Troches, lozenges**, and **dental cones** dissolve slowly in the mouth and provide primarily local effects.

3. **Tablets used to prepare solutions** are dissolved in water prior to administration.
   a. **Effervescent tablets** are prepared by compressing granular effervescent salts or other materials (e.g., citric acid, tartaric acid, or sodium bicarbonate) that have the capacity to release carbon dioxide gas when in contact with water. Commercial alkalinizing analgesic tablets are frequently made to effervesce to encourage fast dissolution and absorption (e.g., Alka-Seltzer).

b. **Other tablets** used to prepare solutions include **dispensing tablets**, **hypodermic tablets**, and **tablet triturates**.

D. **Processing problems**

1. **Capping** is the partial or complete separation of the top or bottom crowns of a tablet from the main body of the tablet. **Lamination** is separation of a tablet into two or more distinct layers. Both of these problems usually result from **air entrapment** during processing.

2. **Picking** is removal of a tablet's surface material by a punch. **Sticking** is adhesion of tablet material to a die wall. These problems may result from **excessive moisture** or **substances with low melting temperatures** in the formulation.

3. **Mottling** is an unequal color distribution on a tablet, with light or dark areas standing out on an otherwise uniform surface. This may result from use of a drug with a color different from that of the tablet excipients or from a drug with colored degradation products. Colorants may solve the problem but may also create other problems.

E. **Tablet evaluation and control**

1. Control of a tablet's **general appearance** is essential for consumer acceptance, lot-to-lot uniformity, tablet-to-tablet uniformity, and monitoring of the manufacturing process.
   a. Tablet appearance includes **visual identity** and **overall appearance**.
   b. **Control of appearance** includes measurement of such attributes as size, shape, color, odor, taste, surface, texture, physical flaws, consistency, and legibility of any markings.

2. Adequate tablet **hardness** and **resistance to friability** are necessary to withstand the mechanical shocks of manufacture, packaging, and shipping, and to ensure consumer acceptance.
   a. **Hardness** relates to both tablet disintegration and to drug dissolution. Certain tablets intended to dissolve slowly are made hard, whereas others intended to dissolve rapidly are made soft.
   b. **Tablet hardness testers** measure the degree of force required to break a tablet.
   c. **Friabilators** determine friability (the tablet's tendency to crumble) by allowing the tablet to roll and fall into a rotating tumbling apparatus. The tablets are weighed before and after a specified number of rotations, and the weight loss is determined.
      (1) **Resistance to weight loss** indicates the tablet's ability to withstand abrasion during handling, packaging, and shipping. Compressed tablets that lose less than 0.5% to 1% of their weight are generally considered acceptable.
      (2) Some chewable tablets and most effervescent tablets are **highly friable** and require special unit packaging.

3. Tablet **weight** is routinely measured to help ensure that the tablet contains the proper amount of drug.
   a. The USP defines a **weight variation standard**, to which tablets must conform.
   b. These standards are applicable for tablets containing **50 mg or more of drug substance** in which the drug substance represents **50% or more (by weight) of the dosage form unit**.

4. **Content uniformity** is evaluated to ensure that each tablet contains the amount of drug substance desired, with little variation among contents within a batch. The USP defines content uniformity tests for tablets containing **50 mg or less of drug substance**.

5. **Disintegration** is evaluated to ensure that the tablet's drug substance is fully available for absorption from the gastrointestinal tract.
   a. All USP tablets must pass an **official disintegration test**, conducted in vitro with special equipment.
      (1) **Uncoated USP tablets** have disintegration times as low as 2 minutes (nitroglycerin) to 5 minutes (aspirin); the majority have a maximum disintegration time of 30 minutes.
      (2) **Buccal tablets** must disintegrate within 4 hours.
      (3) **Enteric-coated tablets** must show no evidence of disintegration after 1 hour in simulated gastric fluid. In simulated intestinal fluid, they should disintegrate in 2 hours plus the time specified.
   b. Newly developed **dissolution requirements** in the USP have replaced earlier disintegration requirements for many drugs.

6. **Dissolution characteristics** are tested to help determine drug absorption and physiologic availability, which depend on the drug in its dissolved state.
   a. The USP gives **standards for tablet dissolution**.
   b. An increased emphasis on **dissolution testing** and **determination of bioavailability** has increased the use of sophisticated systems for the testing and analysis of tablet dissolution.

IX. CONTROLLED-RELEASE DOSAGE FORMS

A. Introduction

1. Controlled-release dosage forms (also known as delayed-release, sustained-action, prolonged-action, sustained-release, prolonged-release, timed-release, slow-release, extended-action, and extended-release forms) are **designed to release drug substance slowly for prolonged action in the body**.

2. Controlled-release forms have the following **advantages**:
   a. Reduction of problems with patient compliance
   b. Employment of less total drug
   c. Minimization or elimination of local or systemic side effects
   d. Minimization of drug accumulation (with chronic dosage)
   e. Reduction of potentiation or loss of drug activity (with chronic use)
   f. Improvement in treatment efficiency
   g. Improvement in speed of control of condition
   h. Reduction in drug level fluctuation
   i. Improvement in bioavailability for some drugs
   j. Improvement in ability to provide special effects (e.g., morning relief of arthritis by bedtime dosing)
   k. Reduction in cost

B. Sustained-release forms. The wide variety of sustained-release forms available can be grouped by the pharmaceutical mechanism employed to provide controlled release.

1. **Coated beads or granules** produce a blood-level profile similar to that obtained with multiple dosing.
   a. A **solution of the drug substance** in a nonaqueous solvent (such as alcohol) is coated onto small, inert beads or granules made of a combination of sugar and starch. (When the drug dose is large, the starting granules may be composed of the drug itself.)
   b. Some of the beads or granules are left **uncoated**, to provide an immediate release of the drug.
   c. **Coats of a lipid material** (such as beeswax) or a **cellulosic material** (such as ethylcellulose) are applied to the remainder of the granules, with some granules receiving few coats and some granules many.
   d. The **various coating thicknesses** produce a sustained-release effect.
   e. **Examples** of coated bead or granule dosage forms include Theo-Dur Sprinkle (Key), Spansules (Smith Kline & French), and Sequels (Lederle).

2. **Microencapsulation** is a process by which solids, liquids, or even gases are encapsulated into microscopic particles by formation of thin coatings of a "wall" material around the substance to be encapsulated.
   a. The most common method of microencapsulation is **coacervation**, which involves addition of a hydrophilic substance to a colloidal drug dispersion.
   b. The **hydrophilic substance**, which acts as the coating material, may be selected from a wide variety of natural and synthetic polymers, including shellacs, waxes, gelatin, starches, cellulose acetate phthalate, ethylcellulose, and others.
   c. Once the **coating material dissolves**, all the drug inside the microcapsule is immediately available for dissolution and absorption. Wall thickness can be varied from less than 1 to 200 μm by changing the amount of the coating material (3% to 30% of total weight).
   d. An **example** of a microencapsulated dosage form is Measurin (Winthrop).

3. **Matrix devices** may employ insoluble plastics (e.g., polyethylene, polyvinyl acetate, or polymethacrylate), hydrophilic polymers (e.g., methylcellulose or hydroxypropyl methylcellulose), or fatty compounds (e.g., various waxes or glyceryl tristearate).
   a. The most common method of preparation is **mixing of the drug with the matrix material** followed by **compression of the material into tablets**.
   b. The **primary dose** (the portion of the drug to be released immediately) is placed on the tablet as a layer or coat.
   c. The **remainder of the dose** is released slowly from the matrix.
   d. **Examples** include Gradumet (Abbott), Lonatabs (Geigy), Dospan (Merrell Dow), and Slow-K (Ciba).

4. **Osmotic systems** include the **Oros system**, an oral osmotic pump composed of a core tablet and a semipermeable coating with a 0.4-mm diameter hole (produced by a laser beam) for drug exit.

a. This system requires only **osmotic pressure** to be effective and is essentially independent of pH changes in the environment.
b. The **drug release rate** can be changed by changing the surface area, the nature of the membrane, or the diameter of the drug-release hole.

5. **Ion-exchange resins** may be complexed to drugs by passage of a cationic drug solution through a column containing the resin. The drug is complexed to the resin by replacement of hydrogen atoms.
   a. After complexing, the **resin–drug complex** is washed and then tableted, encapsulated, or suspended in an aqueous vehicle.
   b. **Drug release** from the complex depends on the ionic environment within the gastrointestinal tract and on the resin's properties. Generally, release is greater in the highly acidic stomach than in the less acidic small intestine.
   c. **Examples** include Biphetamine capsules (Fisons; resin complexes of amphetamine and dextroamphetamine), Ionamin capsules (Fisons; resin complexes of phentermine), and the Pennkinetic system (Fisons), which incorporates a polymer barrier coating and bead technology in addition to the ion-exchange mechanism.

6. **Complex formation** may be used for certain drug substances that combine chemically with other agents. For example, hydroxypropyl-β-cyclodextrin forms a chemical complex that may be only slowly soluble from body fluids, depending on the pH of the environment.

7. **Hydrocolloid systems** (e.g., Valrelease, a slow-release form of diazepam) include a unique, **hydrodynamically balanced drug-delivery system (HBS)** developed by Roche.
   a. The HBS consists of a **matrix** designed so that the dosage form, on contact with gastric fluid, demonstrates a bulk density less than one and, thus, remains buoyant.
   b. When in contact with gastric fluid, the **outermost hydrocolloids swell to form a boundary layer**, which prevents immediate penetration of fluid into the formulation.
   c. This outer hydrocolloid layer **slowly erodes**, with subsequent formation of a new boundary layer.
   d. The **process is continuous**, with each new outer layer eroding slowly. The drug is released gradually through each layer as fluid slowly penetrates the matrix.

C. Transdermal drug delivery systems (TDDS)

1. **TDDS are designed to support the passage of drug substances from the skin surface, through the skin layers, and into the systemic circulation.**

2. A TDDS has these **advantages**:
   a. Bypass of hepatic first-pass metabolism and gastrointestinal incompatibilities
   b. Improvement of patient compliance
   c. Ease of treatment termination (by removal of the TDDS).

3. **Microporous membranes** may be used as rate-controlling barriers in a TDDS. These membranes are a few millimeters thick and have varying pore sizes. They may be made from such materials as regenerated cellulose nitrate or acetate, polypropylene, and others.

4. **Examples** include the Transderm-Scōp (Ciba) and various systems for the delivery of nitroglycerin.
   a. The **Transderm-Scōp** system delivers scopolamine (to prevent and treat motion-induced nausea) without eliciting the side effects that normally accompany oral or intramuscular administration.
   b. **TDDS nitroglycerin forms** include Transderm-Nitro (Ciba), which employs a microporous membrane; Nitrodisc (Searle), which has the drug microsealed in a solid polymer; and Nitro-Dur (Key), which uses a 2% diffusion matrix.
      (1) These devices range from 5 to 20 cm^2 in surface area and are generally **applied to the upper arm or chest**. They release from 2.5 to 22.4 mg/24 hr, depending on the drug content and the surface area.
      (2) TDDS nitroglycerin offers a **significant improvement in sustained-release therapy** over sublingual nitroglycerin and nitroglycerin topical ointments.

X. THE UNITED STATES PHARMACOPEIA (USP) AND THE NATIONAL FORMULARY (NF)

A. The USP and NF are the official compendia, legally recognized by the United States. Since 1975, both compendia are published as a single volume by the United States Pharmacopeial Convention, Inc., Rockville, Maryland.

B. The USP/NF provides standards for drugs and chemicals used in the practice of medicine and pharmacy. The USP provides standards for drugs and their dosage forms and some medical devices; the NF provides standards for pharmaceutical ingredients, including excipients.

1. The monograph for each drug or dosage form establishes the following:
a. Its official **title**
b. A **definition** and **description** of the substance
c. **Standards** for the following characteristics:
(1) Identity
(2) Quality
(3) Strength
(4) Purity
(5) Packaging
(6) Labeling

2. When feasible, the following information is also given:
a. Standards for bioavailability and stability
b. Proper handling and storage procedures
c. Assay procedures
d. Formulas for making the substance or dosage form

3. In addition, the USP provides a wealth of **general information** on such subjects as:
a. Testing and assaying of products
b. Controlled substances regulations
c. FDA requirements
d. Good manufacturing practices
e. Pharmaceutical dosage forms
f. Factors affecting stability
g. Sterilization
h. Reagents and solutions used in tests and assays
i. Container specifications for dispensing
j. Molecular formulas and molecular weights

XI. UNITED STATES PHARMACOPEIAL DRUG INFORMATION (USPDI). The *USPDI System* is a three-volume (four-book) publication by the United States Pharmacopeial Convention, Inc., Rockville, Maryland, which is continually revised and provides drug information for the health care professional and the patient.

A. *Drug Information for the Health Care Professional* (volume I, parts IA and IB) includes information for prescribers, dispensers, and other health care professionals on categories of drug use.

B. *Advice for the Patient* (volume II) contains information for the patient. Monographs correspond directly to monographs in volume I and provide a coordinated approach to patient education, including patient consultation guidelines.

C. *Approved Drug Products and Legal Requirements* (volume III) includes information on bioequivalence and therapeutic equivalence relating to drug product selection available in the FDA Orange Book. In addition, this volume contains information on the federal Controlled Substances Act, Poison Prevention Packaging Act and Regulations, FD&C Act, Good Manufacturing Practices, and other legal information pertaining to pharmacy practice. Furthermore, a medicine chart, which is a drug product identification directory, is printed in color.

STUDY QUESTIONS

Directions: Each question below contains five suggested answers. Choose the **one best** response to each question.

1. In the extemporaneous preparation of a suspension, levigation is used to

A. reduce zeta potential
B. avoid bacterial growth
C. reduce particle size
D. enhance viscosity
E. reduce viscosity

2. A satisfactory suppository base must meet all of the following criteria EXCEPT

A. it should have a narrow melting range
B. it should be nonirritating and nonsensitizing
C. it should dissolve or disintegrate rapidly in the body cavity
D. it should melt below 30° C
E. it should be inert

3. Which of the following capsule sizes has the smallest capacity?

A. 5
B. 4
C. 1
D. 0
E. 000

4. The particle size of the dispersed solid in a suspension is usually greater than

A. 0.5 μm
B. 0.4 μm
C. 0.3 μm
D. 0.2 μm
E. 0.1 μm

5. Cocoa butter (theobroma oil) exhibits all of the following properties EXCEPT

A. it melts at temperatures between 33° and 35° C
B. it is a mixture of glycerides
C. it is a polymorph
D. it is useful in formulating rectal suppositories
E. it is soluble in water

6. All of the following statements concerning syrup NF are true EXCEPT

A. it contains 850 g of sucrose
B. it is made with purified water
C. it has a specific gravity of 1.30
D. it is a supersaturated solution
E. it has a moderately high viscosity

7. Which of the following solutions is used as an astringent?

A. Strong iodine solution USP
B. Aluminum acetate topical solution USP
C. Acetic acid NF
D. Aromatic ammonia spirit USP
E. Benzalkonium chloride solution NF

8. All of the following preparations contain alcohol EXCEPT

A. syrup USP
B. terpin hydrate elixir USP
C. aromatic ammonia spirit USP
D. green soap tincture USP
E. eriodictyon fluidextract NF

9. USP tests for ensuring the quality of drug products in tablet form include all of the following EXCEPT

A. disintegration
B. dissolution
C. hardness and friability
D. content uniformity
E. weight variation

10. The USP content uniformity test is used to ensure which of the following qualities?

A. Bioequivalency
B. Dissolution
C. Potency
D. Purity
E. Toxicity

11. The dispensing pharmacist usually accomplishes the blending of potent powders with a diluent by

A. spatulation
B. sifting
C. trituration
D. geometric dilution
E. levigation

12. Which type of paper will best protect a divided hygroscopic powder?

A. Waxed paper
B. Glassine
C. White bond
D. Blue bond
E. Vegetable parchment

13. Camphor is usually milled by which of the following techniques?

A. Trituration
B. Levigation
C. Pulverization by intervention
D. Geometric dilution
E. Attrition

14. Rectal suppositories intended for adult use usually weigh approximately

A. 1 g
B. 2 g
C. 3 g
D. 4 g
E. 5 g

15. In the fusion method of making cocoa butter suppositories, which of the following substances is most likely to be used for lubricating the mold?

A. Mineral oil
B. Propylene glycol
C. Cetyl alcohol
D. Stearic acid
E. Magnesium silicate

16. The shells of soft gelatin capsules may be made elastic or plastic-like by the addition of

A. sorbitol
B. povidone
C. polyethylene glycol
D. lactose
E. hydroxypropyl methylcellulose

17. A very fine powdered chemical is defined as one that will

A. completely pass through a #80 sieve
B. completely pass through a #120 sieve
C. completely pass through a #20 sieve
D. pass through a #60 sieve and not more than 40% through a #100 sieve
E. pass through a #40 sieve and not more than 60% through a #60 sieve

18. Which of the following compounds is a natural emulsifying agent?

A. Acacia
B. Lactose
C. Polysorbate 20
D. Polysorbate 80
E. Sorbitan monopalmitate

19. Vanishing cream is an ointment that may be classified as

A. a water-soluble base
B. an oleaginous base
C. an absorption base
D. an emulsion base
E. an oleic base

Directions: Each question below contains three suggested answers of which **one or more** is correct. Choose the answer

- **A** if **I only** is correct
- **B** if **III only** is correct
- **C** if **I and II** are correct
- **D** if **II and III** are correct
- **E** if **I, II, and III** are correct

20. Nonionic surface-active agents used as synthetic emulsifiers include

I. tragacanth
II. sodium lauryl sulfate
III. sorbitan esters (spans)

21. A Wedgwood mortar may be preferable to a glass mortar when

I. a volatile oil is added to a powder mixture
II. colored substances (dyes) are mixed into a powder
III. comminution is desired in addition to mixing

22. Substances that may be used to insulate powder components that may liquify when mixed include

I. talc
II. kaolin
III. light magnesium oxide

23. Agents that might be used to coat enteric-coated tablets include

I. hydroxypropyl methylcellulose (HPMC)
II. carboxymethylcellulose (CMC)
III. cellulose acetate phthalate (CAP)

24. True statements about the function of excipients used in tablet formulations include

I. binders promote granulation during the wet granulation process
II. glidants help to promote the flow of the tablet granulation during manufacture
III. lubricants help the patient to swallow the tablets

25. Manufacturing variables that would be likely to affect the dissolution of a prednisone tablet in the body include

I. the amount and type of binder added
II. the amount and type of disintegrant added
III. the force of compression used during tableting

26. Advantages of systemic drug administration by rectal suppository include

I. avoidance of first-pass effects
II. suitability when the oral route is not feasible
III. predictable drug release and absorption

27. Divided powders may be dispensed in

I. individual-dose packets
II. a bulk container
III. a perforated, sifter-type container

28. The amount of nitroglycerin that a transdermal patch delivers within a 24-hour period depends on the

I. occlusive backing on the patch
II. diffusion rate of nitroglycerin from the patch
III. surface area of the patch

29. The sedimentation of particles in a suspension can be minimized by

I. adding sodium benzoate
II. increasing the viscosity of the suspension
III. reducing the particle size of the active ingredient

30. Ingredients that may be used as suspending agents include

I. methylcellulose
II. acacia
III. talc

31. The particles in an ideal suspension should satisfy which of the following criteria?

I. Their size should be uniform
II. They should be stationary or move randomly
III. They should remain discrete

32. Forms of water that are suitable for use in parenteral preparations include which of the following?

I. Purified water USP
II. Water for injection USP
III. Sterile water for injection USP

33. True statements concerning the milling of powders include

I. a fine particle size is essential if the lubricant is to function properly
II. an increased surface area may enhance the dissolution rate
III. milling may cause degradation of thermolabile drugs

34. Mechanisms thought to provide stable emulsions include the

I. formation of interfacial film
II. lowering of interfacial tension
III. presence of charge on the ions

Directions: The groups of questions below consist of lettered choices followed by several numbered items. For each numbered item select the **one** lettered choice with which it is **most** closely associated. Each lettered choice may be used once, more than once, or not at all.

Questions 35–38

For each of the tablet processing problems listed below, select the most likely reason for the condition.

A. Excessive moisture in the granulation
B. Entrapment of air
C. Tablet friability
D. Degraded drug
E. Tablet hardness

35. Picking
36. Mottling
37. Capping
38. Sticking

Questions 39–41

For each description of a comminution procedure below, select the process that it best describes.

A. Trituration
B. Spatulation
C. Levigation
D. Pulverization by intervention
E. Tumbling

39. Rubbing or grinding a substance in a mortar with a rough inner surface

40. Reducing and subdividing a substance by adding an easily removed solvent

41. Adding a suitable agent to form a paste and then rubbing or grinding the paste in a mortar

Questions 42–45

Match the drug product below with the type of controlled-release dosage form that it represents.

A. Matrix device
B. Ion-exchange resin complex
C. Hydrocolloid system
D. Osmotic system
E. Coated granules

42. Biphetamine capsules
43. Thorazine Spansule capsules
44. Valrelease
45. Slow-K

ANSWERS AND EXPLANATIONS

1. The answer is C. (*II E 1*) Levigation is the process of blending and grinding a substance in order to separate the particles, reduce their size, and form a paste. It is performed by adding a small amount of a suitable levigating agent such as glycerin to the solid and then blending the mixture, using a mortar and pestle.

2. The answer is D. (*V C 1*) A satisfactory suppository base should remain firm at room temperature; preferably, it should not melt below 30° C to avoid premature softening during storage and insertion. A satisfactory suppository base should also be inert, nonsensitizing, nonirritating, and compatible with a variety of drugs. Moreover, it should melt just below body temperature and should dissolve or disintegrate rapidly in the fluid of the body cavity in which it is inserted.

3. The answer is A. (*VII B 3 a*) Hard capsules are numbered from 000 (the largest size) to 5 (the smallest size). The approximate capsule capacity ranges from 600 mg to 30 mg; however, the capsule capacity will depend on the density of the contents.

4. The answer is A. (*II A 1*) A suspension is a two-phase system: it consists of a finely powdered solid dispersed in a liquid vehicle. The particle size of the suspended solid should be as small as possible to minimize sedimentation; however, the particle size is usually greater than 0.5 μm.

5. The answer is E. (*V C 3 a*) Cocoa butter is a fat obtained from the seed of *Theobroma cacao.* Chemically, it is a mixture of stearin, palmitin, and other glycerides which are insoluble in water and freely soluble in ether and chloroform. Depending on the fusion temperature, cocoa butter may crystallize into any one of four crystal forms. Cocoa butter is a good base for rectal suppositories but is less than ideal for vaginal or urethral suppositories.

6. The answer is D. (*I C 1*) Syrup NF is a nearly saturated aqueous solution containing, in each liter of syrup, 850 g of sucrose in about 450 ml of purified water. The high sugar content gives syrup a moderately high viscosity and a high specific gravity. The NF does not specify the addition of a preservative; this is perhaps due to the high sugar content of the syrup. Syrups are useful as flavoring vehicles for medicinal agents.

7. The answer is B. (*I D 2*) Aluminum acetate and aluminum subacetate solutions are astringents used as wet dressings for contact dermatitis and as antiperspirants. Strong iodine solution and benzalkonium chloride are topical antibacterial solutions; acetic acid is added to products as an acidifier; and aromatic ammonia spirit is a respiratory stimulant.

8. The answer is A. (*I C 1, E 1, F 1, G 1, H 1*) Syrups are concentrated aqueous sugar solutions; they do not contain alcohol. Elixirs, spirits, tinctures, and fluid extracts are all preparations containing various concentrations of alcohol.

9. The answer is C. (*VIII E*) To satisfy the USP standards, tablets are required to meet a weight variation test (if the active ingredient comprises the bulk of the tablet) or a content uniformity test (if the active ingredient comprises less than 50% of the tablet bulk or if the tablet is coated). Many tablets for oral administration are required to meet a disintegration test, with disintegration times specified in the individual monographs. A dissolution test may be required instead if the active component of the tablet has limited water-solubility. Hardness and friability would affect a tablet's disintegration and dissolution rates, but hardness and friability tests are in-house quality control tests, and are not official USP tests.

10. The answer is C. (*VIII E 4*) The content uniformity test, in effect, is a test of potency. In order to ensure that each tablet or capsule contains the amount of drug substance intended, the USP provides two tests: weight variation and content uniformity. The content uniformity test may be used for any dosage unit, but is required for coated tablets, for tablets in which the active ingredient comprises less than 50% of the tablet bulk, for suspensions in single-unit containers or in soft capsules, and for many solids that contain added substances. The weight variation test may be used for liquid-filled soft capsules, for any dosage-form unit that contains at least 50 mg of a single drug if the drug comprises at least 50% of the bulk, for solids without added substances, and for freeze-dried solutions.

11. The answer is D. (*VI B 3*) When mixing potent substances with a large amount of diluent, the pharmacist uses geometric dilution. The potent drug and an equal amount of diluent are first mixed in a mortar by trituration. A volume of diluent equal to the mixture in the mortar is then added, and the mix is again triturated. The procedure is repeated, each time adding diluent equal in volume to the mixture then in the mortar, until all the diluent has been incorporated.

12. The answer is A. (*VI C 2 d*) Hygroscopic and volatile drugs can be protected best by the use of waxed paper, which is waterproof. The packet may be double-wrapped with a bond paper to improve the appearance of the completed powder.

13. The answer is C. [*VI A 4 b (2)*] Pulverization by intervention is the milling technique used for drug substances that are gummy and tend to reagglomerate or resist grinding (e.g., camphor, iodine). "Intervention" refers to the addition of a small amount of material that aids milling and that can be removed easily after pulverization is complete. For example, camphor can be reduced readily if a small amount of volatile solvent (e.g., alcohol) is added; the solvent is then allowed to evaporate.

14. The answer is B. (*V B 1*) By convention, a rectal suppository for an adult weighs about 2 g; one for an infant or child is smaller. Vaginal suppositories typically weigh about 5 g. Rectal suppositories are usually shaped like a rather elongated bullet, being cylindrical and tapered at one end. Vaginal suppositories are usually ovoid.

15. The answer is A. [*V D 3 a (4)*] In the fusion method of making suppositories, molds made of aluminum, brass, or nickel–copper alloys are used. The mold is lubricated very lightly with mineral oil before a mixture of finely powdered drug in melted cocoa butter is poured in.

16. The answer is A. (*VII C*) The shells of soft gelatin capsules are plasticized by the addition of a polyhydric alcohol (polyol) such as glycerin or sorbitol. An antifungal preservative may also be added. Both hard and soft gelatin capsules may be filled with a powder or other dry substance; soft gelatin capsules also are useful dosage forms for liquids or semisolids.

17. The answer is B. (*VI A 4; Tables 3-7 and 3-8*) The USP definition of a very fine chemical powder is one that will completely pass through a standard #120 sieve (which has 125-μm openings). The USP classification for powdered vegetable and animal drugs differs from that for powdered chemicals. To be classified as very fine, powdered vegetable and animal drugs must pass completely through a #80 sieve (which has 180-μm openings).

18. The answer is A. (*III E 3 a*) Acacia (gum arabic) is the exudate obtained from the stems and branches of various species of Acacia, a woody plant native to Africa. Acacia is a natural emulsifying agent that provides a good stable emulsion of low viscosity. Emulsions consist of droplets of one or more immiscible liquids dispersed in another liquid. Emulsions are inherently unstable: the droplets tend to coalesce into larger and larger drops. The purpose of an emulsifying agent is to keep the droplets dispersed and prevent them from coalescing. Polysorbate 20, polysorbate 80, and sorbitan monopalmitate are also emulsifiers, but are synthetic, not natural, substances.

19. The answer is D. (*IV A, B 3 d*) Ointments are typically used as emollients to soften the skin, or as protective barriers, or as vehicles for medication. To serve these functions, a variety of types of ointment bases are available. Vanishing cream, an emulsion type of ointment base, is an oil-in-water (o/w) emulsion that contains a high percentage of water. Stearic acid is present in the formula to help in the formation of a thin film on the skin when the water evaporates.

20. The answer is B (III). (*III E 4 c*) All of the substances listed in the question are emulsifying agents, but only sorbitan esters are nonionic synthetic agents. Tragacanth, like acacia, is a natural emulsifying agent, and sodium lauryl sulfate is an anionic surfactant. Sorbitan esters (known colloquially as spans by virtue of their trade names) are hydrophobic and form water-in-oil (w/o) emulsions. The polysorbates (known colloquially as tweens) are also nonionic, synthetic sorbitan derivatives, but they are hydrophilic and therefore form oil-in-water (o/w) emulsions. Sodium lauryl sulfate, as an alkali soap, is also hydrophilic and thus forms o/w emulsions.

21. The answer is B (III). (*VI B 2*) In the mixing of powders, if comminution is especially desired, a porcelain or Wedgwood mortar having a rough inner surface is preferred over the smooth working surface of the glass mortar. A glass mortar cleans more easily after use and therefore may be preferable for chemicals that may stain a porcelain or Wedgwood mortar and for simple mixing of substances without the need for comminution.

22. The answer is D (II, III). (*VI B 1 b*) Some solid substances (e.g., aspirin, phenylsalicylate, phenacetin, thymol, camphor) liquify or form eutectic mixtures when in close and prolonged contact with one another. Such substances are best insulated by the addition of light magnesium oxide or magnesium carbonate; other inert diluents that may be used are kaolin, starch, or bentonite.

23. The answer is B (III). (*VIII C 1 d*) An enteric-coated tablet has a coating that remains intact in the stomach but dissolves in the intestines to yield the tablet's ingredients there. Enteric coatings include various fats, fatty acids, waxes, and shellacs. Cellulose acetate phthalate remains intact in the stomach because it dissolves only above pH 6. Other enteric coating materials include povidone (polyvinylpyrrolidone; PVP), polyvinyl acetate phthalate (PVAP), and hyroxypropyl methylcellulose phthalate (HPMCP).

24. The answer is C (I, II). (*VIII B 3 a–d*) Tablets for oral ingestion usually contain excipients that are added to the formulation for their special functions. Binders and adhesives are added to promote granulation or compaction. Diluents are fillers added to make up the required tablet bulk; they may also aid in the manufacturing process. Disintegrants aid tablet disintegration in gastrointestinal fluids. Lubricants, antiadherents, and glidants aid in reducing friction or adhesion between particles or between the tablet and the die. For example, lubricants are used in tablet manufacture to reduce friction when the tablet is ejected from the die cavity in which it was formed. Lubricants are usually hydrophobic substances that can affect the dissolution rate of the active ingredient in a tablet.

25. The answer is E (all). (*VIII B 3 b, c, E 2 a, 5, 6*) Disintegrants are added to tablet formulations to facilitate tablet disintegration in the gastrointestinal fluids. The tablet's disintegration in the body is critical to its dissolution and subsequent absorption and bioavailability. The binder and the compression force used during tablet manufacturing will both affect a tablet's hardness, and this also affects tablet disintegration and drug dissolution.

26. The answer is C (I, II). (*V A 4, C 2*) Rectal suppositories are useful for delivering systemic medication under certain circumstances. Absorption of a drug from a rectal suppository involves release of the drug from the suppository vehicle, followed by diffusion of the drug through the rectal mucosa and transport to the circulation by way of the rectal veins. Because the rectal veins bypass the liver, rapid hepatic degradation of certain drugs (first-pass effect) is avoided. The rectal route is also useful when a drug cannot be given orally (e.g., because of vomiting). However, the extent of drug release and absorption is variable; it depends on the properties of the drug, the suppository base, and the environment in the rectum.

27. The answer is A (I). (*VI C 2*) Powders for oral use may be dispensed by the pharmacist in bulk form or divided into premeasured doses (divided powders). Divided powders are traditionally dispensed in folded paper packets (chartulae) made of parchment, bond paper, glassine, or waxed paper. However, if the powder needs greater protection from humidity or evaporation, the individual doses may be packaged in metal foil or small plastic bags.

28. The answer is E (all). (*IX C 3, 4*) The delivery of drugs through a transdermal drug delivery system (TDDS) depends on the microporous membranes that act as rate-controlling barriers, the mechanism by which the drug diffuses through these barriers (e.g., reservoir, matrix), and the surface area of the patch.

29. The answer is D (II, III). (*II C 2 a, d*) As Stoke's law indicates, the sedimentation rate of a suspension is slowed by reducing its density, reducing the size of the suspended particles, or by increasing its viscosity (achieved by incorporating a thickening agent). Sodium benzoate is an antifungal agent and would not reduce the sedimentation rate of a suspension.

30. The answer is C (I, II). (*II D*) Acacia and methylcellulose are both commonly used as suspending agents. Acacia is a natural product; methylcellulose is a synthetic polymer. By increasing the viscosity of the liquid, these agents enable particles to remain suspended for a longer period of time.

31. The answer is E (all). (*II C 1*) An ideal suspension would have particles of uniform size, minimal sedimentation, and no interaction between particles. These ideal criteria are rarely realized, although they can be approximated by keeping the particle size as small as possible, keeping the densities of the solid and the dispersion medium as similar as possible, and keeping the dispersion medium as viscous as possible.

32. The answer is D (II, III). (*I A 2*) Water for injection USP is water that has been purified by distillation or by reverse osmosis. It is used in preparing parenteral solutions that are subject to final sterilization. For parenteral solutions prepared aseptically and not subsequently sterilized, sterile water for injection USP is used. Sterile water for injection USP is water for injection USP that has been sterilized and suitably packaged; it meets the USP requirements for sterility. Bacteriostatic water for injection USP is sterile water for injection USP that contains one or more antimicrobial agents. It can be used in parenteral solutions if the antimicrobial additives are compatible with the other ingredients in the solution, but it cannot be used in newborn infants. Purified water USP is not used in parenteral preparations.

33. The answer is E (all). (*VI A 4 a*) Milling is the process of mechanically reducing the particle size of solids before formulation into a final product. In order for a lubricant to work effectively, it must coat the surface of the granulation or powder. Hence, fine particle size is essential. Decreasing the particle size increases the surface area, and this may enhance the dissolution rate. Possible degradation of thermolabile drugs may occur as a result of heat buildup during milling.

34. The answer is E (all). (*III D 2*) Emulsifying agents provide a mechanical barrier to coalescence, reducing the natural tendency of the internal-phase (oil or water) droplets in the emulsion to coalesce. Three mechanisms appear to be involved: Some emulsifiers promote stability by forming strong, pliable interfacial films around the droplets. Emulsifying agents also reduce interfacial tension. An electrical charge on the ions in the emulsion can create charge repulsion that causes droplets to repel one another, thereby preventing coalscence.

35–38. The answers are: 35-A, 36-D, 37-B, 38-A. (*VIII D*) Sticking refers to tablet material adhering to a die wall. Sticking may be due to excessive moisture or to ingredients with low melting temperatures. Mottling is uneven color distribution; it is most often due to poor mixing of the tablet granulation, but may also result from a degraded drug that produces a colored metabolite. Capping is the separation of the top or bottom crown of a tablet from the main body of the tablet. Capping implies that compressed powder is not cohesive. Reasons for capping include excessive force of compression, use of insufficient binder, worn tablet tooling equipment, and air entrapment during processing. Picking refers to surface material from a tablet sticking to a punch. Picking may be caused by a granulation that is too damp, by a scratched punch, by static charges on the powder, and particularly by use of a punch tip with engraving or embossing.

39–41. The answers are: 39-A, 40-D, 41-C. (*VI A 4 b, B 1, 2, 5*) Comminution is the process of reducing the particle size of a powder in order to increase the powder's fineness. Several comminution techniques are suitable for small-scale use in a pharmacy. Trituration is used both to comminute and to mix dry powders; if comminution is desired, the substance is rubbed in a mortar with a rough inner surface. Pulverization by intervention is often used for substances that tend to agglomerate or to resist grinding. A small amount of easily removed (e.g., volatile) solvent is added, and after the substance is pulverized, the solvent is allowed to evaporate or is otherwise removed. Levigation is often used to prepare pastes or ointments. The powder is reduced by adding a suitable nonsolvent (levigating agent) to form a paste and then rubbing the paste in a mortar, using a pestle, or on an ointment slab, using a spatula. Spatulation and tumbling are procedures for mixing or blending powders, not for reducing them. Spatulation is blending small amounts of powders together by stirring them with a spatula on a sheet of paper or a pill tile. Tumbling is the process of blending large amounts of powder in a large rotating container.

42–45. The answers are: 42-B, 43-E, 44-C, 45-A. (*IX*) Controlled-release dosage forms are designed to release a drug slowly for prolonged action in the body. A wide variety of pharmaceutical mechanisms are employed to provide the controlled release. Microencapsulation and complex formation are two other mechanisms besides those listed in the question.

4
Biopharmaceutics and Pharmacokinetics

Leon Shargel

I. DEFINITIONS

A. Biopharmaceutics is the study of the relationship of a drug product's physical and chemical properties to its bioavailability.

1. A **drug product** is the finished dosage form (e.g., tablet, capsule, or solution), which contains the active drug ingredient, usually in association with inactive ingredients.

2. **Bioavailability** is a measurement of the rate and extent (amount) of therapeutically active drug that reaches the systemic circulation.

B. Pharmacokinetics is the study of drug movement in the body over time, during the drug's absorption, distribution, and elimination (excretion and biotransformation).

II. DRUG ABSORPTION

A. Transport of drugs across a cell membrane. The cell membrane is a semipermeable structure composed of lipids and proteins. Drugs may be transported by passive diffusion or carrier-mediated transport.

1. **General principles**
   a. **Nonpolar lipid-soluble drugs** traverse cell membranes more easily than **ionic or polar water-soluble drugs**.
   b. **Small molecular weight drugs** diffuse across a cell membrane more easily than **larger** or **higher molecular weight drugs**.
   c. Generally, **proteins and drugs bound to proteins** do not cross cell membranes.

2. **Passive diffusion**
   a. Most drugs cross cell membranes by passive diffusion, moving from an area of high concentration to an area of lower concentration according to **Fick's law of diffusion**:

$$\frac{dQ}{dt} = - \frac{DAK}{h} (C_a - C_p)$$

   where dQ/dt is the rate of drug diffusion, D is the diffusion rate concentration, A is the surface area of the membrane, K is the oil/water partition coefficient of the drug, h is the thickness of the membrane, and $(C_a - C_p)$ is the difference between the drug concentration at the absorption site and in the plasma, respectively.
   b. The **extent of ionization of a weak electrolyte drug** is influenced by the pH of the medium in which the drug is dissolved and the pK_a (see section III A 3) of the drug. The nonionized species is more lipid soluble than the ionized species and diffuses across the cell membrane by passive transport.

3. **Carrier-mediated transport**
   a. **Active transport** of drugs across a membrane is a carrier-mediated transport system with the following characteristics.
      (1) The drug moves **against a concentration gradient**.
      (2) The process **requires energy**.
      (3) The **carrier may be selective** for certain types of drugs resembling natural substrates or metabolites that are normally actively transported.
      (4) The **carrier system may be saturated** at a high drug concentration.
      (5) The **process may be competitive** (drugs with similar structures may compete for the same carrier).

b. Facilitated diffusion is a carrier-mediated transport system similar to active transport. However, facilitated diffusion occurs **with a concentration gradient** and **does not require energy**.

B. Routes of drug administration. Drugs may be administered by parenteral, enteral, inhalation, or topical routes.

1. Parenteral administration

a. For **intravenous (IV) injection**, the drug is injected directly into the bloodstream. Because it is rapidly distributed throughout the body, it acts very rapidly. Any side effects, including an intense pharmacologic response, anaphylaxis, or overt toxicity, will also occur rapidly.

b. For **intra-arterial injection**, the drug is injected into a specific artery to achieve a specific high tissue concentration before distribution throughout the body. Intra-atrial injection is used for diagnostic agents and, occasionally, for cancer chemotherapy.

c. For **IV** infusion, the drug is given intravenously at a constant input rate. IV infusion maintains a relatively constant plasma drug concentration.

d. For **intramuscular injection**, the drug is injected into a muscular area, where it is promptly absorbed. The rate of drug absorption depends upon the vascularity of the muscle site, the drug's lipid solubility, and the vehicle in which the drug is contained.

e. For **subcutaneous injection**, the drug is injected beneath the skin. Because the subcutaneous area is less vascular than muscular areas, absorption may be less rapid. The factors that affect intramuscular absorption also affect subcutaneous absorption.

2. Enteral administration

a. For **buccal and sublingual administration**, a tablet or lozenge is placed under the tongue (sublingual) or in the cheek (buccal). This allows a nonpolar, lipid-soluble drug to be absorbed across the mouth's epithelial lining.

b. For **oral drug administration** (the most common route), the drug is swallowed. It is absorbed from the gastrointestinal tract by way of the mesenteric circulation and proceeds from the hepatic portal vein to the liver and into the systemic circulation.

(1) The oral route is the most convenient for safe drug administration. It is safe, painless, and economical.

(2) The oral route has some disadvantages, however. The drug may not be absorbed from the gastrointestinal tract consistently or completely. It may be digested by enzymes or decomposed by the stomach's acid pH. It may irritate mucosal epithelial cells or complex with gastrointestinal tract contents. In addition, the absorption rate may be erratic because of delayed gastric emptying time or changes in intestinal motility.

(3) The drug is absorbed throughout the gastrointestinal tract, primarily in the **duodenal** region. The large surface area resulting from the presence of villi and microvilli and the large blood supply provided by the mesenteric vessels allow the drug to be absorbed more efficiently by passive diffusion (see section II A 2).

(4) Most drugs are absorbed from the gastrointestinal tract by **diffusion**. Carrier-mediated transport plays a smaller role.

(5) A delay in **gastric emptying** will delay the drug's arrival in the duodenum for systemic absorption. Various factors affect gastric emptying time, including meal content, emotional factors, and anticholinergic drugs.

(6) Normal **intestinal motility** from peristalsis helps bring the drug in contact with the intestinal epithelial cells. A sufficient period of contact, or **residence time**, is needed to allow for drug absorption across the cell membranes from the mucosal to the serosal surface.

c. For **rectal drug administration**, the drug in solution (enema) or suppository form is inserted into the rectum. As the drug diffuses from the solution or is released from the suppository, it is absorbed across the rectum's mucosal surface.

3. Inhalation. The drug is given as an aerosol (liquid or solid particles) into the respiratory tract. Smaller particles reach deeper into the small bronchioles than do larger particles. The drug enters the circulation by diffusion across the alveolar membranes.

4. Topical (percutaneous) administration. The drug (in a lotion, ointment, cream, or patch) is placed on the skin, with or without an occlusive dressing. Lipid-soluble drugs such as nitroglycerin diffuse across the epidermis into the systemic circulation.

C. Local drug activity versus systemic drug absorption. The drug administration route and the bioavailability of the drug from the dosage form are major factors in the design of a drug product.

1. Drugs intended for **local activity**, such as topical antibiotics, anti-infectives, antifungal agents, and local anesthetics, are formulated in dosage forms that minimize systemic drug absorption. The concentration of these drugs at the application site affects their activity.

2. When **systemic drug absorption** is desired, the bioavailability of the drug from the absorption site must be considered. The amount of drug in the dosage form is based on the extent of drug absorption and on the desired systemic drug concentration.

3. An **IV drug** is considered completely (100%) bioavailable because all the drug is placed directly into the systemic circulation. For all other drug administration routes (except the intraarterial route), the drug's bioavailability must be considered.

III. BIOPHARMACEUTIC PRINCIPLES

A. Physicochemical drug properties

1. **Drug dissolution.** For most drugs with limited water solubility, the rate at which the solid drug enters into solution (dissolution) is often the rate-limiting step in the drug's bioavailability.
   a. The **Noyes Whitney equation** describes the rate of drug dissolution:

$$\text{Rate of dissolution} = \frac{dC}{dt} = \frac{DAK}{h}(C_s - C_b)$$

   where D is the diffusion coefficient, A is the surface area of the drug, K is the partition coefficient (water/oil), h is the thickness of the stagnant layer, C_s is the concentration of the drug in the stagnant layer (a saturated solution around the solid drug particle), and C_b is the concentration of the drug in the bulk phase of the solvent.
   b. **Drug solubility** is the maximum concentration of the drug solute dissolved in the solvent (usually water) under specified conditions of temperature, pH, and pressure. The drug's solubility in saturated solution is a static property, whereas the drug dissolution rate is a dynamic property that relates more closely to the bioavailability rate.

2. **Particle size and surface area** are inversely related. As solid drug particle size decreases, more particles (i.e., smaller particles) are needed to preserve the amount of the drug—the overall surface area of the smaller particles is greater than the overall surface area of the larger particles.
   a. As described by the Noyes Whitney equation, the **dissolution rate is directly proportional to the surface area**. An increase in surface area allows for more contact between the solid drug particle and the aqueous solvent, resulting in a faster dissolution rate.
   b. With certain **hydrophobic drugs**, excessive particle size reduction does not always produce an increased dissolution rate. These particles tend to reaggregate into larger particles to reduce the high surface free energy produced by particle size reduction.
   c. To prevent the formation of aggregates, small drug particles may be dispersed (**molecular dispersion**) in polyethylene glycol (PEG), polyvinylpyrrolidone (PVP) [povidone], dextrose, or other agents. For example, a molecular dispersion of griseofulvin in a water-soluble carrier such as PEG 4000 enhances the drug's dissolution and bioavailability.

3. **Partition coefficient and extent of ionization**
   a. The **partition coefficient** of a drug is the ratio of its solubility at equilibrium in an aqueous solvent to its solubility in a nonaqueous solvent. **Hydrophilic drugs** with higher water solubility have a faster dissolution rate than **hydrophobic or lipophilic drugs**, which have very poor water solubility.
   b. Drugs that are **weak electrolytes** exist in both an ionized (salt) form and a nonionized (weak acid or weak base) form. The **extent of ionization** depends upon the pK_a of the weak electrolyte and on the solvent's pH. The drug's ionized or salt forms carry a charge and are more water-soluble than its nonionized forms.
   c. The relationship between ionized and nonionized forms is described by the **Henderson-Hasselbalch** equation.
      (1) For weak acids,

$$pH = pK_a + \log \frac{[\text{salt}]}{[\text{nonionized acid}]}$$

      (2) For weak bases,

$$pH = pK_a + \log \frac{[\text{nonionized base}]}{[\text{salt}]}$$

4. **Salt formation**
   a. The choice of salt form for a drug depends upon the drug's desired physical and chemical properties.
   b. Some soluble salt forms are less stable than the nonionized form. For example, sodium aspirin is less stable than aspirin in the acid form.

c. A solid dosage form containing buffering agents may be formulated with the free acid form of the drug, allowing the drug to dissolve at the site due to the buffering agent's alkaline medium. The dissolved salt form of the drug diffuses into the bulk fluid of the gastrointestinal tract and forms a fine precipitate that redissolves rapidly.

d. Effervescent granules or tablets containing the acid drug along with sodium bicarbonate, tartaric acid, citric acid, and other ingredients are added to water just before oral administration. The excess sodium bicarbonate forms an alkaline solution in which the drug dissolves.

e. For weakly acidic drugs, potassium and sodium salts are more water-soluble than such divalent cation salts as magnesium and aluminum.

f. Common water-soluble salts of weak bases include the hydrochloride, sulfate, citrate, and gluconate salts. The napsylate, stearate and estolate salts of weak bases are less water-soluble.

g. Certain salts are designed to provide slower dissolution, slower bioavailability, and longer duration of activity. Other salts may be chosen for greater stability, less local irritation at the absorption site, or less systemic toxicity.

5. Polymorphism is the ability of a drug to exist in more than one form.

a. Different polymorphs have different physical properties, including melting point and dissolution rate.

b. Amorphous polymorphs (nonrigid, noncrystalline forms) have a faster dissolution rate than the crystalline form of the same drug.

6. Hydrates

a. A drug may exist in a **hydrated (solvated) form** or as an **anhydrous molecule**.

b. The dissolution rates differ for hydrated and anhydrated forms. For example, the anhydrous form of ampicillin dissolves faster and is more rapidly absorbed than the hydrated form.

7. Surfactants are compounds that act at the water/oil interface to lower surface tension and to provide more contact (wetting) of the surface of the solid drug particle by the solvent.

a. A small concentration of surfactant may increase the drug dissolution rate.

b. A larger concentration of surfactant may form a **critical micelle concentration** (CMC), which acts to cause an oil-in-water (o/w) or water-in-oil (w/o) emulsion and retards the drug dissolution rate.

c. A large concentration of surfactant may affect the lipid membranes of the gastrointestinal tract's mucosal cells and may cause a laxative action.

8. Complex formation in drug interaction

a. A complex may be a reversible or irreversible interaction between a drug and another substance. For example, tetracycline and calcium (or some other divalent cation such as magnesium or aluminum) form a complex known as a **chelate**. Many drugs adsorb strongly on charcoal. Drugs may also bind proteins such as albumin to form a drug–protein complex.

b. Complex formation usually alters the drug's physical and chemical characteristics. For example, the chelate of tetracycline with calcium is less water soluble and is poorly absorbed. In contrast, theophylline complexed with ethylene diamine to form aminophylline is more water soluble and is used for parenteral administration.

c. Large drug complexes, such as drug–protein complexes, do not cross cell membranes easily. These complexes must first dissociate to free the drug for absorption at the absorption site, permitting diffusion across cell membranes into tissues or glomerular filtering prior to excretion into the urine.

B. Drug product formulation

1. General considerations

a. Design of the appropriate dosage form depends on the:

(1) Drug's physical and chemical properties
(2) Dose of the drug
(3) Administration route
(4) Desired therapeutic effect
(5) Type of drug product desired
(6) Bioavailability of the drug

b. The more complicated the formulation of the finished drug product (e.g., a controlled-release tablet or an enteric-coated tablet), the greater the potential for a bioavailability problem.

c. The bioavailability of a drug from a solid dosage form depends on a succession of rate processes, including:

(1) Disintegration of the drug product and subsequent release of the drug
(2) Dissolution of the drug in an aqueous environment

(3) **Absorption** of the drug across cell membranes into the systemic circulation (Fig. 4-1)

d. The **rate-limiting step** in the bioavailability of a drug from a drug product is the slowest rate in a series of kinetic processes. For most conventional solid drug products, such as tablets and capsules, the disintegration rate is the slowest, or rate-limiting, step for bioavailability. For a controlled-release or sustained-action drug product, the release of the drug from the dosage form is the rate-limiting step.

2. **Solutions** are homogeneous mixtures of one or more solutes dispersed molecularly in a dissolving medium (solvent).
   a. Compared with other drug formulations, a **drug dissolved in an aqueous solution** has the highest rate of bioavailability and is often used as the reference preparation for other formulations. Because the drug is already dissolved, no dissolution step is necessary before systemic absorption.
   b. A **drug dissolved in a hydroalcoholic solution** (as with an **elixir**) also has good bioavailability. Alcohol aids drug solubility; the drug may form a fine precipitate upon dilution in the bulk contents of the gastrointestinal tract. The precipitate's fine, solid drug particles are well dispersed, have a large surface area, and are rapidly redissolved before systemic absorption.
   c. A **highly viscous syrup** may slow the drug's outward diffusion, slowing the rate of bioavailability. This may occur from both delayed gastric emptying and a slow dissolution rate.

3. **Suspensions** are pharmaceutical dispersions in which finely divided solid particles of a drug are dispersed in a liquid medium that is not a solvent for the drug.
   a. **Drug bioavailability** from a well-prepared suspension may be similar to that from a solution because the small drug particles are dispersed and offer a large surface area for rapid dissolution.
   b. **Suspending agents** (often a cellulose derivative or gum, such as methylcellulose or acacia) are added to suspensions to impart viscosity and prevent the drug particles from settling and agglomerating. Highly viscous suspensions with a large concentration of suspending agent prolong gastric emptying time, slow drug dissolution, and slow the rate of drug bioavailability.

4. **Capsules** are hard or soft gelatin shells in which drugs are contained. A capsule containing a drug is considered a solid dosage form.
   a. A **hard gelatin capsule** is usually filled with a **powder blend** containing the drug. Typically, the powder blend is simpler and less compacted than the blend in a compressed tablet. After ingestion, the gelatin softens, swells, and begins to dissolve in the gastrointestinal tract. The drug is released rapidly, disperses easily, and has good bioavailability. Hard gelatin capsules are the preferred dosage form for early clinical trials of an investigational new drug.
   b. A **soft gelatin capsule** may contain a nonaqueous solution, a powder, or a suspension of a drug. The vehicle may be **water miscible**, as with PEG. A nonionic surfactant such as di-

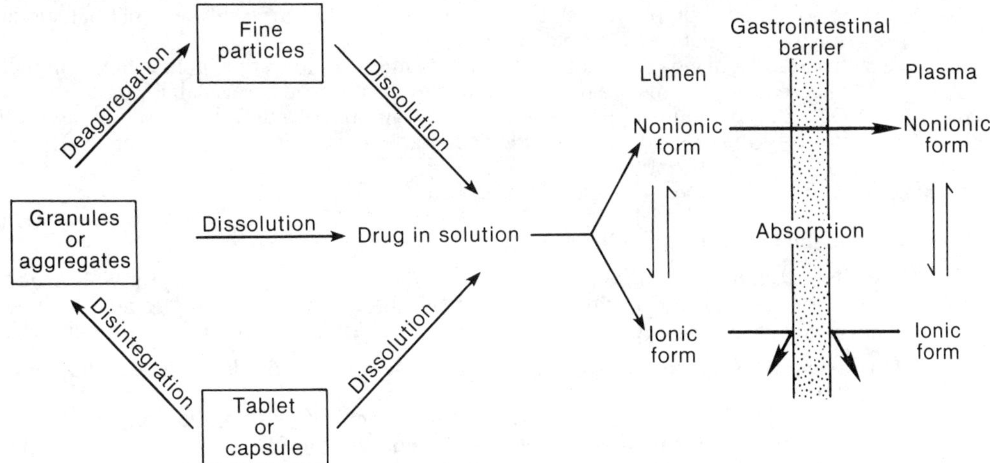

Figure 4-1. Diagrammatic representation of a drug's disintegration, dissolution, and absorption following oral administration in tablet or capsule form. (Adapted with permission from Blanchard J: Gastrointestinal absorption II. Formulation factors affecting bioavailability. *Amer J Pharm* 150:132–151, 1978.)

goxin, dispersed in such a water-miscible vehicle, may have better bioavailability than an equivalent compressed tablet formulation. However, a soft gelatin capsule that contains the drug dissolved in a **hydrophobic vehicle** such as a vegetable oil may have slower bioavailability than a compressed tablet formulation.

c. **Coating** the capsule's gelatin shell (or coating the drug particles within a capsule) alters the drug's bioavailability.

5. **Compressed tablets** are solid dosage forms in which high pressure is used to compress a powder blend or granulation into a solid mass. The powder blend or granulation contains the active drug along with other ingredients or excipients.
   a. **Excipients**, including diluent (filler), binder, disintegrants, lubricants, dye, and flavoring and sweetening agents, provide for the efficient manufacture of compressed tablets, influence the tablets' physical and chemical characteristics, and affect the drug's bioavailability. Generally, the higher the ratio of excipient to active drug (greater than 5:1), the greater the chance that the excipients will affect drug bioavailability.
      (1) **Disintegrants** vary in action, depending on the concentration of the disintegrant, the method of mixing the disintegrant with the powder formulation, and the degree of tablet compaction.
      (2) **Lubricants** are generally hydrophobic, water-insoluble substances such as stearic acid and magnesium stearate. They may reduce wetting of the surface of the solid drug particles, slowing the drug's dissolution rate and bioavailability rate.
      (3) Other excipients such as **surfactants**, **dyes**, and **diluents** may interact with the drug and affect bioavailability.
   b. Disintegration usually is not a major problem in tablet manufacture because it occurs more rapidly than drug dissolution.

6. **Coated compressed tablets** (tablets modified with a sugar coat, a film coat, or an enteric coat, for example) offer a means to affect the drug's disintegration rate, release, and dissolution. Coating can protect the drug from moisture, light, and air; mask the drug's taste or odor; improve the tablet's appearance; and control the drug's release rate.

7. **Modified-release dosage forms** are drug products designed to alter the rate or timing of drug release.
   a. **Extended-release dosage forms** include such drug products as **controlled-release**, **sustained-action**, **long-acting**, and **drug-delivery** systems. These dosage forms allow at least a two-fold reduction in dosing frequency compared to a conventional immediate-release drug product.
      (1) The extended, slow release of controlled-release drug products produces a relatively flat, sustained plasma drug concentration, which avoids toxicity from high concentration peaks.
      (2) Extended-release dosage forms may yield an immediate (initial) release of the drug, followed by a slower sustained release.
   b. **Delayed-release dosage forms** release the active drug at a time other than promptly after administration, at a desired site or location in the gastrointestinal tract. For example, an **enteric-coated** drug product should not dissolve in the stomach's acid pH but should dissolve in the more alkaline pH of the small intestine.
   c. Because modified-release dosage forms are more complex than conventional, immediate-release dosage forms, more stringent quality control and bioavailability tests are required. **Dose dumping** (the abrupt release of a large amount of a drug in an uncontrolled manner) can be a major problem with modified-release dosage forms.

IV. BIOAVAILABILITY AND BIOEQUIVALENCY

A. Bioavailability and therapeutic effect

1. A **pharmacologic response** occurs when a drug combines with a **receptor** within the body. This drug–receptor interaction is usually reversible. As more drug molecules combine with the receptor, the **intensity** of the pharmacologic effect increases up to a maximum (Fig. 4-2).

2. The **time course of the pharmacologic response** depends on drug concentration at the receptor site.
   a. After a drug is administered, it is absorbed systemically. As the drug concentration at the receptor rises to a **minimum effective concentration** (**MEC**), a pharmacologic response is initiated. The time from drug administration to the MEC is known as the **onset time**.
   b. As long as the drug concentration remains above the MEC, pharmacologic activity is observed. The **duration** of the pharmacologic activity is the time for which the drug concentration remains above the MEC.

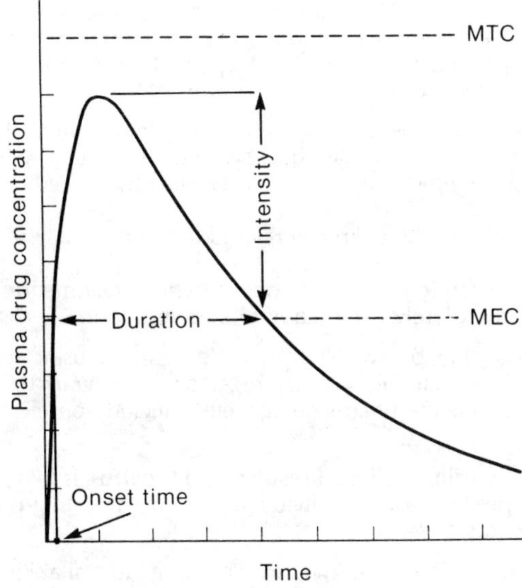

Figure 4-2. Generalized plasma drug concentration versus time curve after oral drug administration. *MEC* = minimum effective concentration; *MTC* = minimum toxic concentration. (Adapted with permission from Shargel L, Yu ABC: *Applied Biopharmaceutics and Pharmacokinetics*, 2nd ed. Norwalk, CT, Appleton-Century-Crofts, 1985.)

c. As the drug concentration increases, other receptors may combine with the drug to exert a toxic or adverse response. This drug concentration is the **minimum toxic concentration (MTC)**. The drug concentration range between the MEC and the MTC is the **therapeutic window**.

B. Methods for measuring bioavailability

1. The **plasma drug concentration versus time curve** measures the bioavailability of a drug from a drug product (Fig. 4-3).
   a. The **time for peak plasma drug concentration** (T_{max}) relates to the rate of systemic drug absorption. If two oral drug products contain the same amount of active drug but different excipients, the dosage form that yields the faster rate of drug absorption will have the shorter T_{max}.
   b. The **peak plasma drug concentration** (C_{max}) is the plasma drug concentration at T_{max} and relates to the intensity of the pharmacologic response. Ideally, C_{max} should be within the therapeutic window.

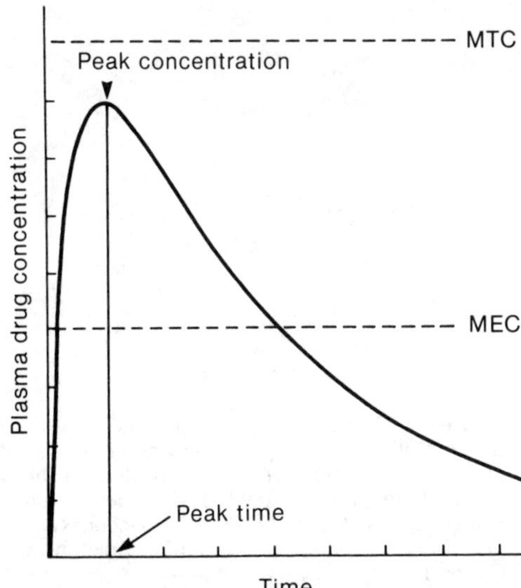

Figure 4-3. Generalized plasma drug concentration versus time curve, showing peak time and peak concentration. The *shaded portion* represents the *area under the curve*; *MEC* = minimum effective concentration; *MTC* = minimum toxic concentration. (Adapted with permission from Shargel L, Yu ABC: *Applied Biopharmaceutics and Pharmacokinetics,* 2nd ed. Norwalk, CT, Appleton-Century-Crofts, 1985.)

c. The **area under the plasma drug concentration versus time curve** (AUC) relates to the amount or extent of drug absorption. The greater the amount of systemic drug absorption, the greater the AUC. The AUC is usually calculated by the **trapezoidal rule** and is expressed in units of concentration multiplied by time (e.g., $\mu g \times hr/ml$).

2. Measurement of **urinary drug excretion** can determine bioavailability from a drug product, if the active therapeutic moiety is excreted unchanged in significant quantity in the urine (Fig. 4-4).
   a. The **cumulative amount** of active drug excreted in the urine (D_U^∞) is directly related to the extent of systemic drug absorption.
   b. The **rate of drug excretion** in the urine (dD_U/dt) is directly related to the rate of systemic drug absorption.
   c. The **time for the drug to be completely excreted** (t^∞) corresponds to the total time for the drug to be systemically absorbed and completely excreted after administration.

3. When no assay for drug concentration is available, bioavailability may be measured using **acute pharmacologic effects**, such as changes in heart rate, blood pressure, electrocardiogram (ECG), or clotting time. Parameters for measuring an acute pharmacologic effect include onset time, duration, and intensity of the effect.

4. Quantitative measurement of bioavailability using a **clinical response to the drug** is less precise than other methods and highly variable because of individual differences in drug pharmacodynamics and subjective measurements.

5. For certain drugs, the **rate of drug dissolution** in vitro correlates with drug bioavailability in vivo. When the dissolution test in vitro is considered statistically adequate to predict drug bioavailability, then it may be used in place of an in vivo bioavailability study.

6. Values for relative bioavailability and absolute bioavailability may also be calculated.
   a. **Relative bioavailability** is the availability of the drug from a dosage form as compared to a reference standard. It is calculated as the ratio of the AUC for the dosage form to the AUC for the reference dosage form. A relative bioavailability of 1 (or 100%) implies that drug

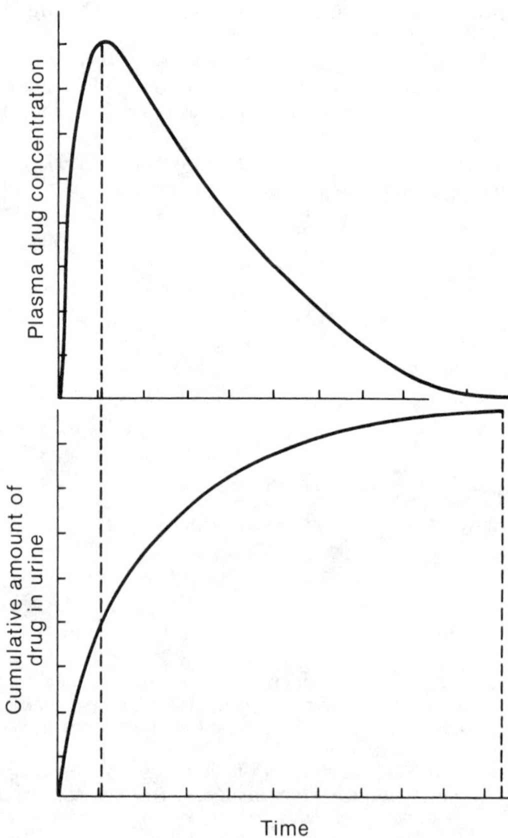

Figure 4-4. These corresponding plots show the relationship of the plasma drug concentration versus time curve to the cumulative amount of drug in the urine versus time curve. (Adapted with permission from Shargel L, Yu ABC: *Applied Biopharmaceutics and Pharmacokinetics*, 2nd ed. Norwalk, CT, Appleton-Century-Crofts, 1985.)

bioavailability from both dosage forms was the same, but it does not indicate the completeness of systemic drug absorption.

b. Absolute bioavailability is the availability of the drug from a dosage form as compared to the availability of the drug after IV administration. It is calculated as the ratio of the AUC for the dosage form given orally to the AUC obtained after IV drug administration. An absolute bioavailability of 0.80 (or 80%) indicates that only 80% of the drug was systemically available from the dosage form.

C. Bioequivalency

1. A generic drug product is considered **bioequivalent** if its rate and extent of systemic absorption (bioavailability) do not show a significant difference from the pioneer drug product when administered at the same molar dose of the therapeutic ingredient, by the same route, and under the same experimental conditions.

2. A **bioequivalency requirement** is imposed by the Food and Drug Administration (FDA) for bioequivalency testing of specified drug products. The requirement must be satisfied as a condition for marketing and is imposed on certain drugs that have a narrow therapeutic window, that demonstrate variable bioavailability, or that have physicochemical properties that would affect bioavailability in vivo, such as poor aqueous solubility, polymorphic forms, or a slow dissolution rate.

3. A **bioequivalency study** permits evaluation of specified drug products.

   a. Usually a **crossover design** (e.g., a **Latin square**) is preferred, because each subject receives each dosage form. Subjects then act as their own controls, reducing individual variation.

   b. The **reference standard** should contain the same active drug as the generic drug product in its most bioavailable form (e.g., a solution or suspension), given in the same molar dose, and by the same administration route.

   c. Data should be presented in both **tabulated and graphic format**, with the proper statistical tests.

   d. The **bioavailability parameters** (C_{max}, T_{max}, and AUC) for each drug product should not differ by more than 20%.

V. PHARMACOKINETICS

A. Introduction

1. Rates and orders of reactions

a. The **rate** of a chemical reaction or process is the velocity with which it occurs. The **order** of a reaction refers to the way in which the concentration of a drug or reactant in a chemical reaction influences the rate.

b. In a **zero-order reaction**, the drug concentration changes with respect to time at a constant rate, according to this equation:

$$\frac{dC}{dt} = -k_0$$

where C is the drug concentration and k_0 is the zero-order rate constant given in units of concentration/time (e.g., mg/ml per hour). Integration of this equation yields the linear (straight-line) equation:

$$C = -k_0t + C_0$$

where k_0 is the slope of the line (see Fig. 2-1) and C_0 is the y-intercept, or drug concentration, when time (t) is equal to zero. The negative sign indicates that the slope is decreasing.

c. In a **first-order reaction**, the drug concentration changes with respect to time as the product of the rate constant and the concentration of drug remaining, according to this equation:

$$\frac{dC}{dt} = -kC$$

where k is the first-order rate constant, given in units of reciprocal time, or $time^{-1}$ (e.g., 1/hr or hr^{-1}).

(1) Integration of the above equation (in section V A 1 c) yields the following mathematically equivalent equations:

$$C = C_0e^{-kt}$$

$$\ln C = -kt + \ln C_0$$

$$\log C = -\frac{kt}{2.3} + \log C_0$$

(2) A graph of the above equation [in section V A 1 c (1)] shown in Figure 2-2 demonstrates the linear relationship of the log of the concentration versus time. In Figure 2-2, the slope of the line is equal to $-k/2.3$ and the y-intercept is C_0. Notice that the values for C are plotted on logarithmic coordinates; the values for t are on linear coordinates.

(3) The **half-life** of a reaction is the time required for the concentration of a drug to decrease by one-half. For a first-order reaction, the half-life is a constant and is related to the first-order rate constant according to this equation:

$$t_{1/2} = \frac{0.693}{k}$$

2. Models and compartments

a. A **model** is a mathematical description of a biologic system and is used as a concise way to express quantitative relationships.

b. A **compartment** is a group of tissues with similar blood flows and drug affinities. A compartment is **not** a real physiologic or anatomical region.

3. Drug distribution

a. Drugs distribute **rapidly** to **tissues with high blood flow** and more **slowly** to **tissues with a smaller blood flow**.

b. Drugs rapidly cross capillary membranes into tissues because of passive diffusion and hydrostatic pressure.

c. Drug permeability across capillary membranes may vary. Generally, drugs cross easily the capillaries of the glomerulus of the kidney and the sinusoids of the liver. The brain's capillaries are surrounded by glial cells, creating a **blood–brain barrier** that acts as a thick lipid membrane, which polar and ionic hydrophilic drugs cross very slowly.

d. Drugs may accumulate in tissues as a result of their physicochemical characteristics and a special affinity of the tissue for the drug. For example, lipid-soluble drugs may accumulate in adipose (fat) tissue from partitioning of the drug. Tetracycline may accumulate in bone from complex formation with calcium.

e. Plasma protein binding of drugs affects drug distribution.

(1) A drug bound to a protein forms a complex that is too large to cross cell membranes.

(2) **Albumin** is the major plasma protein involved in protein binding. **Alpha$_1$-glycoprotein**, also found in plasma, is important for the binding of such basic drugs as propranolol.

(3) Potent drugs such as phenytoin, which are highly bound (>90%) to plasma proteins, may be displaced by other highly bound drugs. The displacement of the bound drug results in more free (nonbound) drug, which rapidly reaches the drug receptors. This causes a more intense pharmacologic response.

B. One-compartment model

1. After a rapid **IV bolus injection**, the entire drug dose enters the body and the rate of absorption is neglected in calculations (Fig. 4-5). The entire body acts as a single compartment, and the drug rapidly equilibrates with all the tissues in the body.

a. Drug elimination is a first-order kinetic process, according to the equations in section V A 1 c).

(1) The **first-order elimination rate constant** (k) represents the sum of all the rate constants for drug removal from the body, including the rate constants for renal excretion and metabolism (biotransformation) as described by this equation:

$$k = k_e + k_m$$

where k_e is the rate constant for renal excretion and k_m is the rate constant for metabolism. This equation assumes all rates are first-order processes.

(2) The **elimination half-life** ($t_{1/2}$) is given by this equation:

$$t_{1/2} = \frac{0.693}{k}$$

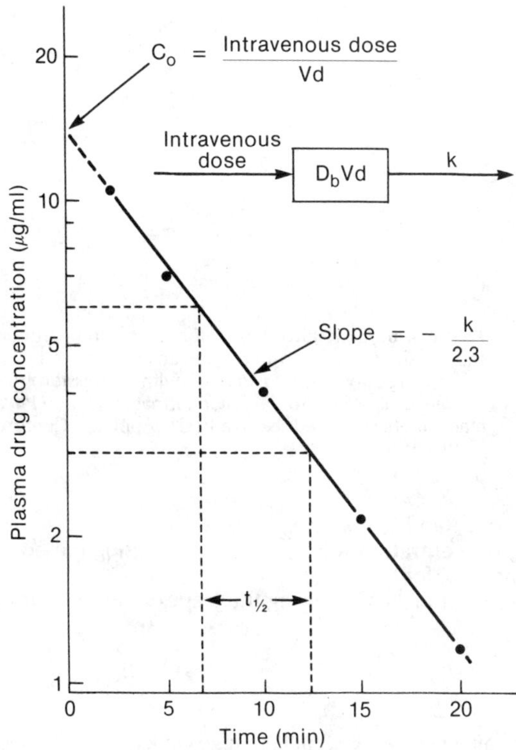

Figure 4-5. Generalized pharmacokinetic model for a drug administered by rapid intravenous (IV) bolus injection. C_o = the extrapolated drug concentration; *Vd* = the apparent volume of distribution; D_b = the amount of drug in the body; *k* = the elimination rate constant; $t_{1/2}$ = the elimination half-life. (Adapted with permission from Gibaldi M, Perrier D: *Pharmacokinetics*. New York, Marcel Dekker, 1982.)

b. The **apparent volume of distribution** (Vd) is the hypothetical volume of body fluid in which the drug is dissolved. This is **not** a true anatomical or physical volume.

(1) The apparent volume of distribution is needed to estimate the amount of drug in the body relative to the concentration of drug in the plasma, as shown in the following relationship:

$$\text{Vd} \times C_p = D_b$$

where Vd is the apparent volume of distribution, C_p is the plasma drug concentration, and D_b is the amount of drug in the body.

(2) To calculate the Vd after an IV bolus injection, the equation above is rearranged to give:

$$\text{Vd} = \frac{D_b{}^0}{C_p{}^0}$$

where $D_b{}^0$ is the dose (D_0) of drug given by IV bolus and $C_p{}^0$ is the extrapolated drug concentration at zero time on the y-axis, after the drug has equilibrated.

(3) According to the above equation, Vd is larger when more drug is distributed extravascularly into the tissues, and $C_p{}^0$ is therefore smaller. When more drug is contained in the vascular space or plasma, $C_p{}^0$ is larger and Vd is smaller.

2. After a **single oral dose** of a drug from a conventional dosage form (e.g, a tablet or capsule), the drug is rapidly absorbed by **first-order kinetics**. Elimination of the drug also follows first-order kinetics (Fig. 4-6).

a. This equation describes the pharmacokinetics of first-order absorbtion and elimination:

$$C_p = \frac{FD_0k_A}{\text{Vd}(k_A - k)}(e^{-kt} - e^{-k_At})$$

where k_A is the first-order absorption rate constant and F is the fraction of drug bioavailable. Changes in F, D_0, Vd, k_A, and k will affect the plasma drug concentration.

b. The **time for maximum or peak drug absorption** is given by this equation:

$$T_{max} = \frac{2.3 \log (k_A/k)}{k_A - k}$$

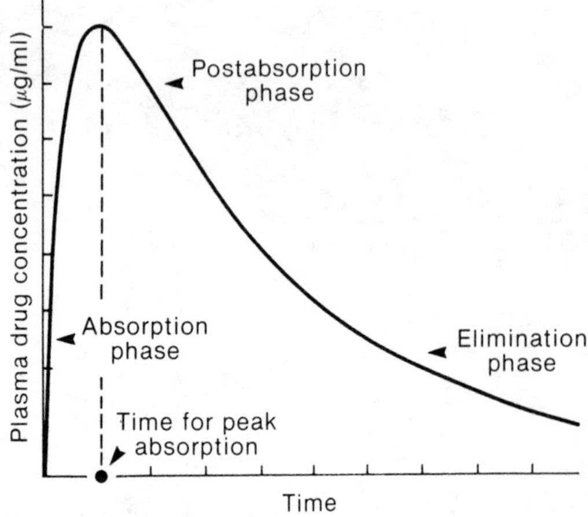

Figure 4-6. Generalized plot for a one-compartment model showing first-order drug absorption and first-order drug elimination. (Adapted with permission from Shargel L, Yu ABC: *Applied Biopharmaceutics and Pharmacokinetics*, 2nd ed. Norwalk, CT, Appleton-Century-Crofts, 1985.)

T_{max} depends only on the rate constants k_A and k, not on F, D_0 or Vd.

c. After T_{max} is obtained, the **peak drug concentration** (C_{max}) is calculated using the equation in section V B 2 a and substituting T_{max} for t.

d. The AUC may be determined by integration of $\int_0^t C_p dt$ using the **trapezoidal rule**, or by this equation:

$$AUC = \frac{FD_0}{Vd\ k}$$

where changes in F, D_0, k, and Vd will affect the AUC. Small changes in k_A will not affect the AUC.

e. Lag time occurs just at the beginning of systemic drug absorption. For some individuals, systemic drug absorption is delayed after oral drug administration from stomach emptying and gastrointestinal mobility.

3. With **IV infusion**, **zero-order absorption** and **first-order elimination** occur (Fig. 4-7).

a. A few **oral controlled-release drug products** release the drug by zero-order kinetics and have zero-order systemic absorption.

b. The **plasma drug concentration** at any time after the start of an IV infusion is given by this equation:

$$C_p = \frac{R}{Vd\ k}(1 - e^{-kt})$$

where R is the zero-order rate of infusion given in units as mg/hr or mg/min.

c. If the IV infusion is stopped, the plasma drug concentration declines by a first-order process and the elimination half-life, or k, may be obtained from the declining plasma drug concentration versus time curve.

d. As the drug is infused, the plasma drug concentration increases to a plateau, or **steady-state concentration**.

(1) Under steady-state conditions, the fraction of drug absorbed equals the fraction of drug eliminated from the body.

(2) The plasma concentration at steady state (C_{ss}) is given by this equation:

$$C_{ss} = \frac{R}{Vd\ k}$$

(3) The **rate of drug infusion** (**R**) may be calculated from a rearrangement of the above equation, provided that the desired C_{ss}, the Vd, and the k are known. The values are often readily obtainable from the drug literature. The rearranged equation is:

$$R = C_{ss}\ Vd\ k$$

e. A **loading dose** is used to give an initial IV bolus injection of drug, producing the C_{ss} as rapidly as possible. The IV infusion is started at the same time.

(1) The **time to reach the C_{ss}** depends on the drug's elimination half-life. To reach 95% or 99% of the C_{ss} would take 4.32 or 6.65 half-lives, respectively.

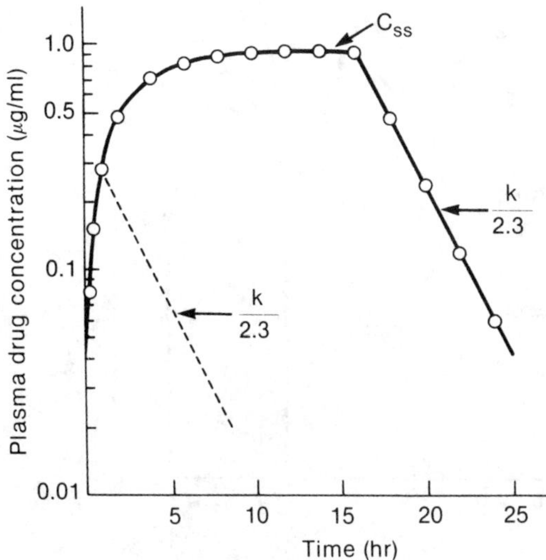

Figure 4-7. Generalized semilogarithmic plot for a drug showing zero-order absorption and first-order elimination. C_{ss} = the steady-state concentration; k = the elimination rate constant. (Adapted with permission from Gibaldi M, Perrier D: *Pharmacokinetics*. New York, Marcel Dekker, 1982.)

(2) The loading dose (D_L) is the amount of drug that, when dissolved in the apparent Vd, produces the desired C_{SS}. Thus, D_L is calculated by these equations:

$$D_L = C_{SS}\,Vd$$

$$D_L = R/k$$

f. For a drug with a narrow therapeutic window, an IV infusion provides a relatively constant plasma drug concentration that does not rise above the MTC or fall below the MEC.

4. Many drugs are given intermittently in a **multiple-dose regimen** for continuous or prolonged therapeutic activity. This regimen is often used in the treatment of a chronic disease.

a. If drug doses are given at frequent intervals before complete elimination of the previous dose, then plasma drug concentrations will **accumulate**, rising to a plateau or steady-state level.

b. At **steady-state**, plasma drug concentration fluctuates between a maximum (C^{∞}_{max}) and a minimum (C^{∞}_{min}) [Fig. 4-8].

c. When calculating a multiple-dose regimen, the **superposition principle** assumes that previous drug doses have no effect on the subsequent doses. Thus, the predicted plasma drug concentration is the total plasma drug concentration obtained by adding the residual drug concentrations found after each previous dose.

d. When designing a multiple-dose regimen, only the **dosing rate** can be easily adjusted.

(1) The dosing rate is based on the **size of the dose** (D_0) and the **time interval between doses or the frequency of dosing** (τ).

(2) The dosing rate is given by this equation:

$$\text{Dosing rate} = D_0/\tau$$

(3) As long as the dosing rate is the same, the **expected average drug concentration at steady state (C^{∞}_{av})** will be the same.

(a) For example, if a 600-mg dose is given every 12 hours, the dosing rate is 600 mg/12 hr, or 50 mg/hr.

(b) A dose of 300 mg every 6 hours, or 200 mg every 4 hours, would also give the same dosing rate (50 mg/hr) with the same expected C^{∞}_{av}.

(c) For a larger dose given over a longer time interval (e.g., 600 mg every 12 hours), the C^{∞}_{max} will be higher and the C^{∞}_{min} lower compared to a smaller dose given more frequently (e.g., 200 mg every 4 hours).

e. A few drugs, such as certain antibiotics, may be given by **multiple rapid IV bolus injections**.

(1) The **peak or maximum serum drug concentration at steady-state** may be estimated by the following equation:

$$C^{\infty}_{max} = \frac{D_0/Vd}{1 - e^{-k\tau}}$$

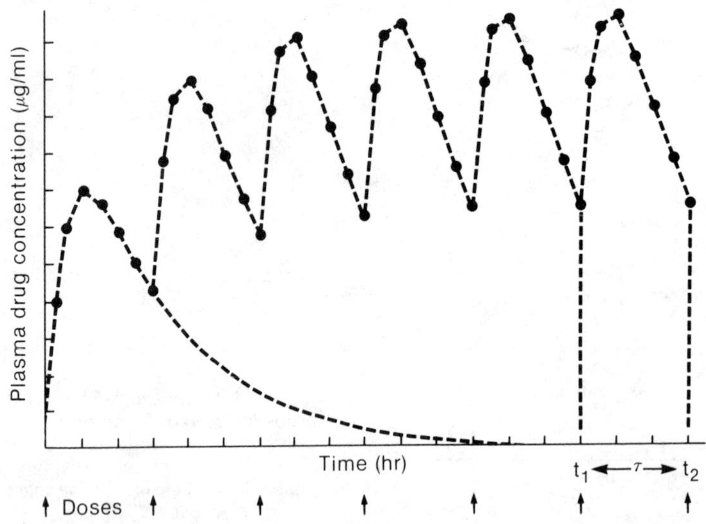

Figure 4-8. Generalized plot showing plasma drug concentration levels after administration of multiple doses and levels of accumulation when equal doses are given at equal time intervals. τ = the time interval between doses (t) or the frequency of dosing. (Adapted with permission from Shargel L, Yu ABC: *Applied Biopharmaceutics and Pharmacokinetics*, 2nd ed. Norwalk, CT, Appleton-Century-Crofts, 1985.)

(2) The **minimum serum drug concentration** (C^{∞}_{min}) at steady-state is the drug concentration after the drug declines one dosage interval. Thus, C^{∞}_{min} is determined by this equation:

$$C^{\infty}_{min} = C^{\infty}_{max}\, e^{-k\tau}$$

(3) The **average drug concentration** (C^{∞}_{av}) at steady-state may be estimated from the same equation as for multiple oral doses:

$$C^{\infty}_{av} = \frac{F\, D_0}{k\, Vd\, \tau}$$

for IV bolus injections, F = 1.

f. Most drugs are given by **multiple oral doses**. For drugs that are very rapidly absorbed and slowly eliminated, $K_A >> k$. These drugs are often contained in immediate-release dosage forms, such as solutions, conventional tablets, and capsules. C^{∞}_{max} and C^{∞}_{min} for these may be approximated by the equations in sections V B 4 e (1) and V B 4 e (2).

(1) For more exact calculations of C^{∞}_{max} and C^{∞}_{min} after multiple oral doses, the following equations may be used:

$$C^{\infty}_{max} = \frac{F\, D_0}{Vd} \quad \frac{1}{1 - e^{-k\tau}}$$

$$C^{\infty}_{min} = \frac{k_A\, F\, D_0}{Vd\, (k_A - k)} \quad \frac{1}{1 - e^{-k\tau}}\, e^{-kt}$$

(2) The calculation of C^{∞}_{av} is the same as for multiple IV bolus injections, using the equation in section V B 4 e (3).

(3) The term $1/(1 - e^{-k\tau})$ is known as the **accumulation rate**.

(4) The **fraction of drug remaining in the body** (f) after a dosage interval is given by this equation:

$$f = e^{-k\tau}$$

(5) An initial large drug dose, or D_L, may be given to obtain a therapeutic **steady-state** drug level quickly.

(a) For multiple oral doses, D_L may be calculated by:

$$D_L = D_M \frac{1}{1 - e^{-k\tau}}$$

where D_M is the maintenance dose.

(b) If D_M is given at a dosage interval equal to the drug's elimination half-life, then D_L will equal twice the maintenance dose.

C. Multicompartment models

1. Introduction

a. Drugs that exhibit **multicompartment pharmacokinetics** distribute into different tissue groups at different rates.

b. Tissues with **high blood flow** equilibrate with a drug more rapidly than tissues with **small blood flow**.

c. Drug concentration in various tissues depends on the drug's physical–chemical characteristics and the nature of the tissue. For example, highly lipid-soluble drugs accumulate slowly in fat (lipid) tissue.

2. Two-compartment model (IV bolus injection)

a. After an IV bolus injection, the drug distributes and equilibrates rapidly into highly perfused tissues (**central compartment**) and more slowly into peripheral tissues (**tissue compartment**) [Fig. 4-9].

b. The initial rapid decline in plasma drug concentration is known as the **distribution phase**. The slower rate of decline in drug concentration after complete equilibration is known as the **elimination phase**.

c. The plasma drug concentration at any time is the sum of two first-order processes, as given in this equation:

$$C_p = Ae^{-at} + Be^{-bt}$$

where a and b are hybrid first-order rate constants and A and B are y-intercepts.

(1) The **hybrid first-order rate constant b** is obtained from the slope of the elimination phase of the curve (see Fig. 6-9) and represents first-order elimination of drug from the body after the drug has equilibrated with all tissues.

(2) The **hybrid first-order rate constant a** is obtained from the slope of the residual line of the distribution phase after subtraction of the elimination phase.

d. The **apparent volume of distribution** depends on the type of pharmacokinetic calculation. Volumes of distribution include the **volume of the central compartment** (V_p), the **volume of distribution at steady-state** (V_{ss}), and the **volume of the tissue compartment** (V_t).

3. Two-compartment model (oral drug administration)

a. A drug with a rapid distribution phase may not demonstrate two-compartment characteristics after oral administration. As the drug is absorbed, it equilibrates with the tissues so that the elimination half-life of the curve's elimination portion equals 0.693/b.

b. Two-compartment characteristics may be observed if the drug is rapidly absorbed and the distribution phase is slower.

4. Models with additional compartments

a. Addition of each new compartment to the model requires an additional first-order plot.

b. Addition of a **third compartment** implies that the drug slowly equilibrates into a deep-tissue space. If the drug is given at frequent intervals, it will begin to accumulate into the third compartment.

c. The **terminal linear phase** generally represents drug elimination from the body after equilibration. The rate constant from the elimination phase is used for dosage regimen calculations.

d. Adequate pharmacokinetic description of multicompartment models is often difficult and depends on proper plasma sampling and drug concentration determination.

D. Nonlinear pharmacokinetics

1. Also termed **capacity-limited**, **dose-dependent**, or **saturation pharmacokinetics**, **nonlinear pharmacokinetics** do not follow first-order kinetics as the dose is increased (Fig. 4-10).

2. These properties are characteristic of nonlinear pharmacokinetics:

a. AUC is not proportional to the dose.

b. **Amount of drug excreted in the urine** is not proportional to the dose.

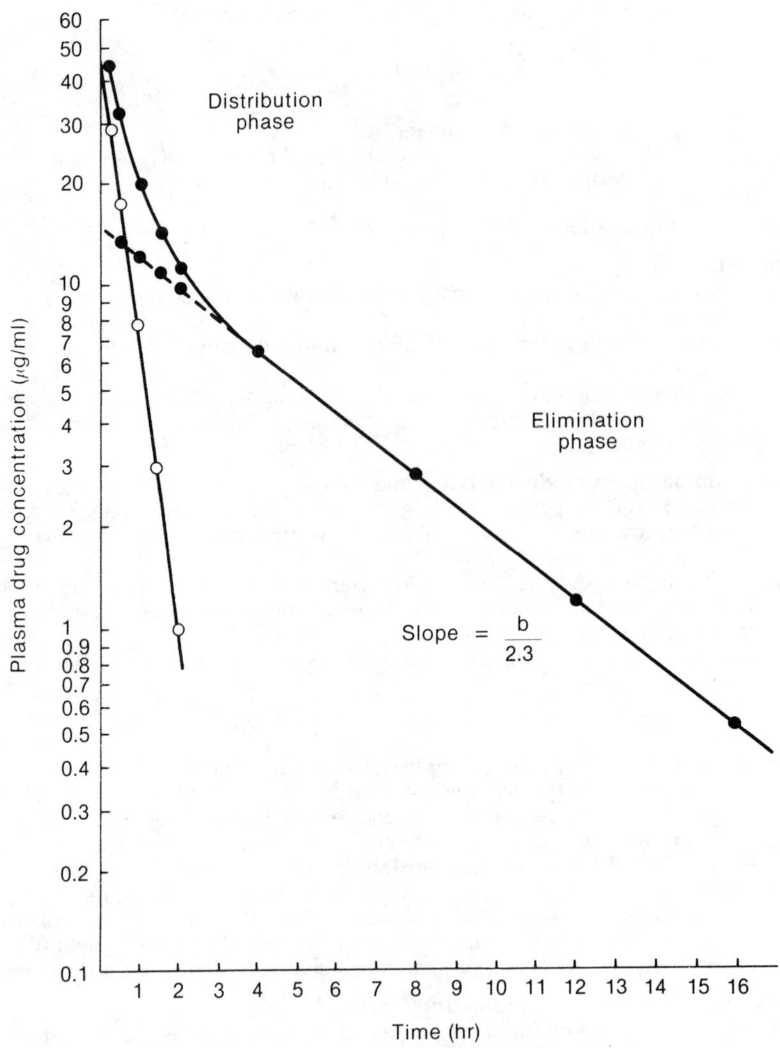

Figure 4-9. Generalized plot showing drug distribution and equilibration for a two-compartment model (IV bolus injection). The distribution phase represents the initial rapid decline in plasma drug concentration. The elimination phase represents the slower rate of decline after the drug's complete equilibration. (Adapted with permission from Shargel L, Yu ABC: *Applied Biopharmaceutics and Pharmacokinetics*, 2nd ed. Norwalk, CT, Appleton-Century-Crofts, 1985.)

c. **Elimination half-life** increases at high doses.

d. The ratio of metabolites formed changes with increased dose.

3. Nonlinear pharmacokinetics may result from **saturation of an enzyme- or carrier-mediated system**.

4. **Michaelis-Menten kinetics**, which describe the velocity of enzyme reactions, are often used to describe nonlinear pharmacokinetics.

   a. The **Michaelis-Menten equation** describes the rate of change (velocity) of plasma drug concentration after an IV bolus injection, as follows:

$$-\frac{dC_p}{dt} = \frac{V_{max}\,C_p}{K_m + C_p}$$

where V_{max} is the maximum velocity of the reaction, C_p is the substrate or plasma drug concentration, and K_m is the rate constant equal to the C_p at 0.5 V_{max}.

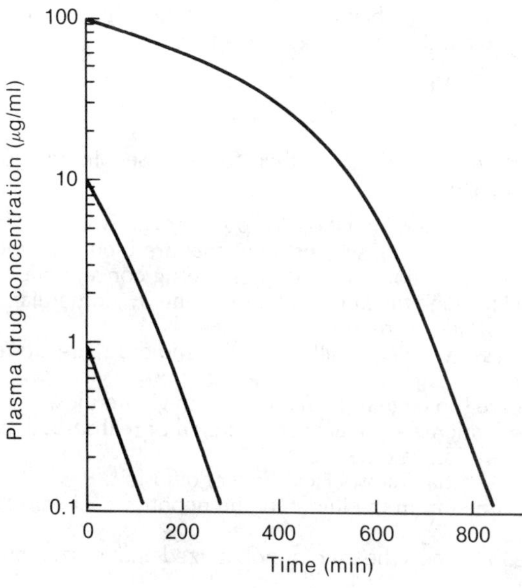

Figure 4-10. Generalized plot showing plasma drug concentration versus time for a drug with Michaelis-Menten (nonlinear) elimination kinetics. For this one-compartment model (IV injection), the doses are 1 mg, 10 mg, and 100 mg, and the apparent in vivo rate constant (K_m) = 10 mg. The maximum velocity of the reaction (V_{max}) = 0.2 mg/min. (Adapted with permission from Gibaldi M, Perrier D: *Pharmacokinetics*. New York, Marcel Dekker, 1982.)

b. At **very low** C_p, where $K_m >> C_p$, the above equation reduces to this first-order rate equation:

$$-\frac{dC_p}{dt} = \frac{V_{max}}{K_m} C_p$$

c. At **high** C_p, where $C_p >> K_m$, the Michaelis-Menten equation becomes a zero-order rate equation:

$$-\frac{dC_p}{dt} = V_{max}$$

5. Drugs that follow nonlinear pharmacokinetics may demonstrate zero-order elimination rates at very high drug concentrations, a mix of zero- and first-order elimination rates at intermediate drug concentrations, and first-order elimination rates at very low drug concentrations (see Fig. 6-10).

E. Clearance

1. Clearance is a measurement of drug elimination from the body.

2. Total body clearance (Cl_T) may be defined as the **drug elimination rate divided by the plasma drug concentration**. It considers the body to contain an apparent volume of distribution in which the drug is dissolved. A constant portion of this volume is assumed to be removed from the body per unit time.

a. These equations express the measurement of total body clearance:

$$Cl_T = \frac{\text{drug elimination}}{\text{plasma drug concentration}} = \frac{dD_e/dt}{C_p}$$

$$Cl_T = V_d\, k$$

$$Cl_T = \frac{FD_0}{AUC}$$

b. For drugs that follow first-order (linear) pharmacokinetics, **total body clearance is the sum of all the clearances in the body**. Thus,

$$Cl_T = Cl_R + Cl_{NR}$$

where Cl_R is renal clearance and Cl_{NR} is nonrenal clearance.

c. The relationship between Cl_T and the $t_{1/2}$ may be obtained by substituting $0.693/t_{1/2}$ for k in the equation in section V E 2 a (2) to obtain the following expression:

$$t_{1/2} = \frac{0.693\ Vd}{\text{clearance}}$$

d. As clearance decreases (as in the case of renal disease), then $t_{1/2}$ increases. In addition, changes in Vd cause a proportional change in $t_{1/2}$.

3. Renal drug excretion is the major route of drug elimination for polar drugs, water-soluble drugs, drugs with low molecular weight (< 500 Mol wt), or drugs that are biotransformed slowly. The relationship between the drug excretion rate and plasma drug concentration is shown in Figure 4-11. Drugs are excreted through the kidney into the urine by glomerular filtration, tubular reabsorption, and active tubular secretion.

a. Glomerular filtration is a passive process by which small molecules and drugs are filtered through the glomerulus of the nephron.

(1) Drugs bound to plasma proteins are too large to be filtered at the glomerulus.

(2) Drugs such as **creatinine** or **inulin**, which are not actively secreted or reabsorbed, are used to measure the **glomerular filtration rate** (GFR).

b. Tubular reabsorption is a passive process that follows Fick's law of diffusion.

(1) Lipid-soluble drugs may be reabsorbed from the lumen of the nephron back into the systemic circulation.

(2) For **weak electrolyte drugs**, urine pH affects the ratio of nonionized and ionized drug species.

(a) If the drug exists primarily in the nonionized or lipid-soluble form, then it will be reabsorbed from the lumen of the nephron more easily.

(b) If the drug exists primarily in the ionized or water-soluble form, then it will be more easily excreted in the urine.

(c) Depending upon the drug's pK_a, alteration of urine pH will alter the ratio of ionized to nonionized drug, affecting the rate of drug excretion. For example, alkalinization of the urine by the administration of sodium bicarbonate will increase the excretion of salicylates (weak acids).

(3) An increase in urine flow resulting from simultaneous administration of a diuretic will decrease the time for drug reabsorption. Consequently, more drug will be excreted.

c. Active tubular secretion is an active transport system that is carrier-mediated and requires energy.

(1) Two active tubular secretion pathways exist in the kidney—one system for weak acids and one system for weak bases.

(2) The active tubular secretion system demonstrates **competition effects**. For example, probenecid (a weak acid) competes for the same system as penicillin, decreasing the rate of penicillin excretion.

(3) The renal clearance of drugs such as **para-aminohippurate** (PAH), which are actively secreted, is used to measure **effective renal blood flow** (ERBF).

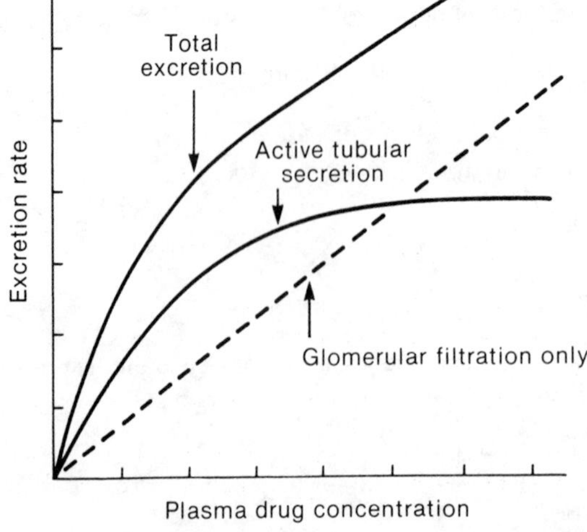

Figure 4-11. Generalized plot showing the excretion rate versus plasma drug concentration for a drug that demonstrates active tubular secretion and for one secreted by glomerular filtration only. (Adapted with permission from Shargel L, Yu ABC: *Applied Biopharmaceutics and Pharmacokinetics*, 2nd ed. Norwalk, CT, Appleton-Century-Crofts, 1985.)

4. **Renal clearance** is the volume of drug-containing plasma that is removed by the kidney per unit time.
   a. **Units for renal clearance** are in volume per time (e.g., ml/min or L/hr).
   b. Renal clearance may be measured by dividing the rate of drug excretion by the plasma drug concentration, as shown:

$$Cl_R = \frac{\text{Rate of drug excretion}}{C_p} = \frac{dDu/dt}{C_p}$$

   c. Measurement of renal clearance may also be expressed by these equations:

$$Cl_R = k_e\, Vd$$

   where k_e is the first-order renal excretion rate constant, and

$$Cl_R = \frac{Du^{\infty}}{AUC}$$

   where Du^{∞} is the total amount of parent (unchanged) drug excreted in the urine.
   d. Renal clearance is measured without regard to the physiologic mechanism of renal drug excretion.
      (1) The probable mechanism for renal clearance may be obtained by using a **clearance ratio**, which relates drug clearance to inulin clearance (a measure of GFR).
      (2) If the clearance ratio is less than 1.0, then the mechanism for drug clearance may result from filtration plus reabsorption. If it is equal to 1.0, the mechanism may be filtration only. If it is greater than 1.0, the mechanism may be filtration plus active tubular secretion.

5. **Hepatic clearance** is the volume of drug-containing plasma that is cleared by the liver per unit time.
   a. Hepatic clearance is usually measured indirectly, as the difference between total body clearance and renal clearance:

$$Cl_H = Cl_T - Cl_R$$

   where Cl_H is the hepatic clearance, which is equivalent to Cl_{NR}, or nonrenal drug clearance.
   b. Hepatic clearance may also be calculated as the product of the blood flow (Q), and the liver and the extraction ratio (ER):

$$Cl_H = Q\ ER$$

      (1) The **extraction ratio** represents the fraction of drug that is irreversibly removed by an organ or tissue as the drug-containing plasma perfuses that tissue.
      (2) The extraction ratio is obtained by measuring the plasma drug concentration entering the liver and the plasma drug exiting the liver:

$$ER = \frac{C_a - C_v}{C_a}$$

      where C_a is the arterial plasma drug concentration entering the liver and C_v is the venous plasma drug concentration exiting the liver.
      (3) Values for ER may range from 0 to 1. For example, if ER equals 0.9, then 90% of the incoming drug is removed by the liver as the plasma perfuses this organ. If ER equals 0, then no drug is removed by the liver.
   c. Hepatic clearance may be affected by blood flow, intrinsic clearance, and protein binding.
      (1) The **blood flow** to the liver is approximately 1.5 L/min and may be altered by exercise, food, disease, or drugs.
         (a) Blood enters the liver by way of the hepatic portal vein and hepatic artery and leaves by way of the hepatic vein.
         (b) After oral drug administration, the drug is absorbed from the gastrointestinal tract into the mesenteric vessels and proceeds to the hepatic portal vein, to the liver, and then to the systemic circulation.
      (2) **Intrinsic clearance** describes the liver's ability to remove the drug independently of blood flow.
         (a) The mechanism of intrinsic drug clearance is primarily the result of the inherent ability of the **biotransformation enzymes** (mixed function oxidases) to metabolize the drug as it enters the liver.

(b) Normally, basal mixed-function oxidase enzymes act to biotransform drugs. These enzymes may be increased by various drugs, such as phenobarbital, or by environmental agents, such as tobacco smoke. Moreover, these same enzymes may be inhibited by other drugs and environmental agents such as cimetidine or acute lead poisoning.

(3) Protein binding prevents hepatic clearance because only the free (or non–plasma protein bound) drug crosses the cell membrane into the liver.

(a) The **free drug** is available to the drug-metabolizing enzymes (mixed function oxidases) for biotransformation.

(b) A **sudden increase in free drug plasma concentration** allows more drug to become available at pharmacologic receptors, producing a more intense effect at organs (e.g., kidney and liver) involved in drug removal.

d. Hepatic clearance is related to blood flow (Q), intrinsic clearance (Cl_{int}), and the free plasma drug concentration (F_U) by the following equation:

$$Cl_H = Q \frac{F_U \, Cl_{int}}{Q + Cl_{int}}$$

(1) The hepatic clearance of drugs such as propranolol, which have high extraction ratios and high Cl_{int} values, is most affected by changes in blood flow and inhibitors of the drug metabolism enzymes.

(2) The hepatic clearance of drugs that have low extraction ratios and low Cl_{int} values, such as theophylline, is most affected by changes in Cl_{int} and is affected only slightly by changes in hepatic blood flow.

(3) Only drugs such as phenytoin, which are highly plasma protein–bound ($> 95\%$) and have a low intrinsic clearance, are affected by a sudden shift to increasing free drug concentration.

e. Hepatic clearance also includes **biliary drug excretion**, an active transport process. Separate active secretion systems exist for both weak acids and weak bases.

(1) Drugs excreted in the bile are usually **high molecular weight compounds** (> 500 Mol wt) or polar drugs such as reserpine, digoxin, and various glucuronide conjugates.

(2) Drugs may be recycled by means of the **enterohepatic circulation**.

(a) Some drugs are absorbed from the gastrointestinal tract by way of the mesenteric and hepatic portal vein, proceeding to the liver. The liver may secrete some of the drug (unchanged or as a glucuronide metabolite) into the bile.

(b) From the bile (stored in the gallbladder), the drug may empty back into the gastrointestinal tract by way of the bile duct.

(c) If the drug is a **glucuronide metabolite**, bacteria in the gastrointestinal tract may hydrolyze the glucuronide moiety, allowing the released drug to be reabsorbed.

f. First-pass effects, or **presystemic elimination**, may occur with drugs given orally. A portion of the drug is eliminated prior to systemic absorption.

(1) The mechanism of first-pass effects generally results from rapid drug biotransformation by the liver enzymes. Other mechanisms may include metabolism of the drug by the gastrointestinal mucosal cells or intestinal flora or biliary secretion.

(2) First-pass effects are usually observed by measuring the **absolute bioavailability** (F) for the drug. If $F < 1$, then some of the drug was eliminated prior to systemic absorption.

(3) Drugs that demonstrate a **high hepatic extraction ratio**, such as propranolol, demonstrate first-pass effects.

(4) If the drug's first-pass effect is extremely high ($> 90\%$), as with nitroglycerin or insulin, then an alternate route of drug administration may be necessary.

VI. CLINICAL PHARMACOKINETICS

A. Clinical pharmacokinetics is the application of pharmacokinetic principles for the rational design of an individualized dosage regimen. The objectives of clinical pharmacokinetics are twofold.

1. An optimum drug concentration at the receptor site must be achieved to produce the desired therapeutic response.

2. The drug's adverse or toxic effects should be minimized.

B. Design factors for an individualized dosage regimen

1. Drug pharmacokinetics in the patient include absorption, distribution, and an elimination profile.

2. The patient's **normal physiologic condition** must be considered, including such characteristics as age, weight, gender, and nutritional status.
3. Pathophysiologic conditions (e.g., renal disease, congestive heart failure, or liver disease) may affect drug pharmacokinetics in the patient.
4. Other interventions may modify the drug's predicted therapeutic activity.
5. Environmental factors may affect drug pharmacokinetics. For example, smoking increases theophylline clearance.
6. The drug's **target concentration** (the desired plasma or serum drug concentration for optimal therapeutic effect) and **therapeutic window** [the range of plasma drug concentration between the maximum therapeutic concentration (MTC) and the minimum effective drug concentration (MEC)] must be considered.
   a. As plasma drug concentration approaches the MTC, the patient has an increased probability of an adverse response to the drug.
   b. As plasma drug concentration approaches the MEC, the probability increases that the drug will lack efficacy (i.e., not produce a therapeutic response).

C. The clinical pharmacist's responsibilities

1. The **appropriate drug must be selected**, usually in conjunction with the clinician.
2. The **dosage regimen** must be designed.
   a. **Target drug concentration** and **dosing rate** must be determined.
      (1) The **dosing rate** (D_0/τ) is the main parameter that the clinical pharmacist may adjust. This rate is based on knowledge of the target drug concentration, the therapeutic window, and the estimated clearance of the drug in the patient, as shown in these equations:

$$\text{target drug concentration} = \text{dosing rate} \times \frac{1}{\text{clearance}}$$

$$C_{av}^{\infty} = \frac{FD_0}{\tau} \times \frac{1}{\text{clearance}}$$

      (2) The **drug dose** should be adjusted to commercially available dosage forms and strengths. For example, if the drug is manufactured in 125-, 250-, and 500-mg tablets, then the calculated dose should be rounded to the nearest strength.
      (3) The **dosage interval** (τ) should be set at intervals convenient for the patient. For example, a dose given every 8 hours is more practical than a dose every 7.3 hours.
      (4) With more drugs available as **controlled-release drug products**, the clinical pharmacist should consider this form rather than an immediate-release dosage form, depending upon the patient's needs.
   b. **Nomograms** are often used to develop dosage regimens. These are based on average, or population, pharmacokinetic parameters. Although easy to use, they may not apply to the patient's special needs.
3. The **patient's response** to the drug and dosage regimen must be evaluated.
4. **Serum or plasma drug concentrations** must be determined as needed.
   a. **Therapeutic drug monitoring** (TDM) can verify the adequacy of the dosage regimen using plasma or drug concentrations.
   b. The **number of blood samples** and the **timing for blood sample collection** are important considerations for TDM.
5. **Drug levels** in plasma or serum must be properly assayed.
6. **Pharmacokinetic interpretation** of the serum drug concentration must be performed.
7. The **dosage must be readjusted**, if necessary, according the results obtained by TDM.
8. **Plasma drug concentrations** must be further monitored.
9. **Special recommendations** or **patient education** must be provided to ensure proper compliance to the dosage regimen. Patients should understand their drug dosage regimen in relation to meals, other drugs, their daily routines, and their sleep habits. They must also understand the need for proper compliance with the dosage.

VII. PHARMACOKINETICS IN RENAL DISEASE

A. Renal disease

1. The patient with renal disease poses a special problem because of the kidneys' role in pharmacokinetics. The kidneys regulate body fluids, electrolyte balance, metabolite waste removal, and drug excretion.
2. **Acute renal failure**, which alters kidney function, may result from a variety of causes, including disease, traumatic injury, and nephrotoxic agents.
3. Renal failure generally results in a **reduction in the GFR** and a decreased ability of the kidneys to remove metabolite wastes, such as urea and drugs.
4. Renal disease may also **decrease plasma drug–protein binding** from competition for binding sites by the accumulating metabolite wastes (including urea, the active drug, and its biotransformation products).

B. Measuring of GFR

1. Several drugs and endogenous substances may be used to measure GFR. The following criteria are necessary for a drug used to measure GFR:
   a. The drug is **filtered at the glomerulus.**
   b. The drug **must not be reabsorbed or actively secreted.**
   c. The drug **should not be metabolized.**
   d. The drug **should not be highly bound to plasma proteins.**
   e. The drug **should be nontoxic and should not affect renal function.**
   f. The drug **should be easily measured in plasma and urine.**
2. **Inulin**, a polysaccharide, meets most of the above criteria. However, it is an exogenous substance that must be administered in addition to any other drug therapy.
3. **Creatinine**, an endogenous substance formed from creatinine phosphate during muscle metabolism, provides an alternative.
   a. Creatinine **production** may vary with gender, age, and body weight.
   b. Creatinine is **filtered** at the glomerulus and is **not reabsorbed**.
   c. A **small fraction may be actively secreted**, so that the creatinine clearance value for measurement of GFR may be slightly higher compared to the inulin clearance value.
4. **Creatinine clearance** is the most common method for obtaining the GFR. It may be estimated by using both urine and serum values or by using only serum creatinine concentration.
   a. Creatinine clearance measurement using **both urine and serum concentrations** is more accurate and is usually estimated by the following equation:

$$Cl_{CR} = \frac{C_U \dot{V} \, 100}{C_{CR} \, 1440}$$

   where C_{CR} is the creatinine serum concentration in mg/dl of the twelfth-hour serum, $\dot{V}$ is the 24-hour urine volume, C_U is the concentration of creatinine in the urine, and Cl_{CR} is the creatinine clearance in ml/min.
   b. Creatinine clearance may be estimated using **only a serum creatinine concentration** because there is usually an inverse relationship between serum creatinine concentration and GFR.
      (1) The nomogram developed by **Siersback-Nielsen** and others may be used to obtain the creatinine clearance, using the serum creatinine concentration (mg/dl) and the patient's body weight and gender (Fig. 4-12).
      (2) The method of **Cockcroft and Gault**, also based on body weight, age, and gender, calculates creatinine clearance from serum creatinine using the following relationship:
         (a) For males,

$$Cl_{CR} = \frac{(140 - \text{age in years}) \text{ body weight in kg}}{72 \, (C_{CR} \text{ in mg/dl})} = \text{ml/min}$$

         (b) For females, use 0.85 of the Cl_{CR} obtained for males.
   c. These methods assume stable renal function. However, renal function may change, depending upon the progress of the renal disease, causing changes in Cl_{CR}.

C. Dosage adjustment in renal disease

1. Dosage adjustment for renal disease is usually based on the following assumptions, which may not be valid for every patient:

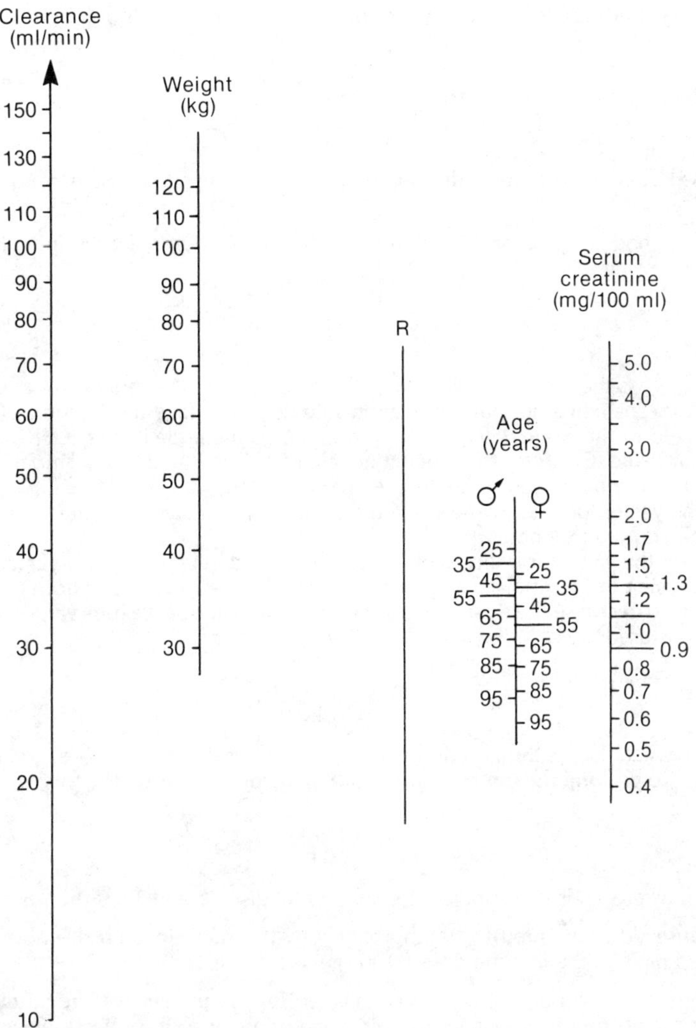

Figure 4-12. Nomogram for evaluation of endogenous creatinine clearance. To use the nomogram, connect with a ruler the patient's weight on the second line from the left with the patient's age on the fourth line. Note the point of intersection on *R* and keep the ruler there. Turn the right part of the ruler to the appropriate serum creatinine value, and the left side will indicate the clearance in ml/min. (Reprinted with permission from Kampmann J, Siersback-Nielsen JM: Rapid evaluation of creatinine clearance. *Acta Med Scand* 196:517–520, 1974.)

a. The **desired plasma or serum drug concentration in a patient with renal disease is the same as that for a patient without renal disease**. A major exception is digoxin dosage adjustment; here, renal disease may alter normal serum potassium concentration, thus altering the target digoxin serum concentration.

b. **Other pharmacokinetic parameters** (including Vd, plasma drug–protein binding, and nonrenal drug elimination, or biotransformation) **are not markedly altered in renal disease.**

c. **Normal GFR is 100 ml/min or greater.** Unless the GFR falls significantly below normal, dosage may not need to be adjusted for a patient with minor renal impairment.

d. **Drugs such as gentamicin** (primarily eliminated by renal excretion) **are more affected by diminished renal function than drugs such as theophylline** (primarily eliminated by biotransformation, as with nonrenal or hepatic clearance).

e. **All drug elimination pathways follow first-order pharmacokinetics.**

2. Dosage adjustment for the renally impaired patient attempts to estimate the fraction of total body drug clearance remaining.

a. **Total body clearance** is the sum of renal clearance and nonrenal clearance, as follows:

$$Cl_T = Cl_R + Cl_{NR}$$

b. Because Vd is assumed to be constant, then:

$$k = k_R + k_{NR}$$

c. As k_R decreases in renal disease, then k (the overall rate constant for drug elimination) also decreases.

3. The method of **Guisti and Hayton** estimates the fraction of k remaining in the patient, using the following equation:

$$\frac{k_U}{k_N} = 1 - f_e \; 1 - \frac{Cl_{CR}{}^U}{Cl_{CR}{}^N}$$

where k_U is the first-order elimination rate constant in the renally impaired (uremic) patient; k_N is the patient's normal elimination rate constant; f_e is the fraction of drug excreted unchanged in the urine; $Cl_{CR}{}^N$ is the normal creatinine clearance (GFR), assumed to be 100 ml/min; and $Cl_{CR}{}^U$ is the creatinine clearance in the renally impaired patient, usually estimated from the serum creatinine concentration.

a. The values for k, k_{NR}, and f_e are the standard population pharmacokinetic parameters obtained from the literature.

b. After the value for k_U/k_N is obtained, the dosage regimen may be calculated by either **decreasing the normal dose, prolonging the dosage interval, or both**.

(1) To **decrease the dose and maintain a constant dosage interval**, the following equation is used:

$$D_U{}^0 = \frac{k_U}{k_N} D_N{}^0$$

where $D_U{}^0$ is the dose in renal disease, $D_N{}^0$ is the normal dose, and k_U/k_N is calculated.

(2) To **prolong the interval and maintain a constant dose**, the following equation is used:

$$T_U = \frac{k_N}{k_U} T_N$$

where T_U is the dosage interval in renal disease and T_N is the normal dosage interval.

4. Because Vd is assumed to be approximately the same in both the normal and renally impaired patient, the loading dose (D_L) is generally the same.

5. Whenever the dosage of a drug is adjusted for the patient with renal disease, **therapeutic drug monitoring** is important to help prevent adverse drug reactions and maintain proper drug therapy.

STUDY QUESTIONS

Directions: Each question below contains five suggested answers. Choose the **one best** response to each question.

1. The term bioavailability refers to the

A. relationship between the physical and chemical properties of a drug and the systemic absorption of the drug
B. measurement of the rate and amount of therapeutically active drug that reaches the systemic circulation
C. movement of a drug into the body tissues over time
D. dissolution of a drug in the gastrointestinal tract
E. amount of drug destroyed by the liver prior to systemic absorption from the gastrointestinal tract

2. The route of drug administration that will give the most rapid onset of the pharmacologic effect is

A. intramuscular injection
B. intravenous injection
C. intradermal injection
D. oral administration
E. subcutaneous injection

3. The route of drug administration that is considered to provide complete (100%) bioavailability is

A. intramuscular injection
B. intravenous injection
C. intradermal injection
D. oral administration
E. subcutaneous injection

4. After oral administration, drugs will generally be absorbed best from the

A. buccal cavity
B. stomach
C. duodenum
D. ileum
E. rectum

5. All of the following are characteristics of an active transport process EXCEPT

A. active transport moves drug molecules against a concentration gradient
B. active transport follows Fick's law of diffusion
C. active transport is a carrier-mediated transport system
D. active transport requires energy
E. active transport of drug molecules may be saturated at high drug concentrations

6. The passage of drug molecules across a cell membrane from a region of high drug concentration to a region of low drug concentration is known as

A. active transport
B. bioavailability
C. biopharmaceutics
D. passive diffusion
E. pinocytosis

7. Creatinine clearance is used as a measurement of

A. renal excretion rate
B. glomerular filtration rate (GFR)
C. active renal secretion
D. passive renal absorption
E. drug metabolism rate

Questions 8–11

A new cephalosporin antibiotic was given by a single intravenous bolus injection to an adult male patient (age, 58 years; weight, 75 kg) at a dose of 5 mg/kg. The antibiotic follows the pharmacokinetics of a one-compartment model and has an elimination half-life of 2 hours. The apparent volume of distribution is 0.28 L/kg, and the drug is 35% bound to plasma proteins.

8. What would be the initial plasma drug concentration (C_p^0) in this patient?

A. 0.24 mg/L
B. 1.80 mg/L
C. 17.9 mg/L
D. 56.0 mg/L
E. 62.6 mg/L

9. The predicted plasma drug concentration (C_p) at 8 hours after the dose would be

A. 0.73 mg/L
B. 1.11 mg/L
C. 2.64 mg/L
D. 4.02 mg/L
E. 15.1 mg/L

10. The amount of drug in the patient's body (D_b) at 8 hours after the dose would be

A. 15.3 mg
B. 23.3 mg
C. 84.4 mg
D. 100.0 mg
E. 112 mg

11. How long after the dose would exactly 75% of the drug be eliminated from the patient?

A. 2 hours
B. 4 hours
C. 6 hours
D. 8 hours
E. 10 hours

12. The equation that describes the rate of drug dissolution from a tablet is known as

A. Fick's law
B. Henderson-Hasselbalch equation
C. Law of mass action
D. Michaelis-Menten equation
E. Noyes Whitney equation

13. Which of the following conditions will generally speed up the rate of drug dissolution from a tablet?

A. An increase in the particle size of the drug
B. A decrease in the surface area of the drug
C. Use of the free acid or free base form of the drug
D. Use of the ionized or salt form of the drug
E. Use of sugar coating around the tablet

14. Dose dumping is a problem in the formulation of

A. compressed tablets
B. modified-release drug products
C. hard gelatin capsules
D. soft gelatin capsules
E. suppositories

15. The rate-limiting step in the bioavailability of a lipid-soluble drug formulated as an immediate-release compressed tablet is the rate of

A. disintegration of the tablet and release of the drug
B. dissolution of the drug
C. transport of the drug molecules across the intestinal mucosal cells
D. blood flow to the gastrointestinal tract
E. biotransformation (metabolism) of the drug by the liver prior to systemic absorption

16. The extent of ionization of a weak electrolyte drug is dependent upon the

A. pH of the media and pK_a of the drug
B. oil/water partition coefficient of the drug
C. particle size and surface area of the drug
D. Noyes Whitney equation for the drug
E. polymorphic form of the drug

Questions 17–22

A physician wishes to give an intravenous (IV) infusion of the antibiotic carbenicillin to a young adult male patient (age, 35 years; weight, 70 kg) with normal renal function. The desired steady-state plasma drug concentration is 15 mg/dl. The physician would like the antibiotic to be infused into the patient for 10 hours. Carbenicillin has an elimination half-life of 1.0 hours and an apparent volume of distribution (Vd) of 9 L in this patient.

17. Assuming no loading dose, what rate of IV infusion would you recommend for this patient?

A. 93.6 mg/hr
B. 135 mg/hr
C. 468 mg/hr
D. 936 mg/hr
E. 1350 mg/hr

18. Assuming that no loading dose was given, how long after the start of the IV infusion would the plasma drug concentration reach 95% of the theoretical steady-state drug concentration?

A. 1 hour
B. 3.3 hours
C. 4.3 hours
D. 6.6 hours
E. 10 hours

19. What loading dose would you recommend?

A. 93.6 mg
B. 135 mg
C. 468 mg
D. 936 mg
E. 1350 mg

20. You would like to infuse the antibiotic as a solution containing 10 g of the drug in 500 ml of 5% dextrose. How many milliliters per hour of this solution would you infuse into the patient?

A. 10 ml/hr
B. 46.8 ml/hr
C. 100 ml/hr
D. 936 ml/hr
E. 1141 ml/hr

21. What is the total body clearance rate for carbenicillin in this patient?

A. 100 ml/hr
B. 936 ml/hr
C. 4862 ml/hr
D. 6237 ml/hr
E. 9000 ml/hr

22. Assuming that the patient's renal clearance for carbenicillin is 86 ml/min, calculate the hepatic clearance for carbenicillin.

A. 108 ml/hr
B. 1077 ml/hr
C. 3840 ml/hr
D. 5160 ml/hr
E. 6844 ml/hr

23. Which of the following would be the earliest evidence that a drug is stored in a tissue?

A. An increase in plasma protein binding
B. A large apparent volume of distribution
C. A decrease in the rate of formation of metabolites by the liver
D. An increase in the number of side effects produced by the drug
E. A decrease in the amount of free drug excreted in the urine

24. The intensity of the pharmacologic action of a drug is most dependent upon the

A. concentration of the drug at the receptor site
B. elimination half-life of the drug
C. onset time of the drug after oral administration
D. minimum toxic drug concentration in the plasma
E. minimum effective concentration (MEC) of the drug in the body

25. Drugs that demonstrate nonlinear pharmacokinetics show which of the following properties?

A. A constant ratio of drug metabolites is formed as the administered dose increases
B. The elimination half-life increases as the administered dose is increased
C. The AUC increases in direct proportion to an increase in the administered dose
D. Both low and high doses follow first-order elimination kinetics
E. The steady-state drug concentration increases in direct proportion to the dosing rate

26. The loading dose of a drug is generally based upon the

A. total body clearance of the drug
B. percent of drug bound to plasma proteins
C. fraction of drug excreted unchanged in the urine
D. apparent volume of distribution (Vd) and the desired drug concentration in plasma
E. area under the plasma level versus time curve (AUC)

27. The renal clearance of insulin is used as a measurement of

A. effective renal blood flow
B. rate of renal drug excretion
C. intrinsic enzyme activity
D. active renal secretion
E. glomerular filtration rate (GFR)

28. All of the following statements are true for plasma protein binding of a drug EXCEPT

A. displacement of a drug from plasma protein binding sites results in a transient enlarged volume of distribution (Vd)
B. displacement of a drug from plasma protein binding sites makes more free drug available for glomerular filtration
C. displacement of a potent drug that is normally > 95% bound may result in an adverse toxicity
D. albumin is the major protein involved in protein binding of drugs
E. drugs highly bound to plasma proteins generally have a larger Vd compared to drugs highly bound to tissue proteins

29. The onset time for a drug given orally is the time for the

A. drug to reach the peak plasma drug concentration
B. drug to reach the minimum effective concentration (MEC)
C. drug to reach the minimum toxic concentration (MTC)
D. drug to begin to be eliminated from the body
E. drug to begin to be absorbed from the small intestine

30. The initial distribution of a drug into the tissues is determined chiefly by the

A. rate of blood flow to the tissue
B. glomerular filtration rate (GFR)
C. stomach emptying time
D. drug affinity for the tissue
E. plasma protein binding of the drug

31. Which of the following tissues has the greatest capacity to biotransform drugs?

A. Brain
B. Kidney
C. Liver
D. Lung
E. Skin

32. The principle of superposition in designing multiple dosage regimens assumes that

A. each dose affects the next subsequent dose, causing nonlinear elimination
B. each dose of drug is eliminated by zero-order elimination
C. steady-state plasma drug concentrations are reached at approximately 10 half-lives
D. early doses of drug do not affect subsequent doses
E. the fraction of drug absorbed is equal to the fraction of drug eliminated

33. The rate of drug bioavailability is most rapid when the drug is formulated as a

A. controlled-release product
B. hard gelatin capsule
C. compressed tablet
D. solution
E. suspension

Questions 34–36

A new cardiac glycoside has been developed for oral and intravenous (IV) administration. The drug has an elimination half-life of 24 hours and an apparent volume of distribution (Vd) of 3 L/kg. The effective drug concentration is 1.5 ng/ml. Toxic effects of the drug are observed at drug concentrations above 4 ng/ml. The drug is bound to plasma proteins at approximately 25%. The drug is 75% bioavailable after an oral dose.

34. Calculate an oral maintenance dose to be given once a day for a 65-kg male patient (age, 68 years) with congestive heart failure and normal renal function. The dose should be

A. 0.125 mg
B. 0.180 mg
C. 0.203 mg
D. 0.270 mg
E. 0.333 mg

35. Calculate a loading dose for this patient. The loading dose should be

A. 0.270 mg
B. 0.293 mg
C. 0.450 mg
D. 0.498 mg
E. 0.540 mg

36. Assume the drug is available in tablets of 0.125 mg and 0.250 mg. What would this patient's plasma drug concentration be if the patient uses a dosage regimen of 0.125 mg every 12 hours?

A. 1.39 ng/ml
B. 1.85 ng/ml
C. 2.78 ng/ml
D. 3.18 ng/ml
E. 6.94 ng/ml

Directions: The question below contains three suggested answers of which **one or more** is correct. Choose the answer

A if **I only** is correct
B if **III only** is correct
C if **I and II** are correct
D if **II and III** are correct
E if **I, II, and III** are correct

37. For a drug, which of the following equations would be true for a zero-order reaction rate?

I. $\frac{dA}{dt} = -k$

II. $t_{1/2} = \frac{0.693}{k}$

III. $A = A_0e^{-kt}$

ANSWERS AND EXPLANATIONS

1. The answer is B. (*I A 2*) Bioavailability is the measurement of the rate and extent (amount) of therapeutically active drug that reaches the systemic circulation. The relationship of a drug's physical and chemical properties to its systemic absorption (i.e., to its bioavailability) refers to its biopharmaceutics. The movement of a drug into body tissues is an aspect of pharmacokinetics, which is the study of drug movement in the body over time. The dissolution of a drug in the gastrointestinal tract is a physiochemical property that affects the drug's bioavailability. Significant destruction of a drug by the liver before it is systemically absorbed (known as the first-pass effect because it occurs during the drug's first passage through the liver) will markedly reduce the drug's bioavailability.

2. The answer is B. (*II B 1 a*) When a drug is given intravenously, it is placed directly into the systemic circulation. The drug is delivered rapidly to all tissues, including the drug receptor sites. For all other routes of drug administration (with the exception of intra-arterial injection), the drug must be systemically absorbed prior to distribution to the drug receptor sites, and therefore the onset of pharmacologic effects is slower.

3. The answer is B. (*II C 3*) When a drug is given by intravenous injection, the entire dose is placed into the systemic circulation. With other routes of administration, drug may be lost prior to reaching the systemic circulation. For example, with first-pass effects, a portion of an orally administered drug is eliminated, usually through degradation by liver enzymes, before the drug reaches its receptor sites.

4. The answer is C. [*II B 2 b (3)*] Drugs given orally are well absorbed from the duodenum. The duodenum has a large surface area due to the presence of villi and microvilli. In addition, the duodenum is well perfused by the mesenteric blood vessels, which helps to maintain a concentration gradient between the lumen of the duodenum and the blood.

5. The answer is B. (*II A 2, 3*) Fick's law of diffusion describes passive diffusion of drug molecules moving from a high concentration to a low concentration. This process is not saturable and does not require energy.

6. The answer is D. (*II A 2*) The transport of a drug across a cell membrane by passive diffusion follows Fick's law of diffusion: the drug moves with a concentration gradient; that is, from an area of high concentration to an area of low concentration. In contrast, drugs that are actively transported move against a concentration gradient.

7. The answer is B. (*VII B 4*) A substance that is used to measure the glomerular filtration rate (GFR) must be filtered only, and not reabsorbed or actively secreted. Although inulin clearance gives an accurate measurement of GFR, creatinine clearance is generally used, since no exogenous drug needs to be given. However, creatinine formation depends upon muscle mass and muscle metabolism, which may change with age and various disease conditions.

8. The answer is C. (*V A 1 c*) Substituting the data for this patient in the equation for the initial plasma drug concentration, one obtains:

$$C_p{}^0 = \frac{D_0}{Vd} = \frac{5\text{ mg/kg}}{0.28\text{ kg}} = 17.9\text{ mg/L}$$

9. The answer is B. (*V B 1 b*) To obtain the patient's plasma drug concentration at 8 hours after the dose, the following calculation is performed:

$$C_p = C_p{}^0 e^{-kt}$$

$$k = \frac{0.693}{t_{1/2}} = \frac{0.693}{2} = 0.347\text{ hr}^{-1}$$

$$C_p = (17.9)\,(0.0623) = 1.11\text{ mg/L}$$

10. The answer is B. (*V B 1 b*) The amount of drug in the patient's body at 8 hours would be calculated as follows:

$$D_B = C_pVd = (1.11)\,(0.28)\,(75) = 23.3$$

11. The answer is B. (*V A 1 c*) For any first-order elimination process, 50% of the initial amount of drug is eliminated at the end of the first half-life, and 50% of the remaining amount of drug (i.e., 75% of the original amount) is eliminated at the end of the second half-life. Since the drug in the present case has an elimination half-life ($t_{1/2}$) of 2 hours, 75% of the dose would be eliminated at two half-lives, or 4 hours.

12. The answer is E. (*III A 1 a*) The Noyes Whitney equation describes the rate at which a solid drug dissolves. Fick's law is similar to the Noyes Whitney equation in that both equations describe drug movement due to a concentration gradient. Fick's law generally refers to the passive diffusion or passive transport of drugs. The law of mass action concerns the rate of a chemical reaction; the Michaelis-Menten equation deals with enzyme kinetics; and the Henderson-Hasselbalch equation gives the pH of a buffer solution.

13. The answer is D. (*III A 1–3*) The ionized or salt form of a drug has a charge and is generally more water-soluble and therefore dissolves more rapidly than the nonionized (free acid or free base) form of the drug. The dissolution rate is directly proportional to the surface area and inversely proportional to the particle size. Therefore, an increase in the particle size or a decrease in the surface area slows the dissolution rate.

14. The answer is B. (*III B 7 c*) A modified-release, or controlled-release, drug product contains two or more conventional doses of the drug, and therefore an abrupt release of the drug, known as dose dumping, may cause some degree of intoxication.

15. The answer is B. (*III A 1, 3 a*) For drugs that are lipid-soluble, the rate of dissolution is the slowest (i.e., rate-limiting) step in drug absorption, and thus in the drug's bioavailability. The disintegration rate of an immediate-release or conventional compressed tablet is usually more rapid than the rate of drug dissolution. Since the cell membrane is a lipoprotein structure, transport of a lipid-soluble drug across the cell membrane is generally rapid.

16. The answer is A. (*III A 3*) The extent of ionization of a weak electrolyte is described by the Henderson-Hasselbalch equation, which relates the pH of the solvent to the pK_a of the drug.

17. The answer is D. (*V B 3*) The equation for the plasma concentration at steady state (C_{ss}) provides the formula for calculating the rate of an intravenous (IV) infusion (R). The equation is:

$$C_{ss} = \frac{R}{kVd}$$

where k is the first-order elimination rate constant and Vd is the apparent volume of distribution. Rearranging the equation and plugging in the data for this patient gives the following calculations:

$$R = C_{ss}kVd = \frac{15 \text{ mg}}{100 \text{ ml}} \times \frac{0.693}{1 \text{ hr}} \times 9000 \text{ ml}$$

$$R = 936 \text{ mg/hr}$$

18. The answer is C. (*V B 3*) The time it takes for an infused drug to reach the C_{SS} depends upon the drug's elimination half-life. The time to reach 95% of the C_{SS} is equal to 4.3 times the half-life, whereas the time to reach 99% of the C_{SS} is equal to 6.6 times the half-life. Since the half-life in the present case is given as 1 hour, the time to reach 95% of the C_{SS} would be 4.3 × 1 hour, or 4.3 hours.

19. The answer is E. (*V B 3*) The proper loading dose (D_L) is calculated as follows:

$$D_L = C_{SS}\, Vd = \frac{15 \text{ mg}}{100 \text{ ml}} \times 9000 \text{ ml} = 1350 \text{ mg}$$

20. The answer is B. (*V B 3*) The answer to question 17 shows that the infusion rate should be 936 mg/hr. Therefore, using a drug solution containing 10 g in 500 ml, the required infusion rate is:

$$\frac{936 \text{ mg}}{1 \text{ hr}} \times \frac{500 \text{ ml}}{10{,}000 \text{ mg}} = 46.8 \text{ ml/hr}$$

21. The answer is D. (*V E 2*) The patient's total body clearance (Cl_T) is calculated as follows:

$$Cl_T = kVd$$

$$Cl_T = \frac{0.693}{1} \times 9000 \text{ ml} = 6237 \text{ ml/hr}$$

22. The answer is B. (*V E 5 a*) The hepatic clearance (Cl_H) is the difference between total clearance (Cl_T) and renal clearance (Cl_R):

$$Cl_H = Cl_T - Cl_R$$

$$Cl_H = 6237 - (86 \text{ ml/min} \times 60 \text{ min/hr}) = 1077 \text{ ml/hr}$$

23. The answer is B. (*V B 1*) A very large apparent volume of distribution is an early sign that a drug is not concentrated in the plasma but is distributed widely in the tissues. An increase in plasma protein binding would signify that the drug is in the plasma rather than in the tissues. A decrease in hepatic metabolism, an increase in side effects, or a decrease in urinary excretion of free drug would be due to a decrease in drug elimination.

24. The answer is A. (*IV A 1*) As more drug is concentrated at the receptor site, more receptors interact with the drug to produce a pharmacologic effect. The intensity of the response will increase up to a maximum response. When all the available receptors are occupied by drug molecules, any additional drug will not produce a more intense response.

25. The answer is B. (*V D*) Nonlinear pharmacokinetics is a term used to indicate that the elimination of a drug is not first-order at all drug concentrations. In the case of some drugs, such as phenytoin, as the plasma drug concentration increases, the elimination pathway for metabolism of the drug becomes saturated and the half-life increases. The AUC of such a drug is not proportional to the dose; neither is the rate of metabolite formation, and the metabolic rate would indeed be related to the effects of the drug.

26. The answer is D. [*V B 3 e; 4 f (5)*] A loading dose of a drug is given in order to obtain a therapeutic plasma drug level as rapidly as possible. The loading dose is calculated on the basis of a drug's apparent volume of distribution (Vd) and the desired plasma level of the drug.

27. The answer is E. (*V E 3 a; VII B 2*) Inulin is neither reabsorbed nor actively secreted and thus is excreted by glomerular filtration only. The inulin clearance rate is used as a standard measure of the glomerular filtration rate (GFR), a test that is useful both clinically and in the development of new drugs.

28. The answer is E. [*V A 3 e; B 1 b (3)*] Drugs that are highly bound to plasma proteins will diffuse poorly into the tissues and thus will have a small apparent volume of distribution (Vd).

29. The answer is B. (*IV A 2 a*) The onset time is the time from drug administration to the time when absorbed drug reaches the minimum effective concentration (MEC). The MEC is the drug concentration in the plasma that is proportional (not necessarily equal) to the minimum drug concentration at the receptor site that elicits a pharmacologic response.

30. The answer is A. (*V A 3*) The initial distribution of a drug is chiefly determined by blood flow, whereas drug affinity for the tissue will determine whether the drug will concentrate at that site. The glomerular filtration rate (GFR) affects the rate of renal clearance of a drug, not its initial distribution. The gastric emptying time and degree of plasma protein binding have an effect on drug distribution but are less important than the rate of blood flow to the tissues.

31. The answer is C. [*V E 5 c (2)*] The kidney, lung, skin, and intestine all have some capacity to biotransform (metabolize) drugs, whereas the brain has very little capacity for drug metabolism. The liver is the major organ with the highest capacity for drug metabolism activity.

32. The answer is D. (*V B 4 c*) The superposition principle, which underlies the design of multiple-dose regimens, assumes that the earlier drug doses do not affect subsequent doses. If any change in the elimination rate constant or total body clearance of the drug occurs during multiple dosing, then the superposition principle is no longer valid. Changes in the total body clearance may be due to enzyme induction, enzyme inhibition, or saturation of an elimination pathway. Any of these would cause nonlinear pharmacokinetics.

33. The answer is D. (*III B 2 a*) A drug in solution is already dissolved and thus no dissolution is needed prior to absorption. Consequently, compared with other drug formulations, a drug in solution has a high rate of bioavailability. A drug in aqueous solution has the highest bioavailability rate and is often used as the reference preparation for other formulations. Drugs in hydroalcoholic solution (e.g., elixirs) also have good bioavailability.

34–36. The answers are: 34-D, 35-E, 36-A. (*V B 4 e, f*) The oral maintenance dose (D_0) should maintain the patient's average drug concentration (C_{av}) at the effective drug concentration. The drug's bioavailability (F), the apparent volume of distribution (Vd), the frequency of dosing (τ), and the excretion rate constant (k) must all be considered in calculating the dose. The equation used is:

$$C_{av} = \frac{FD_0}{kVd\tau}$$

For the drug in question, F = 0.75, k = 0.693/24 hr, Vd = 3L/kg × 65 kg, τ = 25 hr, and C_{av} = 1.5 ng/ml, or 1.5 μg/L. Therefore, by substitution, D_0 = 270 μg, or 0.270 mg. When the maintenance dose is given at a dosage frequency equal to the half-life, then the loading dose is equal to twice the maintenance dose; for the case in question, this would be 540 μg, or 0.540 mg. To determine the plasma drug concentration for a dosage regimen of 0.125 mg every 12 hours, one would again use the C_{av} formula above. This time, F = 0.75, D_0 = 0.125, k = 0.693/24 hr, Vd = 3 L/kg × 65 kg, and τ = 12 hr. Therefore, C_{av} = 1.39 ng/ml.

37. The answer is A (I). (*V A 1*) The first equation in the question describes a zero-order reaction (dA/dt), in which the reaction rate increases or decreases at a constant rate (k). A zero-order reaction will produce a graph of a straight line with the equation of $A = -kt + A_0$ when A is plotted against time (t). The other equations in the question represent first-order reactions.

Part II
Medicinal Chemistry and Pharmacology

David C. Kosegarten
Edward F. LaSala

5 Organic Chemistry and Biochemistry

Edward F. LaSala
Nelson S. Yee

I. ORGANIC CHEMISTRY

A. Introduction. Medicinal chemistry is rooted in organic chemistry—the study of organic (carbon-based) compounds. These compounds are classified by **functional group**—a group of atoms that occurs in many molecules and confers on them a characteristic chemical reactivity, regardless of the carbon skeleton. Functional groups determine such characteristics as water or lipid solubility, reactivity, chemical stability, and in vivo stability, which in turn determine drug properties.

1. Functional groups must be looked on as part of the drug's overall structure.
2. Functional groups that impart **liposolubility** are likely to increase the drug's tendency to cross cellular membranes.
3. Functional group **reactivity** is most important for reactions occurring under **normal environmental conditions**, primarily air oxidation and hydrolysis. For example, benzene's characteristic reactions occur only with special reagents and in special laboratory conditions. Thus, benzene's shelf life is relatively long, and it requires no special storage conditions.
4. Functional groups affect drug reactivity and, hence, **drug shelf life and stability**.
5. Functional groups also affect **in vivo stability**—the susceptibility of the drug to biotransformation and determination of appropriate metabolic pathways.

B. Alkanes

1. Alkanes, which are also called **paraffins** or **saturated hydrocarbons**, have a general formula of $R—CH_2—CH_3$. (R = a radical, or a molecule fragment.)
2. Alkanes are **lipid soluble**.
3. The common reactions of alkanes are **halogenation** and **combustion**.
4. On the shelf, alkanes are **chemically inert** with regard to air, light, heat, acids, and bases.
5. In vivo, alkanes are **stable**; **side-chain hydroxylation may occur**.

C. Alkenes

1. Also called **olefins**, or **unsaturated hydrocarbons**, the alkenes have a general formula of $R—CH{=}CH_2$.
2. Alkenes are **lipid soluble**.
3. The common reactions of alkenes are **addition of hydrogen or halogens**, **hydration** (to form glycols), and **oxidation** (to form peroxides).
4. On the shelf, **volatile alkenes and peroxides may explode** in the presence of oxygen and a spark.
5. In vivo, alkenes are **relatively stable**. **Hydration**, **epoxidation**, **peroxidation**, or **reduction** may occur.

D. Aromatic hydrocarbons

1. Aromatic hydrocarbons are based on **benzene** (Fig. 5-1). These molecules exhibit multicenter bonding, which confers unique chemical properties.

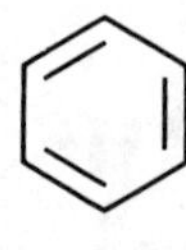
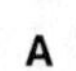
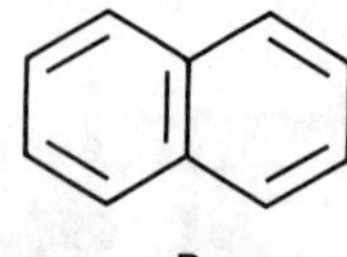

Figure 5-1. Chemical structures of (*A*) benzene and (*B*) naphthalene. Benzene and related compounds, such as naphthalene, are planar molecules in the form of a regular hexagon.

2. Aromatic hydrocarbons are **lipid soluble**.
3. The common reactions of aromatic hydrocarbons are **halogenation**, **nitration**, **sulfonation**, and **Friedel-Crafts alkylation**.
4. On the shelf, aromatic hydrocarbons are **quite stable**.
5. In vivo, aromatic hydrocarbons undergo **hydroxylation**.

E. Alkyl halides

1. Also known as **halogenated hydrocarbons**, the alkyl halides have a general formula of $R—CH_2—X$.
2. Alkyl halides are **lipid soluble**. Their **solubility increases with the extent of halogenation**.
3. The common reactions of alkyl halides are **nucleophilic substitution** and **dehydrohalogenation**.
4. On the shelf, alkyl halides are **stable**.
5. In vivo, alkyl halides **are not readily metabolized**.

F. Alcohols

1. Alcohols contain a **hydroxyl group** (—OH) and may be classified as primary, secondary, or tertiary.
   a. **Primary alcohols** have a general formula of $R—CH_2—OH$.
   b. **Secondary alcohols** have a general formula of $R—CH(CH_3)—OH$.
   c. **Tertiary alcohols** have a general formula of $R—C(CH_3)_2—OH$.
2. Low molecular weight alcohols are **water soluble**; water solubility decreases as hydrocarbon chain length increases. Alcohols are also **lipid soluble**.
3. The common reactions of alcohols are **esterification** and **oxidation**.
   a. **Primary alcohols** are oxidized to **aldehydes** and then to **acids**.
   b. **Secondary alcohols** are oxidized to **ketones**.
   c. **Tertiary alcohols** ordinarily **are not oxidized**.
4. On the shelf, alcohols are **stable**.
5. In vivo, alcohols may undergo **oxidation**, **glucuronidation**, or **sulfation**.

G. Phenols

1. Phenols are **aromatic compounds containing a hydroxyl group** (—OH).
   a. **Monophenols** have **one hydroxyl group** (Fig. 5-2).
   b. **Catechols** have **two hydroxyl groups** (Fig. 5-3).
2. Phenols are **lipid soluble**; phenol itself (carbolic acid) is **fairly water soluble**. Ring substitutions generally decrease water solubility.
3. The common reactions of phenols are **reactions with strong bases** (to form water-soluble salts), **esterification with acids**, and **oxidation** (to form quinones, usually colored).
4. On the shelf, phenols are **susceptible to air oxidation** and to **oxidation on contact with ferric ions**.

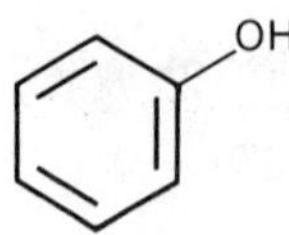

Figure 5-2. Structure of a monophenol functional group.

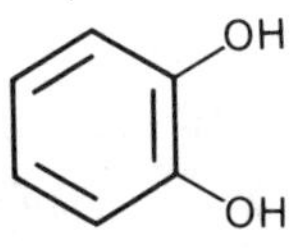

Figure 5-3. Structure of a catechol functional group.

5. In vivo, phenols undergo **sulfation**, **glucuronidation**, **aromatic hydroxylation**, and *O*-**methylation**.

H. Ethers

1. Ethers have a general formula of R—O—R, with an oxygen atom bonded to two carbon atoms.
2. Low molecular weight ethers are **partially water soluble**; water solubility decreases with an increase in the hydrocarbon portion of the molecule. Ethers are also **lipid soluble.**
3. The common reaction of ethers is **oxidation** (to form peroxides).
4. On the shelf, **peroxides may explode**.
5. In vivo, ethers undergo *O*-**dealkylation**. Stability increases with the size of the alkyl group.

I. Aldehydes

1. Aldehydes have a general formula of R—CHO and contain a **carbonyl group** (C=O).
2. **Aldehydes are lipid soluble**; low molecular weight aldehydes are also **water soluble**.
3. The common reactions of aldehydes are **oxidation** and (for those of low molecular weight) **polymerization**.
4. On the shelf, aldehydes **oxidize to acids**.
5. In vivo, aldehydes may also undergo **oxidation to acids**.

J. Ketones

1. Ketones have a general formula of R—CO—R and, like aldehydes, contain a **carbonyl group** (C=O).
2. Ketones are **lipid soluble**. Low molecular weight ketones are also **water soluble**, with solubility decreasing as the hydrocarbon portion of the molecule increases.
3. Ketones are **relatively nonreactive**, although they may exist in equilibrium with their enol forms.
4. On the shelf, ketones are **very stable**.
5. In vivo, ketones may undergo **some oxidation** and **some reduction**.

K. Amines

1. Amines contain an **amine group** ($-NH_2$).
   a. **Primary** amines have a general formula of $R-CH_2-NH_2$.
   b. **Secondary** amines have a general formula of $R-CH_2-NH-R$.
   c. **Tertiary** amines have a general formula of $R-CH_2-N-R_2$.
   d. **Quaternary** amines have a general formula of $R-CH_2-N^+-R_3$.
2. Low molecular weight amines are **water soluble**; solubility decreases with increased branching (e.g., primary amines are more water soluble than secondary amines). However, quaternary amines, being ionic, are quite water soluble, as are most amine salts. Amines are also **lipid soluble**.
3. The common reactions of amines are **oxidation** and, for alkyl amines, **salt formation with acids**. Aromatic amines, which are less basic, have less tendency to react with acids.
4. On the shelf, phenolic amines are susceptible to **air oxidation**.
5. In vivo, amines may undergo minor **glucuronidation**, **sulfation**, and **methylation**. Primary amines also undergo **oxidative deamination**. Primary and secondary amines undergo **acetylation**. Secondary and tertiary amines undergo *N*-**dealkylation**, and tertiary amines undergo *N*-**oxidation**.

L. Carboxylic acids

1. Carboxylic acids have a general formula of R—COOH and contain a **carboxyl group** (—COOH).
2. Low molecular weight carboxylic acids are **water soluble**, as are sodium and potassium salts. Carboxylic acids are also **lipid soluble**.
3. The common reactions of carboxylic acids are **salt formation with bases**, **esterification**, and **decarboxylation**.
4. On the shelf, carboxylic acids are **very stable**.
5. In vivo, carboxylic acids undergo **conjugation** (with glucuronic acid, glycine, and glutamine) and **beta-oxidation**.

M. Esters

1. Esters have a general formula of R—COOR.
2. Esters are **lipid soluble**; low molecular weight esters are slightly **water soluble**.
3. The common reaction of esters is **hydrolysis**.
4. On the shelf, simple or low molecular weight esters are susceptible to hydrolysis, whereas complex, high molecular weight, or water-insoluble esters are resistant.
5. In vivo, esters undergo **enzymatic hydrolysis**.

N. Amides

1. Amides have a general formula of $R—CONH_2$ or R—CONH—R (lactam form).
2. Amides are **lipid soluble**; low molecular weight amides are **fairly water soluble**.
3. Amides have **no common reactions.**
4. On the shelf, amides are **very stable**.
5. In vivo, amides undergo **enzymatic hydrolysis**, primarily in the liver.

II. BIOCHEMISTRY

A. Introduction. Biochemistry is the study of molecular phenomena associated with life processes. It influences drug metabolism, therapeutic effectiveness, and biotransformation. Biochemically significant molecules include amino acids and proteins, carbohydrates, pyrimidines and purines, and biopolymers—enzymes (which are built from amino acids), polysaccharides (which are built from carbohydrates), and nucleic acids (which are built from pyrimidines and purines).

B. Amino acids and proteins

1. **Amino acids** are the monomer units of proteins and have a general formula of

$$\begin{array}{c} R—CH—COOH \\ | \\ NH_2 \end{array}$$

2. The amino acids that form proteins are **α-amino acids**; that is, the amino group ($—NH_2$) and the radical (R) are attached to the first (α) carbon removed from the carboxylic acid group. A protein can be hydrolyzed into its component α-amino acids by acids, bases, or enzymes.
3. Amino acids exist in two **enantiomorphs** (mirror-image forms), also known as **optical isomers**. Optical isomers are designated dextrorotatory (D) or levorotatory (L), depending on whether the molecule rotates polarized light in a clockwise direction (D) or an counterclockwise direction (L). The body synthesizes only **L-amino acids** into proteins.
4. Amino acids have a **zwitterion structure** (both positive and negative regions of charge), which accounts for their high melting point and low water solubility. Amino acids in solution have a general formula of

$$\begin{array}{c} R—CH—COO^- \\ | \\ NH_3^+ \end{array}$$

5. **Ionization** of amino acids to the zwitterion form or other forms depends on pH (Fig. 5-4).

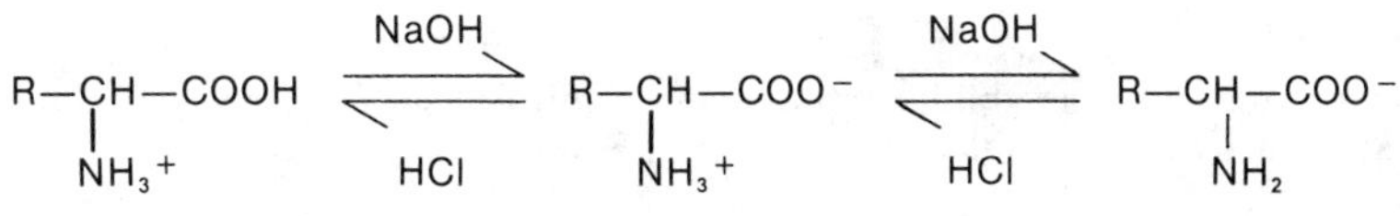

$$\underset{\text{I}}{\underset{|\atop NH_3^+}{R{-}CH{-}COOH}} \underset{HCl}{\overset{NaOH}{\rightleftharpoons}} \underset{\text{II}}{\underset{|\atop NH_3^+}{R{-}CH{-}COO^-}} \underset{HCl}{\overset{NaOH}{\rightleftharpoons}} \underset{\text{III}}{\underset{|\atop NH_2}{R{-}CH{-}COO^-}}$$

Figure 5-4. Amino acid ionization in solution. Form *I* is the dominant form in an acidic solution. Form *II* (the zwitterion form) dominates at the isoelectric point (the pH at which zwitterion formation occurs). Form *III* dominates in an alkaline solution.

6. Amino acids are linked to form proteins by the **peptide bond**—a link between the carbonyl carbon and the amino nitrogen (Fig. 5-5).

7. **Proteins**, which result from amino acids linking by means of peptide bonds, have **four levels of structure**.
   a. **Primary structure** refers to the sequence of amino acids in the protein.
   b. **Secondary structure** refers to the spatial arrangement of sequenced amino acids; for example, α-conformation (helical coil) or β-conformation (pleated sheet).
   c. **Tertiary structure** refers to the coiling and folding of protein chains into compact structures, such as globular shapes.
   d. **Quaternary structure** refers to the arrangement of individual subunit chains into complex molecules.

C. Carbohydrates

1. Carbohydrates are **polyhydroxy aldehydes or ketones**.

2. **Three major classes** of carbohydrates exist: monosaccharides, oligosaccharides, and polysaccharides.
   a. **Monosaccharides** (simple sugars), such as glucose or fructose, consist of a single polyhydroxy aldehyde or ketone unit.
      (1) **Aldehydic monosaccharides** are reducing sugars.
      (2) Monosaccharides can be linked together by **glycosidic bonds**, which are hydrolyzed by acids but not by bases.
   b. **Oligosaccharides**, such as sucrose, maltose, and lactose, consist of short chains of monosaccharides joined covalently.
      (1) **Sucrose** cannot be absorbed by the intestine until it is converted by sucrase into its components, glucose and fructose.
      (2) **Maltose** is hydrolyzed by maltase into two molecules of glucose.
      (3) **Lactose** (or milk sugar) cannot be absorbed by the intestine until it is converted by lactase into its components, galactose and glucose.
   c. **Polysaccharides**, such as cellulose and glycogen, consist of long chains of monosaccharides.

D. Pyrimidines and purines

1. Pyrimidines and purines are **bases** that, when bonded with ribose, form nucleosides, which when subsequently bonded to phosphoric acid form nucleotides—the structural building blocks of nucleic acids.

2. The **pyrimidine bases** include:
   a. **Cytosine** (C), found in deoxyribonucleic acid (DNA) and ribonucleic acid (RNA)
   b. **Uracil** (U), found in RNA only
   c. **Thymine** (T), found in DNA only

3. The **purine bases** include:
   a. **Adenine** (A), found in DNA and RNA

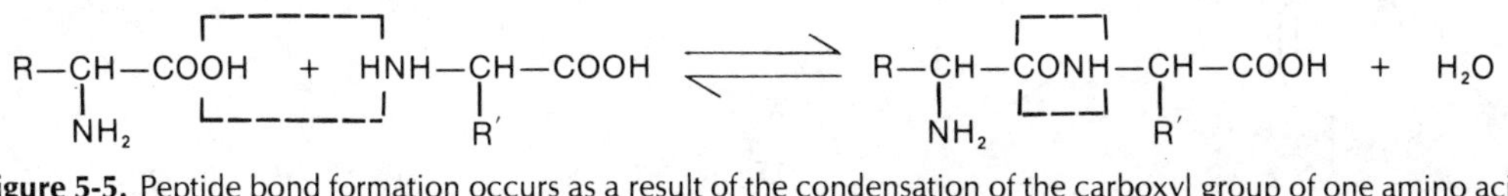

$$\underset{|\atop NH_2}{R{-}CH{-}COOH} + HNH{-}\underset{|\atop R'}{CH}{-}COOH \rightleftharpoons \underset{|\atop NH_2}{R{-}CH{-}CONH{-}}\underset{|\atop R'}{CH}{-}COOH + H_2O$$

Figure 5-5. Peptide bond formation occurs as a result of the condensation of the carboxyl group of one amino acid with the amino group of another. Water is eliminated during this process.

b. Guanine (G), found in DNA and RNA

4. Pyrimidines and purines exhibit **tautomerism** (a form of stereoisomerism) and can exist in either **keto** (lactam) or **enol** (lactim) forms (Fig. 5-6).

E. Bipolymers

1. Enzymes—linked chains of amino acids—are proteins capable of acting as catalysts for biologic reactions. They may be simple or complex and may require cofactors or coenzymes for biologic activity.

a. An enzyme **enhances the rate of a specific chemical reaction** by lowering the activation energy of the reaction. It does not change the reaction's equilibrium point, and it is not used up or permanently changed by the reaction.

b. A **cofactor** may be an inorganic component (usually a metal ion) or a nonprotein organic molecule.

c. A **coenzyme** is an organic cofactor that is actively involved during catalysis.

d. A cofactor may be biologically inactive without an **apoenzyme** (the protein portion of a complex enzyme). A cofactor firmly bound to the apoenzyme is called a **prosthetic group**.

e. A complete, catalytically active enzyme system is referred to as a **holoenzyme**.

f. Enzymes fall into **six major classes**.

(1) Oxidoreductases (e.g., dehydrogenases, oxidases, and peroxidases) are important in the oxidative metabolism of drugs.

(2) Transferases catalyze the transfer of groups, such as phosphate and amino groups.

(3) Hydrolases (e.g., proteolytic enzymes, amylases, and esterases) hydrolyze their substrates.

(4) Lyases (e.g., decarboxylases and deaminases) catalyze the removal of functional groups by means other than hydrolysis.

(5) Ligases (e.g., DNA ligase, which binds nucleotides together during DNA synthesis) catalyze the coupling of two molecules.

(6) Isomerases catalyze various isomerizations, such as the change from D to L forms or the change from cis- to trans-isomers.

2. Polysaccharides (also called **glycans**) are long-chain polymers of carbohydrates and may be linear or branched. They are classified as homopolysaccharides or heteropolysaccharides.

a. Homopolysaccharides (e.g., starch, glucogen, and cellulose) contain only one type of monomeric unit.

(1) Starch (a reserve food material of plants) is composed of two glucose polymers—amylose (linear and water soluble) and amylopectin (highly branched and water insoluble). It yields mainly maltose (a glucose disaccharide) after enzymatic hydrolysis with salivary or pancreatic amylase; only glucose after complete hydrolysis by strong acids.

(2) Glycogen, like amylopectin, is a highly branched, compact chain of D-glucose. The main storage polysaccharide of animal cells, it is found mostly in liver and muscle and can be hydrolyzed by salivary or pancreatic amylase into maltose and D-glucose.

(3) Cellulose (a water-insoluble structural polysaccharide found in plant cell walls) is a linear, unbranched chain of D-glucose. It cannot be digested by humans because the human intestinal tract secretes no enzyme capable of hydrolyzing it.

b. Heteropolysaccharides (e.g., heparin and hyaluronic acid) contain two or more types of monomeric unit.

(1) Heparin (an acid mucopolysaccharide) consists of sulfate derivatives of *N*-acetyl-D-glucosamine and D-iduronate. It can be isolated from lung tissue and is used medically to prevent blood clot formation.

(2) Hyaluronic acid, a component of bacterial cell walls as well as of the vitreous humor and synovial fluid, consists of alternating units of *N*-acetyl-D-glucosamine and *N*-acetylmuramic acid.

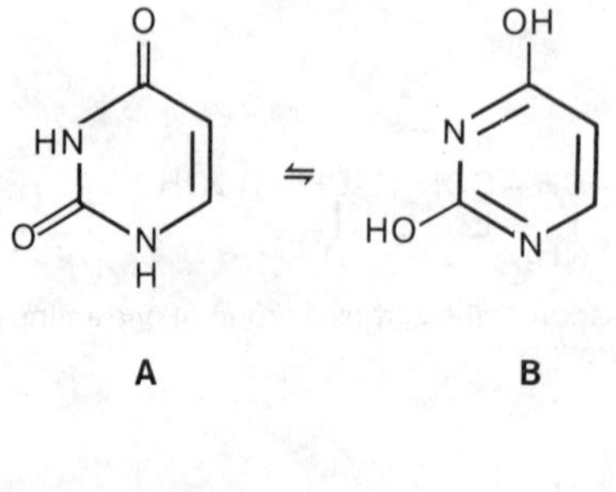

Figure 5-6. Uracil may exist in two tautomeric forms: (*A*) in a **keto** (or lactam) form and (*B*) in an **enol** (or lactim) form.

3. **Nucleic acids** are linear polymers of **nucleotides**—pyrimidine and purine bases linked to ribose or deoxyribose sugars (nucleosides) and bound to phosphate groups. The backbone of the nucleic acid consists of alternating phosphate and pentose units, with a purine or pyrimidine base attached to each.
   a. Nucleic acids are **strong acids**, closely associated with cellular cations and such basic proteins as histones and protamines.
   b. The two main types of nucleic acids are **DNA** and **RNA**. RNA exists in three forms.
      (1) **Ribosomal RNA** (rRNA) is found in the ribosomes, but its functions are not fully understood yet.
      (2) **Messenger RNA** (mRNA) serves as the template for protein synthesis and specifies a polypeptide's amino acid sequence.
      (3) **Transfer RNA** (tRNA) carries activated amino acids to the ribosomes, where the amino acids are incorporated into the growing polypeptide chain.
   c. In both DNA and RNA, the successive nucleotides are joined by **phosphodiester bonds** between the 5′-hydroxy group of one nucleotide's pentose and the 3′-hydroxy group of the next nucleotide's pentose.
   d. **DNA differs from RNA** in that it lacks a hydroxyl group at the pentose's C_2' position, and it contains thymine rather than uracil.
   e. DNA structure consists of two α-helical DNA strands coiled around the same axis to form a double helix. The strands are antiparallel—the 5′, 3′-internucleotide phosphodiester links run in opposite directions.
      (1) **Hydrogen bonding** between specific base pairs—adenine and thymine (A–T) and cytosine and guanine (C–G)—holds the two DNA strands together. The strands are **complementary** (the base sequence of one strand determines the base sequence of the other).
      (2) The **hydrophobic bases** are on the inside of the helix; the **hydrophilic deoxyribose-phosphate backbone** is on the outside.

STUDY QUESTIONS

Directions: Each question below contains five suggested answers. Choose the **one best** response to each question.

1. Monomer units of proteins are known as

A. monosaccharides
B. prosthetic groups
C. amino acids
D. purines
E. nucleosides

2. All of the following carbohydrates are considered to be polysaccharides EXCEPT

A. heparin
B. starch
C. glycogen
D. maltose
E. cellulose

3. Which of the following functional groups is most susceptible to hydrolysis?

A. R—CO—R
B. R—COOR
C. R—O—R
D. R—NH—CH_3
E. R—COOH

4. Enzymes that uncouple peptide linkages are best classified as

A. hydrolases
B. ligases
C. oxidoreductases
D. transferases
E. isomerases

5. Which of the following classes of organic compounds reacts to form salts with hydrochloric acid?

A. Tertiary amines
B. Carboxylic acids
C. Amides
D. Ethers
E. Secondary alcohols

6. The sugar that is inherent in the nucleic acids RNA and DNA is

A. glucose
B. sucrose
C. ribose
D. digitoxose
E. maltose

7. Which of the following formulas represents the zwitterion form of an amino acid?

A. $H_2N—CH(R)—COOH$
B. $\overset{+}{H_3N}—CH(R)—COOH$
C. $H_2N—CH(R)—COOH$
D. $\overset{+}{H_3N}—CH(R)—COO^-$
E. $H_2N—CH(R)—CONH—CH(R)—COOH$

8. Which of the following compounds are considered the building blocks of nucleic acids?

A. Nucleotides
B. Nucleosides
C. Monosaccharides
D. Purines
E. Amino acids

9. Which of the following terms best describes a cofactor that is firmly bound to an apoenzyme?

A. Holoenzyme
B. Prosthetic group
C. Coenzyme
D. Transferase
E. Heteropolysaccharide

10. Which of the following terms best describes the conversion of

$C_6H_5{-}CH_2{-}CH(CH_3){-}NH_2$ to

$C_6H_5{-}CH_2{-}C(=O){-}CH_3$?

A. *N*-dealkylation
B. Oxidative deamination
C. Acetylation
D. Decarboxylation
E. Reductive cleavage

11. Glucose is a carbohydrate that cannot be hydrolyzed into a simpler substance. It is best described as

A. a sugar
B. a monosaccharide
C. a disaccharide
D. a polysaccharide
E. an oligosaccharide

Directions: Each question below contains three suggested answers of which **one or more** is correct. Choose the answer

A if **I only** is correct
B if **III only** is correct
C if **I and II** are correct
D if **II and III** are correct
E if **I, II, and III** are correct

12. When certain functional groups are introduced into a benzene nucleus, they tend to decrease the liposolubility of benzene. These groups include

I. an ethyl group
II. a phenolic group
III. a carboxylic acid group

Questions 13–16

The following questions refer to the drug molecule

$C_6H_4(-OOC{-}CH_3)(-COOH)$

13. The drug molecule is soluble in

I. an aqueous base
II. water
III. an aqueous acid

14. Decomposition of the drug molecule at room temperature most likely would occur by

I. oxidation of the ester
II. reduction of the carboxylic acid
III. hydrolysis of the ester

15. Reactions that would be possible metabolic pathways for the drug molecule include

I. ring hydroxylation
II. enzymatic hydrolysis
III. glucuronide formation

16. Classes of organic compounds that have greater in vitro stability than in vivo stability include

I. carboxylic acids
II. alcohols
III. alkyl halides

ANSWERS AND EXPLANATIONS

1. The answer is C. (*II B 1*) Proteins are large molecules with molecular weights ranging from 5000 to over 1 million daltons. All proteins are composed of chains of amino acids and can be hydrolyzed to yield a mixture of their respective amino acids. There are 20 α-amino acids, which are commonly found in proteins. All the naturally occurring amino acids in proteins are L-enantiomers, with the exception of glycine. All have at least one amino group and one carboxyl group. The amino acids are linked together through the amino group of one amino acid and the carboxyl group of another amino acid, with the splitting out of a water molecule to form an amide linkage, which in a protein is referred to as a peptide.

Monosaccharides are simple, nonhydrolyzable sugars. Purines and pyrimidines are organic bases, while a prosthetic group is a cofactor that is firmly bound to an apoenzyme.

2. The answer is D. (*II C 2 b, c*) Polysaccharides are long-chain polymers of sugars. As the prefix "poly" indicates, there are many sugar units in the molecule. Maltose is composed of two molecules of glucose and is classified as a disaccharide or an oligosaccharide.

3. The answer is B. (*I M*) Hydrolysis is a double decomposition reaction in which water is one of the reactants. Esters, particularly simple esters, commonly undergo hydrolysis. Certain types of ethers such as glycosides also undergo hydrolysis, but they usually require strongly alkaline conditions or a catalyst such as an enzyme. Ketones, amines, or carboxylic acids do not undergo hydrolysis.

4. The answer is A. [*II E 1 f* (3)] A peptide linkage is an amide functional group formed from the loss of a molecule of water from two amino acids. Uncoupling this linkage is the reverse of this reaction, a hydrolysis reaction. A hydrolase is an enzyme that catalyzes hydrolysis reactions. More specific terms for an enzyme that catalyzes the hydrolysis of proteins are amidase or peptidase. A ligase catalyzes the coupling of two molecules. An oxidoreductase catalyzes oxidation reactions. A transferase catalyzes the transfer of groups from one substance to another. An isomerase catalyzes the interconversion of one isomer to another.

5. The answer is A. (*I K 3*) Substances that react with acids to form salts must be bases. Only organic compounds that contain the nitrogen-containing amine group are bases. While amides contain nitrogen, the adjacent carbonyl group decreases the basicity; therefore, they are essentially neutral.

6. The answer is C. (*II E 3*) Nucleic acids are biopolymers consisting of long chains of nucleotides. Nucleotides contain a pentose monosaccharide as one of their three constitutents. Ribonucleic acid (RNA) contains, as the name suggests, the monosaccharide ribose, whereas deoxyribonucleic acid (DNA) contains deoxyribose. The only difference between these two sugars is the absence of oxygen in the 2 position of the ribose ring. Glucose, also known as dextrose, is a hexose. Digitoxose is a deoxyhexose present in the digitalis glycosides. Sucrose and maltose are disaccharides.

7. The answer is D. (*II B 4, 5; Figures 7–4, 7–5*) A zwitterion is a single species containing both negative and positive charges. It sometimes is referred to as an inner salt. Amino acids have an amino group and a carboxyl group in the same molecule. The amino group, which is basic, attracts the proton from the carboxyl group and becomes positively charged, while the carboxyl group becomes negatively charged when it donates its proton to the amino group. Amino acids exist as zwitterions at near neutral pH such as occurs within a cell or in the bloodstream.

8. The answer is A. (*II D, E 3*) Nucleic acids are linear polymers of nucleotides that consist of three different molecules that are covalently linked to form one unit: (1) an organic base of either a purine or a pyrimidine; (2) a 5-carbon sugar (e.g., pentose); and (3) a phosphoric acid group. A nucleoside consists of the organic base and the pentose. A monosaccharide is a simple nonhydrolyzable carbohydrate, which may be considered a building block of polysaccharides. Purines are heterocyclic bases. Adenine and guanine are the two purines found in deoxyribonucleic acid (DNA) and ribonucleic acid (RNA). Amino acids are the building blocks of protein.

9. The answer is B. (*II E 1 d*) Complex, or conjugated, enzymes contain a nonprotein group called a cofactor, which is required for biologic activity. In many cases, the cofactor is quite firmly bound to the protein. In others, the binding occurs only during the reaction that the enzyme catalyzes. Cofactors that are firmly bound to the protein are known as prosthetic groups, whereas those that are actively bound to the protein only during catalysis are referred to as coenzymes.

A holoenzyme is a complete, catalytically active enzyme system. A transferase is an enzyme that catalyzes the transfer of groups from one substance to another, such as catechol O-methyl transferase (COMT). A heteropolysaccharide is a polysaccharide that contains two or more different monomeric units, such as heparin.

10. The answer is B. (*I K 5*) The reactant depicted contains a primary amine that is lost during the reaction; that is, the molecule is deaminated. The resultant product is a ketone formed from the oxidation of the carbon atom. Thus, this reaction would best be termed oxidative deamination.

11. The answer is B. (*II C 2 a*) While glucose is a sugar, it is more specifically a simple sugar that cannot be hydrolyzed into more simple sugars—thus, it is classified as a monosaccharide. Sugars may be simple, such as glucose, or complex, such as sucrose, and are classified as disaccharides or oligosaccharides, respectively. Polysaccharides consist of long chains of monosaccharides such as cellulose and glycogen.

12. The answer is A (I). (*I A 1, 2, G 1, 2, L 1, 2*) The overall solubility of the various classes of organic compounds illustrates a tendency for functional groups containing oxygen or nitrogen to demonstrate a degree of water solubility, whereas functional groups containing only carbon and hydrogen have very little water solubility. The phenolic and carboxylic groups both contain oxygen. In addition, they are acidic groups capable of undergoing ionization. Thus, compared to the ethyl group, they are more likely to increase the water solubility of benzene.

13. The answer is A (I). (*I L 3*) Organic substances generally are nonpolar; thus, they usually are insoluble in water. Since water is a polar solvent, only polar organics are water-soluble. The most common type of polar organic compound is a salt. Since the molecule depicted is a carboxylic acid, it reacts with a base to form a water-soluble salt.

14. The answer is B (III). (*I L 1, 3, 4, M 1, 3, 4*) The molecule contains both a simple ester and a carboxylic acid. Simple esters are susceptible to hydrolysis from moisture in the air but are not susceptible to oxidation. Carboxylic acids are not reduced easily.

15. The answer is E (all). (*I D 5, L 5, M 5*) The molecule, acetylsalicylic acid, contains an aromatic hydrocarbon nucleus (which can undergo ring hydroxylation), a simple acetate ester (which can undergo hydrolysis), and a free carboxyl group (which can undergo glucuronide conjugation as well as glycine conjugation).

16. The answer is E (all). (*I A, E, F, L*) Molecules that have poor in vitro stability are usually those that are susceptible to air oxidation and hydrolysis, or they may be light sensitive. Alcohols undergo oxidation but not without the presence of oxidizing agents. Also, they do not hydrolyze; thus, they are stable in air and moisture. In the body, there are several common metabolic pathways available for their biotransformation. Acids do not hydrolyze, nor are they susceptible to oxidation, thus, are stable in the presence of air and moisture; whereas in vivo, acids easily undergo several common metabolic reactions, particularly conjugation reactions. Alkyl halides are not susceptible to either oxidation or hydrolysis and do not undergo common metabolic reactions in the body. Thus, alkyl halides are equally stable in vitro and in vivo.

6
Medicinal Chemistry

Edward F. LaSala
Nelson S. Yee

I. DRUG SOURCES AND MAJOR CLASSES

A. Natural products are drugs obtained from plant and animal sources.

1. **Alkaloids** are potent nitrogenous bases, obtained primarily from plants through extraction and purification (e.g., **morphine**, from the opium poppy, and **atropine**, from the belladonna plant).
2. **Hormones** are potent organic substances (principally proteins and steroids) primarily obtained from animal sources (e.g., **insulin**, a protein obtained from the pancreas, and **conjugated estrogens**, steroids obtained from the urine of pregnant mares).
3. **Glycosides** are organic substances consisting of a glucose (sugar) moiety bound to an aglycone (nonsugar) moiety by means of an ether bond (e.g., **digitoxin** and **amygdalin**).
4. **Antibiotics** are antimicrobial agents obtained from microorganisms (e.g., **penicillin** and **tetracycline**).

B. Synthetic products are drugs synthesized from organic compounds.

1. Synthetic products may have chemical structures **closely resembling those of active natural products** (e.g., **hydroxymorphone**, which resembles morphine, and **ampicillin**, which resembles penicillin).
2. Synthetic products also may be **completely new products**, obtained by screening synthesized materials for drug activity (e.g., **barbiturates**, **antibacterial sulfonamides**, **thiazide diuretics**, **phenothiazine antipsychotics**, and **benzodiazepine anxiolytics**).

II. DRUG ACTION AND PHYSICOCHEMICAL PROPERTIES

A. Drug action represents an artificial interference with an organism's natural (although not necessarily normal) function.

1. Systemically active drugs must **enter** and **be transported by body fluids**.
   - **a.** The drug must pass various membrane barriers, escape excessive distribution into sites of loss, and **penetrate to the active site**.
   - **b.** At the active site, the drug molecules must orient themselves and interact with the receptors to **alter function**.
   - **c.** The drug must be removed from the active site and must be **metabolized** to a form that is easily **excreted by the body**.
2. Drug absorption, metabolism, utilization, and excretion all depend on the **drug's physicochemical properties** and the **host's physiologic and biochemical properties**. Drug physicochemical properties can be altered; the host's properties cannot be altered.

B. Physicochemical properties of drugs include water solubility, liposolubility, ionization of acids or bases, ionization of salts, and hydrolysis of salts.

1. **Water solubility** depends on the drug's polarity. Polar substances are more water soluble than nonpolar substances; the degree of polarity depends on the extent of the drug's ionic character.
2. **Liposolubility** also depends on drug polarity.
   - **a. Nonpolar substances** are more liposoluble than polar substances.

b. **Non-oxygen-containing functional groups**, such as alkyl and aryl groups, increase the drug's partition coefficient and impart liposolubility (see Chapter 7, section I B 2 and D 2).
c. **Un-ionized molecules** are nonpolar and, hence, liposoluble.

3. **Ionization of acids and bases** plays a role with substances that dissociate into ions.
   a. The **ionization constant (K_a)** indicates the relative strength of the acid or base. An acid with a K_a of 1×10^{-3} is stronger (more ionized) than one with a K_a of 1×10^{-5}.
   b. The **negative log of the ionization constant (pK_a)** also indicates the relative strength of the acid or base. An acid with a pK_a of 5 ($K_a = 1 \times 10^{-5}$) is weaker (less ionized) than one with a pK_a of 3 ($K_a = 1 \times 10^{-3}$).
   c. **Strong acids** (e.g., HCl, H_2SO_4, HNO_3, HBr, HI, and $HClO_4$) are completely ionized. **Almost all other acids**, including organic acids, **are weak. Organic acids** contain one or more of these functional groups:
      (1) Carboxyl group (—COOH)
      (2) Phenolic group (Ar—OH)
      (3) Sulfonic acid group (—SO_2H)
      (4) Sulfonamide group (—SO_2NH—R)
      (5) Imide group (—CO—NH—CO—)
   d. **Strong bases** [e.g., NaOH, KOH, $Mg(OH)_2$, $Ca(OH)_2$, $Ba(OH)_2$, and quaternary ammonium hydroxides] are also completely ionized. **Almost all other bases**, including organic bases, **are weak.**
      (1) **Organic bases** contain a primary, secondary, or tertiary aliphatic or alicyclic amino group (—NH_2, —NHR, or NR_2).
      (2) Most aromatic or unsaturated heterocyclic nitrogens are so weakly basic that they do not readily form salts with acids. Saturated heterocyclic nitrogens, in contrast, are similar to aliphatic amines.
   e. **Ionization of weak acids and bases** is a reversible, dynamic process that conforms to the laws of chemical equilibrium.
      (1) **Ionization of a weak acid** (e.g., acetic acid, which has a pK_a of 4.76) takes place as follows:

$$CH_3COOH \rightleftharpoons CH_3COO^- + H^+$$

         (a) When a weak acid (such as acetic acid) is placed in an **acid medium**, the equilibrium shifts to the left, suppressing ionization. This decrease in ionization conforms to **LeChatelier's principle**, which states that when a stress is placed on an equilibrium reaction, the reaction will move in the direction that tends to relieve the stress.
         (b) When a weak acid is placed in an **alkaline medium**, ionization increases. The H^+ ions from the acid and the OH^- ions from the alkaline medium combine to form water, shifting the equilibrium to the right.
         (c) **Weakly acid drugs** are less ionized in acid media than in alkaline media. When an acidic drug's pK_a is greater than the pH of the medium in which it exists, it will be more than 50% in its nonionized (molecular) form and, thus, more likely to cross lipid cellular membranes.
      (2) **Ionization of a weak base** is the opposite of that for a weak acid.
         (a) Weak bases are less ionized in a **basic (alkaline) medium** and more ionized in an **acid medium**.
         (b) **Weakly basic drugs** are less ionized in alkaline media than in acid media. When a basic drug's pK_a is less than the pH of the medium in which it exists, it will be more than 50% in its nonionized (molecular) form and, thus, more likely to cross lipid cellular membranes.

4. **Ionization of a salt** plays a role with salt forms that dissociate into ions.
   a. **All salts** (with the exceptions of mercuric and cadmium halides and lead acetate) **are strong electrolytes**. Thus, they are very polar and not liposoluble.
   b. Drug salts that do not undergo hydrolysis are ionized in both acid and alkaline media. Thus, they are transported across cell membranes with great difficulty. (**Amphoteric drugs**, containing both acid and basic functional groups, are also ionized in both acid and alkaline media and have the same transportation difficulties.)

5. **Hydrolysis of a salt** plays a role with salt forms that dissociate in aqueous media.
   a. Salts of **strong acids** and **weak bases** hydrolyze in an aqueous medium to yield an **acidic solution**.
   b. Salts of **weak acids** and **strong bases** hydrolyze in an aqueous medium to yield an **alkaline solution**.
   c. Salts of **weak acids** and **weak bases** hydrolyze in an aqueous medium to yield an **acidic**, **basic**, or **neutral solution**, depending on the respective ionization constants involved.

d. Salts of **strong acids** and **strong bases** do not hydrolyze in an aqueous medium; thus, their **solutions are neutral**.

6. A **neutralization reaction** may occur when an acidic solution of an organic salt (a solution of a salt of a strong acid and a weak base) is mixed with a basic solution (a solution of a salt of a weak acid and a strong base). The nonionized organic acid or the nonionized organic base is likely to **precipitate** in this case. This reaction is the basis for many **drug incompatibilities**, particularly when intravenous (IV) solutions are mixed. Neutralization reactions may be avoided by knowing how to predict the approximate pH of the aqueous solutions of common drug salts.
   a. Generally, a drug's **salt form** may be recognized when the generic or trade name consists of two separate words, indicating a **cation** and an **anion**.
   b. Drugs with **nitrate**, **sulfate**, or **hydrochloride anions** (e.g., pilocarpine nitrate, morphine sulfate, or meperidine hydrochloride) are salts of **strong acids**. Thus, their cation portions (pilocarpine, morphine, and meperidine) must be **bases**.
      (1) Because pilocarpine, morphine, and meperidine are neither metal nor quaternary ammonium hydroxides, they must be **weak bases**.
      (2) Salts of weak bases and strong acids are water soluble and form **acidic aqueous solutions**.
   c. Drugs with **sodium** or **potassium cations** (e.g., warfarin sodium or potassium penicillin G) are salts of **strong bases**.
      (1) Because these drugs are organic, they must be **weak acids**.
      (2) Salts of strong bases and weak acids are water soluble and form **basic aqueous solutions**.
   d. Drugs whose **cation name ends with the suffix -onium** or **-inium** and whose anion is a chloride, bromide, iodide, nitrate, or sulfate (e.g., benzalkonium chloride or cetylpyridinium chloride) are salts of **strong bases** and **strong acids** and form **neutral aqueous solutions**.

III. STRUCTURAL FEATURES AND PHARMACOLOGIC ACTIVITY.

Drugs may be classified as those that are structurally nonspecific and those that are structurally specific.

A. **Structurally nonspecific drugs** are those for which the drug's interaction with the cell membrane depends more on the drug molecule's physical characteristics than on its chemical structure.

1. Usually, the interaction is based on the **cell membrane's lipid nature** and the **drug's lipid attraction**.

2. Most **general anesthetics**, as well as some **hypnotics** and some **bactericidal agents**, act through this mechanism.

B. **Structurally specific drugs** are those for which pharmacologic activity is determined by the drug's ability to bind to a **specific endogenous receptor.**

1. The pharmacologic activity of such drugs is described by **receptor site theory**.
   a. The **lock-and-key theory** postulates a complementary relationship between the drug molecule and a specific area on the surface of the enzyme molecule (the **active**, or **catalytic**, **site**) to which the drug molecule is bound as it undergoes the catalytic reaction.
   b. The **occupational theory of response** further postulates that, for a structurally specific drug, the intensity of the pharmacologic effect is directly proportional to the number of receptors occupied by the drug.

2. The drug's **ability to bind to a specific receptor**, while not independent of the drug's physical characteristics, is primarily determined by the drug's **chemical structure**.
   a. In such an interaction, the drug's **chemical reactivity** plays an important role, reflected in its bonding ability and in the exactness of its fit to the receptor.
   b. **Drug interaction** with a specific receptor is analogous to the fitting together of jigsaw puzzle pieces. Only drugs of similar shape (i.e., similar chemical structure) can bind to a specific receptor and initiate a biologic response.

3. Often, only a **critical portion of the drug molecule** (rather than the whole molecule) is involved in receptor site binding.
   a. The functional group making up this critical portion is known as a **pharmacophore**.
   b. Drugs with **similar critical regions** but different other parts may have similar qualitative (although not necessarily quantitative) pharmacologic activity.

4. In general, the better a drug fits the receptor site, the higher the affinity between the drug and

the receptor and the greater the observed biologic response. A drug that fits a receptor well is called an **agonist**.

5. Some drugs lacking the specific pharmacophore for a receptor may nonetheless bind to that receptor. Such a drug will have little or no pharmacologic effect and may also prevent a molecule having the specific pharmacophore from binding, blocking the expected biologic response. A drug that blocks a natural agonist and prevents it from binding to its receptor is called an **antagonist**.

6. The stereochemistry of both the receptor site surface and the drug molecule helps determine the nature and efficiency of the drug–receptor interaction. **Stereoisomers**—compounds in which all the atoms are bonded in the same way but differ in their orientation in space—may differ in their biologic activities and are classified into two major groups.
   a. **Optical isomers** have at least one asymmetric carbon atom, or **chiral center**—a carbon atom with four different groups attached to it.
      (1) This asymmetric carbon atom gives rise to two possible isomers, or **enantiomorphs**, which differ in their spatial orientation (Fig. 6-1). Enantiomorphs usually have identical properties, except that one rotates the plane of polarized light in a clockwise direction (**dextrorotatory**, designated D or +) and the other in an counterclockwise direction (**levorotatory**, designated L or −).
      (2) An equal mixture of D and L enantiomorphs is called a **racemic mixture** and is optically inactive.
      (3) Enantiomorphs may **differ in biologic activity** if their interaction with a receptor involves the asymmetric carbon and its attached groups. For example, **levorphanol** has narcotic, analgesic, and antitussive properties, whereas its mirror image, **dextrorphanol**, has only antitussive activity.
      (4) A molecule with more than one asymmetric carbon gives rise to more than two isomers, only some of which are enantiomorphs. Those isomers that are not enantiomorphs are called **diastereomers**. They may differ in physicochemical and biologic properties.
   b. **Geometric isomers** (also called **cis–trans isomers**) occur as a result of restricted rotation about a chemical bond, owing to double bonds or rigid ring systems in the molecule.
      (1) **Cis–trans isomers** are not mirror images and have very different physicochemical properties and pharmacologic activity.
      (2) Because the functional groups of these isomers are separated by different distances, they generally do not fit the same receptor equally well. If these functional groups are pharmacophores, the isomers will **differ in biologic activity**. For example, cis-diethylstilbestrol has only 7% of the estrogenic activity of trans-diethylstilbestrol (Fig. 6-2).
   c. **Bioisosteres** are molecules containing groups that are spatially and electronically equivalent and, thus, interchangeable without significantly altering the molecules' physicochemical properties. Replacement of a molecule with its isoteric analogue may produce selected biologic effects. For instance, the isostere may act as an antagonist to a normal metabolite (as in an antimetabolite drug).
      (1) The **antibacterial sulfonamides**, for example, are isosteric with para-aminobenzoic acid and act as competitive antagonists to it (Fig. 6-3).
      (2) The anticancer agent **5-fluorouracil** is isosteric with uracil and interferes with the production of DNA (Fig. 6-4).

IV. MECHANISMS OF DRUG ACTION

A. Action on enzymes

1. **Activation**, or increased enzyme activity, may result from induction of enzyme protein synthesis by such drugs as barbiturates, phenytoin and other antiepileptics, rifampin, antihistamines, griseofulvin, and oral contraceptives.
   a. A drug may enhance enzyme activity by **allosteric binding**, which triggers a conformational change in the enzyme system and thus alters its affinity for substrate binding. (This contrasts with the rigid **lock-and-key theory** of enzyme–substrate binding. See section III B 1 a.)

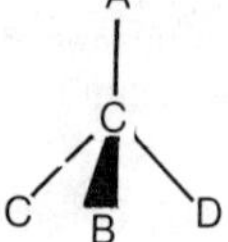

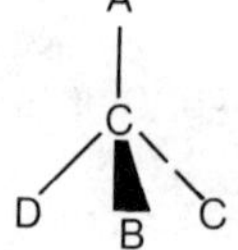

Figure 6-1. A tetrahedral carbon atom bonded to four different groups gives rise to two **enantiomorphs**, or optical isomers, which are mirror images of one another and cannot be superimposed.

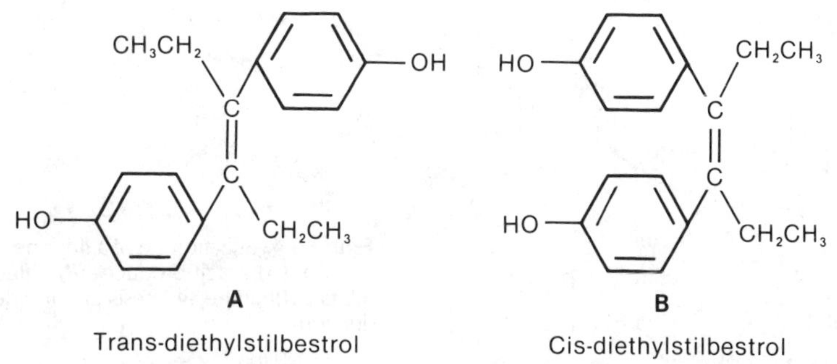

Trans-diethylstilbestrol (A); Cis-diethylstilbestrol (B)

Figure 6-2. These illustrations show (*A*) the trans-isomer of diethylstilbestrol and (*B*) the cis-isomer. Note how the relationship of the functional groups change relative to each other and to the carbon double bond.

b. Coenzymes play a role in optimizing enzyme activity. Coenzymes include **vitamins** (particularly the vitamin B complex) and **cofactors** (mainly metallic ions such as Na^+, K^+, Mg^{2+}, Ca^{2+}, Zn^{2+}, and Fe^{2+}). Coenzymes activate enzymes by complexation and stereochemical interaction.

2. **Inhibition**, or decreased enzyme activity, may result from drugs that interact with the apoenzyme, the coenzyme, or even the whole enzyme complex.
   a. The drug may modify or destroy the apoenzyme's protein conformation, react with the coenzyme (thus reducing the enzyme system's capacity to function), or bind with the enzyme complex (rendering it unable to bind with its substrate).
   b. Inhibition may be reversible or irreversible.
      (1) A **reversible inhibition** is an equilibrium reaction between the enzyme and the drug. Maximum inhibition occurs when equilibrium is reached.
      (2) An **irreversible inhibition** occurs when the drug binds with the enzyme to form a complex that does not dissociate. Inhibition increases with time if the drug is present in sufficient quantity.
   c. Inhibition may also be competitive or noncompetitive.
      (1) In **competitive inhibition**, the drug competes with the natural substrate for the same enzyme site, combining with the site reversibly. If the natural substrate's concentration is increased sufficiently, it will displace the drug from the binding site, reversing the inhibition.
      (2) In **noncompetitive inhibition**, the drug combines with the enzyme or the enzyme–substrate complex at a site other than the catalytic site (where the substrate binds). An excess of natural substrate will not reverse the inhibition.

B. Suppression of gene formation

1. **Inhibition of nucleotide biosynthesis** occurs when folic acid antagonists or purine and pyrimidine analogues interfere with the biosynthesis of the purine and pyrimidine bases (the building blocks of nucleotides).

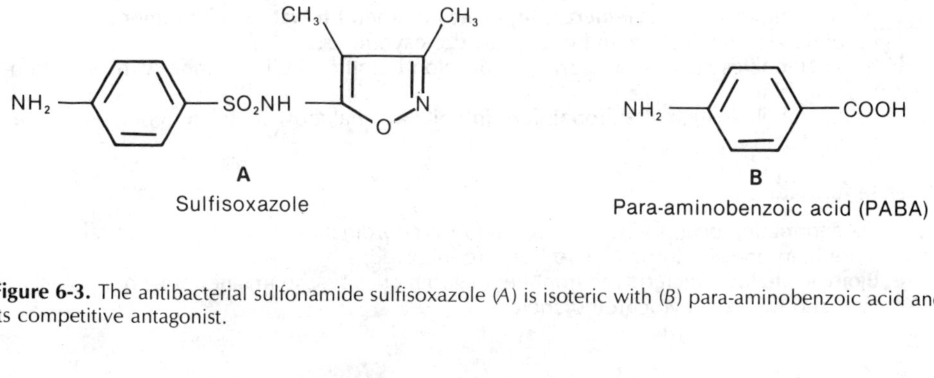

Sulfisoxazole (A); Para-aminobenzoic acid (PABA) (B)

Figure 6-3. The antibacterial sulfonamide sulfisoxazole (*A*) is isoteric with (*B*) para-aminobenzoic acid and acts as its competitive antagonist.

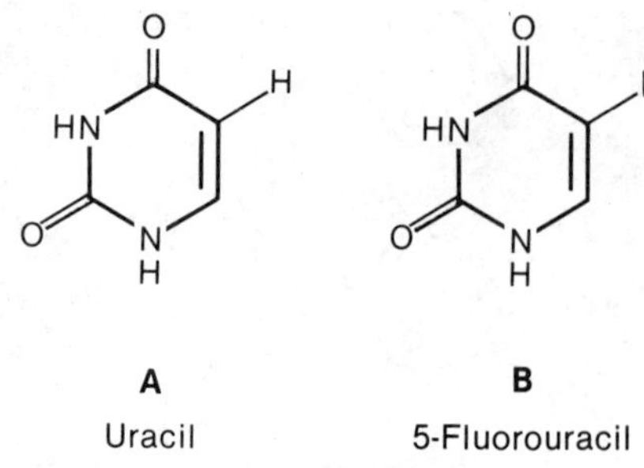

Figure 6-4. Substitution of a fluorine atom for a hydrogen atom of (*A*) uracil produces (*B*) 5-fluorouracil, which inhibits pyrimidine synthesis and interferes with DNA production.

a. **Antifolate drugs** (e.g., methotrexate) inhibit purine and thymidylic acid synthesis by inhibiting folate reductase.
b. **Purine analogue** (e.g., 6-mercaptopurine and 6-thioguanine) act as antagonists in the synthesis of purine bases. These analogues do not act as active inhibitors until they are converted to their respective nucleotides.
c. **Pyrimidine analogues** (e.g., 5-fluorouracil) inhibit the synthesis of thymidylic acid by inhibiting thymidine synthetase.

2. **Inhibition of DNA or RNA biosynthesis** occurs when drugs interfere with nucleic acid synthesis. These drugs are used primarily as antineoplastic agents for cancer chemotherapy.
   a. Drugs that interfere with **DNA replication** include **intercalating agents** (e.g., adriamycin and actinomycin), **alkylating agents** (e.g., the nitrogen mustards and busulfan), and **antimetabolites** (e.g., methotrexate and 6-mercaptopurine).
   b. Drugs that interfere with **transcription** include cisplatin (*cis*-platinum), bleomycin, and rifampicin.
   c. Drugs that interfere with **mitosis** include the **vinca alkaloids** (e.g., vincristine and vinblastine), which interfere with microtubule assembly in the metaphase of cell mitosis.
   d. Drugs that **inhibit DNA polymerase** include cytarabine (ARA-C) and vidarabine (ARA-A), which act as antineoplastic agents as well as antiviral agents.

C. Inhibition of protein synthesis

1. **Tetracyclines** interfere with protein synthesis by inhibiting tRNA binding to the ribosome and blocking the release of completed peptides from the ribosome.

2. **Chloramphenicol** and **erythromycin** (which compete for the same binding site) bind to the ribosome and inhibit peptidyl transferase, blocking formation of the peptide bond and interrupting formation of the peptide chain.

3. **Aminoglycosides** decrease the fidelity of transcription by binding to the ribosome, which permits formation of an abnormal initiation complex and prohibits addition of amino acids to the peptide chain. Additionally, aminoglycosides cause misreading of the mRNA template, so that incorrect amino acids are incorporated into the growing polypeptide chain.

D. Inhibition of enzyme-catalyzed reactions

1. **Antimetabolites** that are structurally similar to normal cellular metabolites can replace these metabolites and react with enzymes to yield abnormal nonfunctional products.

2. These agents are used to inhibit tumor growth, inhibit blood clotting, and inhibit bacterial growth.
   a. Antimetabolites such as **6-mercaptopurine** and **methotrexate** inhibit tumor growth by interfering with nucleotide and nucleic acid biosynthesis.
   b. Antimetabolites such as **warfarin** inhibit blood clotting by interfering with formation of clotting factors.
   c. Antimetabolites such as **sulfonamides** inhibit bacterial growth by interfering with tetrahydrofolic acid formation.

E. Chelate formation

1. Chelate formation occurs when the ligand forms coordination bonds with a central metal ion at more than one site (usually, two sites are involved).
   a. **Biologic chelates** include the iron–hemoglobin chelate, the magnesium–chlorophyll chelate, and the iron–cytochrome chelate.

b. Addition of a ligand with a greater affinity than the natural ligand for the essential metal causes formation of a more stable chelate, accounting for the ligand's medicinal properties. For example, both **isoniazid** and **8-hydroxyquinolone** can chelate with iron to exert antibacterial effects.

2. Chelating agents can also be used as **antidotes for metal poisoning**.

a. Ethylenediaminetetraacetic acid (EDTA, edetate) chelates calcium and lead.

b. Penicillamine (Cuprimine) chelates copper.

c. Dimercaprol (BAL) chelates mercury, gold, antimony, and arsenic.

F. Action on cell membranes

1. Digitalis glycosides inhibit the cell membrane's sodium–potassium pump, inhibiting the influx of K^+ and the outflow of Na^+.

2. Quinidine affects the membrane potential of myocardial membranes by prolonging both the polarized and depolarized states.

3. Local anesthetics block impulse conduction in nerve cell membranes by interfering with membrane permeability to Na^+ and K^+.

4. Antifungal drugs (e.g., amphotericin B and nystatin) affect cell membrane permeability, causing leakage of cellular constituents.

5. Certain **antibiotics** (e.g., polymyxin B and colistin), affect cell membrane permeability through a mechanism that is still unknown.

6. Acetylcholine increases membrane permeability to cations.

G. Nonspecific action

1. Structurally nonspecific drugs form a monomolecular layer over entire areas of certain cells. Because they involve such large surfaces, these drugs are usually given in relatively large doses.

2. Drugs that act by nonspecific action include the **volatile general anesthetic gases** (e.g., ether and nitrous oxide), some **depressants** (e.g., ethanol and chloral hydrate), and many **antiseptic compounds** (e.g., phenol and rubbing alcohol).

STUDY QUESTIONS

Directions: Each question below contains five suggested answers. Choose the **one best** response to each question.

1. All of the following medicinal agents are classified as natural products EXCEPT

A. atropine
B. diazepam
C. digitoxin
D. penicillin
E. morphine

2. Which of the following acids has the highest degree of ionization in an aqueous solution?

A. Aspirin $pK_a = 3.5$
B. Indomethacin $pK_a = 4.5$
C. Warfarin $pK_a = 5.1$
D. Ibuprofen $pK_a = 5.2$
E. Phenobarbital $pK_a = 7.4$

3. Which of the following salts will most likely yield an aqueous solution with a pH below 7?

A. Sodium salicylate
B. Potassium chloride
C. Magnesium sulfate
D. Potassium penicillin
E. Atropine sulfate

4. Which of the following salts forms an aqueous solution that is alkaline to litmus?

A. Sodium chloride
B. Benzalkonium chloride
C. Meperidine hydrochloride
D. Cefazolin sodium
E. Chlordiazepoxide hydrochloride

5. All of the following statements about a structurally specific agonist are true EXCEPT

A. activity is determined more by its chemical structure than by its physical properties
B. the entire molecule is involved in binding to a specific endogenous receptor
C. the drug cannot act unless it is first bound to a receptor
D. a minor structural change in a pharmacophore can produce a loss in activity
E. the higher the affinity between the drug and its receptor, the greater the biologic response

6. The dextro (D) form of β-methacholine (see structure below) is approximately 500 times more active than its levo (L) enantiomer.

$$(CH_3)_3\overset{+}{N}{-}CH_2{-}\underset{\displaystyle CH_3}{\underset{|}{C}}HOOC{-}CH_3 \qquad Cl^-$$

The observed difference in pharmacologic activity between the two isomers is most likely due to differences in the

A. selectivity for a receptor
B. rates of metabolism
C. extent of distribution
D. interatomic distance between pharmacophore groups
E. penetrability to the site of action

Directions: Each question below contains three suggested answers of which **one or more** is correct. Choose the answer

- **A** if **I only** is correct
- **B** if **III only** is correct
- **C** if **I and II** are correct
- **D** if **II and III** are correct
- **E** if **I, II, and III** are correct

7. True statements concerning drugs that act systemically include

I. they must undergo biotransformation into an active form after reaching their active site
II. they must be in a form capable of passage through various membrane barriers
III. they must be converted to a form that is readily excreted from the body

8. Examples of strong electrolytes (i.e., completely dissociated in an aqueous solution) include

I. acetic acid
II. pentobarbital sodium
III. diphenhydramine hydrochloride

9. Precipitation may occur upon mixing aqueous solutions of meperidine hydrochloride with which of the following solutions?

I. Sodium bicarbonate injection
II. Atropine sulfate injection
III. Sodium chloride injection

10. Drugs classified as antimetabolites include

I. 5-fluorouracil
II. sulfisoxazole
III. digoxin

11. The excretion of a weakly acidic drug generally is more rapid in alkaline urine than in acidic urine. This process occurs because

I. a weak acid in alkaline media will exist primarily in its ionized form, which cannot be reabsorbed easily
II. a weak acid in alkaline media will exist in its lipophilic form, which cannot be reabsorbed easily
III. all drugs are excreted more rapidly in an alkaline urine

Questions 12–15

All of the following questions refer to the drug meperidine (see structure below).

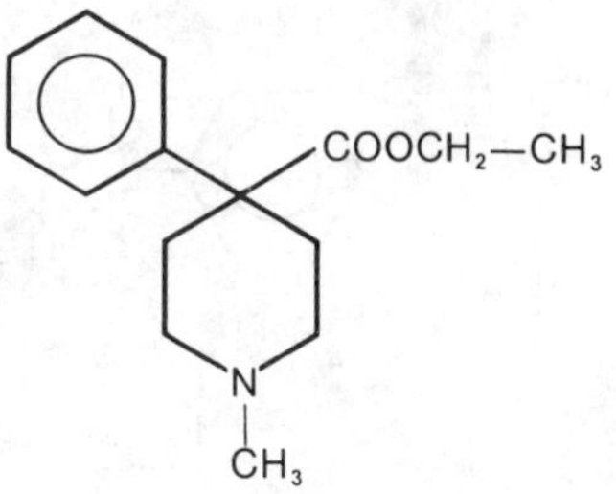

$COOCH_2—CH_3$

N

CH_3

12. Functional groups present in the molecule shown include

I. an ester
II. a tertiary amine
III. a carboxylic acid

13. Meperidine is classified as a

I. weak acid
II. salt
III. weak base

14. Meperidine is soluble in which of the following substances?

I. Dilute hydrochloric acid
II. Dilute sodium hydroxide
III. Water

15. Assuming that meperidine is absorbed after oral administration and that a large percentage of the dose is excreted unchanged, the effect of acidification of the urine will increase its

I. duration of action
II. rate of excretion
III. ionization in the glomerular filtrate

Directions: The group of questions below consists of lettered choices followed by several numbered items. For each numbered item select the **one** lettered choice with which it is **most** closely associated. Each lettered choice may be used once, more than once, or not at all.

Questions 16–19

For each pair of molecules, select the term that best fits the relationship.

A. Geometric isomers
B. Enantiomers
C. Diastereomers
D. Bioisosteres
E. Same compound

16. C_6H_5–C(H)(OH)–C($NHCH_3$)(H)–CH_3 C_6H_5–C(OH)(H)–C($NHCH_3$)(H)–CH_3

17. HO–(I,I)C_6H_2–O–(I,I)C_6H_2–CH_2–C(NH_2)(H)–COONa HO–(I,I)C_6H_2–O–(I,I)C_6H_2–CH_2–C(H)(NH_2)–COONa

18. HO–C_6H_4–C(CH_2–CH_3)=C(CH_2–CH_3)–C_6H_4–OH HO–C_6H_4–C(CH_2–CH_3)=C(CH_2–CH_3)–C_6H_4–OH

19. CH_3–CH_2, CH_3–CH–CH_2–CH_2–CH_3; O, O; HN, NH; S CH_3–CH_2, CH_3–CH–CH_2–CH_2–CH_3; O, O; HN, NH; O

ANSWERS AND EXPLANATIONS

1. The answer is B. (*I A, B*) Diazepam is a benzodiazepine anxiolytic, which, while it is a heterocyclic nitrogen-containing molecule, is not an alkaloid and is prepared synthetically. Natural products refer to those substances biosynthesized in plants or animals. The pure natural products are usually alkaloids, such as morphine or atropine; glycosides, such as digitoxin or digoxin; antibiotics, such as penicillin or streptomycin; or hormones, such as insulin or thyroxine.

2. The answer is A. (*II B 3 b*) The pK_a (the negative log of the acid ionization constant) is indicative of the relative strength of an acidic drug. The lower the pK_a of an acidic drug, the stronger it is as an acid. A strong acid is defined as one that is completely ionized or dissociated in an aqueous solution; therefore, the stronger the acid, the greater the ionization.

3. The answer is E. (*II B 5, 6*) The solution must contain an acidic substance in order to have a pH below 7. Sodium salicylate and potassium penicillin are both salts of strong bases and weak acids; therefore, their aqueous solutions are alkaline. Magnesium sulfate and potassium chloride are salts of strong bases and strong acids; therefore, their aqueous solutions are neutral. Atropine sulfate is a salt of a weak base and a strong acid; therefore, its aqueous solution is acidic.

4. The answer is D. (*II B 3 d, 5, 6*) Sodium chloride and benzalkonium chloride are both salts of strong bases and strong acids, and their aqueous solutions are neutral. Meperidine hydrochloride and chlordiazepoxide hydrochloride are salts of weak bases and strong acids, and their solutions are acidic. Only an aqueous solution of cefazolin sodium, which is a salt of a strong base and a weak acid, may be alkaline.

5. The answer is B. (*III B*) While the whole molecule is attached (bound) to a specific endogenous receptor, the actual binding site may consist of only a specific functional group. For example, a drug containing a hydroxyl group may be attached by hydrogen bonding between the electropositive hydrogen of the hydroxyl group and an electronegative oxygen on the receptor. Binding of drugs to biologic constituents may involve chemical bonds such as covalent, ion–dipole, dipole–dipole, and Van der Waals forces, among others.

6. The answer is A. (*III B 6 a; Figure 8–1*) The term enantiomer and the D and L indicate that the β-methacholine has a chiral center and exhibits optical isomerism. Since the optical isomers have different orientations in space, one orientation will give a better fit than the other and will most likely have greater biologic activity than the other.

7. The answer is D (II, III). (*II A 1, 2*) Generally, drugs must be lipophilic to pass through lipoprotein membranes and hydrophilic to be excreted by the kidney. Drugs do not have to be converted into an active form at their active site, although most drugs must be in their active form when they reach their active site. Many drugs are active in the form in which they are administered. Some drugs, usually referred to as prodrugs, are biotransformed into their active form after administration. Theoretically, drugs that reach their active site and then are metabolically activated should be more specific in their action and have fewer side effects. Currently, research efforts are underway to develop site-specific delivery systems and processes.

8. The answer is D (II, III). (*II B 3 c, 4 a, 6 a*) Acetic acid is a weak acid; therefore, it is a weak electrolyte. Almost all salts (with very few exceptions) are strong electrolytes, and the terminology pentobarbital sodium and diphenhydramine hydrochloride indicate that both compounds are salts.

9. The answer is A (I). (*II B 5, 6*) A neutralization reaction will occur when acidic solutions are mixed with basic solutions, or conversely. No reaction, in terms of acid–base, occurs when solutions are mixed with other acidic or neutral solutions or when basic solutions are mixed with other basic or neutral solutions. There should be no reaction, then, when the meperidine hydrochloride solution, which is acidic, is mixed with the acidic solution of atropine sulfate or the neutral solution of sodium chloride. However, when mixed with the alkaline solution of sodium bicarbonate, a neutralization reaction will occur with the possible precipitation of the water-insoluble free base meperidine.

10. The answer is C (I, II). (*III B 6 c; IV F 1*) Both sulfisoxazole and 5-fluorouracil compete with and antagonize isosteric normal biologic molecules and, therefore, are antimetabolites. Digoxin is a drug that is thought to inhibit Na^+-K^+-ATPase or to affect intracellular influx or utilization of Ca^+. Since digoxin is steroidal, it is not isosteric with either an enzyme, which is a protein, or an ion; therefore, it is not classified as an antimetabolite.

11. The answer is A (I). [*II B 2 c, 3 e (1) (a)–(c)*] A weakly acidic drug will be more ionized in an alkaline urine; therefore, it will be more polar and thus more soluble in the aqueous urine. It would also be less liposoluble, less likely to undergo tubular reabsorption, and thus be more likely to be excreted.

12. The answer is C (I, II). (*II B 3, 4*) The molecule contains a basic nitrogen, which is bonded to three carbon atoms (e.g., a tertiary amine), and an ethyl carboxylate, which is an ester group. An ester is the product of the reaction of an alcohol with a carboxylic acid that forms an alkyl carboxylate. There is no free carboxylic acid present. However, if this molecule is subjected to hydrolysis, it forms a carboxylic acid and ethyl alcohol.

13. The answer is B (III). (*II B 3, 4*) Since meperidine contains a tertiary amine, it is classified as a base; because it is an organic base, it is considered weak. The nitrogen is not protonated. It is not ionic and therefore is not a salt.

14. The answer is A (I). (*II B 3, 4*) Meperidine is an organic base of relatively high molecular weight and therefore is most likely insoluble in water. Water-soluble organic compounds generally must be strongly ionic in order to dissolve in water since water is a highly polar solvent. A salt of meperidine is completely dissociated in water and thus likely to be soluble. Since meperidine is a base, it can form a salt only with an acid.

15. The answer is D (II, III). (*II B 3, 4*) Alkalinization of the urine decreases the ionization of meperidine, making it more liposoluble and thus more likely to undergo reabsorption in the kidney tubule. This results in a decreased rate of excretion and an increased duration of action.

16–19. The answers are: 16-C, 17-B, 18-A, 19-D. (*III B 6 a–c; Figure 8-2*) The first pair of molecules are isomers that have two asymmetric carbon atoms. They are not superimposable and are not mirror images; therefore, they are known as diastereomers.

The second pair of molecules are isomers that have one asymmetric carbon atom. They are nonsuperimposable mirror images; therefore, they are enantiomers.

The third pair of molecules have different spatial arrangements and are isomers. The presence of the double bond, which restricts the rotation of the groups on each carbon atom involved in the double bond, characterizes this type of isomerism as geometric.

The last pair of molecules are neither isomers nor the same compound, since one contains three oxygens whereas the other contains two oxygens and a sulfur. Since oxygen and sulfur are in the same periodic family, they are isosteric, and the two compounds are known as bioisosteres.

7
Drug Metabolism

Edward F. LaSala
Nelson S. Yee

I. INTRODUCTION.
Drug metabolism (also called **biotransformation**) refers to the biochemical changes drugs and other foreign chemicals (**xenobiotics**) undergo in the body, leading to formation of different metabolites with different effects.

A. Inactive metabolites. Some metabolites are inactive—their pharmacologically active parent compounds become inactivated or detoxicated.

1. The hydrolysis of **procaine** to para-aminobenzoic acid results in loss of anesthetic activity.
2. The oxidation of **6-mercaptopurine** to 6-mercaptouric acid results in loss of anticancer activity.

B. Active metabolites. Other metabolites are active—their inactive parent prodrugs undergo bioactivation.

1. The prodrug **enalapril** is hydrolyzed to enalaprilat, a potent antihypertensive.
2. The prodrug **conjugated estrogen** is hydrolyzed to active estrogen hormone.
3. The prodrug **α-methyldopa** is decarboxylated, then β-hydroxylated to α-methylnorepinephrine, an antihypertensive.

C. Metabolites retaining similar activity. Certain metabolites retain the pharmacologic activity of their parent compounds to a greater or lesser degree.

1. **Imipramine** is demethylated to the essentially equiactive antidepressant, desipramine.
2. **Acetohexamide** is reduced to the more active hypoglycemic, L-hydroxyhexamide.
3. **Codeine is demethylated to the more active analgesic, morphine.**

D. Metabolites with altered activity. Some metabolites develop activity different from that of their parent drugs.

1. The antidepressant **iproniazid** is dealkylated to the antitubercular, isoniazid.
2. The vitamin **retinoic acid** (vitamin A) is isomerized to the antiacne agent, isoretinoic acid.

II. BIOTRANSFORMATION PATHWAYS (Table 7-1)

A. Phase I reactions are those in which new functional groups are introduced into the molecule or unmasked by oxidation, reduction, or hydrolysis.

1. **Oxidation** is the most commonly encountered drug reaction.
   a. Many oxidative reactions take place in the **liver**.
   b. Oxidation is catalyzed by a complex of nonspecific enzymes called **NADPH-dependent mixed-function oxidases**, which are bound to the smooth endoplasmic reticulum within liver cells. (NADPH is the reduced form of nicotinamide-adenine dinucleotide phosphate.)
   c. NADPH-dependent mixed-function oxidases catalyze aliphatic hydroxylation; aromatic (or ring) hydroxylation; oxidative *N*-, *O*-, and *S*-dealkylation; oxidative deamination; *N*- and *S*-oxidation (sulfoxidation); desulfuration; dehydrohalogenation; alcoholic oxidation; and aldehydic oxidation (see Table 7-1).
   d. The **increased polarity** of the oxidized products (metabolites) enhances their water solubility and reduces their tubular reabsorption to some extent, thus favoring their excretion in the urine. These metabolites are somewhat **more polar** than their parent compounds and very commonly undergo further biotransformation by phase II pathways (see section II B).

Table 7-1. Major Pathways of Drug Metabolism

Type of Reaction	Reaction Pathway	Examples
Oxidation		
Microsomal oxidations		
Aromatic hydroxylation	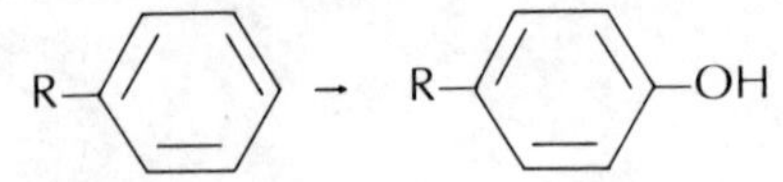 R–C_6H_5 → R–C_6H_4–OH	Phenylbutazone Phenytoin
Aliphatic hydroxylation	$R{-}CH_2{-}CH_3 \rightarrow R{-}CH(OH){-}CH_3$	Pentobarbital Meprobamate
Oxidative deamination	$R{-}CH(CH_3){-}NH_2 \rightarrow R{-}C(CH_3){=}O$	Amphetamine
N-dealkylation	$R{-}NH{-}CH_3 \rightarrow R{-}NH_2$	Ephedrine Morphine
O-dealkylation	$R{-}O{-}CH_3 \rightarrow R{-}OH$	Phenacetin Codeine
Sulfoxidation	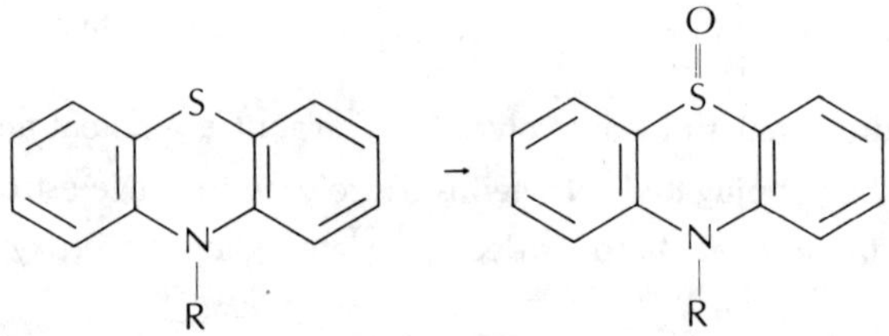 Phenothiazine (S, N–R) → phenothiazine sulfoxide (S=O, N–R)	Chlorpromazine
Desulfuration	$R_2C{=}S \rightarrow R_2C{=}O$	Thiopental
Dehydrohalogenation	$R_2CH{-}CCl_3 \rightarrow R_2C{=}CCl_2$	Halothane
Nonmicrosomal oxidations		
Alcoholic oxidation	$R{-}CH_2OH \rightarrow R{-}CHO$	Ethanol
Aldehydic oxidation	$R{-}CHO \rightarrow R{-}COOH$	Acetaldehyde
Reduction		
Azoreduction	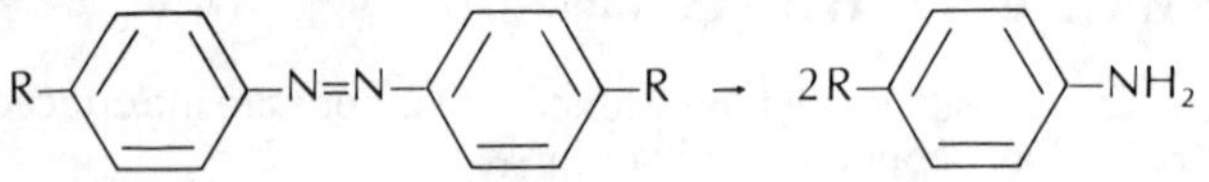 R–C_6H_4–N=N–C_6H_4–R → 2R–C_6H_4–NH_2	Sulfasalazine
Nitroreduction	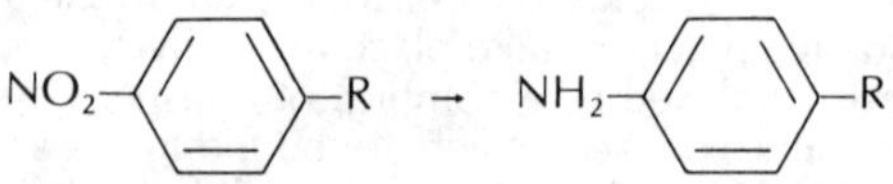 NO_2–C_6H_4–R → NH_2–C_6H_4–R	Chloramphenicol
Hydrolysis		
De-esterification	$R{-}COOR \rightarrow RCOOH + R{-}OH$	Procaine Meperidine
Deamidation	$R{-}CONH{-}R \rightarrow R{-}COOH + NH_2{-}R$	Lidocaine

(continued on next page)

Table 7-1. Continued

Type of Reaction	Reaction Pathway	Examples
Conjugation Glucuronidation	UDP-glucuronic acid (COOH, O, OH, OH, OH; —O—UDP) → glucuronide (COOH, O, OH, OH, OH; —O—X)	
Phenolic OH (X = —Ar)		Salicylates
Alcoholic OH (X = —R)		Oxazepam
Carboxyl (X = —OC—R)		Salicylates
Amine (X = —NH—R)		Sulfamethoxazole
Sulfhydryl (X = —SR)		Disulfiram
Glycine conjugation	C_6H_5—COOH → C_6H_5—CONH—R	Salicylic acid Fenfluramine
Glutathione conjugation	HO—NH—Ar → NH_2—Ar—CH_2—S—CH(NH—OC—CH_3)—COOH	Acetaminophen
Sulfate conjugation	R—OH → R—O—SO_2—OH	Steroids Terbutaline
Methylation Aromatic amines	C_6H_5—R—NH_2 → C_6H_5—R—NH—CH_3	Oxprenolol
Catechols	R—C_6H_3(OH)—OH → R—C_6H_3(OH)—OCH_3	Levodopa
Acetylation Aromatic amines	R—C_6H_4—NH_2 → R—C_6H_4—NHOC—CH_3	Sulfisoxazole Procainamide
Hydrazides	R—NH—NH_2 → R—NH—NHOC—CH_3	Isoniazid

2. **Reduction** is less commonly encountered than oxidation during drug metabolism. Different reductions, such as azoreduction or nitroreduction, lead to different types of polar functional groups (see Table 7-1).

3. **Hydrolysis** (an enzymatic process) results in more polar metabolites (see Table 7-1).
   a. The **esterase enzymes**, usually present in plasma and various tissues, are rather nonspecific and catalyze de-esterification, hydrolyzing relatively nonpolar esters into two polar, more water-soluble compounds—an alcohol and an acid.

b. The **amidase enzymes** hydrolyze amides into amines and acids (deamidation). Deamidation occurs primarily in the liver.

c. Ester drugs susceptible to plasma esterases (e.g., procaine) are usually shorter acting than structurally similar **amide drugs** (e.g., procainamide), which are not significantly hydrolyzed until they reach the liver.

B. Phase II reactions are those in which the functional groups of the original drug (or of a metabolite formed in a phase I reaction) are masked by a **conjugation reaction**. Most phase II conjugates (except for acetylated and methylated metabolites) are very polar, resulting in rapid drug elimination from the body.

1. Conjugation reactions combine the **parent drug** (or its metabolites) with certain **natural endogenous constituents**, such as glucuronic acid, glycine, glutamine, sulfate, glutathione, the two-carbon acetyl fragment, or the 1-carbon methyl fragment.

2. These reactions generally require both a **high-energy molecule** and an **enzyme**.

a. The **high-energy molecule** consists of a **coenzyme** bound to the endogenous substrate, the parent drug, or the drug's phase I metabolite.

b. The **enzymes** (usually called **transferases**) that catalyze conjugation reactions are found mainly in the liver and, to a lesser extent, in the intestines and other tissues.

3. Most conjugates are **highly polar** and **unable to cross cell membranes**, making them almost always **pharmacologically inactive** and of little or no toxicity.

4. Common conjugation reactions in humans are glucuronidation, glycine and glutamine conjugation, glutathione conjugation, sulfation, methylation, and acetylation (see Table 7-1).

a. Glucuronidation is one of the most common drug transformations, because glucuronic acid is readily available in the liver as a product of glucose metabolism.

(1) The high-energy form of glucuronic acid, **uridine diphosphate glucuronic acid** reacts with a large variety of functional groups under the influence of glucuronyl transferase.

(2) Drugs that commonly form glucuronides contain **hydroxyl groups** or **carboxyl groups**, which form ether-type or ester-type glucuronides, respectively. (*N*-glucuronides and *S*-glucuronides are also possible.)

(3) During glucuronidation, a carbohydrate moiety containing several hydrophilic hydroxyl groups and an ionizable carboxyl group is attached to a **lipophilic drug**. This causes formation of a highly polar, water-soluble molecule that is unlikely to penetrate cell membranes and elicit pharmacologic activity. It is also poorly reabsorbed by the renal tubules and, thus, readily excreted.

(4) Glucuronides with **high molecular weight** (> 500) are often excreted into the bile and, eventually, into the intestines. The intestinal enzyme β-glucuronidase may then hydrolyze the conjugate, releasing the unaltered drug (or its primary metabolite) for reabsorption by the intestine.

b. Glycine and **glutamine** can be conjugated with aliphatic or aromatic acids to form amides. The high-energy molecule for this reaction is an ***S*-acyl-coenzyme A(CoA)**; the reaction is catalyzed by a **transacylase**.

c. Glutathione conjugation occurs when glutathione (present in the liver) acts as an endogenous nucleophile and, under the influence of **glutathione transferase**, reacts with electrophilic compounds such as halides or nitrates to form a mercapturic acid derivative.

d. Sulfation depends on the availability of endogenous sulfate, which is usually limited. Unlike glucuronidation, sulfate conjugation can become easily saturated. The high-energy form of sulfate (**3′-phosphoadenosine-5′-phosphosulfate**) reacts with phenols and alcohols under the influence of **sulfotransferase** (also called sulfokinase).

e. Methylation results primarily in *O*-, *N*-, and *S*-methylated products, which are usually less polar than the unaltered drugs. Thus, methylated metabolites may retain their pharmacologic activity, and the pathway is not significant in the elimination of foreign compounds from the body. The high-energy methyl form is ***S*-adenosylmethionine**; **methyltransferase** catalyzes the reaction.

f. Acetylation may occur with primary amines, hydrazides, sulfonamides, and, occasionally amides. It leads to the formation of *N*-acetylated products. These are usually less polar than the unaltered drug and thus may retain pharmacologic activity.

(1) *N*-acetylated metabolites may accumulate in tissues or in the kidneys, as in the case of certain **antibacterial sulfonamides**. Crystalluria and subsequent tissue damage may result.

(2) The high-energy molecule for acetylation is **acetyl-CoA. The reaction is catalyzed by** *N*-acetyltransferase.

III. FACTORS INFLUENCING DRUG METABOLISM

A. A **drug's chemical structure** specifically influences its metabolic pathway.

B. Species differences in metabolism may cause variations in pharmacologic activity in different animals.

1. **Qualitative differences** are differences in the actual metabolic pathway. Such a variation may result from a genetic deficiency of a particular enzyme or from a difference in a particular endogenous substrate. In general, qualitative differences occur primarily with **phase II reactions**.

2. **Quantitative differences** are differences in the extent to which the same type of metabolic reaction occurs. Such a variation may result from a difference in the enzyme level, a difference in the amount of endogenous inhibitor or inducer, or a difference in the extent of competing reactions. In general, quantitative differences occur primarily with **phase I reactions**.

C. The **physiologic or disease state** may influence drug metabolism, usually affecting its rate or extent.

1. Because the liver is the major organ involved in biotransformation, **pathologic factors that alter liver function** can affect a drug's hepatic clearance.

2. **Congestive heart failure** decreases hepatic blood flow by reducing cardiac output, which alters the extent of drug metabolism.

3. An **alteration in albumin production** (the plasma's major drug-binding protein) can alter the fraction of bound to unbound drug. Thus, a decrease in plasma albumin can increase the fraction of unbound (free) drug, which then becomes available to exert a more intense pharmacologic effect. The reverse is true when plasma albumin increases.

D. Genetic variations in drug-metabolizing enzyme activity can affect the metabolism rate. This is particularly common with regard to **acetylation reactions**.

1. The **acetylation rate** depends on the amount of *N*-acetyltransferase present, which is determined by genetic factors.

2. The general population can be divided into **fast acetylators** and **slow acetylators**. For example, fast acetylators are more prone to hepatotoxicity from the antitubercular agent isoniazid than slow acetylators, whereas slow acetylators are more prone to isoniazid's other toxic effects.

E. Drug dosage may influence the metabolism rate or even the metabolic pathway.

1. As the **dosage is increased**, drug concentration in the body may saturate the metabolic enzymes. Because enzyme activity at high drug concentration is already at a maximum, any further increase in the drug level will not increase the rate of metabolism. Thus, the overall metabolism rate no longer follows first-order kinetics.

2. Once the metabolic pathway is **saturated** (either because of an exceedingly high drug level or because the supply of an endogenous conjugated agent is exhausted), an alternative pathway may be pursued. For example, at a low phenol level, phenol is conjugated to sulfate; at a high level, primarily to glucuronide.

F. Nutritional status may influence drug metabolism in numerous ways.

1. The levels of some **conjugating agents** (or endogenous substrates), such as sulfate, glutathione, and (rarely) glucuronic acid, are sensitive to body nutrient levels. For example, a **low-protein diet** may lead to a deficiency of certain amino acids, such as glycine. Low-protein diets also decrease oxidative drug metabolism capacity.

2. Diets **deficient in essential fatty acids** (particularly linoleic acid) reduce the metabolism of ethylmorphine and hexobarbital by decreasing synthesis of certain drug-metabolizing enzymes.

3. A **deficiency of certain dietary minerals** also affects drug metabolism. Calcium, magnesium, and zinc deficiencies decrease drug metabolizing capacity, whereas iron deficiency appears to increase it. A copper deficiency leads to variable effects.

4. **Deficiencies of vitamins** (particularly vitamins A, C, E, and the B group) affect drug metabolizing capacity. For example, a vitamin C deficiency can result in a decrease in oxidative pathways, whereas a vitamin E deficiency can retard dealkylation and hydroxylation.

G. **Age** affects drug metabolism because of differences in the functional level of the metabolizing enzyme systems.

1. In **young children**, particularly **infants**, drugs may be more active than expected because the metabolizing enzyme systems are not fully developed at birth and develop variably. This is particularly significant with glucuronidation.

2. In **older children**, some drugs may be less active than in adults, particularly if the dosage is based on weight. The liver develops faster than the increase in general body weight and thus represents a greater fraction of total body weight.

3. In the **elderly**, metabolizing enzyme systems decline. The lowered level of enzyme activity slows the rate of drug elimination, causing higher plasma drug levels per dose than in young adults.

H. **Gender** also influences drug metabolism. In rats, males have a faster drug metabolism rate after puberty than females. In humans, the same pattern seems to exist with regard to antipyrine, diazepam, and some steroids.

I. **Circadian rhythms** affect the metabolism rate of certain drugs. For example, the **nocturnal plasma levels** of such drugs as theophylline and diazepam are lower than the **diurnal plasma levels**.

J. The **drug administration route** influences the extent of drug metabolism, especially for drugs highly excreted by the liver.

1. With **oral administration**, the drug is absorbed from the gastrointestinal tract and transported to the liver through the hepatic portal vein before entering the systemic circulation. Thus, the drug is subject to hepatic metabolism before it reaches its site of action—an effect known as the **first-pass effect**, or **presystemic elimination**.
   a. The first-pass effect can cause **significant clinical problems**. Because drugs are metabolized in the liver from their active forms to inactive forms, this effect must be counteracted to achieve the desired plasma or tissue drug level.
   b. A common approach is to **increase the oral dose**, offsetting the loss of drug activity from the first-pass effect.

2. **IV administration** bypasses the first-pass effect because the drug is delivered directly to the bloodstream without being metabolized in the liver. Thus, IV doses of drugs undergoing considerable first-pass effects are much smaller than oral doses.

3. **Sublingual administration** and **rectal administration** also bypass first-pass effects, although rectal administration may produce variable effects.

K. **Enzyme induction or inhibition** can pose significant problems for the patient on a multiple-drug regimen, in which drug interactions are likely.

1. **Sequential or concurrent administration** of many structurally diverse drugs and environmental chemicals may increase the metabolism of some drugs—a phenomenon known as **enzyme induction**.
   a. **Drugs** such as phenobarbital and rifampin appear to act as enzyme inducers by increasing the synthesis or decreasing the degradation of drug-metabolizing enzymes. Phenobarbital, for example, induces the enzymes that metabolize theophylline, thus decreasing plasma theophylline levels and activity.
   b. **Environmental chemicals** such as the polycyclic aromatic hydrocarbons and the chlorinated insecticides also act as enzyme inducers. Cigarette smokers, for example, have lower plasma levels of drugs such as theophylline than do nonsmokers. The polycyclic aromatic hydrocarbon components of cigarette smoke appear to induce the *N*-demethylation pathway.

2. Some drugs and xenobiotics can decrease the metabolism of other drugs—a phenomenon known as **enzyme inhibition**. Inhibition may occur by destruction of drug-metabolizing enzymes, inhibition of enzyme synthesis, or complexation and inactivation of the drug-metabolizing enzymes. For example, cimetidine inhibits theophylline metabolizing enzymes, causing an increase in plasma theophylline levels and activity.

3. **Opposite effects** on drug activity occur when **prodrugs** are involved because these are inactive when administered and must be metabolized to their active forms.

4. The **tolerance** that develops with certain drugs, such as barbiturates, is related to enzyme induction. Induction results in increased metabolism and decreased activity compared to the effects of initial doses.

IV. EXTRAHEPATIC METABOLISM

A. **Definition**. Extrahepatic metabolism refers to drug biotransformation that takes place in **tissues other than the liver**. The most common sites include the **portals of entry** (e.g., the skin, lungs, and gut) and the **portals of excretion** (e.g., the kidneys). However, metabolism may occur throughout the body.

B. **Metabolism sites**

1. **Plasma** contains esterases, which are primarily responsible for hydrolysis of esters. Simple esters (e.g., procaine and succinylcholine) are rapidly hydrolyzed in the blood.

2. The **intestinal mucosa** also contains drug-metabolizing enzymes.
   a. As a lipid-soluble drug passes through the intestinal mucosa during drug absorption, it may be metabolized into polar or inactive metabolites before entering the blood. The result is **comparable to a first-pass effect**.
   b. The intestinal mucosa's drug-metabolizing capacity **compares to that of the liver**. However, it shows much greater individual variation because of its greater exposure to the environment.

3. The **intestinal bacterial flora** secrete a number of enzymes capable of metabolizing drugs and other xenobiotics.
   a. Any factor that **modifies the intestinal flora** may also **modify drug activity**. Age, diet, disease state, and exposure to environmental chemicals or drugs may all be important.
      (1) Certain **diseases**, particularly **intestinal disease**, affect intestinal flora. Ulcerative colitis, for example, promotes bacterial growth. Diarrhea reduces the number of bacteria.
      (2) Certain **environmental chemicals and drugs** also act on intestinal flora. Antibiotics, for example, decrease the number of bacteria.
   b. Bacterial flora secrete β-glucuronidase, which hydrolyzes the polar glucuronide conjugates of bile and allows the free, nonpolar bile acids to be reabsorbed. This **enterohepatic circulation** partially maintains the pool of bile acids. This same principle applies to certain glucuronide conjugates of drugs.
   c. Certain bacterial flora **convert vitamin precursors to their active forms**, as with vitamin K.
   d. Bacterial flora may also **convert certain substances to their toxic forms**, as with the conversion of the artificial sweetener cyclamate to cyclohexylamine, a suspected carcinogen.
   e. Intestinal bacteria produce **azoreductase**, which reduces the prodrug sulfasalazine to the active anti-inflammatory aminosalicylic acid and the active antibacterial sulfapyridine. Sulfasalazine is one of the few agents effective in the treatment of ulcerative colitis.

STUDY QUESTIONS

Directions: Each question below contains five suggested answers. Choose the **one best** response to each question.

1. Which of the following statements concerning drug metabolism is true?

A. Generally a single metabolite is excreted for each drug administered
B. Often a drug may undergo a phase-II reaction followed by a phase I reaction
C. Drug metabolizing enzymes are found only in the liver
D. All metabolites are less active pharmacologically than their parent drugs
E. Phase-I metabolites more likely are able to cross cellular membranes than phase-II metabolites

2. Chloramphenicol (see structure below) is considered to be toxic in infants (gray baby syndrome). This is due to tissue cumulation of unchanged chloramphenicol, resulting from an immature metabolic pathway. Which of the following enzymes would most likely be deficient?

NO_2–C₆H₄–CH(OH)–CH(NHOC–$CHCl_2$)–CH_2OH

A. Pseudocholinesterase
B. Glucuronyl transferase
C. *N*-acetyltransferase
D. Azoreductase
E. Methyltransferase

3. Which of the following functional groups would be the least likely urinary excretion product of orally administered aspirin (see structure below)?

Benzene ring with –OOC–CH_3 and –COOH

A. Glycine conjugate
B. Ester glucuronide
C. Unchanged drug
D. Ether glucuronide
E. Hydroxylated metabolite

4. Sulfasalazine (see structure below) is a prodrug that is activated in the intestine by bacterial enzymes. The enzyme most likely responsible is

HO–C₆H₄–N=N–C₆H₄–SO_2NH–(pyridyl, N)

A. azoreductase
B. pseudocholinesterase
C. *N*-acetyltransferase
D. β-glucuronidase
E. methyltransferase

Directions: Each question below contains three suggested answers of which **one or more** is correct. Choose the answer

A if **I only** is correct
B if **III only** is correct
C if **I and II** are correct
D if **II and III** are correct
E if **I, II, and III** are correct

5. Metabolic reactions likely to be affected by a protein deficient diet include

I. glycine conjugation
II. hydrolysis
III. glucuronidation

6. Conditions that tend to increase the action of an orally administered drug that undergoes phase-II metabolism include

I. enterohepatic circulation
II. enzyme saturation
III. first-pass effect

7. Terms that may be used to describe the following metabolic reaction include

$C_6H_5-CH_2-CH(CH_3)-NH_2 \rightarrow C_6H_5-CH_2-C(=O)-CH_3 + NH_3$

I. oxidative *N*-dealkylation
II. oxidative deamination
III. phase-I reaction

8. Phase-II metabolic reactions include which of the following?

I. $C_6H_5-NH_2 \rightarrow C_6H_5-NHOC-CH_3$

II. $C_6H_5-COOH \rightarrow C_6H_5-CONH-CH_2-COOH$

III. $C_6H_5-CH_2-CH_2NH_2 \rightarrow C_6H_5-CH_2-COOH$

Directions: The group of questions below consists of lettered choices followed by several numbered items. For each numbered item select the **one** lettered choice with which it is **most** closely associated. Each lettered choice may be used once, more than once, or not at all.

Questions 9–12

For each drug, select the metabolic pathway that it would most likely follow.

A. Ether glucuronidation
B. Ester glucuronidation
C. Azoreduction
D. Oxidative deamination
E. Hydrolysis

9. Benzoic acid

C_6H_5-COOH

10. Procaine

$NH_2-C_6H_4-COOCH_2-CH_2-N(CH_2-CH_3)_2$

11. Acetaminophen

$CH_3-CONH-C_6H_4-OH$

12. Amphetamine

$C_6H_5-CH_2-CH(CH_3)-NH_2$

ANSWERS AND EXPLANATIONS

1. The answer is E. (*II A 1 d, B*) Phase-I metabolites are often somewhat more polar than their parents. With the exception of acetylated and methylated metabolites, phase-II metabolites are always much more polar than their parents. Thus, phase-I metabolites are more likely to retain some liposolubility and are more likely to cross cellular membranes.

It is unusual for a single metabolite to be excreted for a given drug. Most drugs yield a mixture of metabolites. Because of the high polarity and subsequent high excretion of phase-II metabolites, they are not likely to undergo further metabolism. Phase-I metabolites, on the other hand, are less polar and are very likely to undergo further phase II metabolic reactions.

While the major site of metabolism is the liver, there are many extrahepatic sites that secrete drug metabolizing enzymes. While many metabolites are less pharmacologically active than their parents, there are many drugs whose metabolites have equal or greater pharmacologic activity and sometimes greater toxicity as well. Prodrugs (i.e., drugs inactive in the form administered) always form at least one active metabolite.

2. The answer is B. [*II B 4 a 1; III G 1; Table 7-1*] The chloramphenicol molecule contains an aromatic nucleus, which would be subject to hydroxylation, a nitro group that is subject to reduction, an amide group that is subject to liver hydrolysis, and alcohol groups that are subject to glucuronidation. Of all the enzyme systems responsible for these reactions, the system responsible for glucuronidation is developed poorly in premature infants and infants up to approximately 6 to 8 weeks of age.

3. The answer is C. [*II A 1 c, 3 a, B 4 a (2), b; Table 7-1*] Because of the types of functional groups present, aspirin may undergo a number of different metabolic reactions. These include hydroxylation of the aromatic nucleus, conjugation of the carboxyl group with glycine, conjugation of the carboxyl group with glucuronic acid with the formation of an ester glucuronide, hydrolysis of the acetate ester, and conjugation of the phenol group (resulting from hydrolysis of the acetate ester), with glucuronic acid to form an ether glucuronide.

Since the acetate ester is a simple ester, aspirin is susceptible to hydrolysis in the acid media of the stomach before absorption takes place. In addition, any acetylated molecules that are absorbed are subjected to hydrolysis and are catalyzed by the many esterases present in the circulation. Any acetylated molecules not hydrolyzed in the circulation are subject to hydrolysis in the liver. All of these processes occur before the drug reaches the glomerular filtrate; therefore, excretion of the unchanged acetylated drug is highly unlikely.

4. The answer is A. [*II A 2; IV B 3 e; Table 7-1*] Sulfasalazine has both anti-inflammatory and antibacterial activity when converted to aminosalicylic acid and sulfapyridine in the body. This reaction occurs by reductive cleavage of the "azo" linkage contained in the sulfasalazine molecule and is catalyzed in the intestine by bacterial azoreductase. This is a form of site-specific delivery since the intact drug is not absorbed from the stomach or upper intestine and reaches the colon, where it is metabolized. Sulfasalazine is one of a few drugs that is effective for the treatment of ulcerative colitis.

5. The answer is A (I). (*III F 1*) Phase-II metabolic reactions require natural endogenous substrates, which normally are supplied in the diet. A deficiency of these substances would result in decreasing the biotransformation of drugs that utilize these pathways. Glycine conjugation is such a phase-II reaction. Glycine is an amino acid that requires dietary protein. A diet deficient in protein, therefore, could lead to a deficiency of glycine and thus a decrease in glycine conjugation. Glucuronidation is also a phase-II reaction that requires endogenous glucuronic acid, but this substance is supplied by dietary carbohydrates. Hydroxylation is a phase-I metabolic reaction and does not require dietary protein.

6. The answer is C (I, II). [*III B 4 a (4), E 1, 2; IV B 3 b*] Enterohepatic circulation refers to the process by which glucuronides, which are secreted into the intestine with the bile, are hydrolyzed by intestinal bacterial β-glucuronidase. The hydrolyzed-free drug, which is no longer polar, becomes available for intestinal reabsorption into the system and subsequent penetration to its active site.

If an enzyme system becomes saturated, then the active drug cannot be inactivated by that pathway. If the drug cannot undergo an alternative pathway, the increased plasma levels of an unchanged active drug can result in increased activity or toxicity.

The first-pass effect results in metabolism of a drug by the liver before the drug reaches its site of action, resulting in an overall decrease in its activity. Drugs that undergo first-pass metabolism generally are effective in much smaller intravenous (IV) doses than oral doses.

7. The answer is D (II, III). (*II A; Table 7-1*) The reaction shown in the question involves the conversion of one functional group to another (amine to carbonyl); thus, it is classified as a phase-I reaction. The introduction of oxygen into the molecule indicates oxidation, and the loss of the amino group signifies deamination; thus, the reaction also can be classified as oxidative deamination. Oxidative *N*-dealkylation implies the removal of an alkyl group from a nitrogen. The nitrogen in the parent molecule does not have an alkyl group attached to it.

8. The answer is C (I, II). (*II A, B; Table 7-1*) Phase-II metabolic reactions involve masking of an existing functional group with a natural endogenous constituent. The formulas shown in choices I and II both represent this type of reaction, choice I being an acetylation reaction and choice II being a glycine conjugation reaction. Choice III represents a change in an existing functional group and thus represents a phase-I reaction. It is an oxidative deamination–reaction.

9–12. The answers are: 9-B, 10-E, 11-A, 12-D. [*II A 1 b, B 3 a, 4 a (2); Table 7-1*] A common metabolic pathway of carboxylic acids is conjugation with the endogenous substrate, glucuronic acid, with the net equation involving the splitting out of a molecule of water by combining the hydrogen of the carboxyl group with the anomer OH of glucuronic acid. This essentially is a reaction of an acid and an alcohol, which results in the formation of an ester linkage. Carboxylic acids also undergo glycine or glutamine conjugation, which results in the formation of an amide linkage. Theoretically, it is also possible for benzoic acid to undergo ring hydroxylation, which is a common phase-I pathway for aromatic nuclei.

Procaine is an ester-type local anesthetic. It is a simple ester and, therefore, very susceptible to hydrolysis in the body, due to the wide distribution of esterase enzymes and body water. This susceptibility to hydrolysis is the major reason why local anesthetics of this type have short durations of action when compared to other types of local anesthetics.

One of the principal functional groups in acetaminophen is the phenol, which commonly undergoes glucuronidation. The net result of the reaction is the splitting out of a molecule of water from the loss of the hydrogen atom of the phenol and the hydroxyl group of glucuronic acid, forming an ether linkage. Phenols also commonly undergo sulfate conjugation reactions and occasionally undergo *O*-methylation reactions. They may also undergo ring hydroxylation, due to the aromatic nucleus.

The principal functional group in amphetamine is a primary amine. Amines have a very low in vivo stability. Primary amines commonly undergo phase-I oxidative deamination as well as phase-II acetylation reactions.

8 Drugs Affecting the Autonomic Nervous System and the Neuromuscular Junction

David C. Kosegarten
Edward F. LaSala

I. INTRODUCTION. Drugs affecting the autonomic nervous system and the neuromuscular junction mimic or modify the actions of neurohumoral transmitters. They fall into five major categories: cholinergic agonists, cholinergic antagonists, adrenergic agonists, adrenergic antagonists, and neuromuscular blocking agents. Table 8-1 defines basic pharmacologic concepts.

Table 8-1. Defining Basic Pharmacologic Concepts

Concept	Definition
Drug receptor	A specific cellular site that interacts with a drug molecule, mediating the drug's action. Drug receptors are located in or on the cell membrane or within the cell itself. They are affected by micromolar to nanomolar drug concentrations, demonstrate relative stereospecificity, and can be selectively blocked by drug antagonists.
Affinity	The ability of a drug to combine with a specific receptor.
Agonist	A drug that has both affinity for a receptor and intrinsic activity that produces a pharmacologic effect. A drug that has affinity but very little or low intrinsic activity is considered a partial agonist (or, alternatively, a partial antagonist).
Antagonist	A drug that has affinity for a receptor but lacks intrinsic activity.
Pharmacologic antagonism	The process that occurs when an antagonist combines with a receptor, preventing or limiting an agonist's ability to produce a pharmacologic effect.
Physiologic antagonism	The process that occurs when an agonist and an antagonist act independently on two different receptors for different cellular mechanisms or different physiologic systems. For example, a drug that mimics the activity of the parasympathetic nervous system may be antagonized by a drug that mimics the activity of the sympathetic nervous system.
Drug intrinsic activity	A measure of the drug's ability to produce a pharmacologic effect.
Drug efficacy	A drug's ability to produce a maximum drug effect.
Drug potency	The relative concentrations of two or more drugs that produce the same drug effect.
Drug potentiation	The process that occurs when administration of a second, active drug increases the effectiveness of a first drug that is ineffective when given alone.
Drug synergism	The process that occurs when co-administration of two drugs causes a greater therapeutic effect than administration of each drug individually.
Drug additive effect	The process that occurs when co-administration of two drugs causes a therapeutic effect equal to that obtained by administration of each drug individually.

Continued on next page

Table 8-1. Continued

Concept	Definition
Drug therapeutic index (margin of safety)	The relationship between the dosage that produces an undesirable effect (death) and the dosage that produces a desirable (therapeutic) effect. The greater the ratio of these dosages, the safer the drug and the higher its therapeutic index.
Tolerance	The phenomenon of decreased responsiveness to a drug following chronic administration.
Tachyphylaxis	The rapid development of tolerance.
Anaphylaxis	An acute systemic reaction (commonly characterized by urticaria, respiratory distress, and vascular collapse) that occurs in a previously sensitized individual after exposure to the sensitizing antigen.
Anaphylactoid reaction	A dose-dependent, idiosyncratic reaction, clinically similar to anaphylaxis, that can occur after the first administration of certain drugs.

II. CHOLINERGIC AGONISTS

A. Chemistry

1. **Acetylcholine**, the natural endogenous mediator and the most potent cholinergic agonist, is an ester of acetic acid and choline, a quaternary aminoalcohol (Fig. 8-1). A hygroscopic simple ester, it is unstable and quickly hydrolyzed both in vitro and in vivo. Thus, it is extremely short acting and usually is not a satisfactory therapeutic agent.

2. **Therapeutically useful cholinergic agonists** may be direct acting or indirect acting.
   a. **Direct-acting agonists** may be produced by replacing the acetyl group of acetylcholine with a carbamoyl group or by substituting a methyl group of the β-carbon. These actions decrease the drug's hydrolysis rate, providing such stable, useful agonists as methacholine chloride and bethanechol chloride (Fig. 8-2).
   b. **Indirect-acting agonists** (acetylcholinesterase inhibitors) are divided into two major classes.
      (1) **Reversible** (short-acting) **agents** are principally carbamic esters, such as physostigmine and neostigmine (Fig. 8-3).
      (2) **Irreversible** (long-acting) **agents** are principally organophosphate esters, such as isoflurophate and echothiophate (Fig. 8-4).

B. Pharmacology

1. **Cholinergic responses** are mediated by both muscarinic and nicotinic receptors.
   a. **Muscarinic receptors** are present at parasympathetic postganglionic neuroeffector cell sites (Table 8-2).
   b. **Nicotinic receptors** are present at the ganglia of both the parasympathetic and sympathetic nervous systems and also at the neuromuscular junctions of the somatic nervous system (see section VI A 1).

2. Cholinergic agonists act by **mimicking the activity of endogenous acetylcholine** at muscarinic and nicotinic receptor sites.

$$CH_3\overset{O}{\overset{\|}{C}}OCH_2CH_2\overset{+}{N}(CH_3)_3$$

Figure 8-1. The structural formula of acetylcholine.

$$CH_3\overset{O}{\overset{\|}{C}}OCH_2\underset{CH_3}{\underset{|}{C}}H\overset{+}{N}(CH_3)_3\ Cl^- \qquad NH_2\overset{O}{\overset{\|}{C}}OCH_2\underset{CH_3}{\underset{|}{C}}H\overset{+}{N}(CH_3)_3\ Cl^-$$

A B

Figure 8-2. Clinically useful direct-acting cholinergic agonists include (*A*) methacholine chloride and (*B*) bethanechol chloride.

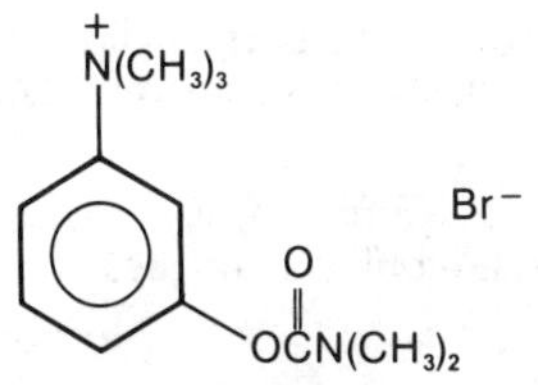

Figure 8-3. The structural formula of neostigmine (Prostigmin), a reversible acetylcholinesterase inhibitor.

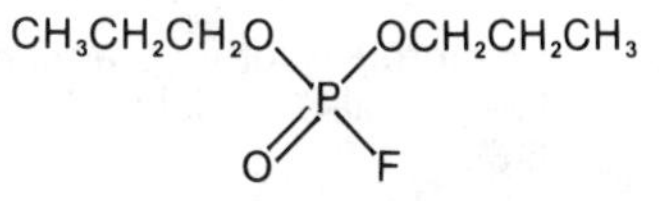

Figure 8-4. The structural formula of isoflurophate (Floropryl), an irreversible acetylcholinesterase inhibitor.

a. **Direct-acting agonists** interact directly with these receptors.

b. **Indirect-acting agonists** inhibit or block the activity of cholinesterase enzymes (e.g., acetylcholinesterase and pseudocholinesterase), which block the action of endogenous acetylcholine. Thus, these agonists allow endogenous acetylcholine to accumulate at cholinergic receptors, producing cholinergic stimulation. Organophosphate cholinesterase inhibitors (e.g., certain agricultural insecticides and so-called nerve gases) bind to the enzyme to form a long-lasting enzyme-inhibitor complex and are extremely toxic.

C. Therapeutic indications

1. **Direct-acting agonists** are indicated to:
   a. **Initiate micturation** in acute nonobstructive urinary retention (bethanechol)
   b. **Produce miosis** in the treatment of glaucoma (pilocarpine)

2. **Indirect-acting agonists** are indicated to:
   a. **Produce miosis** in the treatment of glaucoma (physostigmine, isoflurophate, echothiophate)
   b. **Treat myasthenia gravis** (ambenonium, neostigmine, pyridostigmine)
   c. **Aid in the differential diagnosis of myasthenia gravis and cholinergic crisis** (edrophonium)
   d. **Counteract intoxication or adverse effects from compounds with anticholinergic activity** (physostigmine)

D. Adverse effects

1. **Topical adverse effects** include congested conjunctivae, myopic accommodation, and transient lenticular opacity.

2. **Systemic adverse effects** include headache, syncope, nausea, vomiting, bradycardia, hypotension, bronchospasm, abdominal cramps, diarrhea, epigastric distress, salivation, sweating, lacrimation, flushing, and tremors.

III. CHOLINERGIC ANTAGONISTS

A. Chemistry

1. **Atropine**, an alkaloid obtained from the belladonna plant, is the prototypical cholinergic antagonist (anticholinergic agent). A portion of the atropine molecule is structurally similar to

Table 8-2. Muscarinic Receptor-Mediated Responses to Cholinergic Agonists

Organ	Response
Heart	Decreases conduction velocity Decreases contraction force Decreases contraction rate
Eye	Contracts the iris sphincter muscle and the ciliary muscle, producing miosis
Lung	Contracts tracheal and bronchial muscles
Intestine	Increases peristalsis Increases secretions Relaxes sphincter
Urinary bladder	Relaxes trigone and sphincter muscles Contracts detrusor muscle

acetylcholine (Fig. 8-5), permitting the molecule to bind to postganglionic receptors. However, the molecule has no intrinsic activity, and its bulky shape prevents acetylcholine from binding to the receptor.

2. Numerous **synthetic anticholinergic agents** (e.g., dicyclomine, glycopyrrolate, propantheline) are also available. These agents, like atropine, are bulky analogues of acetylcholine (Fig. 8-6).

B. Pharmacology

1. Cholinergic antagonists **competitively inhibit the activity of endogenous acetylcholine**.
2. Antagonists that inhibit muscarinic receptor-mediated responses are called **antimuscarinic agents**; those that inhibit nicotinic receptor-mediated responses are called **ganglionic blocking agents**.

C. Therapeutic indications

1. **Antimuscarinic agents** are indicated to:
   a. **Reduce glandular and bronchiolar secretions** before anesthesia (atropine, scopolamine)
   b. **Induce sedation** (scopolamine)
   c. **Alleviate motion sickness** (scopolamine)
   d. **Reduce vagal stimulation of the myocardium** (atropine)
   e. **Produce ophthalmic mydriasis and cycloplegia** (homatropine)
   f. **Reduce gastrointestinal smooth muscle spasms** (propantheline)
   g. **Treat bronchospasm** associated with chronic obstructive pulmonary disease (ipratropium)
   h. **Control Parkinson's disease and some neuroleptic-induced extrapyramidal disorders** (benztropine, trihexyphenidyl)
   i. **Treat intoxication by cholinergic agonists or by the rapid form of mushroom poisoning** (atropine)
2. **Ganglionic blocking agents** are indicated to **treat hypertensive crisis** (trimethaphan).

D. Adverse effects

1. **Topical adverse effects** include hyperopic accommodation and increased intraocular pressure.
2. **Systemic adverse effects** include headache, nervousness, drowsiness, dizziness, palpitations, tachycardia, dry mouth, mydriasis, blurred vision, nausea, vomiting, constipation, urinary retention, and fever.

IV. ADRENERGIC AGONISTS

A. Chemistry

1. **Direct-acting adrenergic agonists** include norepinephrine and epinephrine (naturally occurring catecholamines) as well as their derivatives. Catecholamines are biosynthesized from tyrosine, an amino acid (Fig. 8-7).

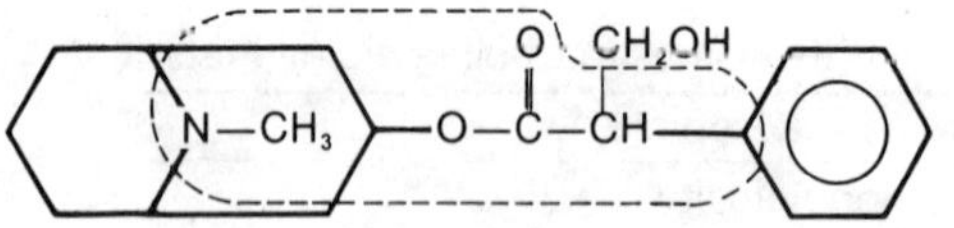

Figure 8-5. Structural formula of atropine, a cholinergic antagonist. The *circled area* resembles acetylcholine.

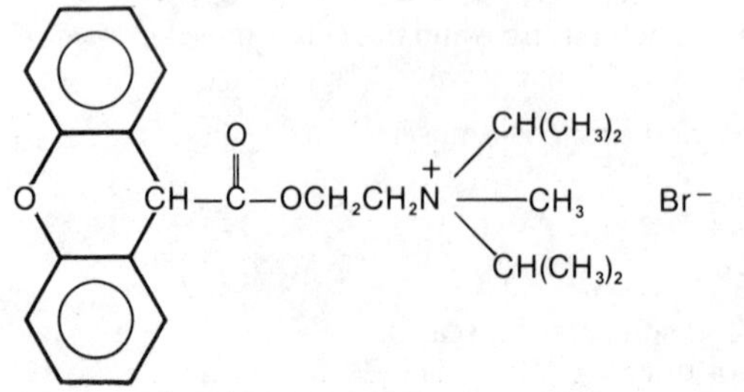

Figure 8-6. Structural formula of propantheline bromide (Pro-Banthine), a synthetic cholinergic antagonist.

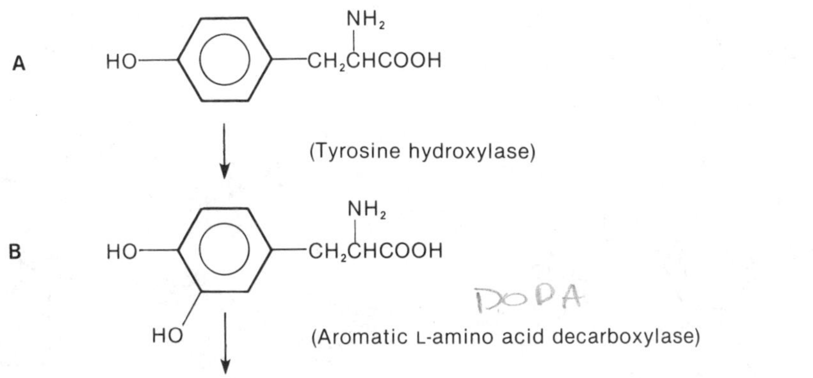

A HO–C_6H_4–$CH_2CH(NH_2)COOH$

(Tyrosine hydroxylase)

B HO, HO–C_6H_3–$CH_2CH(NH_2)COOH$

(Aromatic L-amino acid decarboxylase)

C HO, HO–C_6H_3–$CH_2CH_2NH_2$

(Dopamine β-hydroxylase)

D HO, HO–C_6H_3–$CH(OH)CH_2NH_2$

(Phenylethanolamine *N*-methyltransferase)

E HO, HO–C_6H_3–$CH(OH)CH_2NHCH_3$

Figure 8-7. Synthesis of catecholamines from the amino acid tyrosine. In the presence of tyrosine hydroxylase, (*A*) tyrosine is converted to (*B*) dihydroxyphenylalanine (dopa). Further substitutions permit the synthesis of (*C*) dopamine, (*D*) norepinephrine, and (*E*) epinephrine.

a. The 2-carbon chain common to these agonists is essential to their activity.
b. ***N*-substituents alter drug activity.** Small substituents (e.g., hydrogen or a methyl group) produce α-receptor activity, as with norepinephrine; larger substituents (e.g., an isopropyl group) produce β-receptor activity, as with isoproterenol.
c. Removal of the **para (4) hydroxyl group** leaves only α-receptor activity, as with phenylephrine.
d. The **meta (3) hydroxyl group** is essential for direct α- and β-activity. However, drugs in which the meta hydroxyl is replaced by a sulfonamide or a hydroxymethyl group retain activity.
e. The catecholamines are **inactivated** by methylation of the meta hydroxyl group (catalyzed by catechol *O*-methyltransferase) and by oxidation deamination [catalyzed by monoamine oxidase (MAO)].

2. **Indirect-acting agonists** (usually referred to as **sympathomimetic amines**) are compounds that are chemically related to the catecholamines and have similar effects. These are primarily synthetic compounds; examples include hydroxyamphetamine, ephedrine, tuaminoheptane, naphazoline, methamphetamine, protokylol, terbutaline, and dobutamine (Fig. 8-8).
   a. Sympathomimetic amines may have one, two, or no **hydroxyl groups**. The fewer hydroxyl groups, the less intestinal destruction and the greater the drug's lipophilic character; thus, the greater the absorption and the duration of activity after oral administration.
   b. The **benzene ring** of these drugs may be replaced by cyclohexyl, naphthalene, or other rings or by aliphatic chains.
   c. **Alkyl substitution** at the α-carbon (adjacent to the amino group) retards destruction of

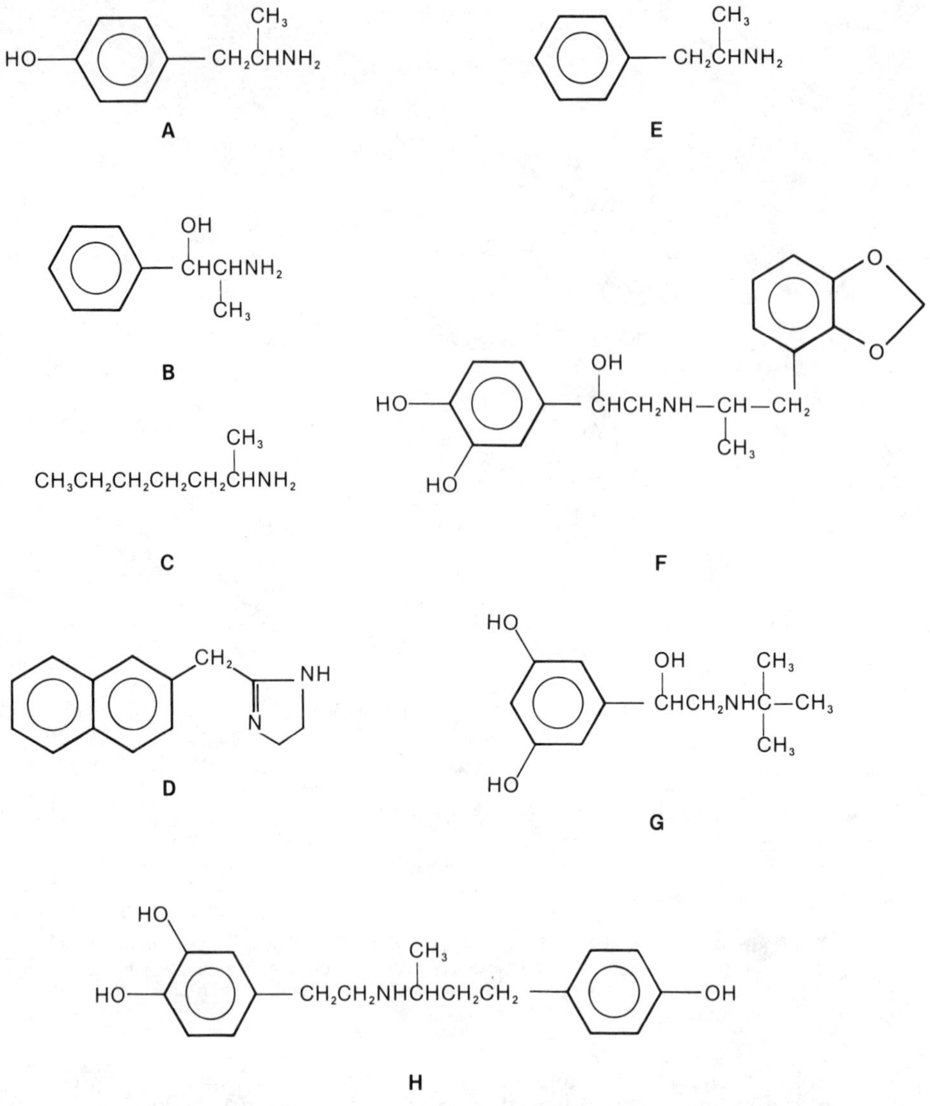

Figure 8-8. Structural formulas of representative sympathomimetic amines. (*A*) Hydroxyamphetamine (Paredrine); (*B*) ephedrine or pseudoephedrine (Sudafed); (*C*) tuaminoheptane (Tuamine); (*D*) naphazoline (Privine); (*E*) methamphetamine (Methedrine); (*F*) protokylol (Ventaire); (*G*) terbutaline (Brethine); (*H*) dobutamine (Dobutrex).

phenol and phenyl compounds and increases lipophilic character, contributing to prolonged activity.

d. ***N*-substituents with bulky groups** increase β-receptor activity, as with direct-acting agents.

B. Pharmacology

1. **Adrenergic peripheral responses** are mediated by both α- and β-receptors (Table 8-3).
   a. **α-Receptors** fall into two groups.
      (1) **Postjunctional α_1-adrenergic** receptors are found in the radial smooth muscle of the iris; in the arteries, arterioles, and veins; in the splenic capsule; and in the gastrointestinal tract. Drugs that are **α_1-selective agonists** include phenylephrine and methoxamine.
      (2) **Prejunctional α_2-adrenergic receptors** mediate the inhibition of release of adrenergic neurotransmitter. Drugs that are **α_2-selective agonists** include α-methylnorepinephrine and clonidine.
   b. **β-Receptors also fall into two groups.**
      (1) **Postjunctional β_1-adrenergic receptors** are found in the myocardium, the intestinal

Table 8-3. Adrenergic Receptor-Mediated Responses to Adrenergic Agonists

Organ/Tissue	Receptor Type	Response
Heart	β_1	Increases conduction velocity
	β_1	Increases contraction force
	β_1	Increases contraction rate
Arterioles	α_1	Constricts cerebral arterioles
	α_1	Constricts cutaneous arterioles
	α_1	Constricts visceral arterioles
	β_2	Dilates skeletal muscle arterioles
Eye	α_1	Contracts iris sphincter muscle, producing mydriasis
Lung	β_2	Relaxes tracheal and bronchial muscles
Intestine	α, β	Decreases peristalsis
	α	Contracts sphincter
Urinary bladder	α_1	Contracts trigone and sphincter muscles
	β_1	Relaxes detrusor muscle
Uterus	α	Excites uterine contractions
	β	Inhibits uterine contractions
Adipose tissue	β_1	Mobilizes fatty acids

smooth muscle, and adipose tissue. Drugs that are **β_1-selective agonists** include dobutamine.

(2) **Postjunctional β_2-adrenergic receptors** are found in bronchiolar and vascular smooth muscle. Drugs that are **β_2-selective agonists** include terbutaline.

2. **Direct-acting adrenergic agonists** (e.g., phenylephrine, clonidine, dobutamine, and terbutaline) produce their effects primarily by direct stimulation of adrenergic receptors. They may be **receptor-selective**, as with the drugs listed above, or they may be **nonselective**. For example, the adrenergic neurotransmitter norepinephrine affects α_1-, α_2-, and β_1-receptors, whereas the adrenal medullary hormone epinephrine affects α_1-, α_2-, β_1-, and β_2-receptors. Isoproterenol affects both β_1- and β_2-receptors.

3. **Indirect-acting adrenergic agonists** work through other routes. For example, tyramine acts by releasing norepinephrine from storage sites in adrenergic neurons. Most (if not all) β-adrenergic responses are mediated by a second messenger—intracellular cyclic adenosine monophosphate (cAMP).

4. Certain agonists (e.g., ephedrine, dopamine, metaraminol, and mephentermine) produce their effects through both **direct and indirect mechanisms**.

C. Therapeutic indications

1. **Epinephrine (an** α- and β-adrenergic agonist) is indicated to treat bronchospasm and hypersensitivity reactions and is the agent of choice for anaphylactic reactions. It is also used to prolong the activity of local anesthetic solutions and to restore cardiac activity in cardiac arrest.

2. **Phenylephrine** (an α_1-selective agonist) is used to provide pressor activity, to prolong the activity of local anesthetic solutions, and to relieve paroxysmal atrial tachycardia.

3. **Clonidine** (an α_2-selective agonist) and the prodrug α-methyldopa (converts to methylnorepinephrine) are used as central-acting sympatholytic antihypertensives.

4. **Isoproterenol** (a β-adrenergic agonist) is used as a bronchodilator and as a cardiac stimulant in shock and cardiac arrest.

5. **Dobutamine** (a β_1-selective agonist) is used to improve myocardial function in congestive heart failure.

6. **Terbutaline** (a β_2-selective agonist) is used as a bronchodilator.

D. Adverse effects. Adrenergic agonists may cause cardiac dysrhythmias, cerebral hemorrhage, pulmonary hypertension and edema, anxiety, headache, and rebound nasal congestion.

V. ADRENERGIC ANTAGONISTS

A. Chemistry

1. **α-Adrenergic antagonists** (α-blockers) have varied structures and bear little resemblance to the adrenergic agonists. Antagonists include the ergot alkaloids (e.g., ergotamine), the dibenzamines (e.g., phenoxybenzamine), the benzolines (e.g. tolazoline), and the quinazolines (e.g., prazosin) [Fig. 8-9.].
2. **β-Adrenergic antagonists** (β-blockers) are structurally similar to β-agonists (Fig. 8-10).
   a. The **catechol ring system** can be replaced by a wide variety of other ring systems, ranging from the prototypical naphthalene (propranolol) to phenylether (oxprenolol), amides (atenolol), indoles (pindolol), and others.
   b. The **side chain** may be either the unchanged isopropyl-aminoethanol or an aryloxyaminopropanol. Side-chain hydroxyl groups are essential for activity.
   c. The *N*-**substituents** must be bulky; an isopropyl group is the minimum effective size.

B. Pharmacology

1. Adrenergic antagonists **inhibit or block adrenergic receptor-mediated responses**.
2. **α-Adrenergic antagonists** may be α_1-selective (e.g., prazosin) or nonselective (e.g., phenoxybenzamine, which forms a covalent irreversible bond with α-receptors).
3. **β-Adrenergic antagonists** may be β_1-selective (e.g., metoprolol) or non-selective (e.g., propranolol).

C. Therapeutic indications

1. **Prazosin** (an α_1-selective antagonist) is used to produce vasodilation and is an important antihypertensive agent.
2. **Phenoxybenzamine** (a nonselective α-antagonist) is used to relieve vasospasm in Raynaud's syndrome and for acute hypertensive emergencies resulting from MAO inhibitors, sympathomimetics, or pheochromocytoma.
3. **Propranolol** (a nonselective β-antagonist) is used for the prophylaxis of angina pectoris, supraventricular and ventricular dysrhythmias, and migraine headache. It's also used as an antihypertensive, as a negative inotropic agent in hypertrophic obstructive cardiomyopathies, and as a negative chronotropic agent in anxiety and hyperthyroidism.
4. **Metoprolol** (a β_1-selective antagonist) is used primarily as an antihypertensive agent.

D. Adverse effects

1. **Prazosin** may cause sudden syncope with the first dose, orthostatic hypotension, dizziness, headache, drowsiness, palpitations, fluid retention, and priapism.
2. **Phenoxybenzamine** may cause orthostatic hypotension, tachycardia, inhibition of ejaculation, miosis, and nasal congestion.
3. **Propranolol** may cause bradycardia and congestive heart failure, increased airway resistance, increased serum triglycerides, decreased high-density lipoprotein cholesterol, blood dyscrasias, psoriasis, depression, hallucinations, organic brain syndrome, and transient hearing loss. Sudden withdrawal may be cardiotoxic.

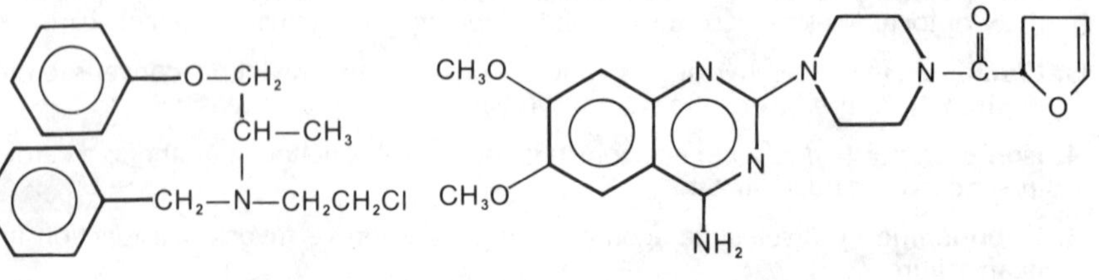

A B

Figure 8-9. The structural formulas of (*A*) phenoxybenzamine (Dibenzyline) and (*B*) prazosin (Minipress), representative α-blockers.

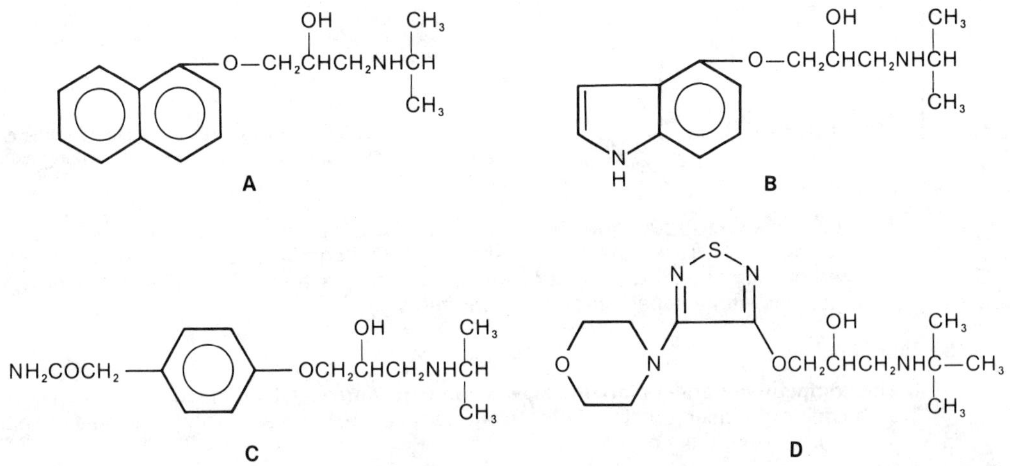

Figure 8-10. The structural formulas of (*A*) propranolol (Inderal); (*B*) pindolol (Visken); (*C*) atenolol (Tenormin); and (*D*) timolol (Blocadren), representative β-blockers.

4. **Metoprolol** has adverse effects similar to those of propranolol, except that it is less likely to increase airway resistance because of its β_1-selectivity.

VI. NEUROMUSCULAR BLOCKING AGENTS

A. Chemistry

1. **Neuromuscular blocking agents** may be competitive (as with the prototypical curare alkaloids) or depolarizing (as with succinylcholine). They act by blocking the effects of acetylcholine at the skeletal neuromuscular junction.
2. The **competitive nondepolarizing agents** are alkaloids of **curare** (the arrow poison of South American Indians) as well as several synthetic analogues. They are primarily bulky, rigid molecules.
   a. The **principal active alkaloids** include tubocurarine chloride and its methyl ether, metocurine iodide (Fig. 8-11). Their most important structural feature appears to be the presence of a **tertiary-quaternary amine** in which the distance between the two cations is rigidly fixed at about 14 A, twice the length of acetylcholine's critical moiety.
   b. The **most common synthetic analogues** are pancuronium bromide, which contains two quaternary nitrogens, and gallamine triethiodide, which contains three quaternary nitrogens.
3. The **noncompetitive depolarizing agents** include decamethonium bromide and succinylcholine chloride (Fig. 8-12).
   a. Unlike the large, bulky competitive agents, noncompetitive agents are **slender aliphatic molecules**. However, they do contain two quaternary nitrogens.

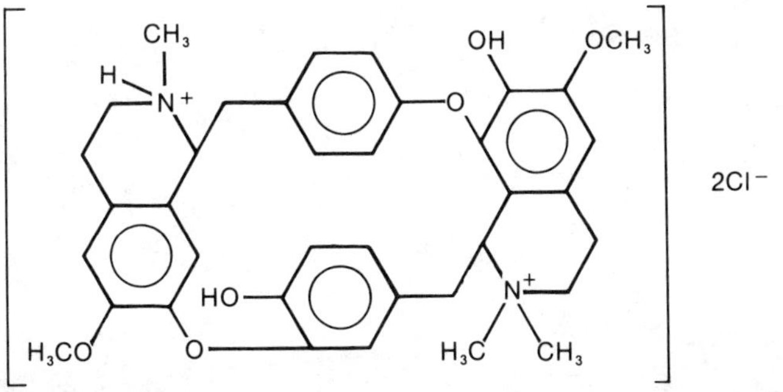

Figure 8-11. Structural formula of tubocurarine chloride (Tubarine), a competitive nondepolarizing agent.

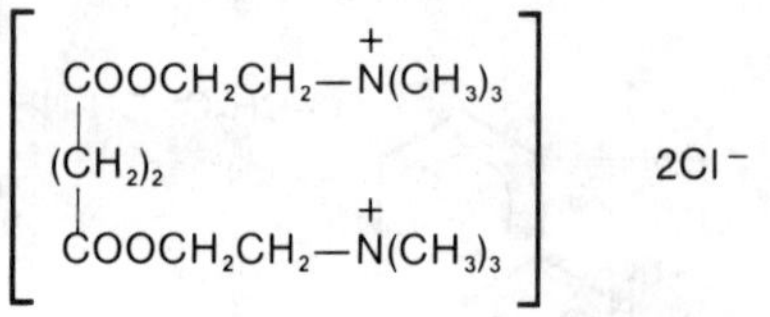

$$\left[\begin{array}{l} \text{COOCH}_2\text{CH}_2\text{—}\overset{+}{\text{N}}(\text{CH}_3)_3 \\ | \\ (\text{CH}_2)_2 \\ | \\ \text{COOCH}_2\text{CH}_2\text{—}\overset{+}{\text{N}}(\text{CH}_3)_3 \end{array}\right] \quad 2\text{Cl}^-$$

Figure 8-12. Structural formula of succinylcholine chloride (Anectine), a noncompetitive depolarizing agent.

b. **Succinylcholine** has a **short duration of action** compared to the other neuromuscular blocking agents. This results from its simple ester functional group, which is rapidly hydrolyzed by plasma and liver pseudocholinesterases. Its action may be prolonged, however, in patients with a genetic pseudocholinesterase deficiency.

B. Pharmacology

1. The **competitive nondepolarizing agents** compete with acetylcholine for nicotinic receptors at the neuromuscular junction. These agents reduce the end-plate potential, so that the depolarization threshold is not reached.

2. The **noncompetitive depolarizing agents** desensitize the nicotinic receptors at the neuromuscular junction. These agents react with the nicotinic receptors, decreasing receptor sensitivity in a manner similar to that of excess released acetylcholine. They depolarize the excitable membrane for a prolonged period (2 to 3 minutes); the membrane then becomes unresponsive (desensitized).

C. Therapeutic indications

1. Neuromuscular blocking agents are used to:
   a. **Promote skeletal muscle relaxation** and **facilitate endotracheal intubation**, as an adjunct to surgical anesthesia
   b. **Limit trauma associated with skeletal muscle contraction during electroconvulsive shock therapy**.

2. These agents cause only **skeletal muscle paralysis**—the patient remains conscious and capable of feeling pain.

D. Adverse effects

1. The **competitive nondepolarizing agents** may cause respiratory paralysis, histamine release, bronchospasm, and hypotension (tubocurarine) or respiratory paralysis, tachycardia, and hypertension (gallamine and pancuronium).

2. The **noncompetitive depolarizing agents** (succinylcholine and decamethonium) may cause respiratory paralysis, muscle fasciculation with pain, extraocular muscle contraction with increased intraocular pressure, and increased intragastric pressure. In addition, succinylcholine may cause muscarinic responses such as bradycardia, increased glandular secretions, and cardiac arrest. In combination with halothane, succinylcholine may cause malignant hyperthermia in genetically predisposed individuals.

STUDY QUESTIONS

Directions: Each question below contains five suggested answers. Choose the **one best** response to each question.

1. Which of the following drugs would most likely be used in the treatment of bronchospasm that is associated with chronic obstructive pulmonary disease?

A. Edrophonium
B. Ipratropium
C. Ambenonium
D. Propantheline
E. Homatropine

2. All of the following adverse effects are manifestations of cholinergic agonists EXCEPT

A. bradycardia
B. bronchoconstriction
C. xerostomia
D. lacrimation
E. myopic accommodation

3. Which of the following drugs is considered to be the agent of choice for anaphylactic reactions?

A. Clonidine
B. Isoproterenol
C. Epinephrine
D. Phenylephrine
E. Terbutaline

4. Which of the following neuromuscular blocking agents may cause muscarinic responses such as bradycardia and increased glandular secretions?

A. Tubocurarine
B. Succinylcholine
C. Pancuronium
D. Decamethonium
E. Gallamine

Directions: Each question below contains three suggested answers of which **one or more** is correct. Choose the answer

A if **I only** is correct
B if **III only** is correct
C if **I and II** are correct
D if **II and III** are correct
E if **I, II, and III** are correct

5. Antimuscarinic agents are used in the treatment of Parkinson's disease and in the control of some neuroleptic-induced extrapyramidal disorders. These agents include

I. ipratropium
II. benztropine
III. trihexyphenidyl

6. True statements concerning therapeutic indications of cholinesterase inhibitors include

I. they may be used as miotic agents in the treatment of glaucoma
II. they may be used to increase skeletal muscle tone in the treatment of myasthenia gravis
III. they decrease gastrointestinal and urinary bladder smooth muscle tone

7. Certain drugs are sometimes incorporated into local anesthetic solutions to prolong their activity and reduce their systemic toxicity. These drugs include

I. dobutamine
II. phenylephrine
III. epinephrine

Directions: The groups of questions below consist of lettered choices followed by several numbered items. For each numbered item select the **one** lettered choice with which it is **most** closely associated. Each lettered choice may be used once, more than once, or not at all.

Questions 8–10

For each of the drug molecules below, select the most appropriate pharmacologic classification.

A. Direct-acting cholinergic agent
B. β-Adrenergic blocker
C. Irreversible acetylcholinesterase inhibitor
D. Anticholinergic agent
E. Indirect sympathomimetic amine

8. $NH_2{-}COOCH_2{-}CH(CH_3){-}\overset{+}{N}(CH_3)_3 \quad Cl^-$

9. (bicyclic ring)N$-CH_3-OOC-CH(CH_2OH)-$(phenyl ring)

10. $CH_3CH_2CH_2{-}O{-}P(=O)(F){-}O{-}CH_2CH_2CH_3$

Questions 11–13

For each of the pharmacologic categories listed below, select the structure that it most likely represents.

A. Benzene ring bearing $\overset{+}{N}(CH_3)_3$ and $-OOC{-}N(CH_3)_2$ (meta) $\quad Br^-$

B. 3,4-(HO)$_2$-phenyl$-CH(OH){-}CH_2{-}NH{-}CH(CH_3)_2$

C. 3-HO-phenyl$-CH(OH){-}CH_2{-}NH{-}CH_3$

D. Quinazoline ring (N, N)$-N$(piperazine ring)$N{-}CO{-}$(furan ring, O)

E. Naphthalene$-O{-}CH_2{-}CH(OH){-}CH_2{-}NH{-}CH(CH_3)_2$

11. β-Adrenergic blocker
12. α-Adrenergic agonist
13. β-Adrenergic agonist

ANSWERS AND EXPLANATIONS

1. The answer is B. (*II C 2 b, c; III C 1 e–g*) Edrophonium and ambenonium are indirect-acting cholinergic agonists and, as such, would be expected to induce bronchospasm. Propantheline and homatropine are antimuscarinic agents used as a gastrointestinal antispasmodic and as a mydriatic, respectively. Ipratropium is a newly approved antimuscarinic agent used to treat bronchospasm.

2. The answer is C. (*II D*) Xerostomia, or dry mouth, results from reduced salivary secretions and therefore is not a manifestation of cholinergic agonist activity. All of the other effects listed in the question are extensions of therapeutic effects of cholinergic agonists to the point of being adverse effects.

3. The answer is C. (*IV C 1*) Of the adrenergic agonists listed in the question, only epinephrine, because of its broad, nonselective α- and β-activity, is an agent of choice for anaphylactic reactions. Epinephrine improves circulatory and respiratory function and counteracts the vascular effects of histamine-related anaphylaxis.

4. The answer is B. (*VI*) Neuromuscular blocking agents interact with nicotinic receptors at the skeletal neuromuscular junction. Succinylcholine is also capable of eliciting autonomic muscarinic responses, such as bradycardia, increased glandular secretions, and cardiac arrest.

5. The answer is D (II, III). (*III C 1 g, h*) All three compounds listed in the question are antimuscarinic agents; however, only benztropine and trihexyphenidyl are used to control parkinsonism and some neuroleptic-induced extrapyramidal disorders. Ipratropium is a newly approved agent for the treatment of bronchospasm.

6. The answer is C (I, II). (*II C 2*) Cholinesterase inhibitors are indirect-acting cholinergic agonists useful in treating myasthenia gravis and glaucoma. Their effects on gastrointestinal and urinary bladder smooth muscle would be to increase smooth muscle tone, not decrease it.

7. The answer is D (II, III). (*IV B 1 b, C*) Dobutamine is a β_1-selective adrenergic agonist. It would be inappropriate to use dobutamine to reduce blood flow at the site of local anesthetic administration. Epinephrine is a nonselective α- and β-agonist, and phenylephrine is an α_1-selective agonist; both of these drugs can be used to limit the systemic absorption of local anesthetics and prolong their activity.

8–10. The answers are: 8-A, 9-D, 10-C. [*II A 2 a, b (2); III A 1; Figures 8-1, 8-2, 8-4, 8-5*] The structure of the direct-acting cholinergic agent in question 8 is very similar to that of acetylcholine, differing only in that it has a carbamoyl group in place of the acetyl group and has a methyl group substituted on the β-carbon atom. Both of these changes decrease the rate of hydrolysis, resulting in an agent that acts directly, as acetylcholine does, but has a significantly longer duration of action.

The structure of the anticholinergic agent in question 9 also resembles that of acetylcholine, but with a significant difference in that the alcohol portion of the ester function is a large bulky group. This agent has no inherent cholinergic activity but can bind to the acetylcholine receptors in the postganglionic fibers, thus preventing acetylcholine molecules from interacting with these sites. This agent, which is atropine, is therefore an anticholinergic.

Because it contains a fluorophosphate group, the structure in question 10 can be recognized as being an organophosphate ester. This agent can bind covalently to the acetylcholine receptor and acts as an irreversible indirect-acting cholinergic agonist.

8. $NH_2—COOCH_2—CH(CH_3)—\overset{+}{N}(CH_3)_3 \quad Cl^-$

9. (bicyclic ring) $N—CH_3—OOC—CH(CH_2OH)—C_6H_5$

10. $CH_3CH_2CH_2—O—P(=O)(F)—O—CH_2CH_2CH_3$

11–13. The answers are: 11-E, 12-C, 13-B. (*IV A 1; V A 2; Figures 8-7, 8-8, 8-9, 8-10*) Structure E resembles the prototype β-agonist isoproterenol. It differs by having isoproterenol's catechol ring replaced by a naphthyloxy group. This substitution destroys the agonist activity, resulting in the formation of a β-adrenergic blocking agent.

Structure C differs from the prototype α-adrenergic agent norepinephrine only in the removal of the parahydroxyl group. While this agent no longer has the catechol structure, it does have inherent α-adrenergic activity.

Structure B possesses the catecholamine moiety typical of adrenergic agonists. The presence of the bulky *N*-isopropyl group characterizes it as a β-agonist.

A.

$\overset{+}{N}(CH_3)_3$

$-OOC-N(CH_3)_2$ Br^-

D.

N, N, N–, N—CO, O

B.

OH

HO—, HO— $-CH-CH_2-NH-CH(CH_3)_2$

E.

OH

$-O-CH_2-CH-CH_2-NH-CH(CH_3)_2$

C.

OH

$-CH-CH_2-NH-CH_3$

HO—

9
Drugs Affecting the Central Nervous System

David C. Kosegarten
Edward F. LaSala

I. INTRODUCTION. Drugs affecting the central nervous system (CNS) provide anesthesia, treat psychiatric disorders, relieve anxiety, provide sleep or sedation, prevent epileptic seizures, suppress movement disorders, and relieve pain. They include general and local anesthetics, antidepressants and antipsychotics, anxiolytics, sedative–hypnotics, antiepileptics, antiparkinsonian agents, and opioid analgesics and antagonists.

II. GENERAL ANESTHETICS

A. Chemistry

1. **Inhalation anesthetics** are drugs inhaled as gases or vapors. These diverse drugs are relatively simple lipophilic molecules, ranging from the inorganic agent nitrous oxide (N_2O) to ethers such as ethyl ether, hydrocarbons such as cyclopropane, and halogenated hydrocarbons such as halothane (F_3C-CHBrCl).

2. **Nonvolatile anesthetics** are also lipophilic molecules. They range from the ultra–short-acting barbiturates, such as thiopental, the cyclohexamines (ketamine), and the opioids (fentanyl), all of which are administered as water-soluble salts, to the benzodiazepines, such as midazolam, which are administered as neutral un-ionized molecules (Fig. 9-1).

B. Pharmacology

1. General anesthetics **depress the CNS**, producing a reversible loss of consciousness and loss of all forms of sensation.

2. Inhalational general anesthetics are **absorbed and primarily excreted through the lungs**. Frequently, they are supplemented with analgesics, a skeletal muscle relaxant, and antimuscarinic agents.
   a. **Analgesics** permit a reduction in the required concentration of inhalational anesthetic.
   b. **Skeletal muscle relaxants** cause adequate muscle relaxation during surgery.
   c. **Antimuscarinic agents** decrease bronchiolar secretions.

3. Nonvolatile general anesthetics are usually **administered intravenously** (thiobarbiturates, benzodiazepines).

C. Therapeutic indications

1. **Inhalation anesthetics** are indicated to provide general surgical anesthesia.

2. **Nonvolatile anesthetics** are indicated to induce drowsiness and provide relaxation prior to induction of inhalational general anesthesia (thiopental, diazepam, midazolam).

D. Adverse effects. General anesthetics **depress respiration and circulation** as well as the CNS. They can also **decrease hepatic and kidney function** (methoxyflurane) and cause **cardiac dysrhythmias** from increased myocardial sensitivity to catecholamines (halothane).

III. LOCAL ANESTHETICS

A. Chemistry

1. Most local anesthetics are structurally similar to the alkaloid **cocaine** (Fig. 9-2). They consist of a hydrophilic amino group linked through an ester or amide connecting group to a lipophilic aromatic moiety. A few phenols and aromatic alcohols also have local anesthetic activity.

2. **Ester-type agents** are short acting and are hydrolyzed by plasma esterases.

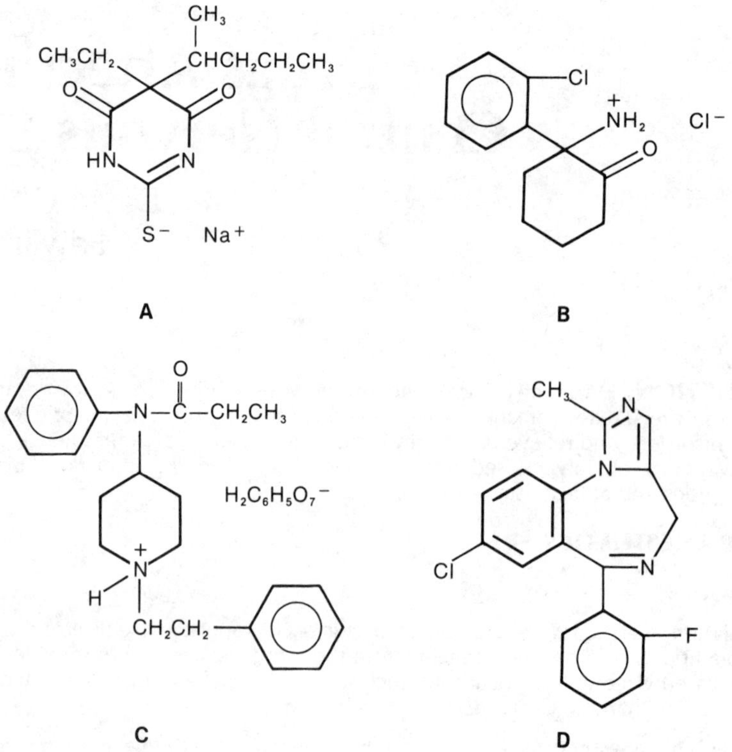

Figure 9-1. Structural formulas of nonvolatile general anesthetics: (A) thiopental sodium (Pentothal), (B) ketamine hydrochloride (Ketaject), (C) fentanyl citrate (Sublimaze), and (D) midazolam (Versed).

3. **Amide-type agents** are long acting and are hydrolyzed in the liver.
4. The drug's **pK_a** influences its state. At tissue pH, the drug can exist either as a lipophilic, uncharged, secondary or tertiary amine that crosses connective tissue and enters nerve cells or as a charged ammonium cation that appears to block the generation of action potentials by means of a membrane receptor complex.

B. Pharmacology

1. Local anesthetics **reversibly block nerve impulse conduction and produce reversible loss of sensation** at their administration site. They do not produce a loss of consciousness.
   a. **Small, nonmyelinated nerve fibers**, which conduct pain and temperature sensations, are affected first.
   b. Local anesthetics appear to become incorporated within the nerve membrane or to bind to specific membrane sodium ion channels, **restricting sodium permeability in response to partial depolarization**.
2. **Local anesthetic solutions** frequently contain the vasoconstrictor **epinephrine**, which re-

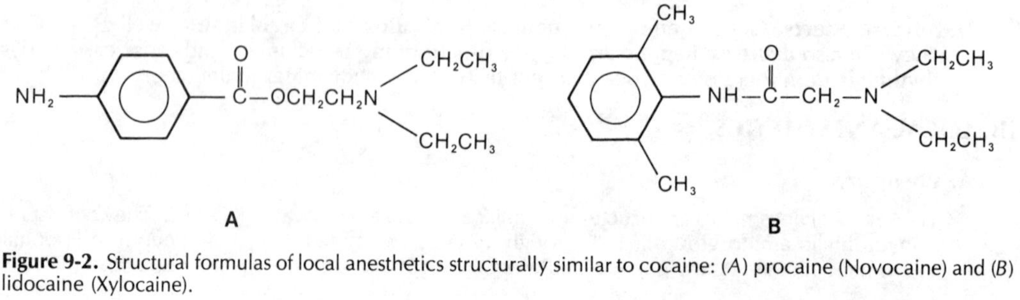

Figure 9-2. Structural formulas of local anesthetics structurally similar to cocaine: (A) procaine (Novocaine) and (B) lidocaine (Xylocaine).

duces vascular blood flow at the administration site. This reduces systemic absorption, prolongs the duration of action, and reduces systemic toxicity.

C. **Therapeutic indications**. Local anesthetics are indicated to:

1. **Produce regional nerve block for the relief of pain**, when injected close to the innervating nerve
2. **Provide anesthesia for minor operations**, when infiltrated around the tissue site
3. **Provide anesthesia for surgery of the lower limbs and pelvis and for obstetric surgery**, when injected into the epidural space or the subarachnoid space of the spinal cord
4. **Provide anesthesia of the skin and mucous membranes**, when applied topically

D. **Adverse effects**

1. **Ester-type local anesthetics** may cause hypersensitivity reactions in susceptible individuals.
2. **Systemic absorption** of toxic concentrations of local anesthetics may cause seizures, CNS depression, respiratory and myocardial depression, and circulatory collapse.

IV. ANTIPSYCHOTICS

A. **Chemistry**

1. The **principal antipsychotics** are phenothiazines, thioxanthenes, and butyrophenones.
2. **Phenothiazines** (e.g., chlorpromazine, triflupromazine, thioridazine, prochlorperazine, trifluoperazine, and fluphenazine) must have a **nitrogen-containing side-chain substituent** on the ring nitrogen for antipsychotic activity (Table 9-1). The ring and side-chain nitrogens must be separated by a **3-carbon chain**; phenothiazines, in which the ring and side-chain nitrogens are separated by a **2-carbon chain**, have antihistaminic or sedative activity only.

Table 9-1. Antipsychotic phenothiazines have the general structure illustrated below. Substituents at the positions marked **X** and **R** result in different drugs.

General Phenothiazine Structure

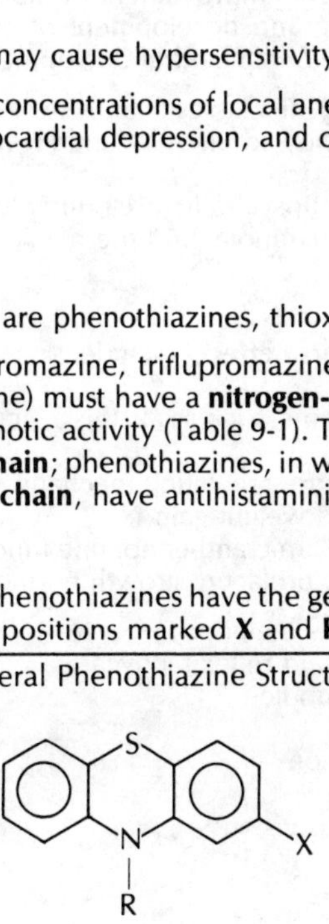

S
N X
R

Drug	X-Substituent	R-Substituent
Chlorpromazine (Thorazine)	—Cl	$-(CH_2)_3-N(CH_3)_2$
Triflupromazine (Vesprin)	$-CF_3$	$-(CH_2)_3-N(CH_3)_2$
Thioridazine (Mellaril)	$-SCH_3$	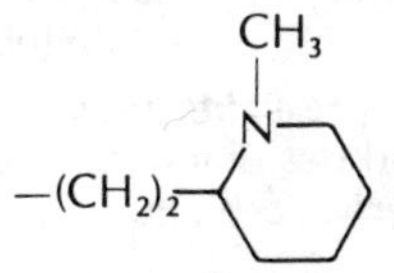 CH_3 N $-(CH_2)_2-$
Prochlorperazine (Compazine)	—Cl	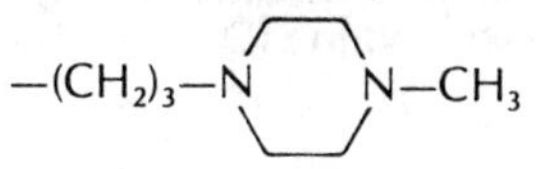 $-(CH_2)_3-N$ $N-CH_3$
Trifluoperazine (Stelazine)	$-CF_3$	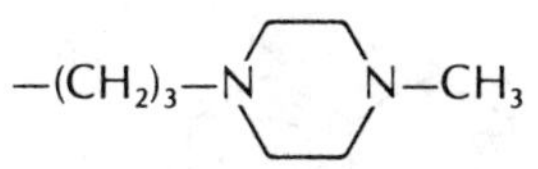 $-(CH_2)_3-N$ $N-CH_3$
Fluphenazine (Prolixin)	$-CF_3$	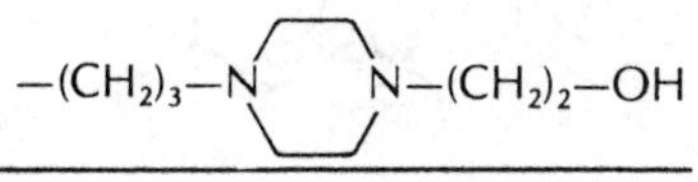 $-(CH_2)_3-N$ $N-(CH_2)_2-OH$

a. The **side chains** are either dimethylaminopropyl, piperazine, or piperidine derivatives. Piperazine side chains confer the greatest potency.
b. The **ring substituent** in position 2 must be electron-attractive for optimum activity. A trifluromethyl substituent confers the greatest activity.

3. **Thioxanthenes** (e.g., chlorprothixene and thiothixene) lack the ring nitrogen of phenothiazines and have a side chain attached by a double bond (Fig. 9-3).

4. **Butyrophenones** (e.g., haloperidol) are chemically unrelated to phenothiazines but have similar activity (Fig. 9-4).

B. Pharmacology

1. Phenothiazines, thioxanthenes, and butyrophenones have similar pharmacologic effects. Their **antipsychotic effects** (improvement of mood and behavior) and their **neuroleptic effects** (emotional quieting and development of extrapyramidal symptoms) appear to result from their ability to antagonize central dopamine-mediated synaptic neurotransmission.

2. Other effects vary among the classes of antipsychotics. These include **antiemetic activity** and **blockade of muscarinic**, **α_1-adrenergic**, and **H_1-histaminergic receptors**.

C. Therapeutic indications.

Antipsychotics are primarily indicated for **treatment of psychosis** associated with schizophrenia, paranoia, and the manic symptoms of manic-depressive illness.

D. Adverse effects

1. **Centrally mediated adverse effects** include:
   a. Drowsiness
   b. Extrapyramidal symptoms, such as akathisia, acute dystonia, akinesia, and tardive dyskinesia
   c. Alteration of temperature-regulating mechanisms, including poikilothermy
   d. Increased appetite and weight gain
   e. Alterations in hypothalamic and endocrine function, such as increased release of corticotropin, gonadotropins, prolactin, growth hormone, and melanocyte-stimulating hormone

2. **Peripheral adverse effects** include:
   a. Postural hypotension and reflex tachycardia
   b. Hepatotoxicity and jaundice
   c. Failure of ejaculation
   d. Bone marrow depression
   e. Photosensitivity
   f. Xerostomia and blurred vision

V. ANTIDEPRESSANTS

A. Chemistry

1. **Antidepressants** are classified into three structurally unrelated groups—the monoamine oxidase (MAO) inhibitors, the tricyclic antidepressants, and the atypical antidepressants.

2. **MAO inhibitors** may be weakly potent **hydrazines** (e.g., phenelzine) or extremely potent **cyclopropylamines** (ring-closed amphetamine derivatives, such as tranylcypromine) [Fig. 9-5].

3. **Tricyclic antidepressants** are secondary or tertiary amine derivatives of **dibenzazepine** (e.g., imipramine and desipramine) or **dibenzocycloheptadiene** (e.g., amitriptyline, nortriptyline, and doxepin) [Figs. 9-6 and 9-7].

4. **Atypical antidepressants** have varied structures. The prototype is a benzotriazole derivative known as **trazodone** (Desyrel) [Fig. 9-8]. Other agents include zimelidine, mianserin, and nomifensine.

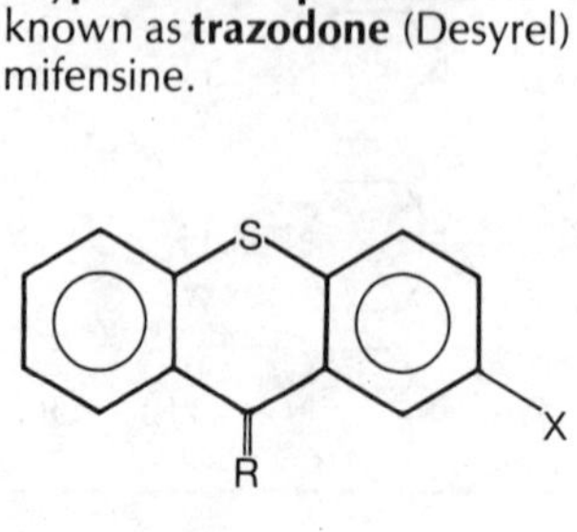

S
X
R

Figure 9-3. Thioxanthenes, similar to phenothiazines, have substituents at *X* and *R* positions that alter drug activity. Chlorprothixene (Taractan) has a—Cl substituent at *X* and the group $-(CH_2)_3-N(CH_3)_2$ at *R*. Thiothixene (Navane) has a $-SO_2N(CH_3)_2$ substituent at *X* and the group:

$(CH_2)_3$—N⟨piperazine⟩N—CH_3 at *R*.

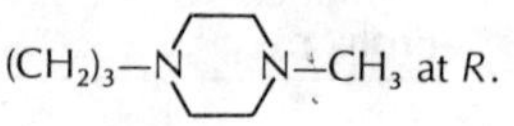

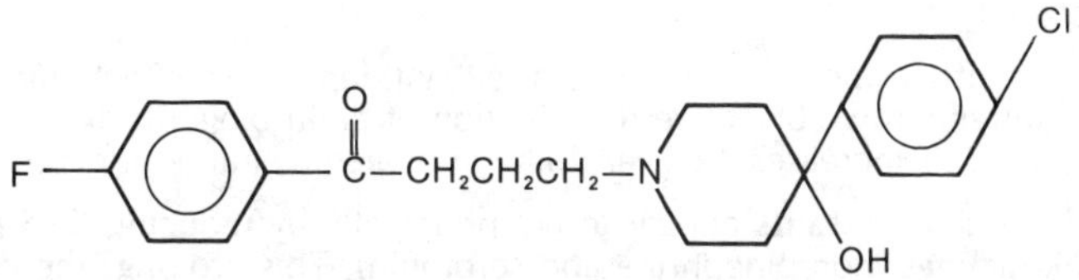

Figure 9-4. Structural formula of haloperidol (Haldol), a butyrophenone antipsychotic.

Figure 9-5. Structural formulas of (*A*) phenelzine (Nardil), a hydrazine derivative monoamine oxidase (MAO) inhibitor, and (*B*) tranylcypromine (Parnate), a cyclopropylamine derivative MAO inhibitor.

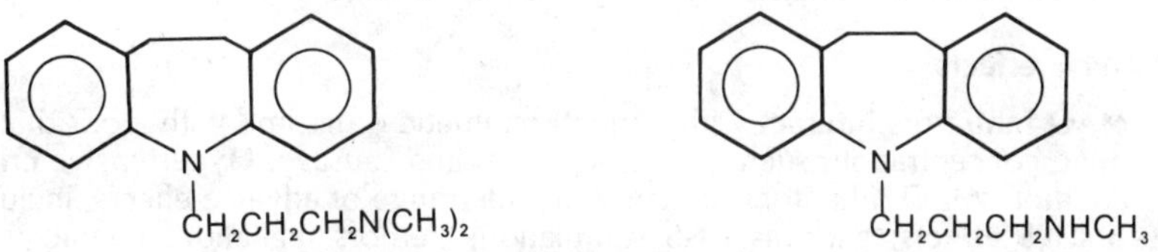

Figure 9-6. Structural formulas of tricyclic antidepressants derived from dibenzazepine: (*A*) imipramine (Tofranil) and (*B*) desipramine (Norpramin).

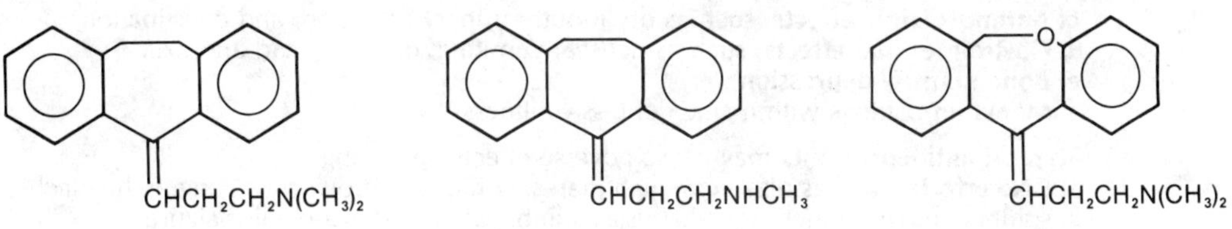

Figure 9-7. Structural formulas of (*A*) amitriptyline (Elavil), (*B*) nortriptyline (Aventyl), and (*C*) doxepin (Sinequan), tricyclic antidepressants derived from dibenzocycloheptadiene.

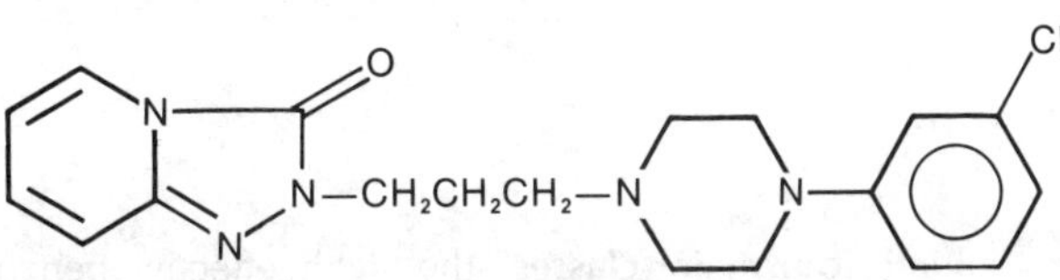

Figure 9-8. Structural formula of trazodone (Desyrel), an atypical antidepressant.

B. Pharmacology

1. **MAO inhibitors** appear to produce their antidepressant effects by blocking the enzyme MAO's intraneuronal oxidative deamination of brain biogenic amines (norepinephrine and serotonin). This increases the availability of biogenic amines at central aminergic receptors.

2. **Tricyclic antidepressants** appear to act principally by reducing CNS neuronal re-uptake of biogenic amines (norepinephrine and serotonin). This prolongs the availability of biogenic amines at central aminergic receptors.

3. **Atypical antidepressants** have varying effects on re-uptake of biogenic amines.
   a. **Trazodone** and **zimelidine** selectively inhibit serotonin re-uptake.
   b. **Mianserin** does not inhibit re-uptake. However, it increases norepinephrine turnover, a response that appears to involve modulation of presynaptic α_2-adrenergic receptors.
   c. **Nomifensine** strongly inhibits re-uptake of both dopamine and norepinephrine.

4. **Other biochemical events** (e.g., the down-regulation of central β-adrenergic and serotoninergic receptors) resulting from chronic inhibition of MAO and re-uptake blockade may also explain the therapeutic action of antidepressants. This explanation is suggested by the latency period of MAO inhibitors, which take 2 to 4 weeks to become effective.

C. Therapeutic indications

1. **MAO inhibitors** are indicated to treat depression, phobic anxiety, and narcolepsy that has not responded to other treatments. However, their use is limited by their adverse effects (see section V D).

2. **Tricyclic** and **atypical antidepressants** are the agents of choice for endogenous depression.

3. The tricyclic **imipramine** is also used to treat enuresis.

D. Adverse effects

1. **MAO inhibitors interact** with sympathomimetic drugs and with foods that have a high tyramine concentration, such as cheese, wine, and sausage. **Hypertensive crisis may result**. In addition, MAO inhibitors can cause a wide range of adverse effects, including:
   a. **CNS effects**, such as CNS stimulation, tremors, agitation, overactivity, hyperreflexia, mania, and insomnia followed by weakness, fatigue, and drowsiness
   b. **Cardiovascular effects**, such as postural hypotension
   c. **Gastrointestinal effects**, such as nausea, abdominal pain, and constipation
   d. **Antimuscarinic effects**, such as dry mouth, urinary retention, and constipation

2. **Tricyclic antidepressants** can cause adverse effects that vary with the drug and may include:
   a. **CNS effects**, such as drowsiness, dizziness, weakness, fatigue, and confusion
   b. **Cardiovascular effects**, such as orthostatic hypotension, tachycardia, and interference with atrioventricular conduction
   c. **Antimuscarinic effects**, such as dry mouth, urinary retention, and constipation
   d. **Gastrointestinal effects**, such as nausea, vomiting, diarrhea, and anorexia
   e. **Bone marrow depression**
   f. **Mania** (in patients with manic-depressive illness)

3. **Atypical antidepressants** may cause adverse effects, including:
   a. **CNS effects**, such as dizziness, nightmares, confusion, drowsiness, fatigue, headache, insomnia, impaired memory, akathisia, numbness, and tonic–clonic seizures
   b. **Cardiovascular effects**, such as hypertension, hypotension, tachycardia, chest pain, and syncope
   c. **Gastrointestinal effects**, such as nausea, vomiting, diarrhea, and constipation
   d. **Blurred vision** and **tinnitus**
   e. **Antimuscarinic effects**, such as urinary retention, dry mouth, and constipation
   f. **Bone marrow depression**
   g. **Priapism** and **menstrual irregularities**

VI. ANXIOLYTICS

A. Chemistry

1. Anxiolytics fall into **four major classes**—the highly effective benzodiazepines and azaspirodecanediones and the less effective propanediol carbamates and diphenylmethanes.

2. Benzodiazepines (e.g., chlordiazepoxide, diazepam, halazepam, oxazepam, lorazepam, and alprazolam) have varying durations of action, which can be correlated with their structures in some cases (Table 9-2).
   a. **Agents with a 3-hydroxyl group** are easily metabolized by phase-II glucuronidation and are **short acting**.
   b. **Agents lacking a 3-hydroxyl group** must undergo considerable phase-I metabolism, including 3-hydroxylation. These agents are **long acting**. Most long-acting agents form the intermediate metabolite desmethyldiazepam, which has a very long half-life. Thus, these agents may have **cumulative action**.
   c. **Triazolobenzodiazepines** undergo a different pattern of metabolism and are **intermediate in activity**.
   d. **Agents lacking an amino side chain** are not basic enough to form water-soluble salts with acids. For example, intravenous (IV) solutions of diazepam contain propylene glycol as a solvent. **Precipitation may occur** if these solutions are mixed with aqueous solutions.
3. **Azaspirodecanediones** (e.g., buspirone) have anxiolytic activity resembling that of the benzodiazepines. However, these agents lack other CNS depressant activity (Fig. 9-9).
4. **Propanediol carbamates** (e.g., meprobamate) and **diphenylmethanes** (e.g., hydroxyzine) **are used much less commonly** than the benzodiazepines for treatment of anxiety (Fig. 9-10).

B. **Pharmacology**

1. **Benzodiazepines** appear to produce their calming effects by depressing the limbic system and reticular formation through potentiation of the inhibitor neurotransmitter gamma-aminobutyric acid (GABA).

Table 9-2. Benzodiazepine anxiolytics have the general structure shown below. Substituents at the positions marked $\mathbf{R_1}$, $\mathbf{R_2}$, $\mathbf{R_3}$, $\mathbf{R_4}$ and **X** result in different drugs.

General Benzodiazepine Structure

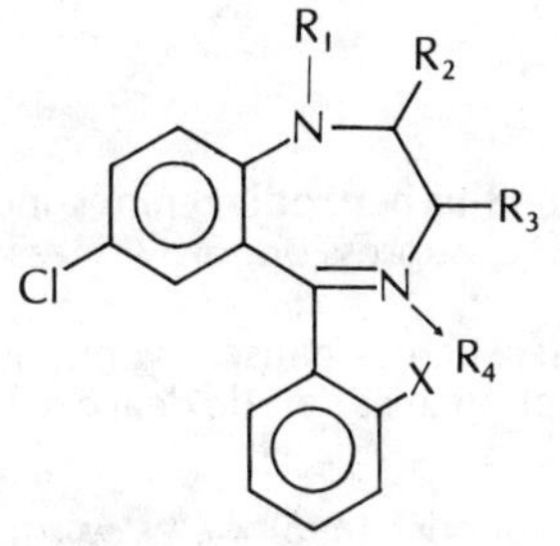

R_1 R_2 N R_3 Cl N R_4 X

Drug	R_1-Substituent	R_2-Substituent	R_3-Substituent	R_4-Substituent	X-Substituent
Chlordiazepoxide (Librium)	=	$-NHCH_3$	. . .	=O	. . .
Diazepam (Valium)	$-CH_3$	=O	. . .	. . .	. . .
Halazepam (Paxipam)	$-CH_2CF_3$	=O	. . .	. . .	. . .
Oxazepam (Serax)	—H	=O	—OH	. . .	. . .
Lorazepam (Ativan)	—H	=O	—OH	. . .	—Cl
Alprazolam (Xanax)	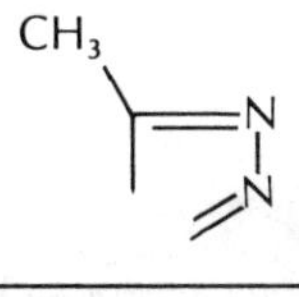 CH_3 =N N		. . .	. . .	. . .

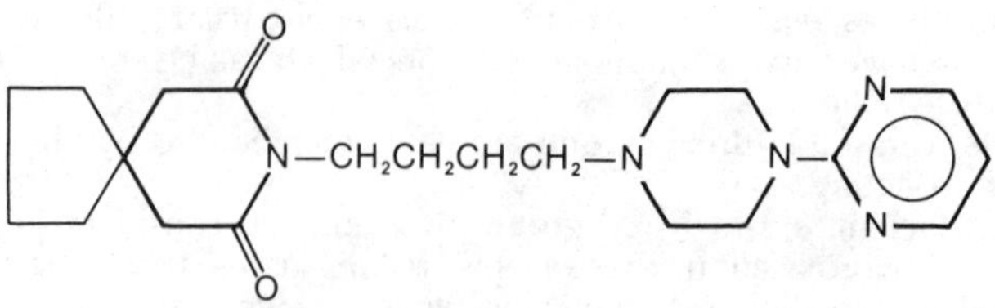

Figure 9-9. Structural formula of buspirone (Buspar), the prototypical azaspirodecanedione anxiolytic.

a. **Anxiolytic activity** correlates with the drug's binding affinity to a macromolecular GABA-chloride ionophore receptor complex.
b. **Hypnotic and anticonvulsant properties** also exist (see sections VII and VIII).
c. Benzodiazepines **increase the depressant effects of alcohol and other CNS depressant drugs**.

2. The azaspirodecanedione **buspirone** has an unknown mechanism of action.
   a. Buspirone **binds to central dopamine and serotonic receptors** rather than to GABA-chloride ionophore receptor complexes.
   b. It possesses **no hypnotic or anticonvulsant properties** and appears **not to add to the depressant effects of alcohol or other CNS depressant drugs**.

C. Therapeutic indications

1. Benzodiazepines and the azaspirodecanedione buspirone are indicated to **treat anxiety**.
2. Benzodiazepines are also indicated for use as a **preanesthetic medication** (see sections II A 2 and C 2), as **sedative–hypnotics** (see section VII), as **anticonvulsants** (see section VIII), and during **acute alcohol withdrawal**.

D. Adverse effects

1. Adverse effects associated with **benzodiazepines** include:
   a. **CNS effects**, such as CNS depression, drowsiness, sedation, ataxia, confusion, and dysarthria
   b. **Gastrointestinal effects**, such as nausea, vomiting, and diarrhea
   c. **Psychiatric effects** (rare), such as paradoxical excitement, insomnia, paranoia, and rage reactions
2. Adverse effects of the azaspirodecanedione **buspirone** are limited to **restlessness**, **dizziness**, **headache**, **nausea**, **diarrhea**, and **paresthesias**. However, **tardive dyskinesia** is possible with long-term therapy.
3. The benzodiazepines have **abuse potential** and may cause **dependence**.

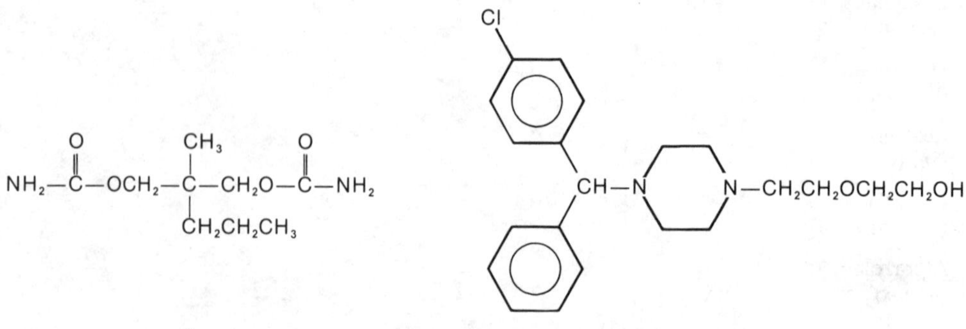

A

B

Figure 9-10. Structural formulas of (*A*) meprobamate (Miltown, Equanil), a propanediol carbamate anxiolytic, and (*B*) hydroxyzine (Atarax, Vistaril), a diphenylmethane anxiolytic.

VII. SEDATIVE–HYPNOTICS

A. Chemistry

1. **Sedatives** are principally long-acting or intermediate-acting barbiturates (e.g., phenobarbital and amobarbital), whereas **hypnotics** may be the widely used benzodiazepines (e.g., flurazepam and alprazolam), short-acting barbiturates (e.g., pentobarbital and secobarbital), piperidinediones (e.g., glutethimide), or aldehydes (e.g., chloral hydrate).
2. **Barbiturates** are 5,5-disubstituted derivatives of barbituric acid, a saturated triketopyramidine (Table 9-3).
   a. **Two side chains in position 5** are essential for sedative–hypnotic activity.
   b. Long-acting agents have **a phenyl and an ethyl group in position 5**.
   c. **Branched side chains, unsaturated side chains,** or **side chains longer than an ethyl group** tend to increase lipophilicity and metabolism rate. Increased lipophilicity leads to a shorter onset of action, a shorter duration of action, and increased potency.
   d. **Replacement of the position-2 oxygen with sulfur** produces an extremely lipophilic molecule that distributes rapidly into lipid tissues outside the brain.
      (1) These **ultra-short-acting barbiturates** are not useful as sedative–hypnotics but do act as effective induction anesthetics (see section II A 2). The action of these drugs is terminated very quickly.
      (2) The prototype ultra-short-acting barbiturate is **thiopental** (Pentothal), the 2-thio isostere of pentobarbital.
   e. The barbiturates and many of their metabolites are **weak acids**, and changes in urinary pH greatly influence their excretion. This is particularly true with overdoses, when a relatively large amount of unchanged drug appears in the glomerular filtrate.
   f. **Phenobarbital** is one of the most powerful and versatile enzyme-inducing agents known. Other barbiturates have less enzyme-inducing effect, except when they are used continuously in higher-than-normal doses.

Table 9-3. Barbiturate sedative–hypnotics have the general structure shown below. Substituents at $\mathbf{R_1}$ and $\mathbf{R_2}$ positions result in different drugs with different durations of action.

General Barbiturate Structure

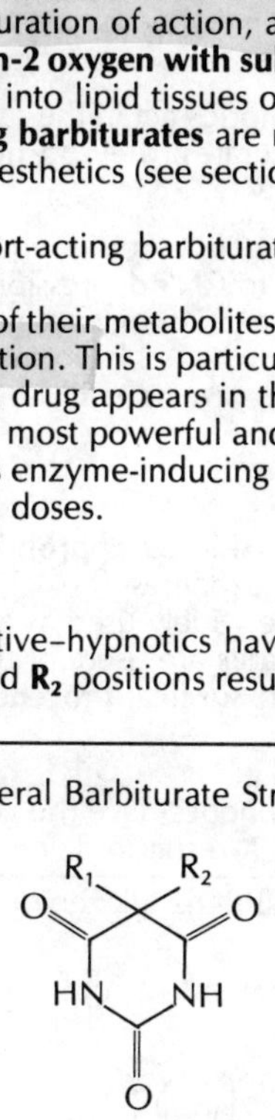

R1, R2, O, O, HN, NH, O

Drug	R_1-Substituent	R_2-Substituent	Duration of Action
Phenobarbital (Luminal)	$-CH_2CH_3$	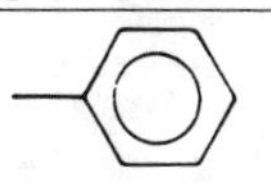 $-C_6H_5$	Long
Amobarbital (Amytal)	$-CH_2CH_3$	$-CH_2CH_2CH_2CH(CH_3)_2$	Intermediate
Butabarbital (Butisol)	$-CH_2CH_3$	$-\underset{\displaystyle CH_3}{\underset{\vert}{C}}HCH_2CH_3$	Intermediate
Pentobarbital (Nembutal)	$-CH_2CH_3$	$-\underset{\displaystyle CH_3}{\underset{\vert}{C}}HCH_2CH_2CH_2CH_3$	Short
Secobarbital (Seconal)	$-CH_2CH\ \ CH_2$	$-\underset{\displaystyle CH_3}{\underset{\vert}{C}}HCH_2CH_2CH_2CH_3$	Short

3. **Benzodiazepine sedative–hypnotics** (e.g., flurazepam, triazolam, and temazepam) have varying durations of action depending on their structures, as is true for the benzodiazepine anxiolytics (Table 9-4). (See also section VI A 2 and Table 9-2.)

4. **Piperidinediones** (e.g., glutethimide) and **aldehydes** (e.g., chloral hydrate) are used less commonly than benzodiazepines as sedative–hypnotics (Fig. 9-11).

B. Pharmacology

1. **Barbiturates** are less selective than benzodiazepines and produce generalized CNS depression.
   a. The barbiturates' **mechanism of action** is unclear. However, barbiturate binding sites have been identified on a macromolecular GABA-chloride ionophore receptor complex, and **barbiturates appear to mimic or enhance GABA's inhibitory actions**.
   b. Barbiturates have a **wide range of dose-dependent pharmacologic actions related to CNS depression**, including sedation, hypnosis, and anesthesia. They also act as potent respiratory depressants and as inducers of hepatic microsomal drug-metabolizing enzyme activity.

2. **Benzodiazepine sedative–hypnotics** act in the same way as benzodiazepine anxiolytics (see section VI B 1). Unlike barbiturates, they do not significantly induce hepatic microsomal drug-metabolizing enzyme activity.

3. **Piperidinediones, aldehydes**, and other nonbarbiturate sedative–hypnotics have similar pharmacologic actions related to CNS depression.
   a. Only **chloral hydrate** is a drug of choice to induce sleep in pediatric or geriatric patients.
   b. Chloral hydrate's activity is mediated by formation of the active metabolite **trichloroethanol**. Chloral hydrate induces hepatic microsomal drug-metabolizing enzyme activity.

C. Therapeutic indications

1. **Barbiturates are no longer considered appropriate as sedative–hypnotics**, in view of the availability of the safer benzodiazepines.
   a. **Long-acting barbiturates** are widely used as **antiepileptics** (see section VIII).
   b. **Ultra-short-acting barbiturates** are used for the **induction of general anesthesia and as general anesthetics for short surgical procedures** (see sections II A 2 and C 2).

Table 9-4. Benzodiazepine sedative–hypnotics have the general structure shown below. Substituents at the positions marked $\mathbf{R_1}$, $\mathbf{R_2}$, $\mathbf{R_3}$, and **X** result in different drugs with different durations of action.

General Benzodiazepine Structure

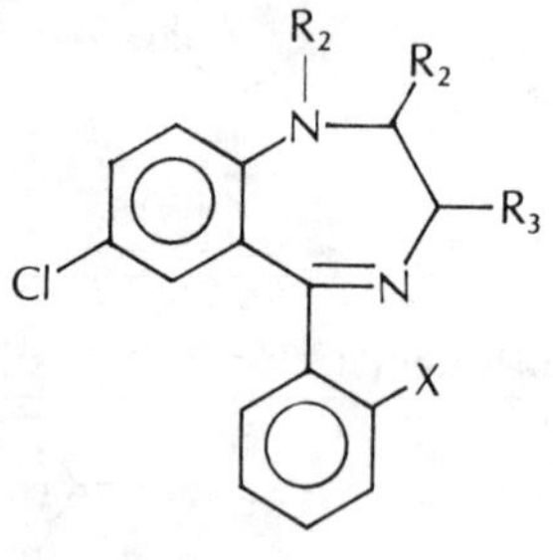

Drug	R_1-Substituent	R_2-Substituent	R_3-Substituent	X-Substituent	Duration of Action
Flurazepam (Dalmane)	$-CH_2CH_2N(CH_3)_2$	$=O$	$-H$	$-F$	Long
Triazolam (Halcion)	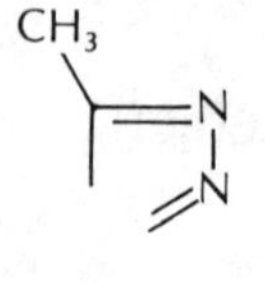	CH_3	$-H$	$-Cl$	Intermediate
Temazepam (Restoril)	$-CH_3$	$=O$	$-OH$	$-H$	Short

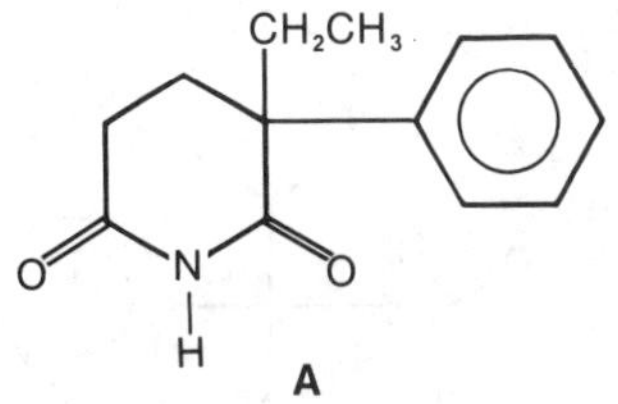

CH$_2$CH$_3$ ... O N O H

A

$Cl_3C{-}CH(OH)_2$

B

Figure 9-11. Structural formulas of (*A*) glutethimide (Doriden), a piperidinedione sedative–hypnotic, and (*B*) chloral hydrate (Noctec), an aldehyde sedative–hypnotic.

2. **Benzodiazepines** are indicated **to produce drowsiness and promote sleep**. They are also indicated for use as a preanesthetic medication (see sections II A 2 and C 2), as anticonvulsants (see section VIII), as anxiolytics (see section VI), and during acute alcohol withdrawal.

3. **Chloral hydrate** is indicated for use as a **pediatric or geriatric hypnotic**.

D. Adverse effects

1. **Barbiturates** may cause a wide variety of adverse effects, including:
   a. **CNS effects**, such as drowsiness, confusion, nystagmus, dysarthria, depressed sympathetic ganglionic transmission, hyperalgesia, impaired judgment, impaired fine motor skills, paradoxic excitement (in geriatic patients), and potentiation of other CNS depressant drugs
   b. **Respiratory and cardiovascular effects**, such as respiratory depression, bradycardia, and orthostatic hypotension
   c. **Gastrointestinal effects**, such as nausea, vomiting, constipation, diarrhea, and epigastric distress
   d. **Exfoliative dermatitis** and **Stevens-Johnson syndrome**
   e. **Headache**, **fever**, **hepatotoxicity**, and **megaloblastic anemia** (with the chronic use of phenobarbital)

2. **Benzodiazepine sedative–hypnotics** have the same adverse effects as benzodiazepine anxiolytics (see section VI D 1).

3. **Chloral hydrate's** adverse effects include:
   a. **Gastrointestinal effects**, such as gastrointestinal irritation and upset, nausea, and vomiting
   b. **CNS effects**, such as CNS depression, disorientation, incoherence, drowsiness, ataxia, headache, and potentiation of other CNS depressants (particularly alcohol)
   c. **Leukopenia**

4. Sedative–hypnotics have **abuse potential** and may cause **dependence**.

VIII. ANTIEPILEPTICS

A. Chemistry

1. Antiepileptics (anticonvulsants) **vary widely in structure** (Fig. 9-12).

2. **Older agents**, which are still widely used, include derivatives of the **long-acting barbiturates** (e.g., phenobarbital and primidone), the **hydantoins** (e.g., phenytoin), the **succinimides** (e.g., ethosuximide), and the **oxazolidinediones** (e.g., trimethadione).

3. **Newer agents**, which are more structurally diverse, include derivatives of the **dibenzazepines** (e.g., carbamazepine), the **benzodiazepines** (e.g., clonazepam), the **dialkylacetates** (e.g., valproic acid), and others.

B. Pharmacology

1. Antiepileptics **prevent or reduce excessive discharge** and **reduce the spread of excitation from CNS seizure foci**.

2. The **mechanisms of action** of antiepileptics appear to be alteration of sodium ion neuronal

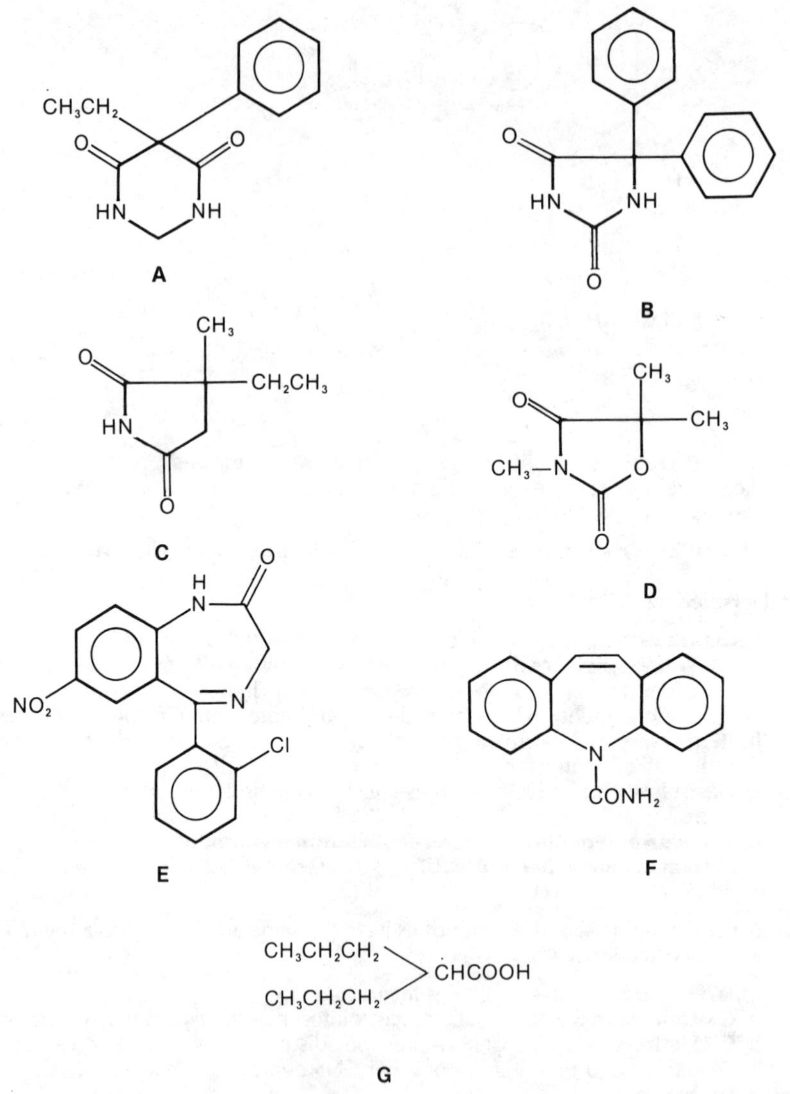

A

B

C

D

E

F

G

Figure 9-12. Structural formulas of the antiepileptic agents: (*A*) primidone (Mysoline), (*B*) phenytoin (Dilantin), (*C*) ethosuximide (Zarontin), (*D*) trimethadione (Tridione), (*E*) clonazepam (Clonopin), (*F*) carbamazepine (Tegretol), and (*G*) valproic acid (Depakene).

concentrations by promotion of sodium efflux (the hydantoins) and restoration or enhancement of GABA-ergic inhibitory neuronal function (the barbiturates, the benzodiazepines, and valproic acid).

C. Therapeutic indications

1. **Phenytoin**, **carbamazepine**, **phenobarbital**, and **primidone** are indicated for treatment of **tonic–clonic** (grand mal) **seizures**.
2. **Ethosuximide**, **valproic acid**, and **clonazepam** are indicated for treatment of **absence** (petit mal) **seizures**.
3. **Clonazepam** is indicated for treatment of **myoclonic seizures**.
4. **IV diazepam**, **phenytoin**, and **phenobarbital** are indicated for treatment of **status epilepticus**.

D. Adverse effects

1. **Barbiturate antiepileptics** have the same adverse effects as barbiturate sedative–hypnotics

(see section VII D 1). **IV use of barbiturates** may cause **cardiovascular collapse** and **respiratory depression**.

2. **Hydantoins** are associated with these adverse effects:
   a. **Gastrointestinal effects**, such as gastrointestinal irritation, nausea, and vomiting
   b. **CNS effects**, such as nystagmus, diplopia, and ataxia
   c. **Blood dyscrasias**, **osteoporosis**, and **gingival hyperplasia**
   d. **Stevens-Johnson syndrome**
   e. **Cardiovascular collapse** and **respiratory depression** (with IV administration)
3. **Succinimides** are associated with these adverse effects:
   a. **Gastrointestinal effects**, such as gastrointestinal irritation, nausea, and vomiting
   b. **CNS effects**, such as CNS depression, drowsiness, headache, and confusion
   c. **Blood dyscrasias**
   d. **Stevens-Johnson syndrome**
4. **Dibenzazepines** are associated with these adverse effects:
   a. **Gastrointestinal effects**, such as nausea and vomiting
   b. **CNS effects**, such as drowsiness and dizziness
   c. **Blood dyscrasias**, such as aplastic anemia
   d. **Renal failure**, **hepatotoxicity**, and **congestive heart failure**
   e. **Stevens-Johnson syndrome**
5. **Benzodiazepine antiepileptics** have the same adverse effects as benzodiazepine anxiolytics (see section VI D 1). **IV administration** may cause **cardiovascular collapse** and **respiratory depression**.
6. **Dialkylacetates** are associated with these adverse effects:
   a. **Gastrointestinal effects**, such as gastrointestinal irritation, nausea, and vomiting
   b. **CNS effects**, such as sedation, headache, ataxia, and dysarthria
   c. **Pancreatitis**, **hepatotoxicity**, **prolonged bleeding time**, and **blood dyscrasias**

IX. ANTIPARKINSONIAN AGENTS

A. **Chemistry**. The principal antiparkinsonian agents are structurally related to atropine (e.g., **benztropine** and **trihexyphenidyl**), to the antihistamines (e.g., **ethopropazine** and **orphenadrine**), or to the catecholamines (e.g., **levodopa**) [Fig. 9-13].

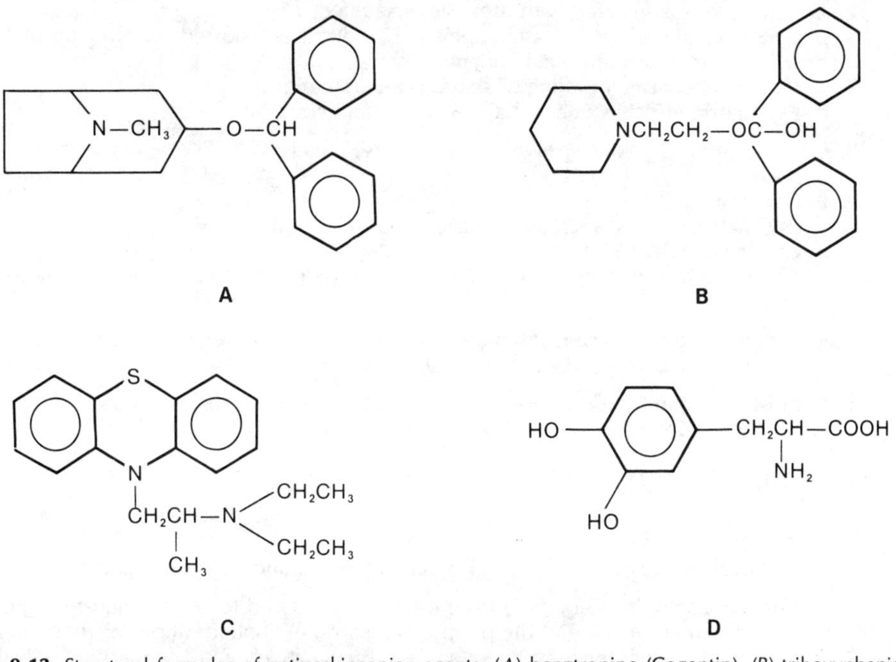

Figure 9-13. Structural formulas of antiparkinsonian agents: (*A*) benztropine (Cogentin), (*B*) trihexyphenidyl (Artane), (*C*) ethopropazine (Parsidol), and (*D*) levodopa (Larodopa).

B. Pharmacology. Antiparkinsonian agents act by **restoring the striatal balance of dopaminergic and cholinergic neurotransmitters**, which are disturbed in parkinsonism.

1. **Levodopa**, which can cross the blood–brain barrier, is the immediate precursor of the striatal inhibitory neurotransmitter dopamine and is converted to dopamine in the body.
2. **Amantadine**, an antiviral agent, appears to stimulate the release of dopamine from intact striatal dopaminergic terminals.
3. **Bromocriptine**, a dopaminergic receptor agonist, mimics the activity of striatal dopamine.
4. Anticholinergics such as **trihexyphenidyl** and **benztropine** block the excitatory cholinergic striatal system.
5. Antihistamines such as **diphenhydramine** possess anticholinergic properties.

C. Therapeutic indications

1. **Levodopa** is indicated to treat idiopathic, postencephalitic, or arteriosclerotic parkinsonism.
2. **Amantadine** is indicated to treat idiopathic, postencephalitic, or arteriosclerotic parkinsonism, as well as extrapyramidal symptoms induced by antipsychotic drugs (with the exception of tardive dyskinesia).
3. **Bromocriptine is indicated to treat idiopathic or postencephalitic parkinsonism.**
4. **Anticholinergics and antihistamines** are indicated for use as adjunctive therapy for all types of parkinsonism, including drug-induced extrapyramidal symptoms (with the exception of tardive dyskinesia).

D. Adverse effects

1. **Levodopa is associated with these adverse effects:**
   a. **Gastrointestinal effects**, such as gastrointestinal upset, nausea, vomiting, anorexia, and excessive salivation
   b. **Cardiovascular effects**, such as orthostatic hypotension, tachycardia, and dysrhythmias
   c. **CNS effects**, such as headache, dizziness, and insomnia
   d. **Abnormal involuntary movements**, such as dyskinesia and choreiform or dystonic movements
   e. **Psychiatric effects**, such as delusions, hallucinations, confusion, psychoses, and depression
2. **Amantadine** is associated with these adverse effects:
   a. **CNS effects**, such as drowsiness, insomnia, dizziness, slurred speech, and nightmares
   b. **Urinary retention** and **ankle edema**
   c. **Livedo reticularis** (mottling of skin on the extremities)
   d. **Psychiatric effects**, such as hallucinations and confusion
3. **Bromocriptine** is associated with these adverse effects:
   a. **Nausea**
   b. **Hypotension**
   c. **Psychiatric effects**, such as confusion and hallucinations
   d. **Livedo reticularis**
   e. **Abnormal involuntary movements**, such as dyskinesia and choreiform or dystonic movements
4. **Anticholinergic antiparkinsonian agents** have the same adverse effects as other cholinergic antagonists (see Chapter 8, section III D).
5. **Antihistaminic antiparkinsonian agents** have the same adverse effects as other antihistamines (see Chapter 10, section II A).

X. OPIOID ANALGESICS

A. Chemistry

1. Opioid analgesics consist of **natural opiate alkaloids** and their **synthetic derivatives**.
2. The opiate alkaloids are derived from **opium**, considered to be the oldest drug on record. Opium (the dried exudate of the poppy seed capsule) contains about 25 different alkaloids. Of these, **morphine** is the most important both quantitatively and pharmacologically (Fig. 9-14).
   a. The **morphine molecule** can be altered in a variety of ways; related compounds may also be synthesized from other starting materials.

Figure 9-14. Structural formula of morphine.

b. Morphine's **phenolic OH group** is extremely important; however, analgesic activity appears to depend on a *p*-**phenyl-N-alkylpiperidine moiety**, in which the piperidine ring is in the chair form and is perpendicular to the aromatic ring. The alkyl group is usually methyl. Morphine's amphoteric character (phenolic OH and tertiary amine) contributes to its erratic absorption when administered orally.

c. The **piperidine moiety** of morphine is common to most opioid analgesics, including the **morphine analogues** (e.g., codeine, heroin, hydromorphone, oxycodone, and others), and the **piperidines** (meperidine, diphenoxylate, and others). The **methadones** (e.g., methadone and propoxyphene) appear to assume a pseudopiperidine ring configuration in the body (Fig. 9-15).

B. Pharmacology

1. Opioid analgesics **mimic endogenous enkephalins and endorphins at CNS opiate receptors**, raising the pain threshold and increasing pain tolerance.

2. Opioid analgesics also **cause chemoreceptor trigger zone stimulation** and **decrease α-adrenergic receptor responsiveness**.

C. Therapeutic indications. Opioid analgesics are indicated to **relieve moderate-to-severe pain**, such as the pain associated with myocardial infarction. They are also used as **preanesthetic medications**, as **analgesic adjuncts during anesthesia**, as **antitussives**, and as **antidiarrheals**.

D. Adverse effects. Opioid analgesics are associated with these adverse effects:

1. **CNS effects**, including CNS depression, miosis, dizziness, sedation, confusion, disorientation, and coma

2. **Gastrointestinal effects**, including nausea, vomiting, constipation, biliary spasm, and increased biliary tract pressure

3. **Cardiovascular effects**, such as orthostatic hypotension, peripheral circulatory collapse, dysrhythmias, and cardiac arrest

4. **Respiratory depression**

5. **Bronchoconstriction**

6. **Psychiatric effects**, such as euphoria, dysphoria, and hallucinations

7. **Abuse potential** and **dependence**

8. **Precipitation of withdrawal symptoms in opioid-dependent patients** (when opioid agonist–antagonists, such as pentazocine or nalbuphine, are used as analgesics)

XI. OPIOID ANTAGONISTS

A. Chemistry. Replacement of the N-methyl group of morphine or a morphine derivative (see section X A 2) with an allyl or cycloalkyl group results in drugs that are **pure opioid antagonists** (e.g., naloxone and naltrexone) or **mixed opioid agonists–antagonists** (e.g., pentazocine and butorphanol) [Fig. 9-16].

B. Pharmacology

1. The pure opioid antagonist **naloxone** reverses or prevents the effects of opioids but has no opioid-receptor agonist activity.

2. The mixed opioid agonist–antagonist **pentazocine** has both opioid agonistic actions (e.g., analgesia, sedation, and respiratory depression) and weak opioid antagonistic activity.

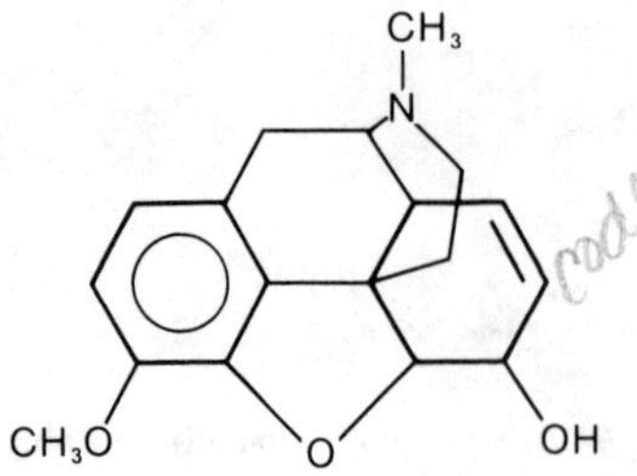

A

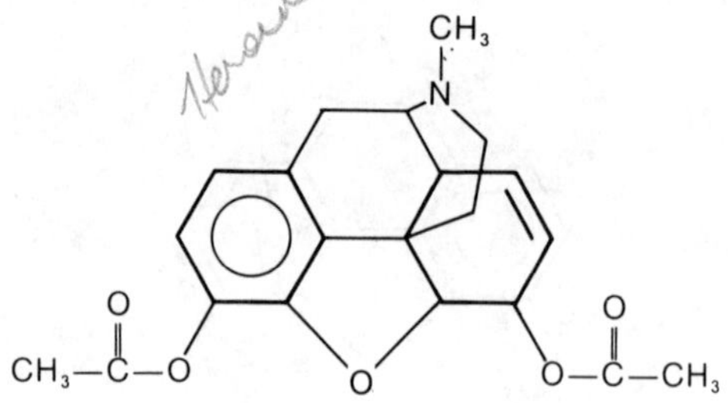

B

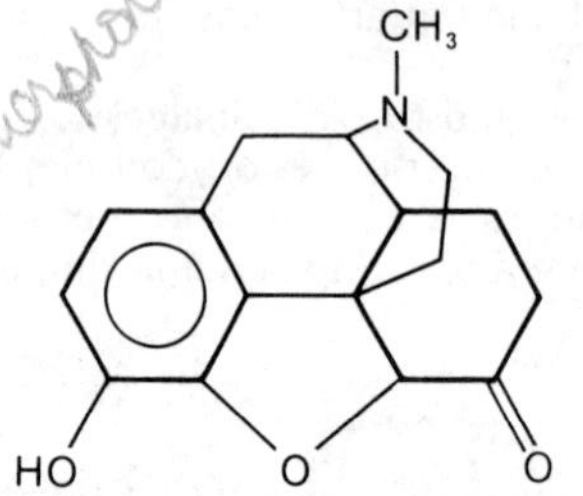

C

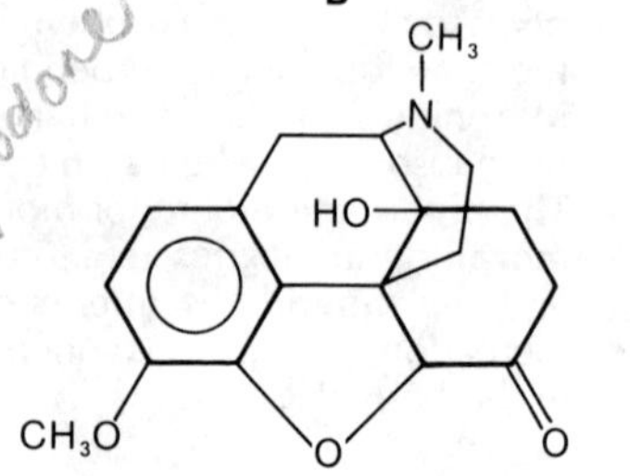

D

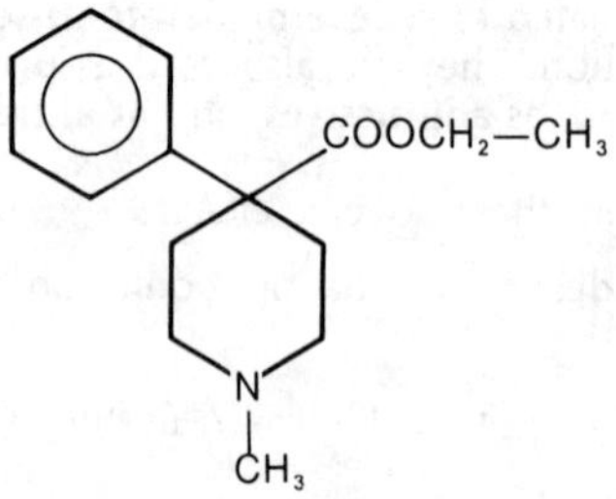

E

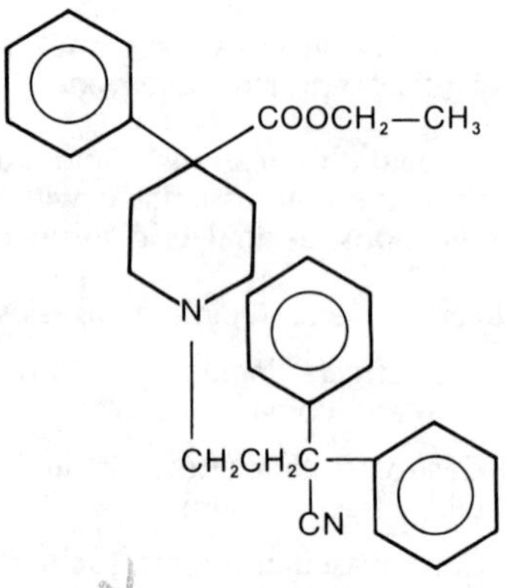

F

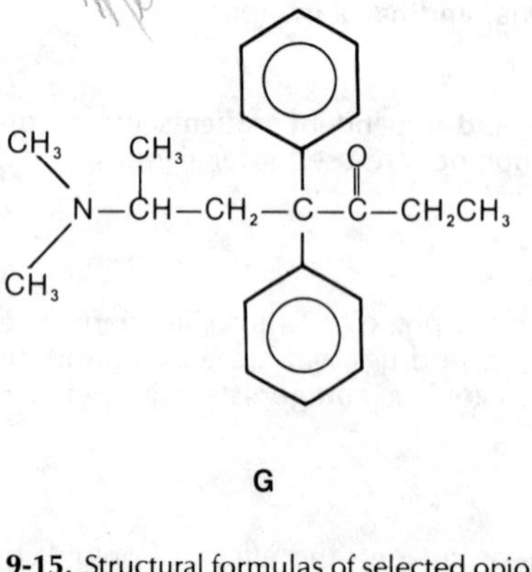

G

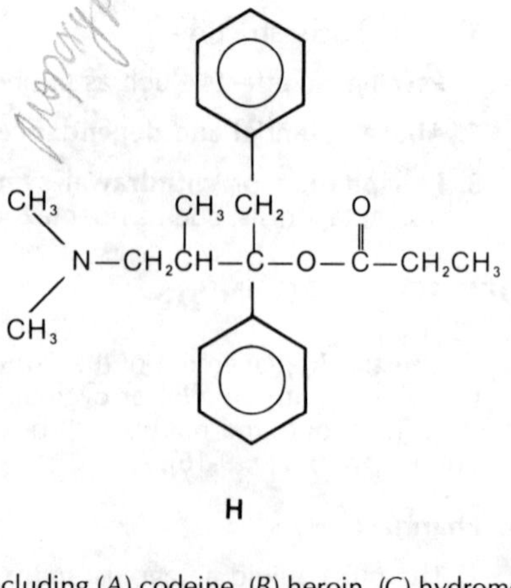

H

Figure 9-15. Structural formulas of selected opioid agonists, including (*A*) codeine, (*B*) heroin, (*C*) hydromorphone (Dilaudid), and (*D*) oxycodone (Percodan), morphine analogues; (*E*) meperidine (Demerol) and (*F*) diphenoxylate (Lomotil), piperidine analgesics; and (*G*) methadone (Dolophine) and (*H*) propoxyphene (Darvon), methadone analgesics.

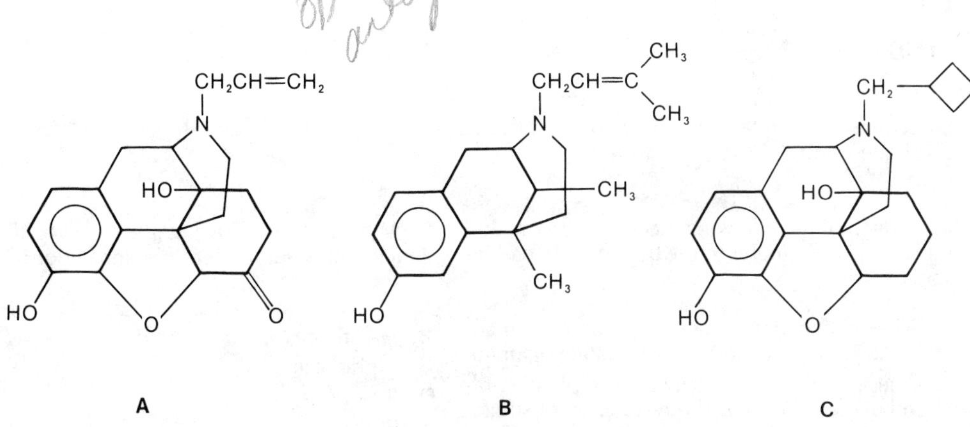

Figure 9-16. Structural formulas of opioid antagonists: (*A*) naloxone (Narcan), (*B*) pentazocine (Talwin), and (*C*) butorphanol (Stadol).

C. Therapeutic indications

1. **Pure opioid antagonists** are used as antidotes to reverse the adverse effects of opioid agonists (e.g., respiratory depression, cardiovascular depression, and sedation).
2. The **mixed agonist–antagonists** are used as analgesics.

D. Adverse effects

1. **Pure opioid antagonists** can precipitate withdrawal syndrome in opioid-dependent patients.
2. In the absence of opioids, **mixed agonist–antagonists** will produce opioid-like effects, such as respiratory depression (see section X D).

STUDY QUESTIONS

Directions: Each question below contains five suggested answers. Choose the **one best** response to each question.

1. Which of the following mechanisms of action most likely contributes to the treatment of parkinsonism?

A. The direct-acting dopaminergic agonist amantadine mimics the activity of striatal dopamine
B. The antimuscarinic activity of diphenhydramine contributes to the restoration of striatal dopaminergic–cholinergic neurotransmitter balance
C. Striatal H_1 receptors are blocked by the antihistaminic trihexyphenidyl
D. The ergoline bromocriptine stimulates the release of striatal dopamine from intact terminals
E. The ability of dopamine to cross the blood–brain barrier allows it to restore striatal dopaminergic–cholinergic neurotransmitter balance

2. Opioids are used as all of the following agents EXCEPT

A. antitussives
B. analgesics
C. anti-inflammatories
D. antidiarrheals
E. preanesthetic medications

3. All of the following adverse effects are associated with the use of levodopa EXCEPT

A. sialorrhea
B. orthostatic hypotension
C. delusions, confusion, and depression
D. dyskinesia and dystonia
E. livedo reticularis

4. The activity of which of the following drugs is dependent upon a *p*-phenyl-*N*-alkylpiperidine moiety?

A. Phenobarbital
B. Chlorpromazine
C. Diazepam
D. Imipramine
E. Meperidine

5. Which of the following drugs is a volatile substance that is administered by inhalation?

A. Thiopental
B. Halothane
C. Alprazolam
D. Buspirone
E. Phenytoin

6. The brief duration of action of an ultra-short-acting barbiturate is due to a

A. slow rate of metabolism in the liver
B. low lipid solubility, resulting in a minimal concentration in the brain
C. high degree of binding to plasma proteins
D. rapid rate of redistribution from the brain due to its high liposolubility
E. slow rate of excretion by the kidneys

7. The structure of the drug prochlorperazine is shown below. Which of the following medications, because of its chemical relationship to prochlorperazine, would most likely cause similar side effects?

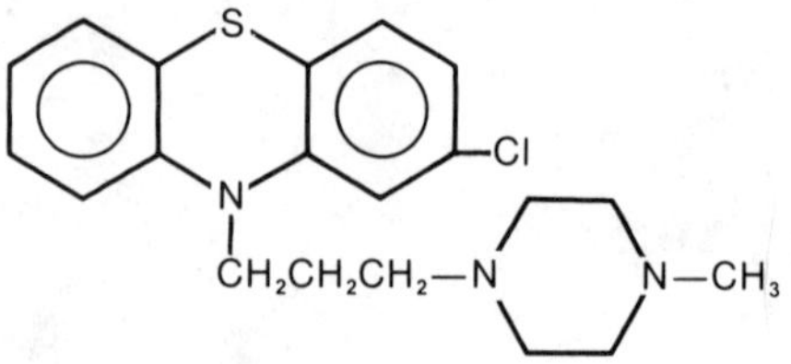

S
Cl
N
$CH_2CH_2CH_2$—N N—CH_3

A. Fluphenazine
B. Thioridazine
C. Alprazolam
D. Buspirone
E. Pentobarbital

Directions: Each question below contains three suggested answers of which **one or more** is correct. Choose the answer

A if **I only** is correct
B if **III only** is correct
C if **I and II** are correct
D if **II and III** are correct
E if **I, II, and III** are correct

8. Improper administration of local anesthetics can cause toxic plasma concentrations that may result in

I. seizures and central nervous system depression
II. respiratory and myocardial depression
III. circulatory collapse

9. In addition to their anxiolytic properties, benzodiazepines are indicated for use

I. as preanesthetic medications
II. as anticonvulsants
III. during acute withdrawal from alcohol

Directions: The groups of questions below consist of lettered choices followed by several numbered items. For each numbered item select the **one** lettered choice with which it is **most** closely associated. Each lettered choice may be used once, more than once, or not at all.

Questions 10–12

For each statement below, choose the drug that it most closely describes.

A. Tranylcypromine
B. Imipramine
C. Buspirone
D. Trazodone
E. Phenelzine

10. An anxiolytic drug that does not possess either hypnotic or anticonvulsant properties

11. A prototype tricyclic antidepressant with antimuscarinic properties that make it useful in the treatment of enuresis

12. An antidepressant that inhibits serotonin reuptake and may cause adverse effects such as impaired memory, akathisia, and menstrual irregularities

Questions 13–15

For each of the following structures, select the most appropriate pharmacologic category.

A. General anesthetic
B. Local anesthetic
C. Antidepressant
D. Anxiolytic
E. Opioid antagonist

13.

NH_2 —(benzene ring)— $COOCH_2CH_2N(CH_2CH_3)_2$

14.

CH_3 O N Cl N

15.

N
$CH_2CH_2CH_2NH-CH_3$

ANSWERS AND EXPLANATIONS

1. The answer is B. (*IX B*) The H_1 antagonist diphenhydramine possesses antimuscarinic activity, which allows it to be of use in the restoration of striatal dopaminergic–cholinergic neurotransmitter balance. Amantadine appears to stimulate the release of striatal dopamine; it does not mimic the action of dopamine. Trihexyphenidyl is an antimuscarinic agent, not antihistaminic; it blocks cholinergic, not H_1, receptors. Bromocriptine is a dopaminergic agonist and mimics the activity of striatal dopamine. The neurotransmitter dopamine is not able to cross the blood–brain barrier and is therefore not effective as an antiparkinsonian drug.

2. The answer is C. (*X C*) Unlike the salicylates, opioids do not possess anti-inflammatory activity. Opioids do suppress the cough reflex and are preeminent analgesics. Opioids cause constipation and are thus effective antidiarrheal agents. When used as preanesthetic medication, opioids permit a reduction in the amount of general anesthetic required for surgical anesthesia.

3. The answer is E. (*IX D 1*) Livedo reticularis is a circulatory disorder characterized by large, bluish, discolored areas on the extremities. It is an adverse effect associated with the use of amantadine and bromocriptine but not with the use of levodopa.

4. The answer is E. (*X A 2 b, c; Figure 9-15, E*) The *p*-phenyl-*N*-alkylpiperidine moiety is common to the structurally specific opioid analgesics. Meperidine is an opioid analgesic and is an *N*-methyl-*p*-phenyl-piperidine derivative. Its chemical name is ethyl 1-methyl-4-phenyl-piperidine-4-carboxylate. Phenobarbital is a barbiturate sedative. Chlorpromazine is a phenothiazine antipsychotic. Diazepam is a benzodiazepine anxiolytic. Imipramine is a tricyclic dibenzazepine antidepressant.

5. The answer is B. (*II A 1*) The general anesthetics are divided into two major classes of drugs: those that are gases or volatile liquids, which are administered by inhalation, and those that are nonvolatile salts, which are administered as intravenous solutions. Halothane is a halogenated hydrocarbon, which belongs to the former class. It has the advantage over older volatile anesthetics (e.g., ethyl ether and cyclopropane) of being nonflammable. Thiopental sodium, alprazolam, buspirone, and phenytoin are all nonvolatile substances that are administered orally or parenterally. Thiopental is a general anesthetic; it is sometimes referred to as a basal anesthetic since it does not produce significant third-stage surgical anesthesia. Alprazolam and buspirone are anxiolytics, whereas phenytoin is an anticonvulsant.

6. The answer is D. (*VII A 2 c, d; Figure 9-1*) Ultra–short-acting barbiturates are characterized by having branched and/or unsaturated 5,5-side chains and by having a sulfur atom in place of oxygen in the 2 position of the barbituric acid molecule. These modifications of barbituric acid result in an extremely liposoluble molecule that is very soluble in lipid tissues. After administration, an ultra–short-acting barbiturate readily crosses the blood–brain barrier but then is quickly redistributed into extra-cerebral tissue, resulting in a rapid loss of activity. While these agents do remain in the body for a long time and may appear to have slow rates of metabolism and excretion, their long retention time is due more to their slow rate of leaching out of lipid tissue.

7. The answer is A. (*IV A 2; Table 9-1*) Fluphenazine, like prochlorperazine, is a piperazinyl phenothiazine antipsychotic and would be likely to cause similar side effects. While thioridazine is also a phenothiazine antipsychotic, it is a piperidyl derivative rather than a piperazinyl derivative. Alprazolam, phenytoin, and pentobarbital are not phenothiazines; therefore, structurally, they are not similar to prochlorperazine.

8. The answer is E (all). (*III D 2*) Careful administration of a local anesthetic by a knowledgeable practitioner is essential to prevent systemic absorption and consequent toxicity. This is especially important when the patient has cardiovascular disease, poorly controlled diabetes, thyrotoxicosis, or peripheral vascular disease.

9. The answer is E (all). (*VII C 2*) Benzodiazepines may serve as induction agents for general anesthesia; they also have anxiolytic properties. In addition, intravenous diazepam is used to treat status epilepticus, while clonazepam is used orally for myoclonic and absence (petit mal) seizures. Benzodiazepines also diminish alcohol withdrawal symptoms.

10–12. The answers are: 10-C, 11-B, 12-D. (*V B 3, C 3, D 2 c; VI B 2*) Buspirone's mechanism of anxiolytic action is unknown. Unlike the benzodiazepines, buspirone lacks hypnotic and anticonvulsant properties. The tricyclic antidepressant imipramine is useful in the treatment of enuresis because the compound blocks muscarinic receptors mediating micturition. Trazodone is categorized as an atypical antidepressant that selectively blocks serotonin re-uptake.

13–15. The answers are: 13-B, 14-D, 15-C. (*III A 1; V A 3; VI A 1, 2; Figures 9-2 and 9-6; Table 9-2*) The structure shown in question 13 is that of procaine, which is a diethylaminoethyl-*p*-aminobenzoate ester. It contains a hydrophilic amino group in the alcohol portion of the molecule and a lipophilic aromatic acid connected by the ester linkage. The procaine molecule is typical of ester-type local anesthetics.

The structure in question 14 is that of diazepam, which has a benzo-1,4-diazepine as its base nucleus. The widely used benzo-1,4-diazepine derivatives have significant anxiolytic, hypnotic, and anticonvulsant activities.

The structure in question 15 is that of desipramine, which has a dibenzazepine as its base nucleus. Dibenzazepine derivatives that have a methyl- or a dimethylaminopropyl group attached to the ring nitrogen have significant antidepressant activity. Similarly substituted dibenzocycloheptadienes also have antidepressant activity. Together these two chemical classes make up the majority of the tricyclic antidepressants.

10

Autacoids and Their Antagonists, Nonnarcotic Analgesic–Antipyretics, and NSAIDs

David C. Kosegarten
Edward F. LaSala

I. INTRODUCTION

A. Autacoids, which are also referred to as autopharmacologic agents or local hormones, have widely differing structures and pharmacologic actions. The two most important autacoids are histamine and the prostaglandins. Their **antagonists** also have important pharmacologic roles.

B. Nonnarcotic analgesic–antipyretics have dissimilar structures but share certain therapeutic actions, including relief of pain, fever, and, sometimes, inflammation. They appear to work in large part by inhibiting synthesis of prostaglandins and related autacoids.

C. Nonsteroidal anti-inflammatory drugs (NSAIDs) differ in structure and activity from the nonnarcotic analgesic–antipyretics, but they all have anti-inflammatory properties and also appear to inhibit prostaglandin synthesis.

II. AUTACOIDS AND THEIR ANTAGONISTS

A. Histamine and antihistaminics

1. Chemistry

a. Histamine is a bioamine derived principally from dietary histidine, which is decarboxylated by L-histidine decarboxylase (Fig. 10-1).

b. Antihistaminics—histamine antagonists—may be classified as H_1-receptor antagonists or H_2-receptor antagonists.

(1) H_1-receptor antagonists, the classic antihistaminic agents, are chemically classified as **ethylenediamines** (e.g., tripelennamine and pyrilamine), **alkylamines** (e.g., chlorpheniramine and brompheniramine), **ethanolamines** (e.g., diphenhydramine and dimenhydrinate), **piperazines** (e.g., cyclizine and meclizine), and **phenothiazines** (e.g., promethazine and trimeprazine) [Fig. 10-2].

(2) H_2-receptor antagonists are heterocyclic methylthioalkyl derivatives. These include cimetidine (Tagamet), ranitidine (Zantac), famotidine (Pepcid), and nizatidine (Axid) [Fig. 10-3].

2. Pharmacology

a. Histamine has powerful pharmacologic actions, mediated by two specific receptor types.

(1) H_1 receptors mediate typical allergic and anaphylactic responses to histamine, such as **bronchoconstriction**, **vasodilation**, **increased capillary permeability**, and **spasmodic contractions of gastrointestinal smooth muscle**.

(2) H_2 receptors mediate other responses to histamine, such as **increased secretion of gastric acid, pepsin, and Castle's factor** (also known as intrinsic factor).

b. H_1-receptor antagonists (antihistaminics) competitively block H_1 receptors and thus **limit histamine's effects on bronchial smooth muscle, capillaries, and gastrointestinal smooth muscle**. They also **prevent histamine-induced pain and itching of the skin and mucous membranes**.

$CH_2CH_2NH_2$ HN N

Figure 10-1. Structural formula of histamine, an autacoid.

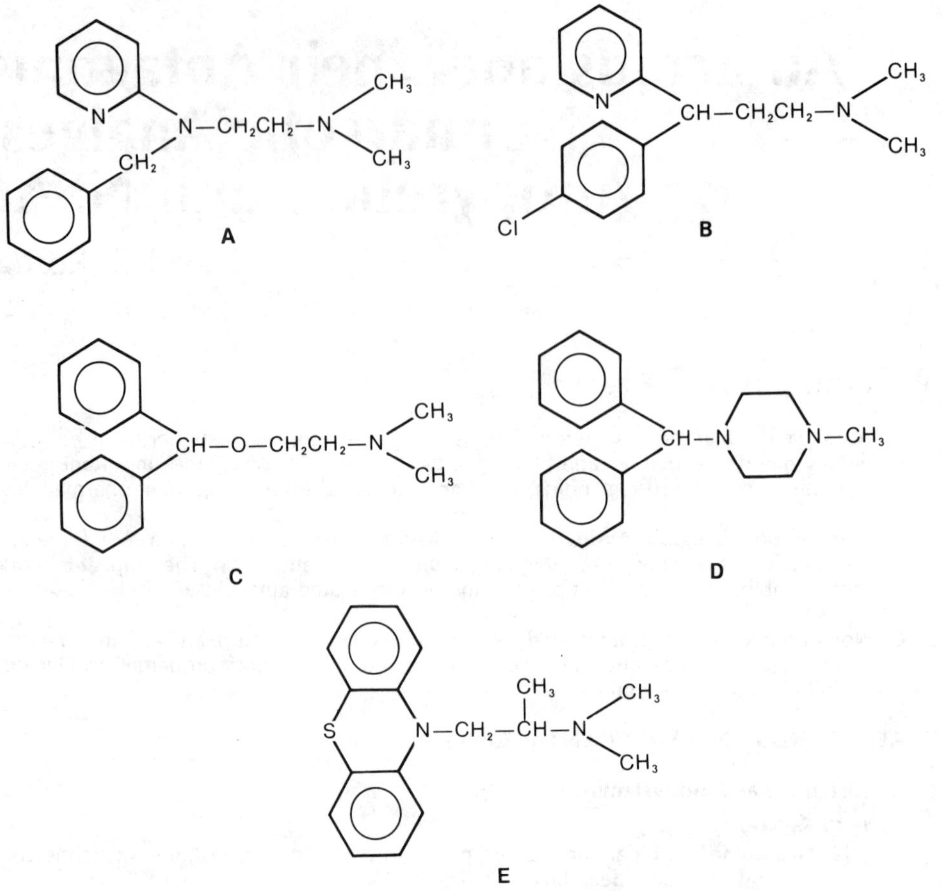

Figure 10-2. Structural formulas of (*A*) tripelennamine, (*B*) chlorpheniramine, (*C*) diphenhydramine, (*D*) cyclizine, and (*E*) promethazine, H_1-receptor antagonists.

c. **H_2-receptor antagonists** competitively block H_2 receptors and thus **limit histamine's effects on gastric secretions.**

3. Therapeutic indications

a. **Exogenous histamine** may be used as a **diagnostic agent for testing gastric function.** However, other stimulants of gastric secretion usually prove more suitable and safer.

b. **H_1-receptor antagonists** are used to provide **symptomatic relief of allergic symptoms,** such as seasonal rhinitis and conjunctivitis. Their anesthetic and antipruritic effects also make them useful for **symptomatic relief of urticaria.**

c. **H_2-receptor antagonists** are used to treat **gastric hypersecretory conditions,** such as duodenal ulcer and Zollinger-Ellison syndrome.

4. Adverse effects

a. **Histamine** may cause **numerous adverse effects** related to its basic pharmacology (see section II A 2 a).

b. **H_1-receptor antagonists** are associated with these adverse effects:

(1) **Central nervous system (CNS) effects,** such as CNS depression, sedation, fatigue, tinnitus, hallucinations, and ataxia

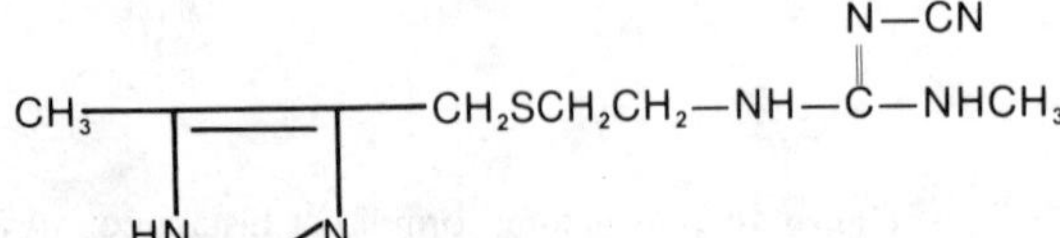

Figure 10-3. Structural formula of cimetidine, an H_2-receptor antagonist.

    (2) **Gastrointestinal effects**, such as nausea and vomiting
    (3) **Antimuscarinic effects**, such as dry mouth, urinary retention, and constipation
    (4) **Teratogenic effects** (possible with piperazine compounds)

  c. **H_2-receptor antagonists** are associated with these adverse effects:

    (1) **CNS effects**, such as confusion and dizziness
    (2) **Hepatic and renal dysfunction**
    (3) **Inhibition of the hepatic microsomal drug-metabolizing enzyme system** (with cimetidine)
    (4) **Androgenic effects** (with high doses of cimetidine), such as impotence and gynecomastia in men and galactorrhea in women

B. Prostaglandins

1. Chemistry

a. Prostaglandins are **derivatives of prostanoic acid**, a 20-carbon fatty acid containing a 5-carbon ring (Fig. 10-4). In the body, prostaglandins are principally synthesized from **arachidonic acid**, a component of membrane phospholipids.

b. **Classification** of prostaglandins as prostaglandin A (PGA), prostaglandin B (PGB), prostaglandin E (PGE), and so forth relates to the presence or absence of keto or hydroxyl groups at positions 9 and 11 (see Fig. 10-4). Subscripts (PGE_1 and so forth) relate to the number and position of double bonds in the aliphatic chains (Fig. 10-5).

2. Pharmacology

a. **Endogenous prostaglandins** appear to affect virtually every body function. They are released in response to many chemical, bacterial, mechanical, and other insults, and they **appear to contribute to the signs and symptoms of the inflammatory process, including pain and edema.**

b. When given clinically, **PGE_1 inhibits platelet aggregation, stimulates intestinal and uterine smooth muscle, produces vasodilation**, and **relaxes the smooth muscle of the ductus arteriosus.**

3. Therapeutic indications.

PGE_1 is used for **temporary maintenance of a patent ductus arteriosus** in infants awaiting corrective surgery for congenital heart defects.

4. Adverse effects

Adverse effects associated with PGE_1 include:

a. **CNS effects**, such as CNS irritability, fever, and seizures
b. **Cardiovascular effects**, such as hypotension, dysrhythmias, vasodilation, and cardiac arrest
c. **Respiratory effects**, such as respiratory depression and distress
d. **Hematologic effects**, such as anemia, thrombocytopenia, and disseminated intravascular coagulation (DIC)
e. **Diarrhea**
f. **Decreased renal function**

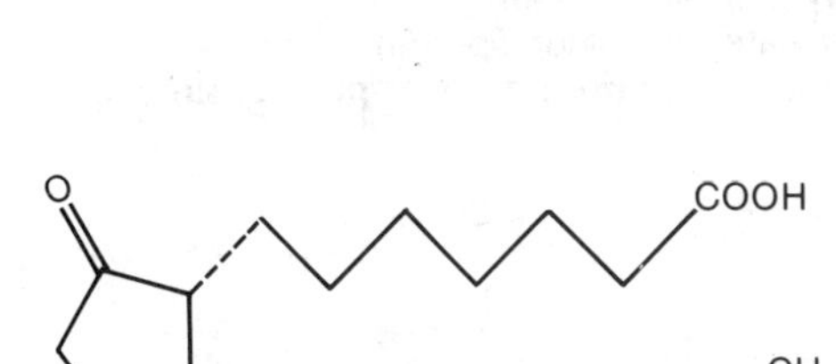

Figure 10-4. Structural formula of prostanoic acid, from which the prostaglandins are derived.

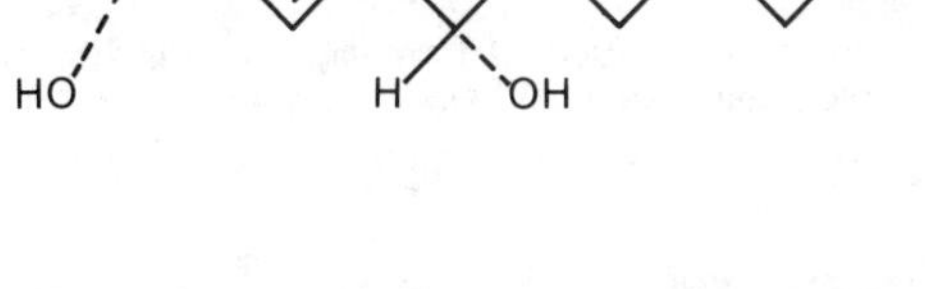

Figure 10-5. Structural formula of alprostadil, a derivative of prostaglandin E_1 (PGE_1).

III. NONNARCOTIC ANALGESIC–ANTIPYRETICS AND NONSTEROIDAL ANTI-INFLAMMATORY AGENTS

A. Salicylates

1. Chemistry

a. Salicylates are **derivatives of salicylic acid**, which is found as the glycoside salicin in willow bark. The prototypical drug is **aspirin**, the acetyl ester of salicylic acid (Fig. 10-6). A simple ester, aspirin **hydrolyzes easily**, is **unstable in aqueous media**, and is **affected by moisture**.

b. More **stable** salicylates include **diflunisal** and the topical agent **methyl salicylate** (oil of wintergreen) [Fig. 10-7].

c. Most salicylates are **weak acids**. Their excretion is influenced by changes in **urinary pH**.

2. Pharmacology

a. Salicylates **inhibit the enzyme cyclooxygenase** and thus **inhibit local prostaglandin synthesis** (see section II B 2 a). As a result, they are **analgesic** for low-intensity integumental pain, **antipyretic**, and **anti-inflammatory**.

b. Salicylates also **block platelet cyclooxygenase** and subsequent formation of thromboxane A_2. As a result, they **inhibit platelet aggregation and eventual thrombus formation**.

3. Therapeutic indications

a. Salicylates are indicated for use as:

(1) Analgesics, for relief of skeletal muscle pain, headache, neuralgias, myalgias, and spasmodic dysmenorrhea

(2) Anti-inflammatory agents, for relief of rheumatoid arthritis symptoms and acute rheumatic fever

(3) Antipyretic agents, for relief of fever. (**Children with varicella or influenza-type viral infections should not be given salicylates** because of the observed association between salicylate use in these situations and Reye's syndrome.)

b. Aspirin is also indicated for **prophylaxis of myocardial infarction**.

c. Methyl salicylate (oil of wintergreen) is used topically as a **counter-irritant**.

4. Adverse effects

a. Salicylates are associated with the following effects:

(1) Gastrointestinal effects, such as nausea, vomiting, and gastrointestinal irritation, discomfort, ulceration, and hemorrhage

(2) Increased depth of respirations

(3) Antagonism of vitamin K, with associated **hypoprothrombinemia**

(4) Uncoupling of oxidative phosphorylation, **hyperglycemia**, **glycosuria**, and **reduced lipogenesis**

(5) Delayed onset of labor

(6) Salicylism (salicylate toxicity, usually marked by tinnitus, nausea, and vomiting)

b. In addition, **low daily doses** of salicylates (< 2 g) **decrease renal urate excretion and increase serum uric acid levels. High daily doses** (> 5 g) have the **opposite effect**.

c. Ingestion of one teaspoonful of the topical agent **methyl salicylate** (oil of wintergreen) can cause **fatal intoxication**.

B. Para-aminophenol derivatives

1. Chemistry. The prototypical para-aminophenol derivative is **acetaminophen**, an active metabolite of phenacetin and acetanilid (Fig. 10-8).

2. Pharmacology

a. Para-aminophenol derivatives **inhibit central prostaglandin synthesis** (see section II B 2 a). They are **analgesic for low-intensity pain** and are **antipyretic**.

b. Because they are less effective than salicylates in blocking peripheral prostaglandin synthesis, they have **no anti-inflammatory activity** and **do not affect platelet function**.

Figure 10-6. Structural formula of aspirin, the prototypical salicylate analgesic–antipyretic.

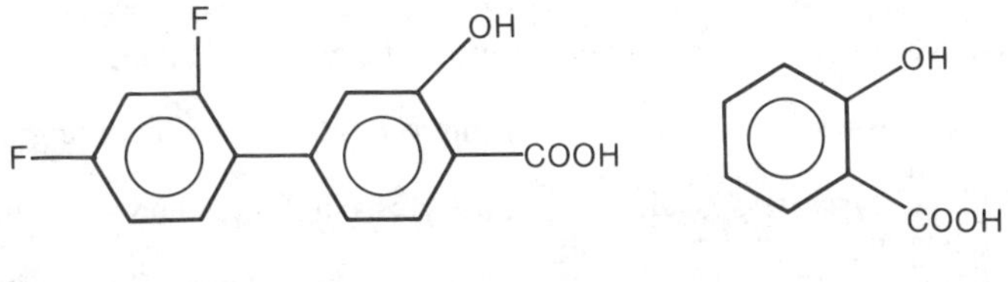

Figure 10-7. Structural formulas of (*A*) diflunisal and (*B*) methyl salicylate (oil of wintergreen), salicylate derivatives.

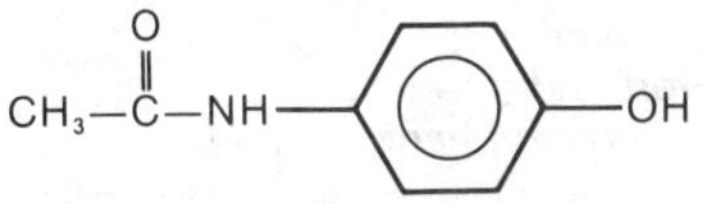

Figure 10-8. Structural formula of acetaminophen, the prototypical para-aminophenol derivative.

3. Therapeutic indications

a. **Acetaminophen** and **phenacetin** are indicated for use as **analgesics** and **antipyretics**, particularly in the patient unable to tolerate salicylates.

b. **Acetaminophen** may be safely used as an **alternative antipyretic** in the child with varicella or an influenza-type viral infection [see section III A 3 a (3)].

4. Adverse effects

a. When given in **therapeutic doses**, adverse effects are limited to:
   (1) **Skin rash**
   (2) **Hemolytic anemia** (with long-term phenacetin use)
   (3) **Methemoglobinemia**
   (4) **Renal dysfunction and tubular necrosis**

b. **Acute overdose** causes **severe hepatotoxicity** with necrosis and liver failure.

C. Pyrazolone derivatives

1. Chemistry. The most important pyrazolone derivatives are **phenylbutazone**, its metabolite **oxyphenbutazone**, and the uricosuric agent **sulfinpyrazone**. Phenylbutazone is the prototypical agent (Fig. 10-9).

2. Pharmacology

a. **Phenylbutazone** and **oxyphenbutazone** inhibit prostaglandin synthesis (see section II B 2 a) and stabilize lysosomal membranes. As a result, they have **analgesic**, **antipyretic**, and **anti-inflammatory effects**.

b. **Sulfinpyrazone** inhibits proximal tubular absorption of urate and has a **uricosuric effect**. However, it is devoid of analgesic, antipyretic, or anti-inflammatory effects.

3. Therapeutic indications

a. **Phenylbutazone** and **oxyphenbutazone** are used for **short-term treatment of acute rheumatoid arthritic conditions and acute gout**. However, they should be given **only after other therapeutic measures have failed**.

b. **Sulfinpyrazone** is used to **control hyperuricemia** in the treatment of intermittent and chronic gout.

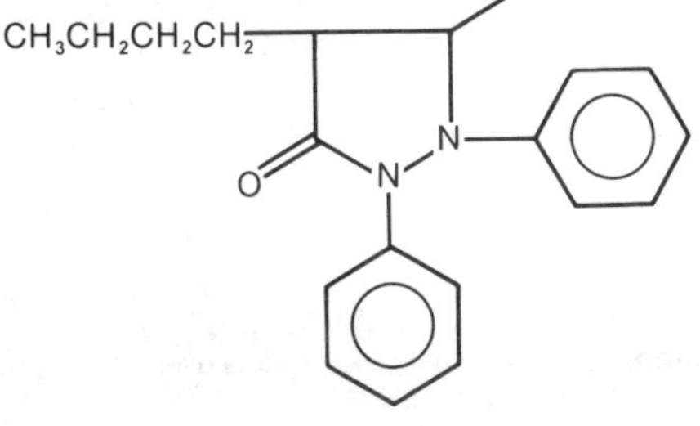

Figure 10-9. Structural formula of phenylbutazone, a pyrazolone derivative.

4. Adverse effects

a. The adverse effects of **phenylbutazone** and **oxyphenbutazone** often limit their use and include:

(1) **Gastrointestinal effects**, such as discomfort, nausea, vomiting, dyspepsia, and peptic ulceration

(2) **Blood dyscrasias**, such as agranulocytosis, aplastic anemia, hemolytic anemia, thrombocytopenia, and petechiae

(3) **Cardiovascular effects**, such as congestive heart failure (CHF) with edema and dyspnea

(4) **Renal effects**, such as nephrotic lithiasis, renal necrosis, impaired renal function, and renal failure

(5) **CNS effects**, such as drowsiness, agitation, confusion, headache, lethargy, numbness, weakness, tinnitus, and hearing loss

(6) **Hyperglycemia**

(7) **Skin rash**

b. Sulfinpyrazone is associated with these adverse effects:

(1) **Gastrointestinal effects**, such as discomfort and upset

(2) **Blood dyscrasias**, as for phenylbutazone and oxyphenbutazone

(3) **Renal failure**

D. Agents used for the treatment of gout

1. Chemistry

a. Acute attacks of **gout** result from an **inflammatory response to joint depositions of sodium urate crystals**. Therapeutic agents counter this response by reducing plasma uric acid concentrations or inhibiting the inflammatory response.

b. Agents used for the treatment of gout have widely varying structures and include the pyrazolone derivative **sulfinpyrazone** (see section III C 2 b, C 3 b, and C 4 b), the alkaloid **colchicine**, isopurines such as **allopurinol**, and benzoic acid derivatives such as **probenecid** (Fig. 10-10).

2. Pharmacology

a. Although **colchicine's** exact mechanism of action is unknown, it appears to **reduce the inflammatory response to deposited urate crystals** by inhibiting leukocyte migration and phagocytosis. It also interferes with kinin formation and reduces leukocyte lactic acid production.

b. Allopurinol reduces serum urate levels by blocking uric acid production. It competitively inhibits the enzyme xanthine oxidase, which converts xanthine and hypoxanthine to uric acid.

c. Probenecid, a uricosuric agent, inhibits the proximal tubular reabsorption of uric acid, increasing uric acid excretion and thus **reducing plasma uric acid concentrations**.

3. Therapeutic indications

a. Colchicine is used principally for the treatment of **acute gout attacks**.

b. Allopurinol, which reduces uric acid synthesis and facilitates the dissolution of tophi (chalky urate deposits), is used to **prevent the development or progression of chronic tophaceous gout**.

c. Probenecid is used to treat **chronic tophaceous gout**. It is also used in smaller doses to prolong the effectiveness of penicillin-type antibiotics, by inhibiting their tubular secretion.

4. Adverse effects

a. Chronic use of **colchicine** is associated with these adverse effects:

(1) **Agranulocytosis**, **aplastic anemia**, **myopathy**, **hair loss**, and **peripheral neuritis**

(2) **Nausea**, **vomiting**, **abdominal pain**, and **diarrhea** (indications of impending toxicity)

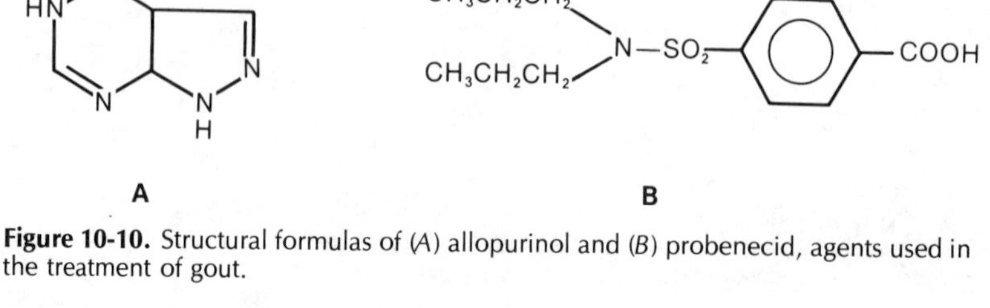

OH
HN
N
N
N
H

A

$CH_3CH_2CH_2$
N—SO_2—⌬—COOH
$CH_3CH_2CH_2$

B

Figure 10-10. Structural formulas of (*A*) allopurinol and (*B*) probenecid, agents used in the treatment of gout.

b. Allopurinol is associated with these adverse effects:

(1) Gastrointestinal effects, such as gastrointestinal distress, nausea, vomiting, and diarrhea

(2) Skin rash, Stevens-Johnson syndrome, and **hepatotoxicity**

(3) Precipitation of an acute gout attack (with initial allopurinol therapy)

c. Probenecid is associated with these adverse effects:

(1) Headache, nausea, vomiting, urinary frequency, sore gums, and **dermatitis**

(2) Dizziness, anemia, hemolytic anemia, and **renal lithiasis**

E. Nonsteroidal anti-inflammatory drugs

1. Chemistry. The **NSAIDs** consist of a large number of structurally diverse acids. These include **arylacetic acids** (e.g., ibuprofen and naproxen), **indene derivatives** (e.g., indomethacin and sulindac), **fenamic acids** (e.g., mefenamic acid and diclofenac), and other structurally unrelated agents (e.g., piroxicam) [Fig. 10-11].

2. Pharmacology

a. NSAIDs have **anti-inflammatory effects** resulting from their ability to inhibit the cyclooxygenase enzyme system and thus reduce local prostaglandin synthesis (see section II B 2 a).

b. NSAIDs also have **analgesic** and **antipyretic effects**.

3. Therapeutic indications. NSAIDs, like aspirin, are agents of choice for the treatment of **rheumatoid arthritis, osteoarthritis**, and **ankylosing spondylitis**.

4. Adverse effects. NSAIDs are associated with these adverse effects:

a. Gastrointestinal effects, such as gastrointestinal distress and irritation, erosion of gastric mucosa, nausea, vomiting, and dyspepsia

b. CNS effects, such as CNS depression, drowsiness, headache, dizziness, visual disturbances, ototoxicity, and confusion

c. Hematologic effects, such as thrombocytopenia, altered platelet function, and prolonged bleeding time

d. Skin rash

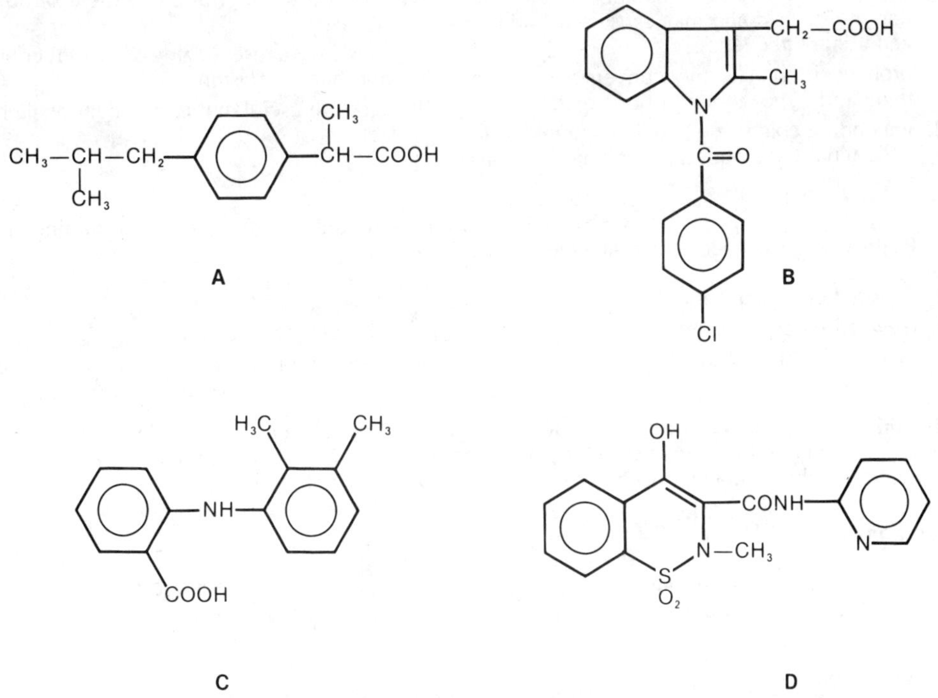

Figure 10-11. Structural formulas of (*A*) ibuprofen, (*B*) indomethacin, (*C*) mefenamic acid, and (*D*) piroxicam, representative nonsteroidal anti-inflammatory drugs (NSAIDs).

STUDY QUESTIONS

Directions: Each question below contains five suggested answers. Choose the **one best** response to each question.

1. All of the following are therapeutic indications for salicylates EXCEPT

A. rheumatoid arthritis
B. fever in children with influenza or varicella
C. fever in adults with influenza
D. spasmodic dysmenorrhea
E. prophylaxis against myocardial infarction

2. All of the following statements describing acetaminophen are true EXCEPT

A. it has anti-inflammatory activity similar to or greater than that of salicylates
B. it acts as an analgesic and antipyretic
C. it may cause skin rash
D. it may be used in children with varicella or influenza-type viral infections
E. acute overdose is characterized by severe hepatotoxicity

Directions: Each question below contains three suggested answers of which **one or more** is correct. Choose the answer

A if **I only** is correct
B if **III only** is correct
C if **I and II** are correct
D if **II and III** are correct
E if **I, II, and III** are correct

3. Correct statements regarding agents used in the treatment of gout include

I. allopurinol inhibits proximal tubular reabsorption of uric acid and may cause renal lithiasis and urinary frequency
II. probenecid blocks the conversion of xanthine and hypoxanthine to uric acid
III. impending colchicine toxicity is heralded by abdominal pain, nausea, vomiting, and diarrhea

4. Pharmacologic properties of histamine include

I. constriction of capillaries
II. elevated blood pressure
III. increased gastric secretions

5. True statements concerning cimetidine and ranitidine include

I. they are useful in the treatment of duodenal ulcers
II. they may cause dizziness, mental confusion, and hepatic dysfunction
III. they are useful in the treatment of allergic reactions

6. The antihistaminic drug famotidine is classified as a

I. classic antihistamine
II. H_1-receptor antagonist
III. H_2-receptor antagonist

Directions: The group of questions below consists of lettered choices followed by several numbered items. For each numbered item select the **one** lettered choice with which it is **most** closely associated. Each lettered choice may be used once, more than once, or not at all.

Questions 7–11

For each characteristic given below, select the drug that most appropriately corresponds to it.

A. Acetaminophen
B. Indomethacin
C. Aspirin
D. Diphenhydramine
E. Ibuprofen

7. Hydrolyzed in the bloodstream
8. An active metabolite of another drug
9. Classified as a salicylate
10. Excretion somewhat increased in an acidified urine
11. Classified as an arylacetic acid

ANSWERS AND EXPLANATIONS

1. The answer is B. (*III A 3*) The association of Reye's syndrome with the use of salicylates in febrile children with varicella or influenza-type viral infections warrants that a nonsalicylate antipyretic be used if needed in such circumstances.

2. The answer is A. (*III B 2 b, 3, 4*) Acetaminophen has a limited peripheral effect on prostaglandin synthesis and therefore lacks anti-inflammatory capability. Acetaminophen is a nonsalicylate alternative antipyretic, which may be used in children with varicella or influenza-type viral infections. Adverse effects include skin rash or other allergic reactions, and acute overdose is accompanied by severe liver damage.

3. The answer is B (III). [*III D 2 b, c, 4 a (2), b, c*] Gastrointestinal upset, with adverse effects such as nausea, vomiting, and diarrhea, is associated with the early stages of colchicine toxicity. Probenecid inhibits the proximal tubular reabsorption of uric acid, while allopurinol inhibits the formation of uric acid from xanthine and hypoxanthine. Probenecid, not allopurinol, may cause renal lithiasis and urinary frequency.

4. The answer is B (III). (*II A 2 a*) While gastric secretions are stimulated by histamine, the autacoid causes increased capillary permeability, capillary dilation, vasodilation, and hypotension.

5. The answer is C (I, II). (*II A 3, 4 c*) Cimetidine and ranitidine are examples of H_2-receptor antagonists. They restrict H_2-mediated gastric secretions. They are ineffective in the treatment of allergic reactions since they are not H_1-receptor antagonists. Adverse effects that limit their duration of use include altered hepatic and renal function, as well as dizziness and confusion.

6. The answer is B (III). [*II A 1 b (2)*] The generic name famotidine more closely resembles those of the widely used H_2-receptor antagonists, cimetidine and ranitidine—all three have the common suffix -tidine. The generic names of most of the H_1 antagonists end in the suffix -amine, such as diphenhydramine and chlorpheniramine. The H_1 antagonists, which are much older drugs, now often are referred to as the classic antihistamines.

7–11. The answers are: 7-C, 8-A, 9-C, 10-D, 11-E. (*III A 1 a, b, B 1, E 1; Figures 10-2, 10-6, 10-8, 10-11*) Esters, particularly simple esters, readily undergo in vivo hydrolysis both with and without the aid of catalytic enzymes. Amides also undergo hydrolysis but require the aid of catalytic enzymes. There are a number of specific and nonspecific esterases circulating in the bloodstream but few, if any, amidases. Aspirin (acetylsalicylic acid) is the phenolic acetyl ester of *p*-hydroxybenzoic acid (i.e., salicylic acid) and thus is classified as a salicylate. Aspirin is readily hydrolyzed in the bloodstream and is the only drug listed that contains an ester linkage.

Acetaminophen is a metabolite of phenacetin. Phenacetin (*N*-acetyl-*p*-ethoxyaniline) undergoes oxidative *O*-dealkylation in the body, forming *N*-acetyl-*p*-aminophenol (acetaminophen).

In order for its excretion to be increased in an acidic urine, a drug must be a weak base. Aspirin, indomethacin, and ibuprofen are all weak acids, as are the other nonsteroidal anti-inflammatory agents (NSAIDs). Acetaminophen is a neutral molecule. Diphenhydramine, as the generic name implies, has an amino group present in its molecule. As can be seen in its structure (see Fig. 10-2C), it contains a tertiary amine. Amines are weak bases; thus, diphenhydramine would be more ionized in acidic media and less likely to undergo tubular reabsorption from the glomerular filtrate. It would therefore be more easily excreted in acidic urine.

The NSAIDs are all acids, which contributes to their ability to penetrate synovial fluids. The NSAIDs are often classified as arylacetic acids or heteroarylacetic acids. Ibuprofen does not contain any hetero atoms and thus is classified as an arylacetic acid. Indomethacin, an indene derivative, contains a nitrogen in the pyrrole ring and thus is a heteroarylacetic acid. Aspirin, although an acid, is a salicylic acid derivative. Diphenhydramine is a base, and acetaminophen is neutral.

11
Drugs Affecting the Cardiovascular System

David C. Kosegarten
Edward F. LaSala

I. INTRODUCTION. Numerous categories of drugs affect the cardiovascular system. Certain drugs can treat heart failure (the **cardiac glycosides**), relieve angina pectoris (the **antianginal agents**), and control dysrhythmias (the **antiarrythmic agents**). Others can reduce hypertension (the **antihypertensives**, including a wide variety of diuretics, β-blocking agents, arteriolar smooth muscle dilators, and others); treat the hyperlipidemias (the **antihyperlipidemic agents**); reduce clotting and treat such conditions as venous thrombosis and pulmonary embolism (the **anticoagulants**); and treat anemias (the **antianemic agents**).

II. CARDIAC GLYCOSIDES

A. Chemistry

1. Almost all the cardiac glycosides (also called **cardiotonics**) are naturally occurring steroidal glycosides obtained from plant sources. **Digitoxin** is obtained from *Digitalis purpura*, **digoxin** from *Digitalis lanata*, and **ouabain** from *Strophanthus gratus*.
2. The **digitalis-like agents** are closely related structurally, consisting of one or more sugars (the **glycone** portion) and a steroidal nucleus (the **aglycone** or **genin** portion) bonded through an **ether** (glycosidic) **linkage**. These agents also have an **unsaturated lactone substituent** (cyclic ester) on the genin portion. The prototypical agent is **digitoxin** (Fig. 11-1).
   a. **Digoxin** has an additional OH group at position 12 (see Fig. 11-1).
   b. **Ouabain** has a rhamnose glycone portion and additional OH groups at positions 1, 5, 11, and 19 (see Fig. 11-1).
3. **Removal of the glycone portion** causes decreased activity and increased toxicity from changes in polarity that cause erratic absorption from the gastrointestinal tract.
4. The **duration of action** of a cardiac glycoside is indirectly proportional to the **number of hydroxyl groups**, which increase polarity. Increased polarity results in decreased protein binding, liver biotransformation, and tubular reabsorption.
   a. Thus, **digitoxin** has a long duration of action and may act cumulatively.
   b. **Ouabain**, in contrast, has an extremely short duration of action and is effective only when given intravenously.
5. The one non-naturally occurring glycoside is **amrinone**, a bipyridine derivative (Fig. 11-2).

B. Pharmacology. Cardiac glycosides **increase myocardial contractility and efficiency, improve**

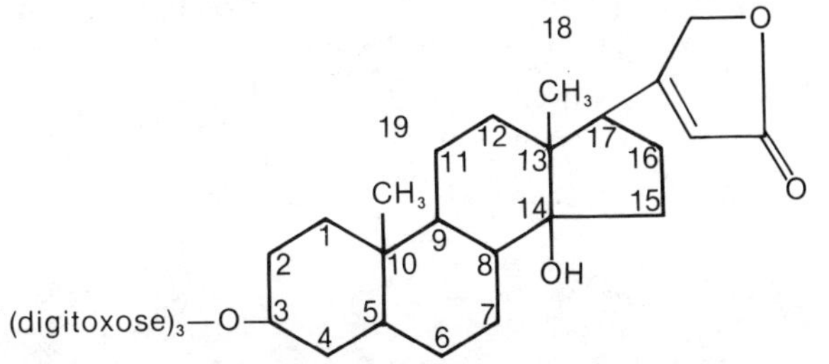

Figure 11-1. Structural formula of digitoxin, the prototypical digitalis-like cardiac glycoside.

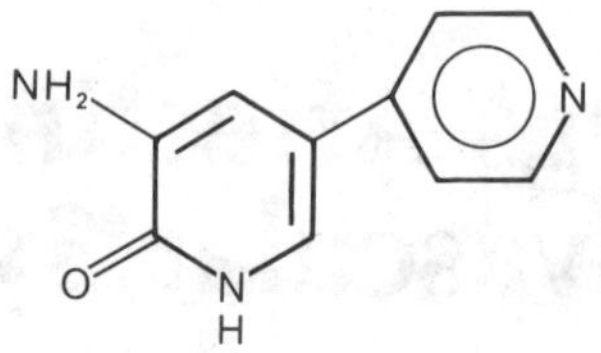

Figure 11-2. Structural formula of amrinone (Inocor), the bipyridine derivative cardiac glycoside.

systemic circulation, **improve renal perfusion**, and **reduce edema**. They act through a variety of mechanisms (Table 11-1).

1. When given in therapeutic doses, cardiac glycosides have these **direct actions** on the heart and its conduction system:
   a. A **positive inotropic effect** (thought to involve either enhanced calcium entry into myocardial cells during depolarization or enhanced calcium release from intracellular sarcoplasmic reticulum binding sites)
   b. An **increase in systolic contraction velocity** [probably initiated by inhibition of membrane-bound sodium, potassium (Na^+, K^+)-activated adenosinetriphosphatase]
   c. An **increase in the refractory period of the atrioventricular (AV) node**
2. Therapeutic doses of glycosides also have these **indirect effects**:
   a. A **negative chronotropic effect**, from increased vagal tone of the sinoatrial (SA) node
   b. **Diminished central nervous system (CNS) sympathetic outflow**, from increased carotid sinus baroreceptor sensitivity
3. In addition, therapeutic doses of cardiac glycosides cause **systemic arteriolar and venous constriction**, which increases venous return and, thus, increases cardiac output.

C. **Therapeutic indications**. Cardiac glycosides are used to treat:

1. **Congestive heart failure**
2. **Atrial fibrillation**
3. **Atrial flutter**
4. **Paroxysmal atrial tachycardia**

D. **Adverse effects**

1. **Early adverse effects** of cardiac glycosides represent the **early stages of toxicity** and include:
   a. **Gastrointestinal effects**, such as anorexia, nausea, vomiting, and diarrhea
   b. **CNS effects**, such as headache, visual disturbances (green or yellow vision), confusion, delirium, neuralgias, and muscle weakness
2. Adverse effects occurring later represent **intoxication** and include such **serious cardiac disturbances** as premature ventricular contractions, paroxysmal and nonparoxysmal atrial tachycardia, AV dissociation or block, ventricular tachycardia, and ventricular fibrillation.

Table 11-1. Effects of Cardiac Glycosides on the Heart

	Atria	AV Node	Ventricles
Direct effects	Contractility↑ ERP↑ Conduction velocity↓	ERP↑ Conduction velocity↓	Contractility↑ ERP↓ Automaticity↑
Indirect effects	ERP↓ Conduction velocity↑	ERP↑ Conduction velocity↓	No effect
Effects on electrocardiogram	P changes	P-R interval↑	Q-T↓; T and ST depressed
Adverse effects	Extrasystole Tachycardia	AV depression or block	Fibrillation Extrasystole Tachycardia

ERP = Effective refractory period. Arrows indicate changes: ↑ = increased; ↓ = decreased.
Reprinted with permission from Jacob LS: *Pharmacology*, 2nd ed. Media, Pennsylvania, Harwal, 1987, p 90.

III. ANTIANGINAL AGENTS AND PERIPHERAL VASODILATORS

A. Chemistry

1. **Antianginal agents** include **nitrites** (organic esters of nitrous acid, such as amyl nitrite); **nitrates** (organic esters of nitric acid, such as nitroglycerin and isosorbide); **β-blockers**, such as propranolol; and **calcium antagonists**, such as verapamil and nifedipine (Fig. 11-3).
   a. **Amyl nitrite** is a very volatile and flammable liquid, administered by inhalation. It requires special precautions (especially restriction of smoking) during administration.
   b. **Nitroglycerin** is also a very volatile and flammable liquid and requires great care during storage. It must be dispensed from its original glass containers and protected from body heat.
      (1) When given **intravenously**, nitroglycerin requires the use of special plastic administration sets to avoid absorption and loss of potency.
      (2) Nitroglycerin is **metabolically unstable** and undergoes extensive first-pass metabolism.
2. **Peripheral vasodilators** include the dipiperidino-dipyrimidine **dipyridamole** (see Fig. 11-3).

B. Pharmacology

1. **Nitrites** and **nitrates** are fast-acting antianginal agents that **directly relax vascular smooth muscle**. This causes peripheral pooling of the blood, diminished venous return (reduced preload), decreased systemic vascular resistance, and decreased arterial pressure (reduced afterload).
   a. These vascular effects **reduce myocardial oxygen demand**.
   b. They also cause redistribution of coronary blood flow along the collateral coronary arteries, **improving perfusion of the ischemic myocardium**.
2. **β-Adrenergic blockers** decrease sympathetic-mediated myocardial stimulation (see Chapter 8, sections V A 2 and V C 3). The resulting negative inotropic and negative chronotropic effects reduce myocardial oxygen requirements.
3. **Calcium antagonists** (also known as calcium channel blockers) block calcium entry through the membranous calcium ion channels of cardiac and vascular smooth muscle.

$$\begin{array}{l} CH_2-ONO_2 \\ | \\ CH-ONO_2 \\ | \\ CH_2-ONO_2 \end{array}$$

A

CH_2; $CH-ONO_2$; O; CH; CH; O; O_2NO-CH; CH_2

B

CH_3; NO_2; HN; CH_3; $C-OCH_3$; O

C

N; CH_2CH_2OH; N; N; CH_2CH_2OH; N; $HOCH_2CH_2$; N; N; N; $HOCH_2CH_2$; N

D

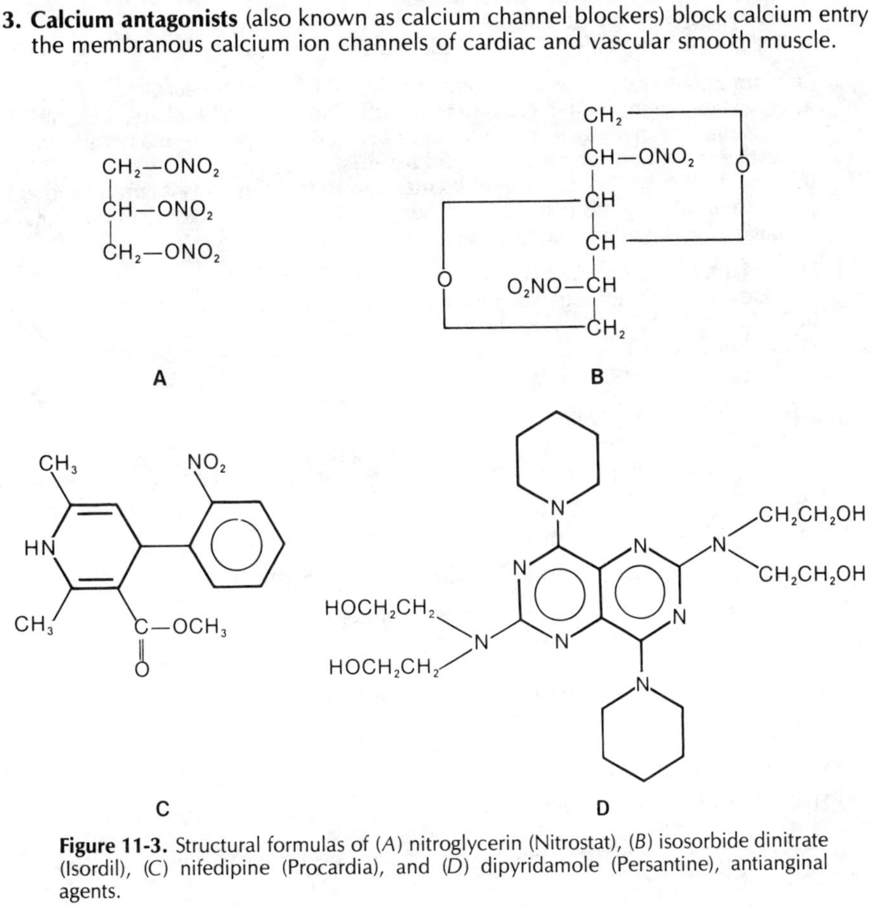

Figure 11-3. Structural formulas of (*A*) nitroglycerin (Nitrostat), (*B*) isosorbide dinitrate (Isordil), (*C*) nifedipine (Procardia), and (*D*) dipyridamole (Persantine), antianginal agents.

a. Peripheral arterioles dilate, and total peripheral resistance decreases, reducing afterload and **reducing myocardial oxygen requirements**.

b. Calcium antagonists also **increase oxygen delivery to the myocardium** by dilating coronary arteries and arterioles.

4. **Dipyridamole** relaxes smooth muscles, **decreasing coronary vascular resistance** and **increasing coronary blood flow**.

C. Therapeutic indications

1. **Nitrites** and **nitrates** are used to **relieve acute anginal attacks**, as **prophylaxis during anticipation of an acute anginal attack**, and for **long-term management of recurrent angina pectoris**.

2. **β-Adrenergic blockers** are used for **adjunctive prophylaxis of chronic stable angina pectoris**, in combination with nitrites or nitrates.

3. **Calcium antagonists** are used to treat **chronic stable angina pectoris** and **variant (Prinzmetal's) angina**.

4. **Dipyridamole** is used primarily for **prophylaxis of angina pectoris**, although its beneficial effects are not well understood.

D. Adverse effects

1. **Nitrites** and **nitrates** are associated with these adverse effects:
   a. **CNS effects**, such as headache, apprehension, dizziness, and weakness
   b. **Cardiovascular effects**, such as hypotension, tachycardia, palpitations, and syncope
   c. **Skin effects**, such as rash and dermatitis
   d. **Methemoglobinemia**

2. **β-Adrenergic blockers** are associated with these adverse effects:
   a. **Worsening of congestive heart failure**
   b. **Bradycardia** and **hypotension**
   c. **Reduced kidney blood flow and glomerular filtration**

3. **Calcium antagonists** generally produce only mild adverse effects.
   a. However, when given **in conjunction with β-adrenergic blockers**, their cardiovascular effects may be enhanced, resulting in **bradycardia**, **hypotension**, **peripheral edema**, **congestive heart failure**, **AV block**, and **asystole**.
   b. **Verapamil** may also cause **sleeplessness**, **muscle fatigue**, **nystagmus**, and **emotional depression**. During the first week of therapy, verapamil increases serum digitalis levels and may cause **digitalis toxicity**.

4. **Dipyridamole** is associated with these adverse effects:
   a. **Gastrointestinal effects**, such as nausea, vomiting, and diarrhea
   b. **CNS effects**, such as headache and dizziness
   c. **Cardiovascular effects**, such as hypotension (with excessive doses)

IV. ANTIARRHYTHMIC AGENTS

A. Chemistry. Antiarrhythmic agents have widely diverse chemical structures. They include representatives of these groups:

1. **Cinchona alkaloids** (e.g., quinidine, an optical isomer of quinine)

2. **Amides** (e.g., procainamide, flecainide, and disopyramide)

3. **Xylyl** derivatives (e.g., lidocaine and mexiletine)

4. **Quaternary ammonium salts** (e.g., bretylium)

5. **Diiodobenzyloxyethylamines** (e.g., amiodarone)

6. **β-Blockers** (e.g., nadolol, propranolol, and acebutolol)

7. **Calcium antagonists** (e.g., diltiazem and verapamil)

8. **Hydantoins** (e.g., phenytoin)

B. Pharmacology. Antiarrhythmic agents are classified according to their ability to **alter the action potential of cardiac cells** (Tables 11-2 and 11-3).

Table 11-2. Effects of Antiarrhythmic Drugs on Electrophysiologic Properties of the Heart

	Automaticity		Effective Refractory Period		Membrane Responsiveness
Drug	**Sinus Node**	**Purkinje Fibers**	**AV Node**	**Purkinje Fibers**	**(Purkinje Fibers)**
Quinidine Procainamide Disopyramide	→	↓	↑→↓	↓	↓
Lidocaine Phenytoin	→	↓	↑→↓	↓	↓
Propranolol	↓	↓	↑	↑	↓

Arrows indicate changes: ↑ = increased; ↓ = decreased; → = no change.

Reprinted with permission from Jacob LS: *Pharmacology*, 2nd ed. Media, Pennsylvania, Harwal, 1987, p 94.

1. **Class IA** compounds (e.g., quinidine, procainamide, and disopyramide) slow the rate of rise of phase 0 (the phase of rapid depolarization and reversal of transmembrane voltage) and prolong repolarization.
2. **Class IB** compounds (e.g., lidocaine, tocainide, mexiletine, and phenytoin) have a minimal effect on the rate of rise of phase 0 and shorten repolarization.
3. **Class II** compounds (e.g., propranolol, nadolol, and acebutolol) are β-adrenergic antagonists that competitively block catecholamine-induced stimulation of cardiac β-receptors and depress phase-4 depolarization.
4. **Class III** compounds (e.g., bretylium) prolong repolarization.
5. **Class IV** compounds (e.g., verapamil) are calcium antagonists that block the slow inward current carried by calcium during phase 2 (long-sustained depolarization, or the plateau of the action potential) and increase the effective refractory period.

C. Therapeutic indications. Antiarrhythmic agents are used to **reduce abnormalities of impulse generation** (ectopic pacemaker automaticity) and to **modify the disturbances of impulse conduction within cardiac tissue**. For indications for specific agents, see Table 11-4.

D. Adverse effects

1. **Class IA** compounds are associated with these adverse effects:
   a. **Cardiovascular effects**, such as myocardial depression, AV block, ventricular dysrhythmias, asystole, and hypotension

Table 11-3. Major Effects of Antiarrhythmic Drugs on Electrocardiogram

Drug	**QRS**	**Q-T**	**P-R**
Quinidine Procainamide	↑	↑	→↑
Disopyramide	↑	↑	→
Lidocaine Phenytoin	→	↓	→↑↓*
Propranolol	→	↓	→↑*

Arrows indicate changes: ↑ = increased; ↓ = decreased; → = no change.

*P-R intervals: All antiarrhythmics have a variable response, usually with little observable effect. However, lidocaine hardly ever affects the P-R interval, while phenytoin and propranolol usually increase the P-R interval.

Reprinted with permission from Jacob LS: *Pharmacology*, 2nd ed. Media, Pennsylvania, Harwal, 1987, p 95.

Table 11-4. Uses of Antiarrhythmic Drugs in Common Cardiac Arrhythmias

Arrhythmia	Treatment of Choice	Alternatives
Supraventricular		
Atrial fibrillation or flutter	Digitalis to control ventricular rate, DC shock for conversion	Quinidine to suppress recurrences after DC shock
Paroxysmal atrial or nodal tachycardia	Vagotonic maneuver; digitalis	Verapamil (quinidine, procainamide, disopyramide, and propranolol may all be useful, especially prophylactically)
Ventricular		
Ventricular premature depolarization	Lidocaine	Procainamide, quinidine, or disopyramide for prolonged suppression
Ventricular tachycardia	DC shock	Lidocaine or procainamide

Reprinted with permission from Jacob LS: *Pharmacology*, 2nd ed. Media, Pennsylvania, Harwal, 1987, p 95.

b. **Gastrointestinal effects**, such as gastrointestinal upset, nausea, vomiting, and diarrhea
c. **Blood dyscrasias**
d. In addition, **quinidine** may also cause **cinchonism**, with tinnitus, confusion, photophobia, headache, and psychosis.
e. **Procainamide** may also cause **systemic lupus erythematosus–like syndrome**.
f. **Disopyramide** may also cause **congestive heart failure** and **antimuscarinic effects**.

2. **Class IB** compounds are associated with these adverse effects.
   a. **CNS effects** include CNS depression, drowsiness, disorientation, and paresthesias.
   b. **Cardiovascular effects** include hypotension and circulatory collapse.
   c. **Hepatitis** may occur.
   d. **Lidocaine** may also cause **seizures** and **respiratory arrest**.
   e. **Tocainide** may also cause **pneumonitis** and **blood dyscrasias**.
   f. **Mexiletine** may also cause **hepatic injury** and **blood dyscrasias**.
   g. **Phenytoin** may also cause **nystagmus**, **decreased mental function**, and **blood dyscrasias**.
3. **Class II** compounds are associated with these adverse effects:
   a. **Cardiovascular effects**, such as hypotension, AV block, and asystole
   b. **Respiratory effects**, such as bronchospasm
4. The **class III** compound **bretylium** is associated with these adverse effects:
   a. **Cardiovascular effects**, such as hypotension and initially increased dysrhythmias
   b. **Gastrointestinal effects**, such as nausea and vomiting.
5. The **class IV** compound **verapamil** is associated with **cardiovascular adverse effects**, such as hypotension, bradycardia, AV block, congestive heart failure, and asystole.

V. ANTIHYPERTENSIVE AGENTS

A. **Chemistry**. Antihypertensive agents vary so widely in chemical structure that they are usually classified by **mechanism of action** rather than chemical class (Table 11-5).

B. **Pharmacology**. Antihypertensive agents lower blood pressure by **reducing total peripheral resistance or cardiac output** through a variety of mechanisms (see Table 11-5).

1. **Diuretics** (thiazides) create a negative sodium balance, reduce blood volume, and decrease vascular smooth muscle responsiveness to vasoconstrictors (see Chapter 12, section IV).
2. **Vasodilators** (e.g., hydralazine) relax arteriolar smooth muscle, decreasing arterial resistance.
3. **Peripheral sympatholytics** interfere with adrenergic function by blocking postganglionic adrenergic receptors (e.g., propranolol and prazosin), limiting the release of neurotransmitters from adrenergic neurons (e.g., guanethidine) or depleting intraneuronal catecholamine storage sites (e.g., reserpine).
4. **Central α_2-sympathomimetics** (e.g., clonidine and methyldopa) appear to mediate their effects by stimulation of presynaptic α_2-inhibitory receptors, resulting in a negative sympathetic outflow and lowered peripheral resistance.
5. **Angiotensin-converting enzyme inhibitors** (e.g., captopril) block the conversion of inactive

Table 11-5. Classification of Antihypertensive Agents by Their Mechanism of Action

Mechanism of Action	Drug	Chemical Class
Diuretic	Hydrochlorothiazide (Hydrodiuril)	Benzothiadiazide
Vasodilators		
Arteriolar	Diazoxide (Hyperstat)	Benzothiadiazide
	Hydralazine (Apresoline)	Phthalazine
	Minoxidil (Loniten)	Guanidine (cyclic)
Arteriolar and venous	Sodium nitroprusside (Nipride)	Nitroprusside
Peripheral sympatholytics	Atenolol (Tenormin)	β-blocker (selective)
	Guanadrel (Hylorel)	Guanidine (open-chain)
	Guanethidine (Ismelin)	Guanidine (open-chain)
	Labetalol (Trandate)	β-blocker (nonselective)
	Metoprolol (Lopressor)	β-blocker (selective)
	Nadolol (Corgard)	β-blocker (nonselective)
	Pindolol (Visken)	β-blocker (nonselective)
	Prazosin (Minipress)	Guanidine (cyclic)
	Propranolol (Inderal)	β-blocker (nonselective)
	Reserpine (Serpasil)	Rauwolfia alkaloid
Central α_2-sympathomimetics	Clonidine (Catapres)	Guanidine (cyclic)
	Guanabenz (Wytensin)	Guanidine (open-chain)
	Guanfacine (Tenex)	Guanidine (open-chain)
	Methyldopa (Aldomet)	Catecholaminoacid
Angiotensin-converting enzyme inhibitors	Captopril (Capoten)	Pyrrolidine
	Enalapril (Vasotec)	Pyrrolidine

angiotensin I to the potent vasoconstrictor angiotensin II. The reduced angiotensin II level also lowers aldosterone levels, which limits sodium retention.

C. Therapeutic indications

1. Antihypertensive agents are used separately or in combination to **treat high blood pressure**.
2. These agents may also be administered **parenterally** to **treat hypertensive emergencies**, such as malignant hypertension, eclampsia, or the severe hypertension associated with excess catecholamines. Parenteral therapy may include some combination of these agents:
   a. **Arteriolar and venous vasodilator**, such as nitroprusside
   b. **Arteriolar vasodilator**, such as diazoxide or hydralazine
   c. **α-Adrenergic blocking agent and β-adrenergic blocking agent**, such as labetalol
   d. **β-Blocking agent**, such as propranolol
   e. **Ganglionic blocking agent**, such as trimethaphan

D. Adverse effects

1. **Diuretics** (thiazides) may cause these adverse effects:
   a. **Fluid and electrolyte imbalances**, such as hypokalemia, hypercalcemia, hyperuricemia, hypomagnesemia, hyponatremia, and hyperglycemia
   b. **Increased serum low-density lipoprotein cholesterol and triglyceride levels**
   c. **Other effects** (see Chapter 12, section IV D)
2. **Vasodilators** are associated with these adverse effects:
   a. **Gastrointestinal effects**, such as gastrointestinal upset
   b. **CNS effects**, such as headache and dizziness
   c. **Cardiovascular effects**, such as tachycardia, fluid retention, and aggravation of angina
   d. **Other effects**, such as nasal congestion, hepatitis, glomerulonephritis, and systemic lupus erythematosus–like syndrome.
3. **Peripheral sympatholytics** are associated with a variety of adverse effects, depending on the specific agent.
   a. **β-Blockers** (e.g., propranolol) are associated with:
      (1) **Cardiovascular effects**, such as bradycardia, congestive heart failure, and Raynaud's phenomenon

(2) **Gastrointestinal effects**, such as gastrointestinal upset
(3) **Blood dyscrasias**
(4) **CNS effects**, such as depression, hallucinations, organic brain syndrome, and transient hearing loss
(5) **Other effects**, such as increased airway resistance, increased serum triglyceride levels, decreased high-density lipoprotein cholesterol levels, and psoriasis
(6) **Withdrawal syndrome** if withdrawal is abrupt

b. **Prazosin** is associated with these adverse effects:
(1) **Cardiovascular effects**, such as sudden syncope with the first dose, palpitations, and fluid retention
(2) **CNS effects**, such as headache, drowsiness, weakness, dizziness, and vertigo
(3) **Antimuscarinic effects** and **priapism**

c. **Guanethidine** is associated with these adverse effects:
(1) **Cardiovascular effects**, such as bradycardia, orthostatic hypotension, and sodium and water retention
(2) **Diarrhea**
(3) **Aggravation of bronchial asthma**

d. **Reserpine** is associated with these adverse effects:
(1) **CNS effects**, such as nightmares, depression, and drowsiness
(2) **Cardiovascular effects**, such as bradycardia
(3) **Gastrointestinal effects**, such as gastrointestinal upset
(4) **Nasal stuffiness**

4. **Central α_2-sympathomimetics** also have adverse effects that vary with the specific agent.

a. **Clonidine** is associated with these adverse effects:
(1) **CNS effects**, such as sedation and drowsiness
(2) **Dry mouth** and **severe rebound hypertension**
(3) **Insomnia**, **headache**, and **cardiac dysrhythmias** (with sudden withdrawal)

b. **Methyldopa** is associated with these adverse effects:
(1) **Cardiovascular effects**, such as orthostatic hypotension and bradycardia
(2) **CNS effects**, such as sedation and fever
(3) **Gastrointestinal effects**, such as colitis
(4) **Other effects**, such as hepatitis, cirrhosis, Coombs-positive hemolytic anemia, and systemic lupus erythematosus–like syndrome

5. **Angiotensin-converting enzyme inhibitors** are associated with these adverse effects:

a. **Cardiovascular effects**, such as hypotension
b. **Hematologic effects**, such as neutropenia and agranulocytosis
c. **Other effects**, such as anorexia, polyuria, oliguria, acute renal failure, and cholestatic jaundice

VI. ANTIHYPERLIPIDEMIC AGENTS

A. Chemistry. Antihyperlipidemic agents vary in chemical structure and are usually classified by their **site of action—locally** in the intestine (nonabsorbable agents) or **systemically** (absorbable agents).

1. The major **nonabsorbable agents** are **bile acid sequestrants**. These agents are hydrophilic, water-insoluble resins that bind to bile acids in the intestine. Examples include **cholestyramine chloride**, a basic anion-exchange resin consisting of trimethylbenzylammonium groups in a large copolymer of styrene and divinylbenzene, and **colestipol hydrochloride**, a copolymer of diethylpentamine and epichlorohydrin (Fig. 11-4).

2. The major **absorbable agents** include **nicotinic acid** (but not the structurally similar nicotinamide), the aryloxyisobutyric acid derivatives **clofibrate** (a prodrug ester) and **gemfibrozil**, the sulfur-containing *bis*-phenol **probucol**, the human menopausal gonadotropin coenzyme A (CoA) reductase inhibitor **lovastatin**, and the fatty fish oils containing large amounts of **eicosapentaenoic acid** (EPA) and **docosahexaenoic acid** (DHA) [Fig. 11-5].

B. Pharmacology. Antihyperlipidemic agents help **reduce lipoprotein production** (e.g., clofibrate and gemfibrozil) or **increase the efficiency of lipoprotein removal** (e.g., cholestyramine and colestipol).

C. Therapeutic indications. These agents are used (in conjunction with appropriate diet and exercise) to **reduce plasma lipoprotein levels.**

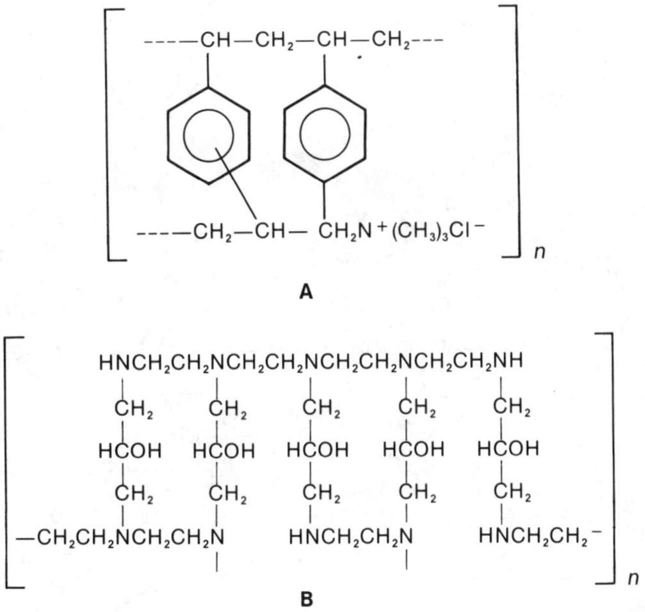

A

B

Figure 11-4. Structural formulas of (*A*) cholestyramine chloride (Questran) and (*B*) colestipol hydrochloride (Colestid), nonabsorbable antihyperlipidemic agents.

D. Adverse effects

1. **Nonabsorbable agents** (e.g., cholestyramine and colestipol) are associated with **gastrointestinal distress**, including abdominal bloating, nausea, dyspepsia, steatorrhea, and constipation or diarrhea.

2. **Absorbable agents** (e.g., clofibrate and gemfibrozil) are associated with **gastrointestinal distress, skin rash**, and **leukopenia**.
   - **a.** In addition, **clofibrate** may cause nausea, vomiting, dysphagia, weight gain, alopecia, and breast tenderness.
   - **b. Gemfibrozil** may also cause skeletal muscle pain, blurred vision, and anemia.

VII. ANTICOAGULANT AGENTS

A. Chemistry. The major anticoagulant agents are heparin and the oral anticoagulants.

1. **Heparin** is a large, highly acidic **mucopolysaccharide** composed of sulfated D-glucosamine and D-glucuronic acid molecules (Fig. 11-6).
   - **a.** Because it is **highly acidic**, it exists as an anion at physiologic pH and is very poorly absorbed from the gastrointestinal tract. Thus, it is **usually administered parenterally as the sodium salt**.
   - **b.** The action of heparin is quickly terminated by **protamine sulfate**, a highly basic protein that combines chemically with heparin in approximately equal amounts (mg:mg).

2. **Oral anticoagulants** consist of the highly effective coumarin derivatives and the relatively unimportant indanedione derivatives.
   - **a.** The **coumarin derivatives** (e.g., warfarin and dicumarol) are water insoluble, weakly acidic **4-hydroxycoumarin lactones** (Fig. 11- 7).
     - **(1)** These agents are **chemically related to vitamin K**, and their mechanism of action is directly related to their antagonism of this vitamin.
     - **(2)** These agents are also highly protein-bound and extensively metabolized in the liver. These characteristics, in addition to their relatively narrow therapeutic index, make them **very susceptible to significant drug interactions**.
   - **b. Phenindione** represents a typical indanedione derivative (Fig. 11-8).

B. Pharmacology

1. **Heparin** activates antithrombin III (heparin cofactor), which in turn **inhibits the conversion of prothrombin to thrombin**. In combination with antithrombin III, heparin also **inactivates**

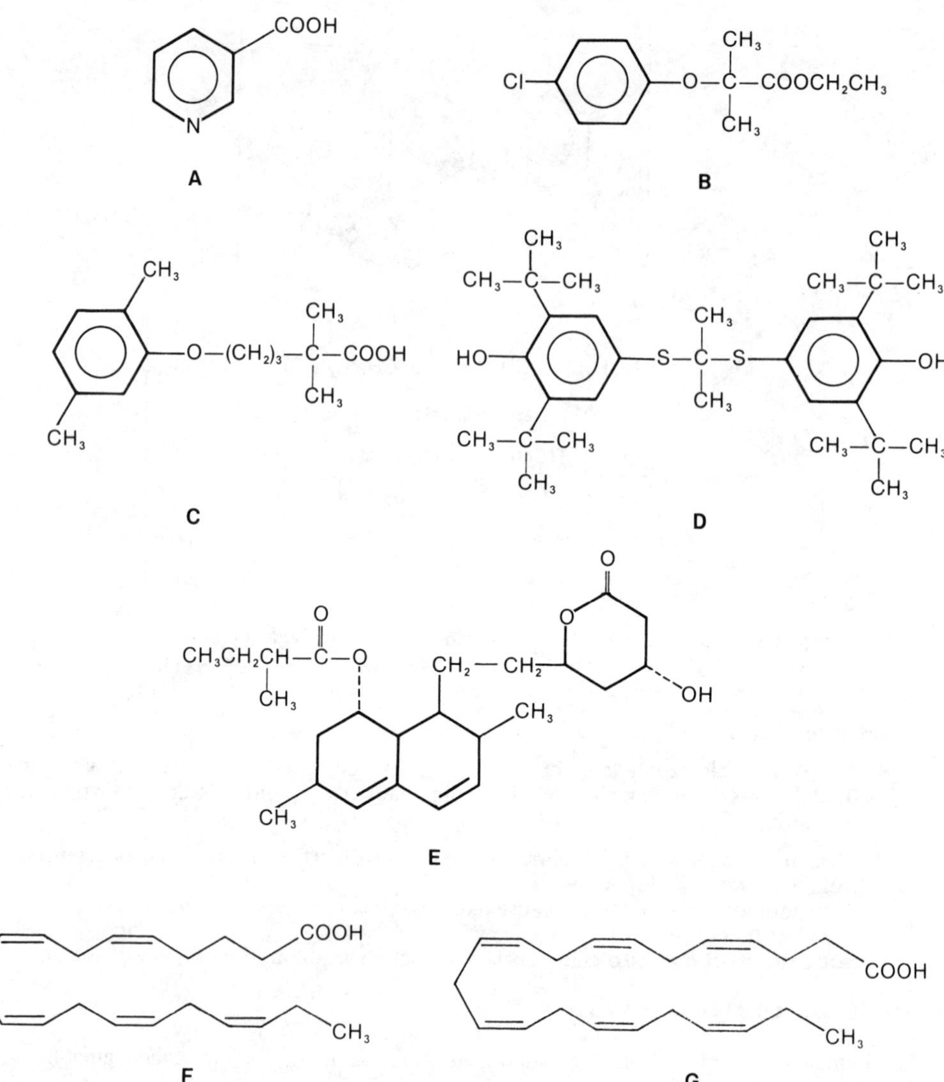

Figure 11-5. Structural formulas of (*A*) nicotinic acid (niacin), (*B*) clofibrate (Atromid-S), (*C*) gemfibrozil (Lopid), (*D*) probucol (Lorelco), (*E*) lovastatin (Mevacor), (*F*) eicosapentaenoic acid (found in Promega, Proto-Chol, and others), and (*G*) docosahexaenoic acid (found in Promega, Proto-Chol, and others). These agents are absorbable antihyperlipidemics.

Figure 11-6. Structural formula of heparin, a mucopolysaccharide anticoagulant agent.

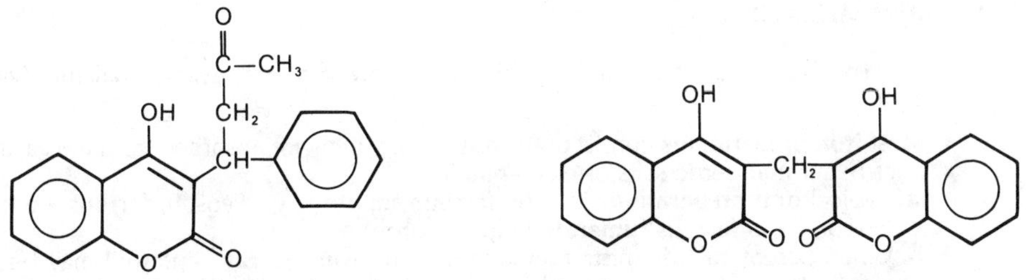

Figure 11-7. Structural formulas of (A) warfarin (Coumadin) and (B) dicumarol, coumarin-derivative oral anticoagulants.

thrombin, inhibiting the conversion of fibrinogen to fibrin. It **prolongs blood clotting time** both in vivo and in vitro.

2. **Oral anticoagulants interfere with** the vitamin K-dependent **hepatic synthesis of the active clotting factors** II (prothrombin), VII, IX, and X. These agents **prolong blood clotting time** in vivo only.

C. Therapeutic indications

1. **Heparin** is indicated:
   a. For the **prophylaxis and treatment of venous thrombosis, pulmonary embolism, peripheral arterial embolism**, and **atrial fibrillation with embolization**
   b. To **prevent clotting** during arterial surgery and cardiac surgery
   c. To **diagnose and treat disseminated intravascular coagulation**
   d. To **prevent postoperative venous thrombosis and pulmonary embolism** (in low-dose form)
   e. To **prevent cerebral thrombosis** during an evolving stroke
   f. As adjunct therapy to **prevent coronary occlusion** with acute myocardial infarction

2. The oral anticoagulant **warfarin sodium** is indicated:
   a. For the **prophylaxis and treatment of venous thrombosis, pulmonary embolism**, and **atrial fibrillation with embolization**
   b. As adjunct therapy to **prevent coronary occlusion** with acute myocardial infarction

D. Adverse effects

1. **Heparin**
   a. Heparin is associated with these adverse effects:
      (1) **Hematologic effects**, such as hemorrhage, local irritation, thrombocytopenia, hematoma, ulceration, erythema, and pain
      (2) **Other effects**, such as hypersensitivity reactions, fever, chills, and urticaria
   b. Severe adverse effects may be treated by administration of **protamine sulfate**, the specific antidote for heparin.

2. **Warfarin**
   a. The oral anticoagulant warfarin sodium is associated with these adverse effects:
      (1) **Hemorrhage**
      (2) **Other effects**, such as anorexia, urticaria, purpura, and alopecia
   b. Severe adverse effects may be treated by administration of **vitamin K_1**(phytonadione), the specific antidote for warfarin sodium.

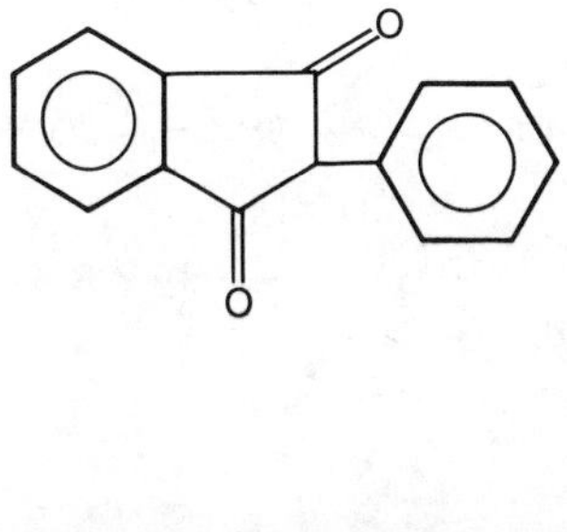

Figure 11-8. Structural formula of phenindione (Danilone), an indanedione-derivative oral anticoagulant.

VIII. ANTIANEMIC AGENTS

A. Chemistry. The major antianemic agents are iron preparations, cyanocobalamin (vitamin B_{12}), and folic acid.

1. Most **iron preparations** consist of **ferrous salts**, which are absorbed from the gastrointestinal tract better than ferric salts or elemental iron.
   a. Typical **oral preparations** include **ferrous sulfate** (e.g., Feosol), **ferrous gluconate** (e.g., Fergon), and **ferrous fumarate** (e.g., Femiron).
   b. When parenteral administration is indicated, **iron dextran** (Imferon) may be used. This preparation consists of a complex of ferric hydroxide and low molecular weight dextrans, forming a colloidal solution.

2. **Cyanocobalamin** (vitamin B_{12}) is a **nucleotide-like macromolecule** with a modified porphyrin unit (a **corrin ring**) containing a **trivalent cobalt atom**. A cyanide ion is also coordinated to the cobalt atom, as is a benzimidazole group. The benzimidazole group is bonded to an α-ribosyl phosphate.

3. **Folic acid** consists of three major components: a **pteridine nucleus** bonded to the nitrogen of *p*-aminobenzoic acid, which is bonded through an amide linkage to **glutamic acid** (Fig. 11-9).

B. Pharmacology

1. **Iron preparations** (ferrous salts) are readily absorbed from the gastrointestinal tract and stored in the bone marrow, liver, and spleen as **ferritin** and **hemosiderin**. They are subsequently incorporated as needed into **hemoglobin**, where the iron reversibly binds molecular oxygen. A **lack of body iron** causes **iron-deficiency anemia**, with hypochromic, microcytic red blood cells, which transport oxygen poorly.

2. **Cyanocobalamin** is readily absorbed from the gastrointestinal tract in the presence of intrinsic factor (Castle's factor), a glycoprotein produced by gastric parietal cells, which is necessary for gastrointestinal absorption of cyanocobalamin.
   a. Cyanocobalamin is transported to tissue by transcobalamin II. It is **essential for cell growth, for maintenance of normal nerve cell myelin**, and **for the metabolic functions of folate**.
   b. **Lack of dietary cyanocobalamin** (or lack of intrinsic factor) causes a vitamin B_{12} deficiency and **megaloblastic anemia**, with hyperchromic, macrocytic, immature red blood cells. Demyelination of nerve cells also occurs, causing **irreversible CNS damage**.

3. **Folic acid** is readily absorbed from the gastrointestinal tract, transported to tissue, and stored intracellularly. It is a precursor of several coenzymes (derivatives of tetrahydrofolic acid) that are involved in single carbon atom transfers. A **lack of dietary folic acid** causes folic acid deficiency and **megaloblastic anemia**, with hyperchromic, macrocytic, immature red blood cells. However, folic acid deficiency causes no neurologic impairment.

C. Therapeutic indications

1. **Iron preparations** (ferrous salts) are used to **treat iron-deficiency anemia**.
2. **Cyanocobalamin** is used to **treat vitamin B_{12}-deficiency megaloblastic anemia**.
3. **Folic acid** is used to **treat folic acid–deficiency megaloblastic anemia**.

D. Adverse effects

1. **Iron preparations** are associated with **gastrointestinal effects**, such as gastrointestinal distress, nausea, heartburn, diarrhea, and constipation.
2. **Cyanocobalamin** has only **rare adverse effects**.
3. **Folic acid** is associated only with **rare allergic reactions after parenteral administration**.

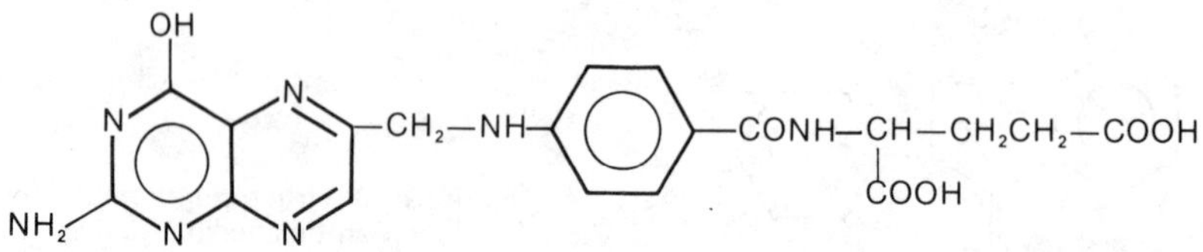

Figure 11-9. Structural formula of folic acid, an antianemic agent.

STUDY QUESTIONS

Directions: Each question below contains five suggested answers. Choose the **one best** response to each question.

1. Calcium channel blockers have all of the following characteristics EXCEPT

A. they block the slow inward current carried by calcium during phase 2 of the cardiac action potential
B. they dilate peripheral arterioles and reduce total peripheral resistance
C. they constrict coronary arteries and arterioles and decrease oxygen delivery to the myocardium
D. they are useful in treating stable angina pectoris and Prinzmetal's angina
E. their adverse effects include aggravation of congestive heart failure

2. The termination of heparin activity by protamine sulfate is due to

A. a chelating action
B. the inhibition of gastrointestinal absorption of heparin
C. the displacement of heparin–plasma protein binding
D. an acid–base interaction
E. the prothrombin-like activity of protamine

3. Which of the following cardiovascular agents is classified chemically as a glycoside?

A. Nifedipine
B. Digoxin
C. Flecainide
D. Cholestyramine
E. Warfarin

4. Cardiac glycosides may be useful in treating all of the following conditions EXCEPT

A. atrial flutter
B. paroxysmal atrial tachycardia
C. congestive heart failure
D. ventricular tachycardia
E. atrial fibrillation

5. Ingestion of which of the following vitamins should be avoided by a patient taking the oral anticoagulant warfarin?

A. Vitamin A
B. Vitamin B
C. Vitamin D
D. Vitamin E
E. Vitamin K

Directions: Each question below contains three suggested answers of which **one or more** is correct. Choose the answer

A if **I only** is correct
B if **III only** is correct
C if **I and II** are correct
D if **II and III** are correct
E if **I, II, and III** are correct

6. In the oral treatment of iron-deficiency anemias, iron is preferably administered as

I. ferrous iron
II. ferric salts
III. elemental iron

7. Parenterally administered antihypertensive agents used in the treatment of hypertensive emergencies include the

I. centrally acting antiadrenergic clonidine
II. arteriolar and venous vasodilator nitroprusside
III. ganglionic-blocking agent trimethaphan

SUMMARY OF DIRECTIONS

A	B	C	D	E
I only	III only	I, II only	II, III only	All are correct

8. Certain factors contribute to the longer duration of action of digitoxin when compared to that of digoxin. These include

I. greater protein binding
II. reduced polarity
III. greater tubular reabsorption

9. Correct statements concerning the properties of oral anticoagulants include

I. oral anticoagulants interfere with vitamin K-dependent synthesis of active clotting factors II, VII, IX, and X
II. adverse effects associated with oral anticoagulants are hemorrhage, urticaria, purpura, and alopecia
III. oral anticoagulants prolong the clotting time of blood both in vivo and in vitro

Directions: The group of questions below consists of lettered choices followed by several numbered items. For each numbered item select the **one** lettered choice with which it is **most** closely associated. Each lettered choice may be used once, more than once, or not at all.

Questions 10–12

For each adverse effect, select the class of drug that most closely relates to it.

A. Cardiac glycosides
B. Calcium channel blockers
C. Angiotensin converting enzyme (ACE) inhibitors
D. β-adrenergic blockers
E. Nitrites and nitrates

10. Bradycardia, hypotension, increased airway resistance, and congestive heart failure

11. Visual disturbances (yellow or green vision), confusion, anorexia, vomiting, atrioventricular block, and ventricular tachycardia

12. Hypotension, acute renal failure, cholestatic jaundice, and agranulocytosis

ANSWERS AND EXPLANATIONS

1. The answer is C. (*III B 3, C 3, D 3*) Calcium channel blockers are used in the treatment of angina because they dilate coronary arteries and arterioles, thus decreasing coronary vascular resistance and increasing coronary blood flow.

2. The answer is D. (*VII A 1, D 1; Figure 11-6*) Heparin is a highly acidic mucopolysaccharide, whereas protamine is a highly basic protein. When administered subsequently to heparin, protamine chemically combines with it (presumably by an acid–base interaction) and inactivates its anticoagulant effect. Hence, it is an effective antidote for heparin. Caution must be employed in the use of protamine since an excess of protamine can cause an anticoagulant effect itself.

3. The answer is B. (*II A*) Most glycosides are natural products obtained from plant material. While there are very few medicinal agents that are glycosides, the group known as the cardiac glycosides are extremely important and are widely used in the treatment of congestive heart failure. Digoxin is a cardiac glycoside obtained from *Digitalis lanata*. Other cardiac glycosides include digitoxin, which is obtained from *Digitalis purpurea* and ouabain, which is obtained from *Strophanthus gratus*.

4. The answer is D. (*II C; Table 11-4*) Ventricular tachycardia is produced by toxic cardiac glycoside dosage and would not be a therapeutic indication for the agents. Cardiac glycosides increase systolic contraction velocity and increase the refractory period of the atrioventricular (AV) node. They also have a positive inotropic effect.

5. The answer is E. [*VII A 2 a (1), D 2*] The oral anticoagulants such as warfarin act by inhibiting the liver biosynthesis of prothrombin, which is the precursor of the enzyme thrombin that catalyzes the conversion of soluble fibrinogen to the insoluble polymer fibrin, which results in clot formation. One of the principal factors in the biosynthesis of prothrombin is vitamin K, with which warfarin competes to inhibit this process. Since this is a reversible competition, vitamin K acts as an antagonist to the oral anticoagulants.

6. The answer is A (I). (*VIII A 1*) Absorption of orally administered iron is significantly more complete with ferrous iron than with either ferric salts or elemental iron, presumably because of its better solubility characteristics. Iron preparations (ferrous salts) are more readily absorbed from the gastrointestinal tract and are stored in the bone marrow, liver, and spleen as ferritin and hemosiderin.

7. The answer is D (II, III). (*V B 4, C 2 a, e*) Clonidine is not recognized as a drug of choice for hypertensive emergencies, possibly because of its central mechanism of action and the latent period required for its effect compared with other peripheral agents.

8. The answer is E (all). (*II A; Figure 11-1*) Structurally, digitoxin has only one alcohol group on its steroidal nucleus, whereas digoxin has two. This slight difference in structure has a significant effect on the polarity of the molecule. Due to its greater liposolubility, digitoxin is more likely to undergo tubular reabsorption, to undergo enterohepatic cycling, to penetrate into the liver microsomes and undergo metabolism, and to be protein-bound, all of which contribute to its longer duration of action and potential cumulative effects.

9. The answer is C (I, II). [*VII A 2 a (1), D 2*] Oral anticoagulants are only effective in vivo since they block hepatic synthesis of vitamin K-dependent coagulation factors (factors II, VII, IX, and X). This also explains the latency period associated with initiation of oral anticoagulant therapy.

10–12. The answers are: 10-D, 11-A, 12-C. (*II D; III D 2; V B 5*) Nonselective β-adrenergic blockers (e.g., propranolol) produce adverse effects associated with their mechanism of action on the autonomic nervous system. Thus, bronchospasm, lowering of blood pressure, and reduced heart rate result from blockade of autonomic β-adrenergic receptors. Visual disturbances (yellow or green vision) are peculiar to cardiac glycoside overdose. Atrioventricular (AV) dissociation and ventricular tachycardia are obviously more significant adverse effects. Angiotensin converting enzyme (ACE) inhibitors reportedly may cause blood dyscrasias in addition to cholestatic jaundice and acute renal failure.

12 Diuretics

David C. Kosegarten
Edward F. LaSala

I. INTRODUCTION. Diuretics increase the rate of urine formation, increasing urine volume and water and solute excretion. They fall into five major categories: osmotic diuretics, carbonic anhydrase inhibitors, benzothiadiazide diuretics, loop diuretics, and potassium-sparing diuretics.

II. OSMOTIC DIURETICS

A. Chemistry. Osmotic diuretics (e.g., mannitol and urea) are **highly polar**, **water-soluble** agents with a **low renal threshold** (Fig. 12-1).

B. Pharmacology

1. Osmotic diuretics are relatively inert chemicals that are **freely filtered at the glomerulus** and **poorly absorbed**. By increasing the osmolarity of the glomerular filtrate, they limit tubular reabsorption of water and thus **promote diuresis**.
2. Because these agents increase water, sodium, chloride, and bicarbonate excretion, they cause an **increase in urinary pH**.

C. Therapeutic indications. Osmotic diuretics are used to:

1. **Help prevent and treat oliguria and anuria**
2. **Reduce cerebral edema** and **decrease intracranial pressure**
3. **Reduce intraocular pressure**

D. Adverse effects. Osmotic diuretics are associated with the following adverse effects:

1. **Headache** and **blurred vision**
2. **Increased blood volume** (aggravates congestive heart failure)

III. CARBONIC ANHYDRASE INHIBITORS

A. Chemistry. Carbonic anhydrase inhibitors are **aromatic or heterocyclic sulfonamides** with a prominent thiadiazole nucleus. **Acetazolamide** is the prototypical agent (Fig. 12-2).

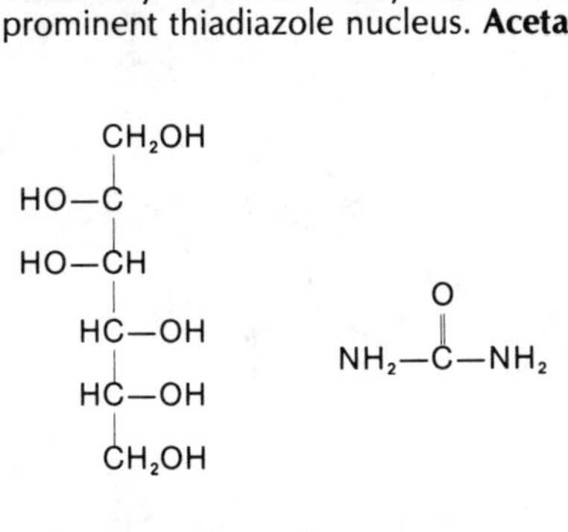

Figure 12-1. Structural formulas of (*A*) mannitol (Osmitrol) and (*B*) urea (Ureaphil), osmotic diuretics.

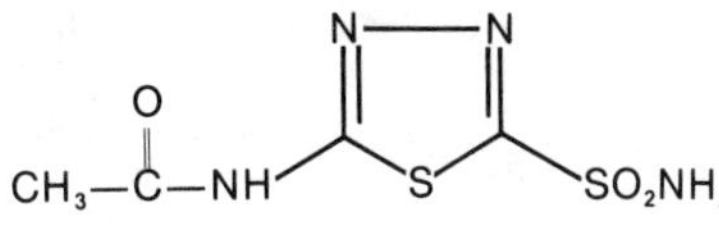

Figure 12-2. Structural formula of acetazolamide (Diamox), the prototypical carbonic anhydrase inhibitor.

B. Pharmacology

1. Carbonic anhydrase inhibitors **noncompetitively inhibit the enzyme carbonic anhydrase.** This prevents the enzyme from providing the tubular hydrogen ions needed for exchange with sodium, reducing sodium reabsorption in the proximal tubule and enhancing sodium's subsequent exchange with potassium in the distal tubule.
2. Because these agents increase water, sodium, potassium, and bicarbonate excretion, they cause an **alkaline urinary pH**.

C. Therapeutic indications.
Carbonic anhydrase inhibitors are used:

1. To **reduce edema** (as adjunct diuretic therapy)
2. To **reduce intraocular pressure** (retard aqueous humor formation)
3. To **alkalinize the urine**, enhancing excretion of acidic drugs and their metabolites
4. As **anticonvulsant agents** in the treatment of petit mal epilepsy

D. Adverse effects.
Carbonic anhydrase inhibitors are associated with the following adverse effects:

1. **Central nervous system (CNS) effects**, such as CNS depression, drowsiness, sedation, fatigue, disorientation, and paresthesias
2. **Gastrointestinal effects**, such as gastrointestinal upset, nausea, vomiting, and constipation
3. **Hematologic effects**, such as bone marrow depression, thrombocytopenia, hemolytic anemia, leukopenia, and agranulocytosis
4. **Hyperchloremic acidosis**

IV. BENZOTHIADIAZIDE DIURETICS

A. Chemistry

1. The commonly used benzothiadiazide diuretics (**also called thiazides**) are primarily closely related **benzothiadiazines with variable substituents**. The prototypical agent is **chlorothiazide** (Fig. 12-3; see Fig. 12-3*A*).

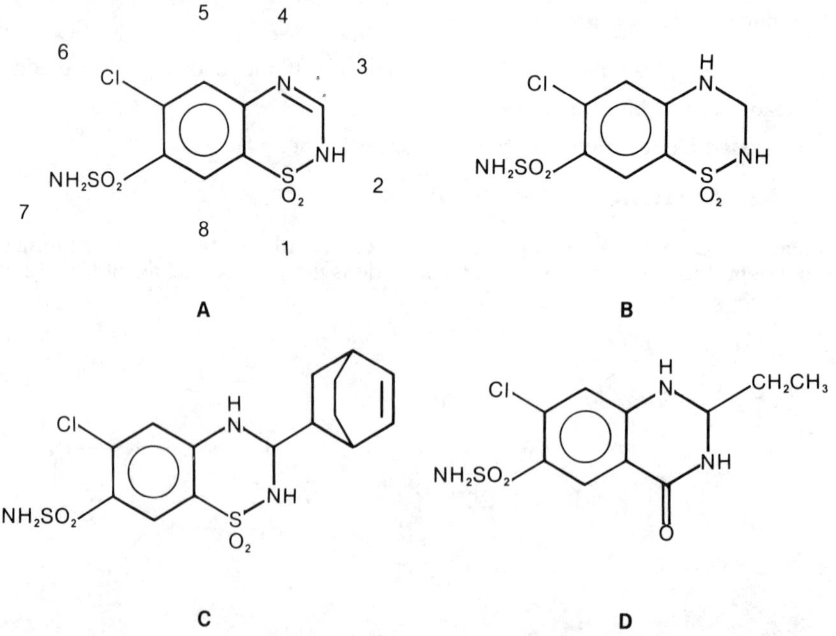

Figure 12-3. Structural formulas of (*A*) chlorothiazide (Diuril), the prototypical benzothiadiazide diuretic, and (*B*) hydrochlorothiazide (Hydrodiuril) as well as (*C*) cyclothiazide (Anhydron) and (*D*) quinethazone (Hydromox), related compounds with substituents that prolong activity and enhance potency.

2. Optimal diuretic activity depends on certain **structural features**.
   a. The benzene ring must have a **sulfonamide group** (preferably unsubstituted) in position 7 and a **halogen** (usually a chloro group) or a **trifluoromethyl group** in position 6 (see Fig. 12-3).
   b. **Saturation of the 3,4-double bond** increases potency, as with hydrochlorothiazide (see Fig. 12-3*B*).
   c. **Lipophilic substituents** at position 3 or **methyl groups** at position 2 enhance potency and prolong activity, as with cyclothiazide and bendroflumethiazide (see Fig. 12-3C).
   d. **Replacement of the sulfonyl group** in position 1 by a **carbonyl group** results in prolonged activity, as with quinethazone (see Fig. 12-3*D*).
3. A few **sulfamoylbenzamides** (e.g., indapamide and chlorthalidone) have activity similar to that of the benzothiadiazines (Fig. 12-4).
4. **Benzothiadiazines without the sulfonamide group** (e.g., diazoxide) retain antihypertensive activity but lack diuretic activity (Fig. 12-5).

B. Pharmacology

1. Benzothiadiazides **directly inhibit sodium and chloride reabsorption** at the proximal portion of the distal convoluted tubule.
2. These agents increase water, sodium, chloride, potassium, and bicarbonate excretion and decrease calcium excretion and uric acid secretion. They cause an **alkaline urinary pH**.

C. Therapeutic indications. Benzothiadiazides are used to:

1. **Treat chronic edema**
2. **Treat hypertension**
3. **Treat congestive heart failure** (as adjunctive edema therapy)

D. Adverse effects. Benzothiadiazides are associated with these adverse effects:

1. **CNS effects**, such as headache, dizziness, paresthesias, drowsiness, and restlessness
2. **Gastrointestinal effects**, such as gastrointestinal irritation, nausea, vomiting, abdominal bloating, and constipation
3. **Cardiovascular effects**, such as orthostatic hypotension, palpitations, hemoconcentration, and venous thrombosis
4. **Hematologic effects**, such as blood dyscrasias, leukopenia, thrombocytopenia, agranulocytosis, aplastic anemia, hemolytic anemia, and rash
5. **Fluid and electrolyte imbalances**, such as hypokalemia, hypercalcemia, and hyperuricemia
6. **Muscular cramps**
7. **Acute gout attacks**

V. LOOP DIURETICS

A. Chemistry. Loop diuretics are **anthranilic acid derivatives** with a sulfonamide substituent (e.g., furosemide and bumetanide) or **aryloxyacetic acids** without a sulfonamide substituent (e.g., ethacrynic acid) [Fig. 12-6].

Figure 12-4. Structural formula of indapamide (Lozol), a sulfamoylbenzamide with pharmacologic activity similar to that of the benzothiadiazide diuretics.

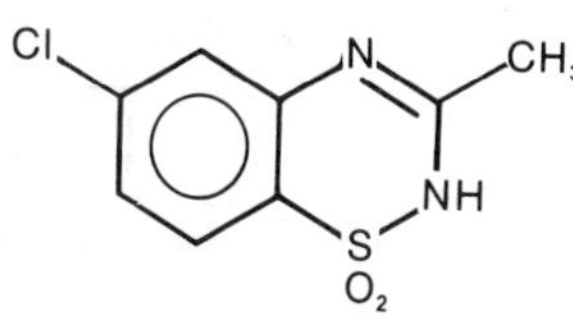

Figure 12-5. Structural formula of diazoxide (Hyperstat), a benzothiadiazine lacking a sulfonamide group.

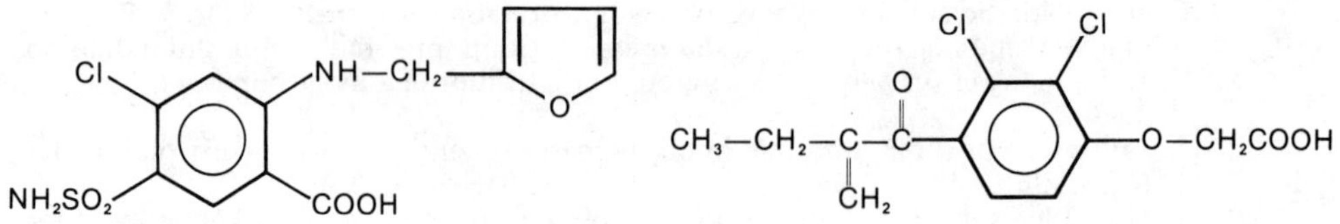

Figure 12-6. Structural formulas of (A) furosemide (Lasix) and (B) ethacrynic acid (Edecrin), loop diuretics.

B. Pharmacology

1. These agents act principally at the ascending limb of the loop of Henle, where they **inhibit the cotransport of sodium and chloride from the luminal filtrate.**
2. Loop diuretics increase excretion of water, sodium, and chloride, decrease uric acid secretion, and cause **no change in urinary pH.**

C. Therapeutic indications. Loop diuretics are used to:

1. **Treat edema** from congestive heart failure, hepatic cirrhosis, and renal disease
2. **Treat pulmonary edema** and **ascites**

D. Adverse effects. Loop diuretics are associated with these adverse effects:

1. **Fluid and electrolyte imbalances**, such as hypokalemia, azotemia, dehydration, hyperuricemia, and hypercalciuria
2. **CNS effects**, such as headache, vertigo, blurred vision, tinnitus, and (rarely) irreversible hearing loss
3. **Hematologic effects**, such as thrombocytopenia and agranulocytosis
4. **Cardiovascular effects**, such as orthostatic hypotension
5. **Gastrointestinal effects**, such as nausea, vomiting, and diarrhea
6. **Leg cramps**

VI. POTASSIUM-SPARING DIURETICS

A. Chemistry. The potassium-sparing diuretics are **pteridine or pyrazine derivatives** (e.g., triamterene and amiloride) or **steroid analogue antagonists of aldosterone** (e.g., spironolactone) [Fig. 12-7].

B. Pharmacology

1. **Spironolactone** acts as a **competitive inhibitor of aldosterone** at receptors in the distal

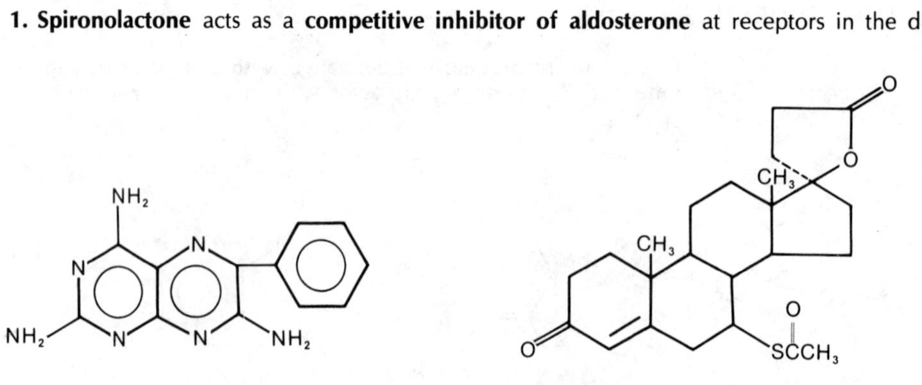

Figure 12-7. Structural formulas of (A) triamterene (Dyrenium) and (B) spironolactone (Aldactone), potassium-sparing diuretics.

tubule. It interferes with aldosterone-mediated sodium–potassium exchange, decreasing potassium secretion.

2. **Triamterene**, which is not an aldosterone antagonist, **acts directly on the distal tubule** through an unknown mechanism. It interferes with sodium reabsorption and potassium transport, decreasing potassium secretion.

3. **Amiloride**, which also is not an aldosterone antagonist, appears to **inhibit sodium–potassium ATPase**. Thus, it inhibits active transport of sodium and potassium at the distal tubule, decreasing potassium secretion.

4. The potassium-sparing diuretics increase bicarbonate excretion and cause an **alkaline urinary pH**.

C. Therapeutic indications. Potassium-sparing diuretics are used:

1. As adjunctive therapy, to **treat edema** from congestive heart failure, hepatic cirrhosis, nephrotic syndrome, and hyperaldosteronism

2. As adjunctive therapy (with thiazides and loop diuretics), to **treat hypertension**

3. To **treat or prevent hypokalemia**

D. Adverse effects

1. **Spironolactone** is associated with these adverse effects:
   a. **Hyperkalemia**
   b. **Gastrointestinal effects**, such as gastrointestinal upset, nausea, abdominal cramps, and diarrhea
   c. **Endocrine effects**, such as gynecomastia, menstrual irregularities, and hirsutism
   d. **CNS effects**, such as mental confusion and lethargy

2. **Triamterene** and **amiloride** are associated with these adverse effects:
   a. **Hyperkalemia**
   b. **Gastrointestinal effects**, such as gastrointestinal upset, nausea, and vomiting
   c. **CNS effects**, such as headache and dizziness
   d. **Increased uric acid levels in patients with gouty arthritis** (with triamterene)
   e. **Methemoglobinemia in patients with alcoholic cirrhosis** (with triamterene, which inhibits dihydrofolate reductase)

STUDY QUESTIONS

Directions: Each question below contains five suggested answers. Choose the **one best** response to each question.

1. The structure shown below is characteristic of which of the following agents?

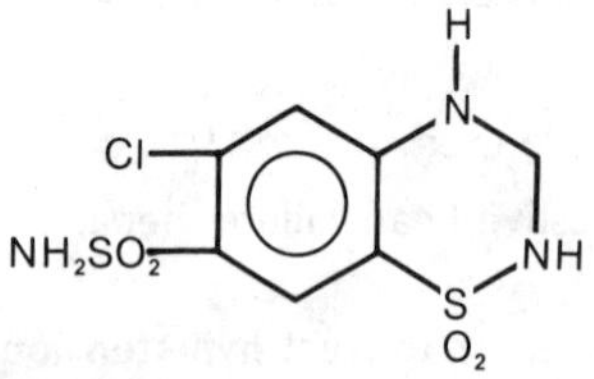

A. Osmotic diuretics
B. Carbonic anhydrase inhibitors
C. Thiazides
D. Loop diuretics
E. Potassium-sparing diuretics

2. Which of the following diuretics is most similar in chemical structure to the antihypertensive agent diazoxide?

A. Furosemide
B. Spironolactone
C. Mannitol
D. Acetazolamide
E. Chlorothiazide

Directions: The group of questions below consists of lettered choices followed by several numbered items. For each numbered item select the **one** lettered choice with which it is **most** closely associated. Each lettered choice may be used once, more than once, or not at all.

Questions 3–5

For each statement listed below, select the drug that it most closely characterizes.

A. Furosemide
B. Hydrochlorothiazide
C. Spironolactone
D. Mannitol
E. Acetazolamide

3. It interferes with distal tubular aldosterone-mediated sodium–potassium exchange, renders the urine alkaline, and may cause hyperkalemia, gynecomastia, and menstrual irregularities

4. Freely filtered, this drug limits tubular reabsorption of water and is useful in reducing cerebral edema and intracranial pressure

5. The principal site of action of this drug is on the thick ascending limb of Henle's loop; it is useful in treating pulmonary edema and ascites

ANSWERS AND EXPLANATIONS

1. The answer is C. (*IV A; Figure 12-3*) The structure can be recognized as a benzothiadiazine, which is known also as a thiazide. It represents the structure of hydrochlorothiazide, a sulfonamide diuretic. Other sulfonamide diuretics include the carbonic anhydrase inhibitors, such as acetazolamide, and the loop diuretics, such as furosemide. Neither of these subclasses contains drugs with a benzothiadiazine nucleus.

2. The answer is E. (*IV A; Figures 12-3, 12-5*) Diazoxide is a benzothiadiazine derivative; therefore, it would be most similar to chlorothiazide, which is also a benzothiadiazine. While both the thiazides and the diazoxides have antihypertensive activity, only the thiazides have significant diuretic activity. One of the structural requirements of the thiazide diuretics is an electron-withdrawing group, such as a halogen, ortho to the sulfonamide group on the benzene nucleus. The diazoxide molecule lacks such a group.

3–5. The answers are: 3-C, 4-D, 5-A. (*VI B, D; II B, C; V B, C*) Spironolactone reduces the amount of potassium excreted and is often used with other diuretics that promote the excretion of potassium, such as the benzothiadiazides. Mannitol increases the osmolarity of the glomerular filtrate since it is reabsorbed poorly. Furosemide is a diuretic of choice in the treatment of acute congestive heart failure because it promotes a significant rapid excretion of water and sodium.

13
Hormones and Related Drugs

David C. Kosegarten
Edward F. LaSala

I. INTRODUCTION. Hormones—substances secreted by specific tissues and transported to other specific tissues, where they exert their effects—may be classified pharmacologically as drugs. They may be obtained from **natural substances** (animal preparations), or they may be **synthetic or semisynthetic compounds** resembling the natural products. They are often used for **replacement therapy** (e.g., exogenous insulin for treatment of diabetes mellitus). However, they can also be used for a variety of other therapeutic and diagnostic purposes. Certain drugs (e.g., thyroid hormone inhibitors and oral antidiabetic agents), while not hormones themselves, influence the synthesis or secretion of hormones. Therapeutically useful hormones and related drugs include the **pituitary hormones**, the **gonadal hormones**, the **adrenocorticosteroids**, the **thyroid hormones and inhibitors**, and the **antidiabetic agents**.

II. PITUITARY HORMONES

A. Chemistry. Pituitary hormones are divided into two groups by their site of secretion.

1. The two **posterior pituitary hormones—oxytocin** (Pitocin) and **vasopressin** (Pitressin)—are closely related octapeptides. They differ from each other in only two of their eight amino acids but have different biologic actions.
2. The **anterior pituitary hormones used therapeutically** are protein molecules.
   a. **Corticotropin** (Acthar)—commonly referred to as **adrenocorticotropic hormone**, or **ACTH**—is a single-chain polypeptide containing 39 amino acids. It has a molecular weight of 4600.
   b. **Thyrotropin** (Thytropar)—commonly referred to as **thyroid-stimulating hormone (TSH)**—is a glycoprotein with a molecular weight of 28,000.
   c. **Thyrotropin-releasing hormone (TRH)** [Relefact]—commonly known as **protirelin**—is a tripeptide with a molecular weight of 363.
   d. **Growth hormone** (Asellacrin)—commonly known as **somatotropin**—consists of 191 amino acids and has a molecular weight of 21,500.
3. The anterior pituitary hormones known as the **pituitary gonadotropins** are **not available for therapeutic use**. These include **follicle-stimulating hormone (FSH)**, **luteinizing hormone (LH)**, and **prolactin** (commonly known as luteotropic hormone, or LTH). However, several related **nonpituitary gonadotropins** have FSH-like or LH-like actions and are **used therapeutically**.
   a. **Menotropins** (Pergonal)—commonly known as **HMG**—are high in FSH-like and LH-like activity and are obtained from the urine of postmenopausal women.
   b. **Urofollitropin** (Metrodin) is high in FSH-like activity and is obtained from the urine of postmenopausal women.
   c. **Human chorionic gonadotropin** (Follutein)—commonly known as **HCG**—has LH-like activity and is obtained from the urine of pregnant women.

B. Pharmacology. The therapeutically important pituitary hormones include the anterior pituitary agents **corticotropin**, **growth hormone** (somatotropin), and **menotropins** (gonadotropin), and the posterior pituitary agents **vasopressin** and **oxytocin**.

1. **Corticotropin** is secreted from the anterior pituitary, stimulating the adrenal cortex to produce and secrete **adrenocorticosteroids** (see section IV).
2. **Growth hormone** stimulates protein, carbohydrate, and lipid metabolism to promote increased cell, organ, connective tissue, and skeletal growth, causing a **rapid increase in the overall rate of linear growth**.

3. **Menotropins** produce **ovarian follicular growth** and **induce ovulation** by means of FSH-like and LH-like actions.

4. **Vasopressin** has vasopressor and antidiuretic hormone (ADH) activity. It acts primarily on the distal renal tubular epithelium, where it **promotes the reabsorption of water**.

5. **Oxytocin stimulates uterine contraction** and plays an important role in the **induction of labor**.

C. **Therapeutic indications**

1. **Corticotropin** is used primarily for the **diagnosis and differentiation of primary and secondary adrenal insufficiency**.

2. **Growth hormone** is used for the **long-term treatment of children whose growth failure is the result of lack of endogenous growth hormone secretion**.

3. **Menotropins** are used to **induce ovulation and pregnancy** in anovulatory infertile women whose anovulation is not the result of primary ovarian failure. In men, menotropins are used to **induce spermatogenesis**.

4. **Vasopressin** is used to **treat neurogenic diabetes insipidus** and to **treat postoperative abdominal distention**.

5. **Oxytocin** is used to **promote delivery** by initiating and improving uterine contractions and to **control postpartum bleeding or hemorrhage**.

D. **Adverse effects**

1. **Corticotropin** is **only rarely associated** with adverse effects, which represent hypersensitivity reactions or corticosteroid excess.

2. **Growth hormone** is associated with adverse effects primarily related to the **development of antibodies to growth hormone**. The antibodies are nonbinding in most cases and do not interfere with continued growth hormone treatment.

3. **Menotropins** are associated with these adverse effects:
   a. In **women**—hypersensitivity, arterial thromboembolism, febrile reactions, ovarian enlargement hyperstimulation syndrome, hemoperitoneum, and (rarely) birth defects
   b. In **men**—gynecomastia

4. **Vasopressin** is associated with these adverse effects:
   a. **Gastrointestinal effects**, such as abdominal cramps, flatulence, nausea, and vomiting
   b. **Central nervous system (CNS) effects**, such as tremor, sweating, vertigo, and headache
   c. **Other effects**, such as urticaria, bronchoconstriction, and anaphylaxis

5. **Oxytocin** is associated with these adverse effects:
   a. **Severe water intoxication** with convulsions and coma, after slow (24-hour) infusion
   b. **Uterine hypertonicity**, with spasm, tetanic contractions, or uterine rupture
   c. **Postpartum hemorrhage**
   d. **Nausea, vomiting**, and **anaphylaxis**
   e. **Fetal effects**, such as bradycardia, neonatal jaundice, cardiac dysrhythmias, and premature ventricular contractions

III. GONADAL HORMONES

A. **Chemistry**. Most natural and synthetic gonadal hormones are derivatives of **cyclopentanoperhydrophenanthrene** (Fig. 13-1). All hormones having this fused reduced 17-carbon-atom ring system are classified as **steroids**.

1. The basic nucleus of the **natural estrogens** has a methyl group designated as C 18 on position C 13 cyclopentanoperhydrophenanthrene. This basic nucleus is known as **estrane**.

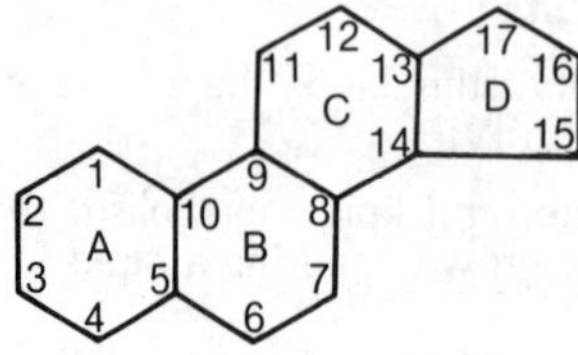

Figure 13-1. Structural formula of cyclopentanoperhydrophenanthrene, from which the gonadal hormones are derived. The letters *A* through *D* indicate the rings, which may be modified during subsequent conversions; the numbers *1* through *17* refer to carbon atom positions on the rings.

a. Unlike other steroid hormones, all **estrogens have an aromatic A ring** (see Fig. 13-1).

b. Estradiol (Estrace), the principal estrogenic hormone, exists in the body in equilibrium with **estrone**, which is converted to **estriol** prior to excretion (Fig. 13-2).

(1) Several **estradiol esters** [e.g., estradiol 17-cypionate (Depo-Estradiol) and estradiol 17-valerate (Delestrogen)] **are prepared** as intramuscular injections **in oil, to prolong their action.**

(2) These estradiol esters are **slowly hydrolyzed in muscle tissues** before absorption, and thus are considered to be prodrugs.

(3) Addition of an α-ethynyl group (—C≡CH) at position C 17 of estradiol increases resistance to first-pass metabolism and enhances oral effectiveness. Two of these **estradiol derivatives, ethinyl estradiol** and its 3-methyl ether **mestranol**, are used principally as the estrogenic components of serial-type **oral contraceptives** (Fig. 13-3). Another, **quinestrol** (Estrovis), is used principally for **estrogen replacement therapy**.

c. The **synthetic estrogens** (e.g., diethylstilbestrol and chlorotrianisene) are **nonsteroidal stilbene derivatives** that appear to assume an estradiol-like conformation in vivo (Fig. 13-4).

d. The **antiestrogens** clomiphene and tamoxifen citrate are stilbene derivatives that are structurally related to chlorotrianisene (Fig. 13-5). However, these agents have different in vivo binding sites and activities.

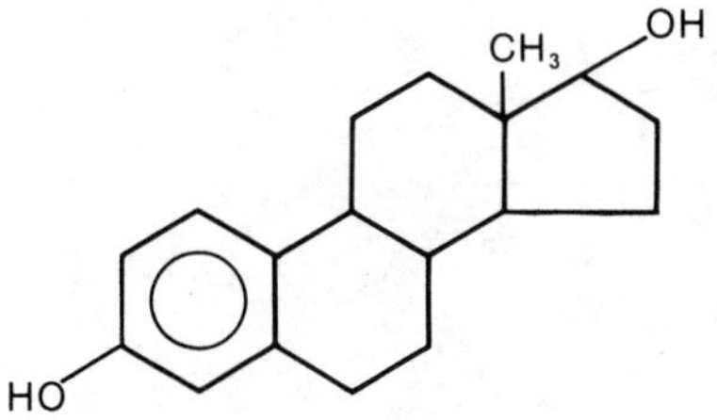

A (HO; CH_3; OH) ⇌ B (HO; CH_3; O) →

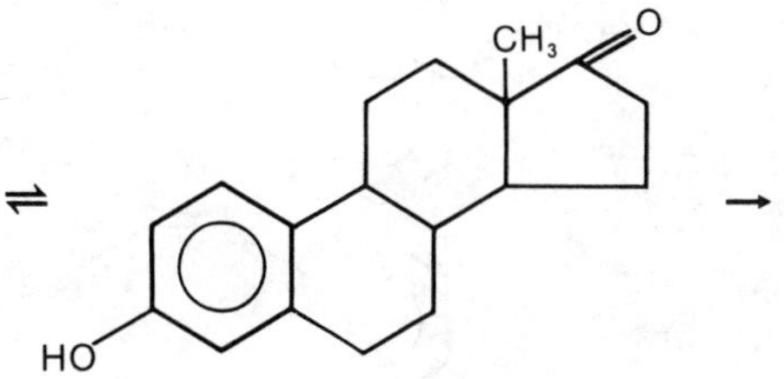

C (HO; CH_3; OH; —OH)

Figure 13-2. Structural formulas of (*A*) estradiol, which exists in the body in equilibrium with (*B*) estrone, which in turn is converted to (*C*) estriol before excretion.

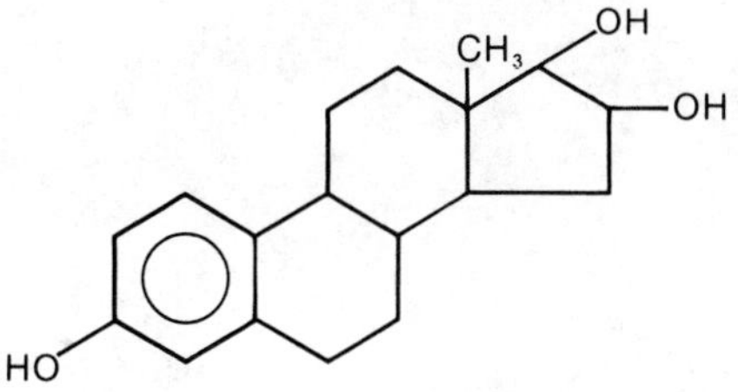

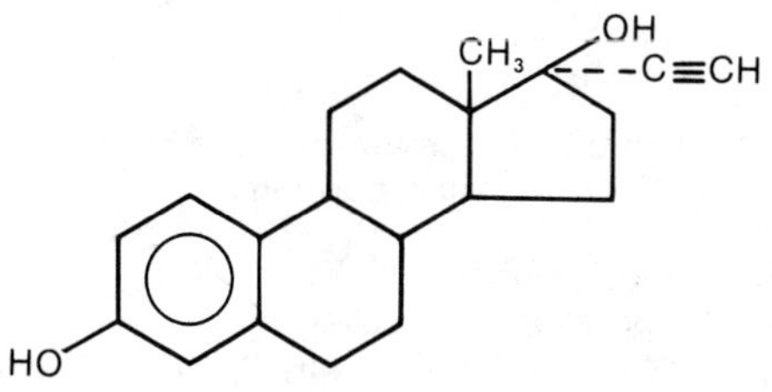

A (HO; CH_3; OH; --C≡CH)

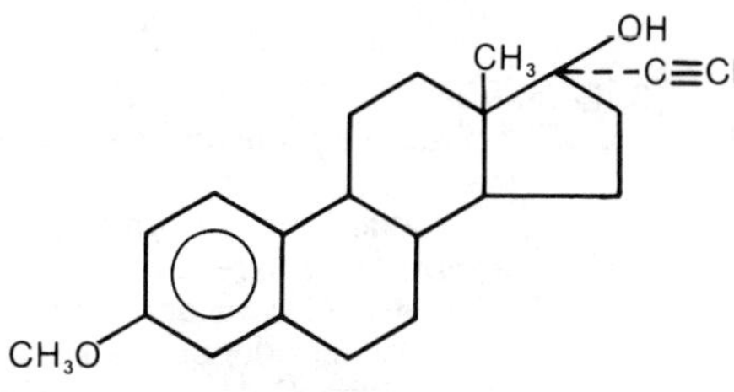

B (CH_3O; CH_3; OH; --C≡CH)

Figure 13-3. Structural formulas of (*A*) ethinyl estradiol and (*B*) mestranol, estradiol derivatives used principally as the estrogenic components of serial-type oral contraceptives.

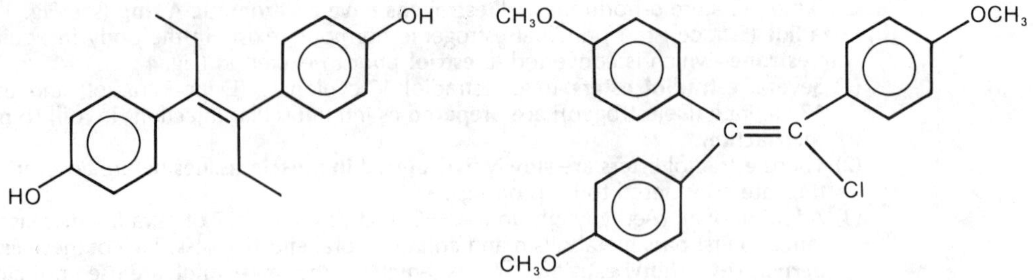

Figure 13-4. Structural formulas of (A) diethylstilbestrol (DES) and (B) chlorotrianisene (Tace), synthetic estrogens derived from stilbene.

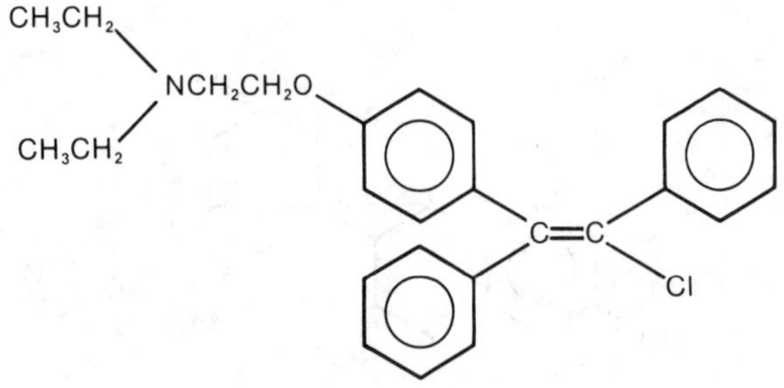

Figure 13-5. Structural formulas of (A) clomiphene (Clomid) and (B) tamoxifen (Nolvadex), antiestrogens that are structurally similar to chlorotrianisene.

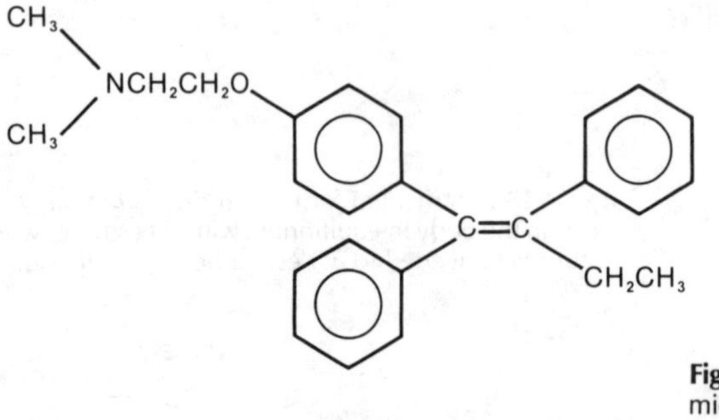

2. Progestins

a. The **naturally occurring progestin** progesterone is a C 21 steroid with a methyl group designated C 19 at position C 10 of estrane and a C 20–C 21 chain at position C 17 (see Fig. 13-1). Its basic nucleus is known as pregnane (Fig. 13-6).

b. The **synthetic progestins**, which are also steroids, consist of two types.

(1) The **progesterone derivatives** (e.g., medroxyprogesterone acetate and megestrol acetate) typically introduce a methyl group at position C 6 of progesterone and an acetoxy group at position C 17. These substitutions increase lipid solubility and decrease first-pass metabolism, **enhancing oral activity and the progestin effect** (Fig. 13-7).

(2) The **19-norprogestins** replace the C 19 methyl group of progesterone with a hydrogen; they also replace the C 17 acetyl group with a hydroxyl group and an ethynyl group. The prototypical agent of this type is **norethindrone** (Fig. 13-8).

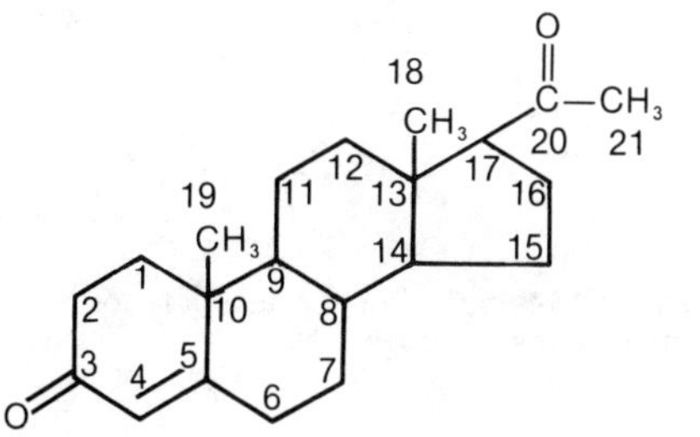

Figure 13-6. Structural formula of progesterone, which is a derivative of pregnane. The numbers 1 through 21 refer to carbon atom positions on the rings.

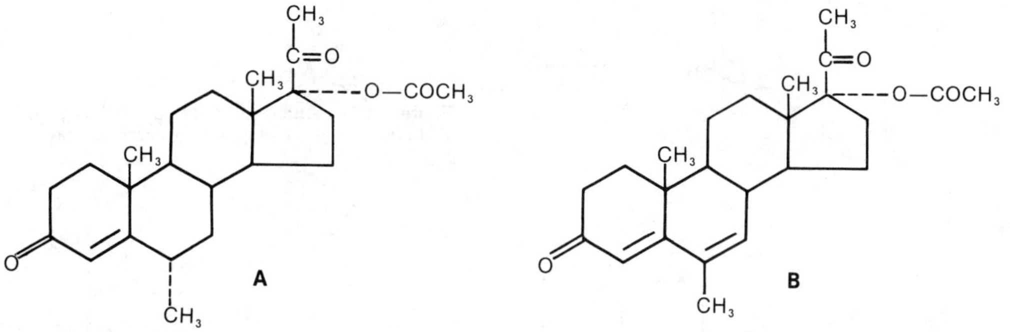

Figure 13-7. Structural formulas of (A) medroxyprogesterone acetate (Provera) and (B) megestrol acetate (Megace), synthetic progestins.

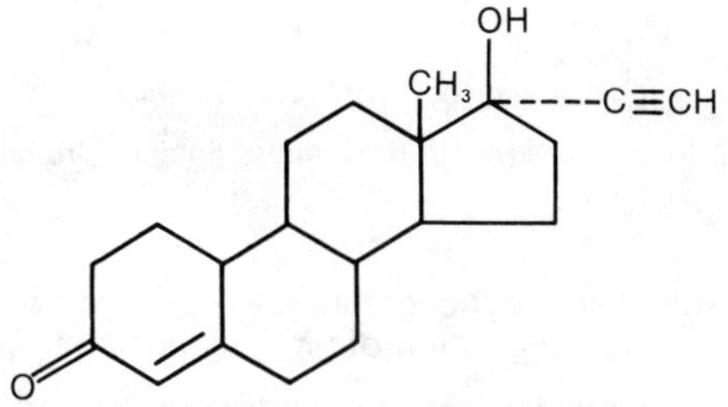

Figure 13-8. Structural formula of norethindrone, the prototypical 19-norprogestin.

(a) The 19-norprogestins are more liposoluble than progesterone and undergo less first-pass metabolism.
(b) These agents have **potent oral activity** and are extensively used as **oral contraceptives**.
(c) Other 19-norprogestins include the positional isomer of norethindrone, **norethynodrel**, its 18-methyl homologue **norgestrel**, and its 3, 17-diacetate analogue **ethynodiol diacetate**.

3. The **primary natural androgen is testosterone**, a C 19 steroid structurally similar to progesterone (Fig. 13-9). It differs from progesterone in having a hydroxyl group at position C 17, rather than a C 20– C 21 chain (see Fig. 13-6).
   a. **Esters of testosterone**, such as testosterone 17-enanthate (Delatestryl), resemble estradiol esters in that they provide **increased duration of action when administered intramuscularly** [see section III A 1 b (1)].
   b. Introduction of a methyl group at position C 17 results in potent, orally active androgens such as **fluoxymesterone** (Fig. 13-10).
   c. Other structural modifications of testosterone result in drugs with a **much-enhanced anabolic-to-androgenic activity ratio** (e.g., oxandrolone and dromostanolone) [Fig. 13-11]. Agents with 17-methyl groups are orally active.

B. Pharmacology. Gonadal hormones are steroids that require cytoplasmic receptors for transport

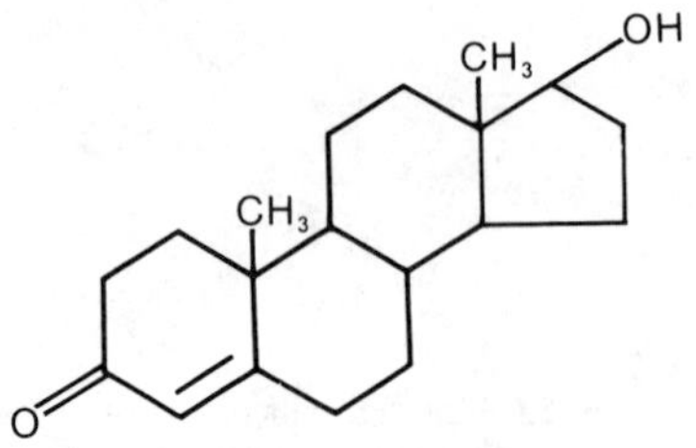

Figure 13-9. Structural formula of testosterone, the primary natural androgen.

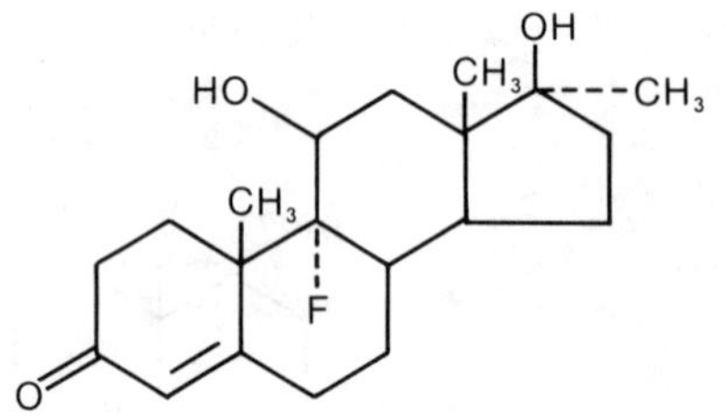

Figure 13-10. Structural formula of fluoxymesterone (Halotestin), a modified testosterone with potent androgenic activity.

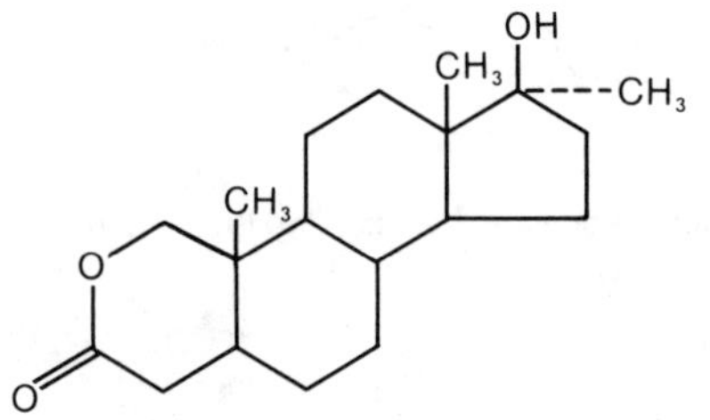

Figure 13-11. Structural formulas of (*A*) oxandrolone (Anavar) and (*B*) dromostanolone (Drolban).

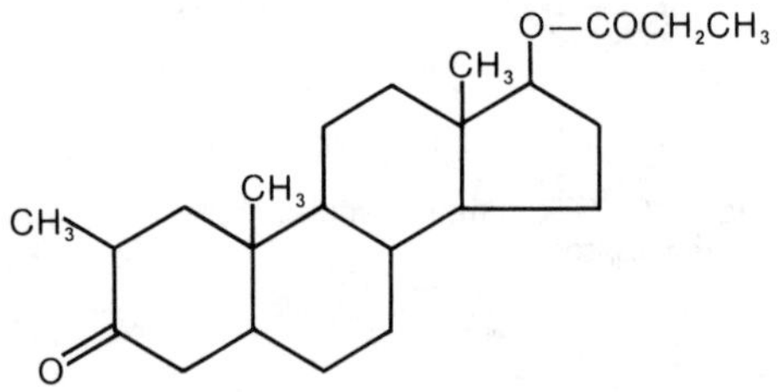

to the nuclei of target-tissue cells, where they stimulate production of messenger and ribosomal ribonucleic acid (RNA). They also act in the feedback regulation of pituitary gonadotropins.

1. **Estrogens** and **progestins** mimic the activities of the female gonadal hormones (estradiol and progesterone), which initiate and control sexual development and maintain the integrity of the female reproductive system.
2. **Androgens** mimic the activity of the male gonadal hormone (testosterone), which initiates and controls sexual development and maintains the integrity of the male reproductive system.

C. Therapeutic indications

1. **Estrogens are used:**
   - **a.** In **oral contraceptives**
   - **b.** For replacement therapy, to **treat menopause and female hypogonadism** (Turner's syndrome)
   - **c.** To **treat prostatic carcinoma** and **breast carcinoma**
2. **Progestins** are used:
   - **a.** In **oral contraceptives**
   - **b.** To **treat dysfunctional uterine bleeding**
   - **c.** To **treat endometriosis with dysmenorrhea**
   - **d.** To **treat endometrial carcinoma**
3. **Androgens** are used to:
   - **a. Treat male hypogonadism**
   - **b. Treat osteoporosis associated with hypogonadism**
   - **c. Aid in the treatment of acute renal failure**, by decreasing the rate of urea formation and, thus, decreasing the frequency of dialysis

d. **Stimulate erythropoiesis**
e. **Treat hereditary angioneurotic edema**

D. Adverse effects

1. **Estrogens** are associated with these adverse effects:
   a. **Gastrointestinal effects**, such as gastrointestinal distress, nausea, vomiting, anorexia, and diarrhea
   b. **Cardiovascular effects**, such as hypertension and an increased incidence of thromboembolic diseases, stroke, and myocardial infarction
   c. **Fluid and electrolyte disturbances**, such as increased fluid retention and increased triglyceride levels
   d. An **increased incidence of endometrial cancer** and **hepatic adenomas** (associated with long-term use)
2. **Progestins** are associated with these adverse effects:
   a. **Gynecologic effects**, such as irregular menses, breakthrough bleeding, and amenorrhea
   b. **Weight gain** and **edema**
   c. **Exacerbation of breast carcinoma**
3. **Androgens** are associated with these adverse effects:
   a. **Hepatic effects**, such as hepatic toxicity, jaundice, and hepatic adenocarcinoma
   b. **Urogenital effects**, such as prostatic enlargement, urinary retention, priapism, and azoospermia
   c. **Edema**
   d. **Paradoxical gynecomastia**

IV. ADRENOCORTICOSTEROIDS

A. Chemistry. The adrenal cortex synthesizes **nongonadal steroids** (adrenocorticosteroids), which may be classified as **mineralocorticoids**, possessing sodium-retaining and potassium-excreting effects, and **glucocorticoids**, possessing anti-inflammatory, protein-catabolic, and immunosuppressant effects. However, most naturally occurring adrenocorticosteroids have some degree of both mineralocorticoid and glucocorticoid activity. All adrenocorticosteroids are derived from the **C 21-pregnane steroidal nucleus**.

1. The **prototypical glucocorticoids** are **cortisone** and **hydrocortisone**, which are formed in the middle (fascicular) layer of the adrenal cortex (Fig. 13-12).
   a. The 17 β-ketol side chain ($-COCH_2OH$), the 4-ene, and the 3-ketone structures are found in all clinically useful adrenocorticosteroids (see Fig. 13-12).
   b. Many natural, semisynthetic, and synthetic glucocorticoids are available. **Modifications** of the prototypes cortisone and hydrocortisone represent attempts to **increase glucocorticoid activity while decreasing mineralocorticoid activity**.
      (1) The **oxygen atom** at position C 11 is essential for glucocorticoid activity.
      (2) A **double bond** between positions C 1 and C 2 increases glucocorticoid activity without increasing mineralocorticoid activity, as with **prednisolone** (Fig. 13-13).
      (3) **Fluorination** at position C 9 greatly increases both mineralocorticoid and glucocorticoid activity, as with **fludrocortisone**; whereas fluorination at position C 6 increases glucocorticoid activity with less effect on mineralocorticoid activity, as with **fluprednisolone** (see Fig. 13-13).
      (4) A **hydroxyl group** at position C 17 and a **hydroxyl group** (as with **triamcinolone**) or a **methyl group** (as with **dexamethasone**) at position C 16 enhance glucocorticoid activity and abolish mineralocorticoid activity (see Fig. 13-13).

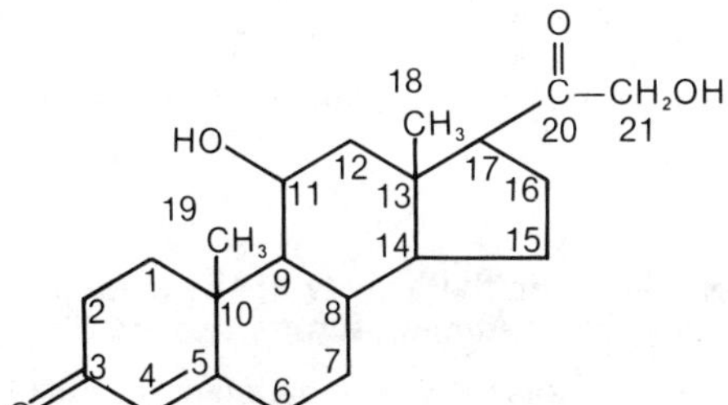

Figure 13-12. Structural formula of hydrocortisone, a prototypical glucocorticoid. The numbers *1* through *21* refer to carbon atom positions on the rings.

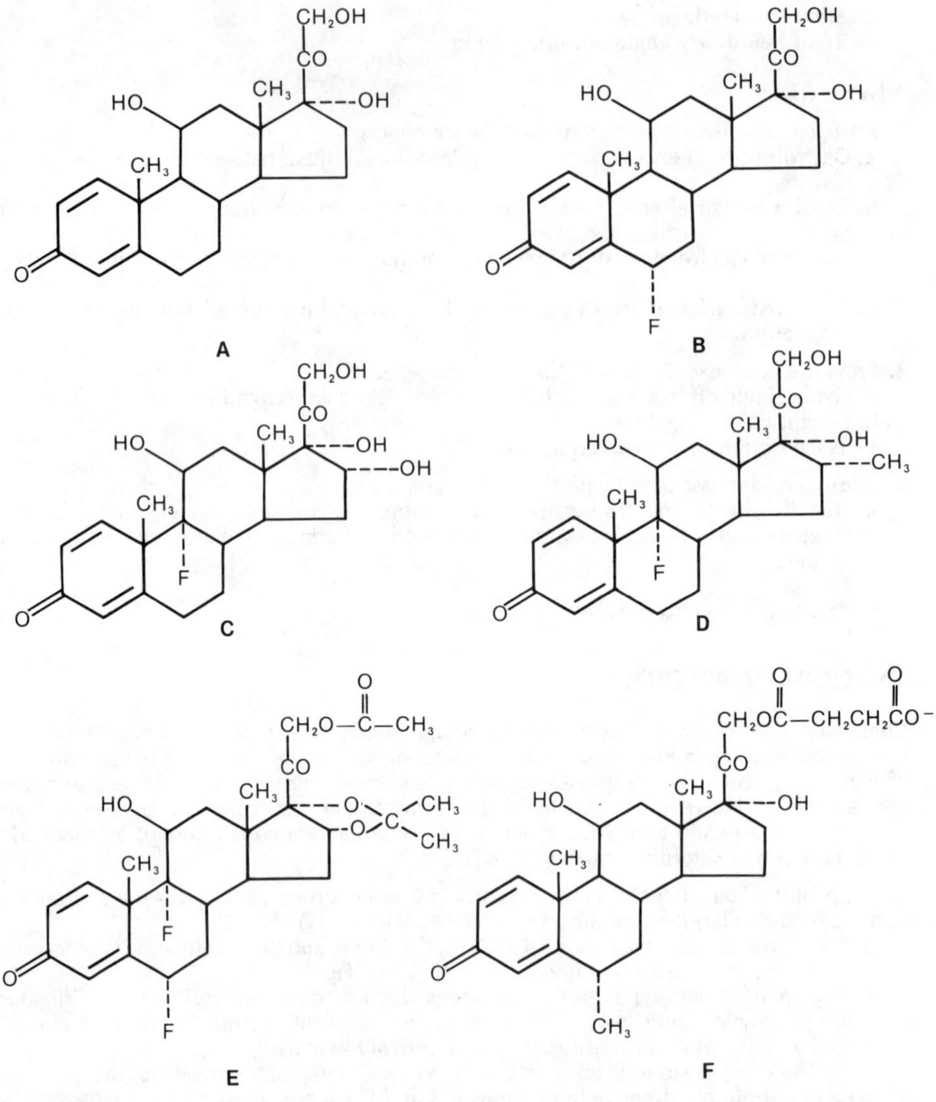

Figure 13-13. Structural formulas of (*A*) prednisolone (Delta-Cortef), (*B*) fluprednisolone (Alphadrol), (*C*) triamcinolone (Aristocort), (*D*) dexamethasone (Decadron), (*E*) fluocinonide (Lidex), and (*F*) methylprednisolone sodium succinate (Solu-Medrol), clinically important glucocorticoids.

(5) An **acetate ester** or a **16α**, 17**α-isopropylidenedioxy group** (also known as an **acetonide group**) at position C 21 enhances topical absorption, as with **fluocinonide** (see Fig. 13-13).

(6) Sodium salts of 21-succinate or phosphate esters result in water-soluble compounds, as with **methylprednisolone sodium succinate** and **betamethasone sodium phosphate** (see Fig. 13-13).

2. The **prototypical mineralocorticoid is aldosterone**, which is formed in the outer (glomerular) layer of the adrenal cortex. The two clinically useful mineralocorticoids are **desoxycorticosterone** and **fludrocortisone acetate** (Fig. 13-14).

B. Pharmacology

1. Therapeutically useful adrenocorticosteroids **mimic the activity of the natural glucocorticoids** and have **metabolic, anti-inflammatory**, and **immunosuppressive activity**.

2. Adrenocorticosteroids require cytoplasmic receptors for transportation to the nuclei of target

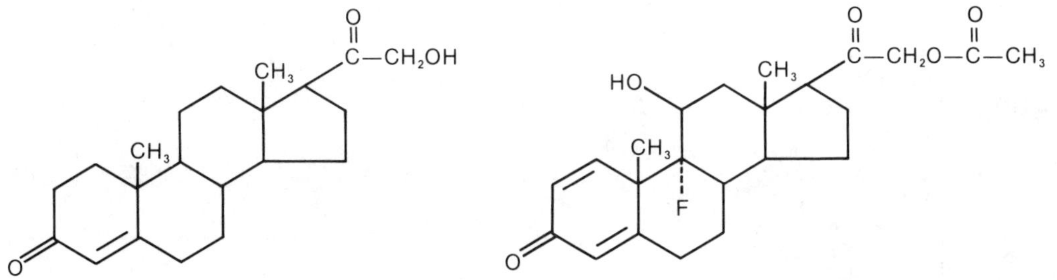

Figure 13-14. Structural formulas of (*A*) desoxycorticosterone (Percorten) and (*B*) fludrocortisone acetate (Florinef Acetate), the clinically useful mineralocorticoids.

tissue cells, where they **stimulate production of messenger and ribosomal RNA**. Adrenocorticosteroids also **act in the feedback regulation of pituitary corticotropin**.

C. Therapeutic indications. Adrenocorticosteroids are used:

1. As replacement therapy, to **treat acute and chronic adrenal insufficiency**
2. As the therapy of last resort, to **treat severe, disabling arthritis**
3. To **treat severe allergic reactions**
4. To **treat chronic ulcerative colitis**
5. To **treat rheumatic carditis**
6. To **treat renal diseases**, including nephrotic syndrome
7. To **treat collagen vascular diseases**
8. To **treat cerebral edema**
9. As topical agents, to **treat skin disorders and inflammatory ocular disorders**

D. Adverse effects. Adrenocorticosteroids are associated with these adverse effects:

1. **Suppression of pituitary-adrenal integrity**
2. **Gastrointestinal effects**, such as peptic ulcer, gastrointestinal hemorrhage, ulcerative esophagitis, and acute pancreatitis
3. **CNS effects**, such as headache, vertigo, increased intraocular and intracranial pressures, muscle weakness, and psychological disturbances (euphoria or dysphoria, depression, and suicidal tendencies)
4. **Cardiovascular effects**, such as edema and hypertension
5. **Other effects**, including weight gain, osteoporosis, hyperglycemia, flushed face and neck, acne, hirsutism, cushingoid "moon face" and "buffalo hump," and increased susceptibility to infection

V. THYROID HORMONES AND INHIBITORS

A. Chemistry

1. The **active thyroid hormones thyroxine** (T_4) and **triiodothyronine** (T_3; also known as liothyronine) are synthesized in the thyroid gland. Their precursor **thyroglobulin** (Proloid) is a large protein (molecular weight about 650,000) obtained from partial purification of bovine or porcine thyroid gland extracts.
   a. **T_3 and T_4 are used therapeutically. These agents contain aromatic rings and iodine**, an essential component that must be obtained in the diet (Fig. 13-15).
   b. A 4:1 mixture of T_4 and T_3, known as **liotrix** (Euthroid), is also employed therapeutically.
2. **Thyroid inhibitors** directly or indirectly interfere with the synthesis of thyroid hormones. These agents include the **iodides** (potassium and sodium salts), **radioactive iodine** (primarily

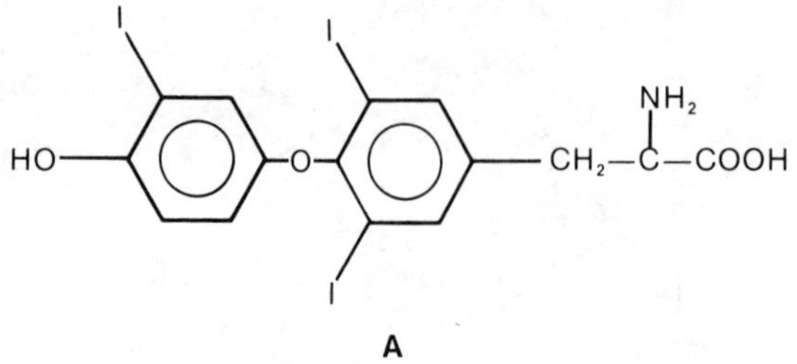

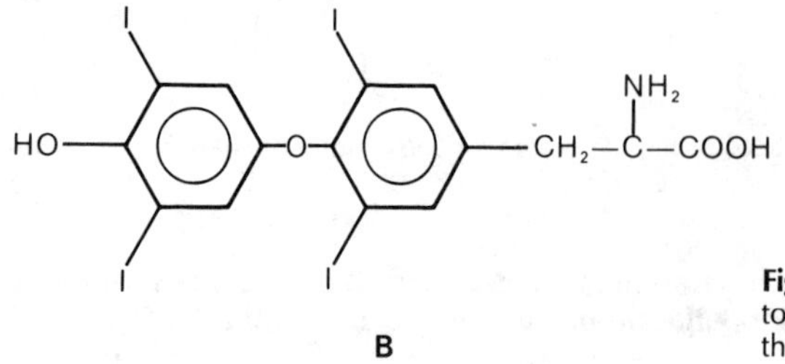

A

B

Figure 13-15. Structural formulas of (A) liothyronine (Cytomel) and (B) levothyroxine (Synthroid), clinically useful thyroid hormone preparations.

sodium iodide 131), and the **thioamides** (e.g., methimazole and propylthiouracil) [Fig. 13-16].

B. Pharmacology

1. **Thyroid hormone preparations** mimic the activity of endogenous thyroid hormones. These hormones regulate growth and development, have calorigenic and metabolic activity, and (through sensitization of β-adrenergic receptors) have positive inotropic and chronotropic effects on the myocardium. Thyroid hormones also act in the feedback regulation of pituitary thyrotropin.
2. **Thyroid inhibitors** act in various ways.
   a. **Iodides in high concentrations** acutely inhibit synthesis of iodotyrosine and iodothyronine. They also antagonize the effect of thyrotropin on endocytosis, proteolysis, and thyroid hormone secretion.
   b. **Radioactive iodine** is rapidly trapped by the thyroid gland and incorporated into the colloid of the follicles. Its ionizing radiation, which is slowly released, is toxic to thyroid cells.
   c. **Thioamides** interrupt the synthesis of thyroid hormones by preventing iodine incorporation into the tyrosyl residues of thyroglobulin.

C. Therapeutic indications

1. **Thyroid hormone preparations** are used to **treat myxedema**, **myxedema coma**, **hypothyroidism**, **simple goiter**, and **thyrotropin-dependent carcinoma**.
2. **Thyroid inhibitors** are indicated for the **treatment of hyperthyroidism**.
   a. **High concentrations of iodide** (Lugol's solution) are used before thyroid surgery to make the thyroid gland firmer and reduce its size.

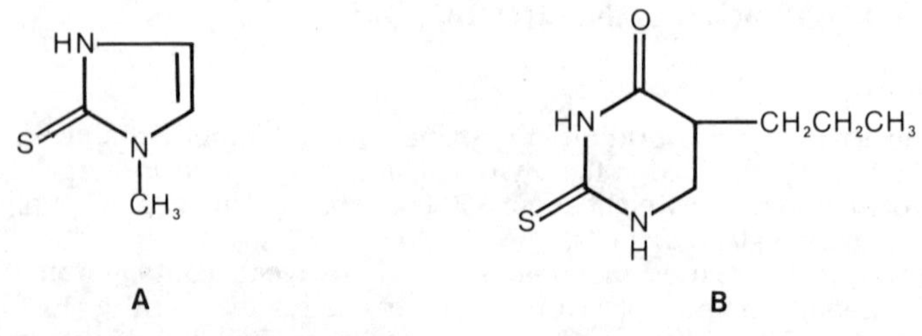

A

B

Figure 13-16. Structural formulas of (A) methimazole (Tapazole) and (B) propylthiouracil, thioamide thyroid hormone inhibitors.

b. Radioactive iodine (^{131}I) is especially useful to treat hyperthyroidism in older patients and in patients with heart disease.
c. Thioamides (e.g., methimazole and propylthiouracil) are used to treat hyperthyroidism—to control the disorder in mild cases, in conjunction with ^{131}I, or to prepare the patient before thyroid surgery.

D. Adverse effects

1. **Thyroid hormone preparations** are only **rarely associated** with adverse effects. Overdosage may cause palpitations, nervousness, insomnia, and weight loss.

2. **Thyroid inhibitors** are associated with adverse effects that depend on the agent used.
   a. Iodides are associated with these adverse effects:
   (1) **Iodism**, including increased salivation, brassy taste, sore teeth and gums, swollen eyelids, inflamed larynx and pharynx, frontal headache, skin lesions, and skin eruptions
   (2) **Hypersensitivity reactions**, with fever, arthralgia, eosinophilia, and angioedema
   b. ^{131}**I** is associated with these adverse effects:
   (1) **Delayed hypothyroidism** (relatively high incidence)
   (2) **Possible effects on the future offspring of young adults**
   c. Thioamides are associated with these adverse effects:
   (1) **CNS effects**, such as drowsiness, headache, and paresthesias
   (2) **Gastrointestinal effects**, such as gastrointestinal distress, nausea, and vomiting
   (3) **Hematologic effects**, such as leukopenia, thrombocytopenia, and agranulocytosis
   (4) **Dermatologic effects**, such as urticaria, rash, dermatitis, and alopecia
   (5) **Other effects**, such as hepatitis, nephritis, jaundice, myalgia, arthralgia, edema, and systemic lupus erythematosus–like syndrome

VI. ANTIDIABETIC AGENTS

A. Chemistry. Antidiabetic agents include **insulin preparations** and **oral hypoglycemic agents**.

1. **Insulin** is an endocrine hormone secreted by the beta cells of the pancreas. It is composed of two polypeptide chains: an **A chain** of 21 amino acids and a **B chain** of 30 amino acids. Two **disulfide bonds** connect the A and B chains, and a third disulfide bond is found within the A chain.
   a. Insulin is available as **bovine insulin** (differs from human insulin by three amino acids), **porcine insulin** (differs from human insulin only in the terminal amino acid), and **human insulin**.
   (1) **Single-species insulins** contain **only bovine** or **only porcine** insulin.
   (2) **Mixed insulins** contain **both bovine and porcine** insulin.
   (3) **Human insulins** are prepared either by enzymatic conversion of the terminal amino acid of porcine insulin (Novolin) or by means of recombinant deoxyribonucleic acid (DNA) technology (Humulin).
   (4) **Purified insulins** (also called single-peak insulins) are preparations containing less than 10 ppm of the insulin precursor proinsulin.
   b. Insulins are classified by their **duration of action** as well as by their source and purity.
   (1) **Short-acting insulins** include crystalline zinc insulin and semilente insulin.
   (a) **Crystalline zinc insulin** (also called **regular insulin**, or **CZI**) is a soluble insulin prepared at neutral pH. It is the only type of insulin that can be mixed with all other insulins and also the only type forming a clear solution, which can be given intravenously.
   (b) **Semilente insulin** is a finely divided, amorphous preparation also known as **prompt insulin zinc suspension**. The lente insulins [see sections VI A 1 b (2) (b) and (3) (b)] contain no modifying protein and are prepared with an acetate buffer. Lente insulins **can be mixed with each other** but **cannot be mixed with either isophane insulin (NPH) or protamine zinc insulin (PZI)**. Semilente insulin has a duration of action comparable to that of CZI.
   (2) **Long-acting insulins** include PZI and ultralente insulin.
   (a) **PZI** consists of insulin complexed with zinc and an excess of protamine in a phosphate buffer.
   (b) **Ultralente insulin** is a large, crystalline form, also known as **extended insulin zinc suspension**. Its duration of action is comparable to that of PZI.
   (3) **Intermediate-acting insulins** include NPH and lente insulin.
   (a) **NPH** is similar to PZI but contains less protamine.

(b) **Lente insulin**, also known as **insulin zinc suspension**, is a mixture of 70% ultralente crystals and 30% semilente powder. Its duration of action is comparable to that of NPH.

2. **Oral hypoglycemic agents** are classified chemically as **sulfonylureas** and are derivatives of the phenylsulfonylurea nucleus. Therapeutically useful agents include **tolbutamide, chlorpropamide, tolazamide, acetohexamide, glyburide,** and **glipizide** (Table 13-1).

B. Pharmacology

1. **Insulin preparations** mimic the activity of endogenous insulin, which is required for the proper utilization of glucose in normal metabolism. Insulin interacts with a specific cell-surface receptor to facilitate the transport of glucose and amino acids.

2. **Oral hypoglycemic agents** stimulate insulin secretion from functioning pancreatic beta cells. These agents may also sensitize pancreatic beta cells to the insulin-releasing effects of glucose, and they may increase cell-surface receptors or increase the affinity of these receptors for insulin.

C. Therapeutic indications

1. **Insulin preparations** are used to **treat diabetes mellitus** that cannot be controlled by diet alone.

2. **Oral hypoglycemic agents** are used as an adjunct to diet—to **treat non-insulin–dependent diabetes mellitus** that cannot be controlled by diet alone.

Table 13-1. The sulfonylurea oral hypoglycemic agents have the general structure illustrated below. Substituents at the positions marked $\mathbf{R_1}$ and $\mathbf{R_2}$ result in different drugs.

General Sulfonylurea Structure

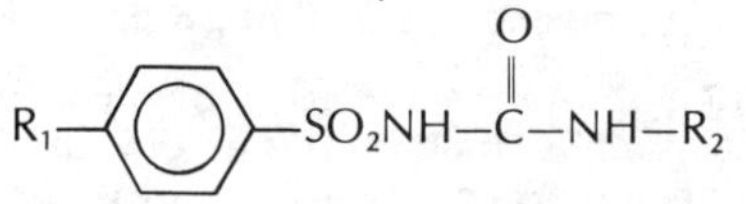

R_1–(benzene ring)–$SO_2NH–C(=O)–NH–R_2$

Drug	R_1-Substituent	R_2-Substituent
First-generation drugs		
Tolbutamide (Orinase)	CH_3—	—$CH_2CH_2CH_2CH_3$
Chlorpropamide (Diabinese)	Cl—	—$CH_2CH_2CH_3$
Tolazamide (Tolinase)	CH_3—	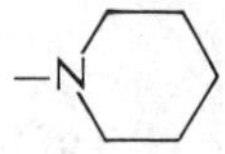 —N(azepane ring)
Acetohexamide (Dymelor)	CH_3CO—	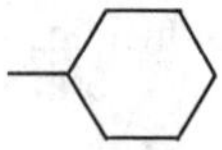 —(cyclohexyl)
Second-generation drugs		
Glyburide (DiaBeta, Micronase)	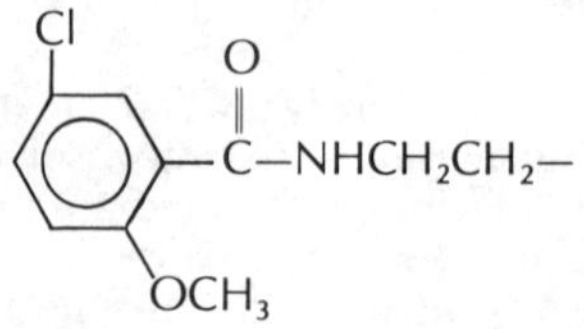 (5-Cl, 2-OCH_3 phenyl)—C(=O)—$NHCH_2CH_2$—	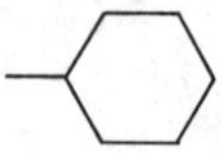 —(cyclohexyl)
Glipizide (Glucotrol)	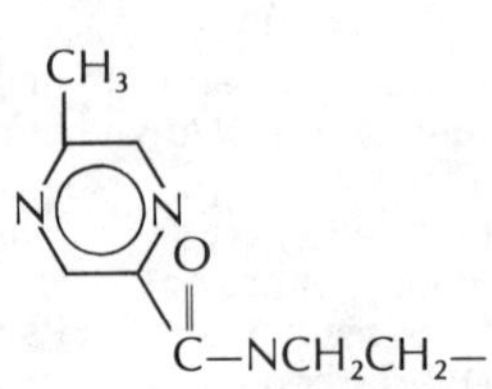 (CH_3-pyrazine, N, N)—C(=O)—NCH_2CH_2—	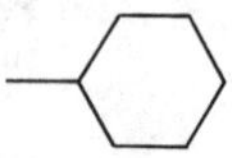 —(cyclohexyl)

D. Adverse effects

1. **Insulin preparations** are associated with these adverse effects:
   a. **Hypoglycemia**, with sweating, tachycardia, and hunger; possibly progressing to insulin shock with hypoglycemic convulsions
   b. **Hypersensitivity reactions**
   c. **Local irritation** at the injection site
2. **Oral hypoglycemic agents** are associated with these adverse effects:
   a. **Hypoglycemia**, particularly in patients with renal or hepatic insufficiency
   b. **Gastrointestinal effects**, such as gastrointestinal disturbances, nausea, and vomiting
   c. **Blood dyscrasias**, such as leukopenia, thrombocytopenia, agranulocytosis, and hemolytic anemia
   d. **Hypersensitivity reactions**, with skin rash and photosensitivity
   e. **Cholestatic jaundice**

STUDY QUESTIONS

Directions: Each question below contains five suggested answers. Choose the **one best** response to each question.

1. The following structure is a hormone. It would be classified best as

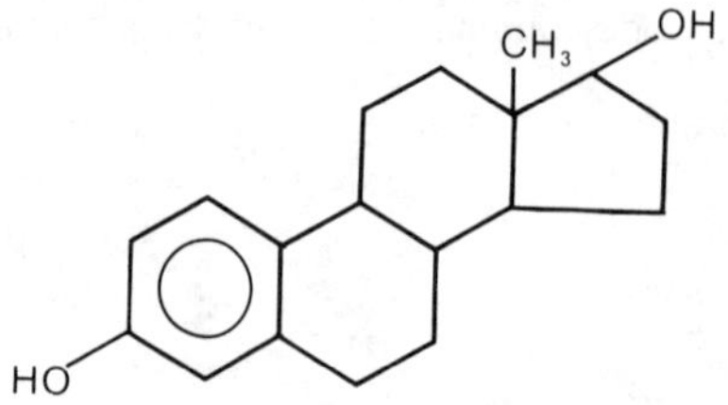

A. an estrogen
B. a progestin
C. an androgen
D. a gonadotropin
E. an adrenocorticosteroid

2. All of the following substances are endogenous tropic hormones secreted by the pituitary gland EXCEPT

A. somatotropin
B. human chorionic gonadotropin (HCG)
C. follicle-stimulating hormone (FSH)
D. thyroid-stimulating hormone (TSH)
E. corticotropin (ACTH)

3. Which of the following substances when present in urine is the most likely positive sign of pregnancy?

A. Thyroid-stimulating hormone (TSH)
B. Corticotropin (ACTH)
C. Human chorionic gonadotropin (HCG)
D. Interstitial cell-stimulating hormone (ICSH)
E. Protamine zinc insulin (PZI)

4. All of the following hormonal drugs possess a steroidal nucleus EXCEPT

A. ethinyl estradiol
B. norethindrone
C. liothyronine
D. prednisolone
E. fluoxymesterone

5. Which of the following glucocorticoids produces the least sodium retention?

A. Cortisone
B. Hydrocortisone
C. Prednisolone
D. Dexamethasone
E. Fludrocortisone

6. Which of the following insulins can be administered intravenously?

A. Regular insulin
B. Isophane insulin (NPH)
C. Protamine zinc insulin (PZI)
D. Semilente insulin
E. Ultralente insulin

Directions: Each question below contains three suggested answers of which **one or more** is correct. Choose the answer

A if **I only** is correct
B if **III only** is correct
C if **I and II** are correct
D if **II and III** are correct
E if **I, II, and III** are correct

7. Hormones that form lipophilic esters without prior structural modifications include

I. hydrocortisone
II. testosterone
III. progesterone

8. Water-soluble adrenocorticoid derivatives include

I. hydrocortisone acetate
II. fluocinonide
III. methylprednisolone sodium succinate

9. Insulin preparations that contain a modifying protein include

I. lente insulin
II. regular insulin
III. isophane insulin (NPH)

Directions: The groups of questions below consist of lettered choices followed by several numbered items. For each numbered item select the **one** lettered choice with which it is **most** closely associated. Each lettered choice may be used once, more than once, or not at all.

Questions 10–12

For each pharmacologic property, select the hormone that most closely relates to it.

A. Testosterone
B. Insulin
C. Corticotropin
D. Estradiol
E. Vasopressin

10. Secreted by pancreatic beta cells to facilitate glucose and amino acid transport for normal cellular metabolic processes

11. Initiates and controls male sexual development and maintains the integrity of the male reproductive system

12. Promotes the resorption of water at the renal distal convoluted tubule

Questions 13–15

For each adverse effect select the class of drug that most closely relates to it.

A. Antithyroid agents
B. Sulfonylurea oral hypoglycemics
C. Adrenocorticosteroids
D. Progestins
E. Androgens

13. Peptic ulceration and gastrointestinal hemorrhage; hyperglycemia, hypertension, and edema; "buffalo hump" and "moon face"; psychological disturbances; and increased susceptibility to infection

14. Agranulocytosis and other blood dyscrasias; cholestatic jaundice; nausea and vomiting; hypoglycemia; and photosensitivity

15. Hepatotoxicity and jaundice; urinary retention and azoospermia; prostatic hypertrophy and priapism; and paradoxical gynecomastia

ANSWERS AND EXPLANATIONS

1. The answer is A. (*III A 1; Figure 13-2*) Ring A is aromatic. Since the only type of steroidal hormone that has an aromatic A ring is an estrogen, this structure represents an estrogen. Other structural characteristics of estrogens include the fact that the structure contains 18 carbon atoms; thus, it is an estrane and contains a β-alcohol group in position 17.

2. The answer is B. (*II A 2, 3*) Human chorionic gonadotropin (HCG) is produced by placental tissue and serves to stimulate the secretion of progesterone during pregnancy. Growth hormone (somatotropin), follicle-stimulating hormone (FSH), thyroid-stimulating hormone (TSH), and corticotropin (ACTH) are all secreted by the anterior pituitary gland.

3. The answer is C. (*II A 3 c*) Human chorionic gonadotropin (HCG) is a proteinaceous tropic hormone that is secreted by chorionic (e.g., placental) tissue. Thus, HCG is present in the urine only after conception has occurred.

4. The answer is C. (*V A 1; Figures 13-3, 13-8, 13-13, 13-15*) Liothyronine is a thyroid hormone. Thyroid hormones consist of iodinated aromatic amino acids and are not steroidal in nature. Ethinyl estradiol is a steroidal estrogen, norethindrone is a steroidal 19-norprogestin, prednisolone is an adrenocorticosteroid, and fluoxymesterone is a steroidal androgen.

5. The answer is D. [*IV A 1 b (4); Figure 13-13*] Glucocorticoids have varying degrees of mineralocorticoid activity. This mineralocorticoid activity, which can result in sodium and fluid retention, can be blocked by the introduction of a methyl or hydroxyl group in position 16 of the steroidal nucleus. Dexamethasone has a 16 α-methyl substituent.

6. The answer is A. (*VI A 1 b*) Most insulin preparations are suspensions; thus, they contain particulate matter. Only clear solutions may be administered intravenously. Regular insulin, which consists of water-soluble crystalline zinc insulin, is therefore suitable for intravenous administration. Insulin preparations normally are injected subcutaneously.

7. The answer is C (I, II). (*Figures 13-6, 13-12*) Hydrocortisone has a 21-hydroxyl group, and testosterone has a 17-hydroxyl group; therefore, both of these agents can form esters (e.g., hydrocortisone acetate and testosterone propionate). Progesterone does not have any alcohol groups in its molecule; therefore, it cannot directly form any esters.

8. The answer is B (III). [*IV A 1 b (6); Figure 13-13*] Methylprednisolone sodium succinate is the sodium salt of the succinate ester of methylprednisolone; thus, it is water-soluble. Hydrocortisone acetate is an ester, and fluocinonide is an acetonide; neither of which is water-soluble.

9. The answer is B (III). (*VI A 1 b*) Regular insulin, which is a rapid-acting insulin preparation, contains only zinc insulin crystals. All lente insulins are free of modifying proteins, which contributes to their hypoallergenic properties. Isophane insulin is NPH insulin, which contains protamine, a strongly basic protein. The protamine reduces the water solubility of zinc insulin and lengthens its duration of action. Isophane insulin is classified as an intermediate-acting insulin preparation, having a duration of action of about 24 hours.

10–12. The answers are: 10-B, 11-A, 12-E. (*II B 4; III B 2; VI B*) Insulin is required for the proper utilization of glucose and the transport of glucose and amino acids across cell membranes. Testosterone, which is produced principally from the Leydig cells of the testes, is responsible for male sexual characteristics. Vasopressin is secreted from the posterior pituitary and is sometimes referred to as an antidiuretic hormone.

13–15. The answers are: 13-C, 14-B, 15-E. (*III D 3; IV D; VI D 2*) Exogenously administered adrenocorticosteroids are effective anti-inflammatory agents but give rise to a wide range of metabolic and immunosuppressive effects that result in severe adverse effects. Oral antidiabetic agents of the sulfonylurea type may cause blood dyscrasias, impaired liver function, and photosensitivity. Exogenously administered androgens suppress sperm formation and cause paradoxical gynecomastia. Most significant is the hepatotoxicity produced by alkyl-substituted androgen compounds.

14
Antineoplastic Agents

Edward F. LaSala

I. INTRODUCTION. Chemotherapeutic agents used in the treatment of cancer are referred to by a number of terms, including antineoplastics, cytotoxic agents, carcinostatic agents, and anticancer agents.

A. Uses

1. As a group, these agents can, in certain cases, **relieve pain**, **prevent or delay metastasis after surgery**, **cause temporary remission**, and **significantly increase survival time**. However, they provide relatively few cures.

2. Common cancers that can be cured effectively by drugs include **Hodgkin's disease**, **acute lymphocytic and myelogenous leukemia**, **testicular cancer**, and **non-Hodgkin's lymphomas**. Other forms of human cancer, such as lung cancer and colon cancer, are more resistant to chemotherapy.

B. Mechanism of action

1. Antineoplastic agents work by **destroying cancer cells**. Many of the most potent agents act at specific phases of the cell cycle and are thus **effective only against dividing cells**.

2. Malignancies most susceptible to drugs are those that **grow rapidly** (those with a high percentage of cells in the process of division). Slow-growing tumors are often unresponsive to these drugs.

3. Antineoplastic agents are **selectively more toxic to cancer cells than to normal cells**. However, this selectivity is narrow, and these agents are **very toxic**.
   a. Toxicity is most evident in tissues with a high turnover rate, such as **bone marrow**, **hair follicles**, and **intestinal epithelium**.
   b. Common **adverse effects** of these drugs include bone marrow depression, alopecia, and severe nausea and vomiting.
   c. Such toxicity often **limits the use** of antineoplastic agents.

4. Greater effectiveness of action and reduced toxicity are often obtained by **combination therapy**—the use of two or more drugs with differing fundamental actions.
   a. In many cases, combination therapy permits **greater effect against a tumor** without a corresponding increase in toxicity.
   b. Combination therapy also **delays the development of resistance to a single agent** and **increases survival time**.

C. Classification. Antineoplastic agents are classified by their mechanism of action or physicochemical properties. Classes include alkylating agents, antimetabolites, hormones, antibiotics, plant products and derivatives, and miscellaneous agents.

II. ALKYLATING AGENTS. These highly reactive chemicals can alkylate, or **bind covalently**, with the cellular components of deoxyribonucleic acid (DNA).

A. Nitrogen mustards

1. **Chemistry**. These agents, which include mechlorethamine (Mustargen), cyclophosphamide (Cytoxan), melphalan (Alkeran), and chlorambucil (Leukeran), are characterized by a *bis*-2-chloroethylamine substituent, $R{-}NH(CH_2CH_2Cl)_2$.

2. **Pharmacology**. In vivo, this substituent acts as a **bifunctional alkylating agent** on guanine bases in both DNA strands. This results in **cross-linking** (interstrand linking).

a. Cross-linking **prevents division of the helical DNA strands** and, thus, subsequent reproduction of daughter cells.
b. These agents act as **cell-growth inhibitors**.

3. **Therapeutic indications**. Nitrogen mustards are indicated for use with a variety of neoplastic diseases, including Hodgkin's disease, non-Hodgkin's lymphomas, acute and chronic lymphocytic leukemias, breast cancer, ovarian cancer, and others.

4. **Adverse effects**. Major adverse effects include leukopenia, anemia, thrombocytopenia, nausea, vomiting, hyperuricemia, dermatitis, and alopecia.

B. Ethylenimines

1. **Chemistry**. The prototypical agent is **triethylenethiophosphoramide** (Thiotepa) [Fig. 14-1].

2. **Pharmacology**. This agent acts as a **bifunctional alkylating agent**, as a result of the in vivo opening of the ethylenimine rings.

3. **Therapeutic indications**
   a. Ethylenimines are **seldom employed clinically** today. Nitrogen mustards often are used instead.
   b. On occasion, triethylenethiophosphoramide may be indicated for treatment of Hodgkin's disease, non-Hodgkin's lymphomas, and breast, lung, and ovarian cancer.

4. **Adverse effects.** Major adverse effects include leukopenia, thrombocytopenia, neutropenia, nausea, vomiting, amenorrhea, decreased spermatogenesis, dermatitis, and hyperuricemia.

C. Alkyl sulfonates

1. **Chemistry. Busulfan** (Myleran) is the only clinically used agent in this group (Fig. 14-2).

2. **Pharmacology**. In vivo, cleavage of busulfan's C—O bonds produces a bifunctional alkylating butyl carbonium ion, which **cross-links strands of DNA**.

3. **Therapeutic indications**. Busulfan has well-established beneficial effects when used to treat chronic granulocytic leukemia.

4. **Adverse effects**
   a. **Major adverse effects** include thrombocytopenia, anemia, nausea, vomiting, diarrhea, amenorrhea, impotence, sterility, and hyperuricemia.
   b. **Less common effects** include gynecomastia, alopecia, anhidrosis, generalized skin pigmentation, and pulmonary fibrosis.

D. Nitrosoureas

1. **Chemistry**. These agents, which include carmustine (BCNU, BICNU), lomustine (CCNU, CeeNU), and streptozocin (Zanosar), have the general structure shown in Figure 14-3.

2. **Pharmacology**. These agents appear to act as **bifunctional alkylating agents**, cross-linking strands of DNA as monofunctional carbamoylating agents.

3. **Therapeutic indications**
   a. **Carmustine** and **lomustine** cross the blood–brain barrier, making them useful agents for the treatment of brain tumors. These agents are also indicated for use with Hodgkin's disease, non-Hodgkin's lymphomas, and renal cell, stomach, colon, and lung cancers.
   b. **Streptozocin** is used for metastatic pancreatic islet-cell cancer.

4. **Adverse effects**
   a. **Carmustine** and **lomustine** may cause leukopenia, thrombocytopenia, nausea, and vomit-

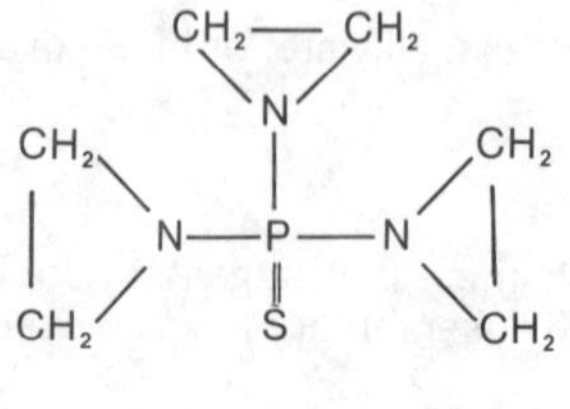

Figure 14-1. Structural formula of triethylenethiophosphoramide (Thiotepa), an ethylenimine alkylating agent.

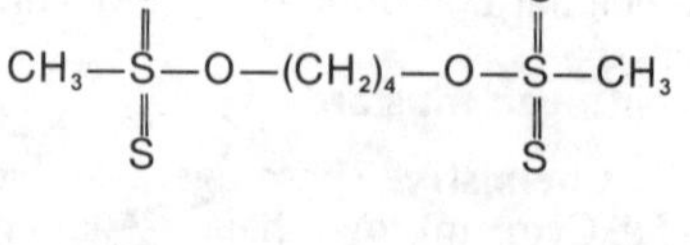

$$CH_3-\overset{O}{\overset{\|}{\underset{\underset{S}{\|}}{S}}}-O-(CH_2)_4-O-\overset{O}{\overset{\|}{\underset{\underset{S}{\|}}{S}}}-CH_3$$

Figure 14-2. Structural formula of busulfan (Myleran), an alkyl sulfonate alkylating agent.

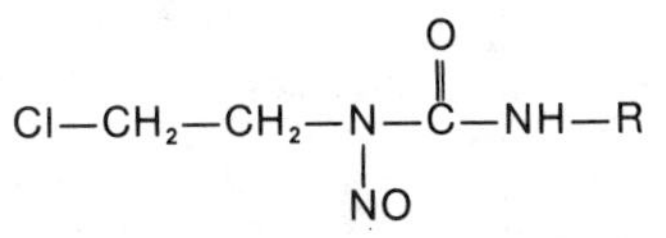

$$Cl-CH_2-CH_2-N(NO)-C(=O)-NH-R$$

Figure 14-3. General structural formula of the nitrosourea alkylating agents.

ing. **Carmustine** may also cause hepatotoxicity, hyperuricemia, and pulmonary fibrosis. **Lomustine** may also cause nephrotoxicity and alopecia.

b. Streptozocin may cause aplastic anemia, nausea, vomiting, diarrhea, nephrotoxicity, and hepatotoxicity.

E. Triazenes

1. **Chemistry. Dacarbazine** (DTIC) is the only clinically used agent in this group. It closely resembles the metabolite 5-aminoimidazole-4-carboxamide (AIC), which can be converted to inosinic acid.
2. **Pharmacology**. Dacarbazine appears to act as a **monofunctional alkylating agent**.
3. **Therapeutic indications**. Dacarbazine is used principally for the treatment of malignant melanoma. It also may be used in combination with other drugs to treat Hodgkin's disease and various sarcomas.
4. **Adverse effects**. Major adverse effects include severe nausea and vomiting, anorexia, leukopenia, thrombocytopenia, alopecia, fever, malaise, and myalgia.

III. ANTIMETABOLITES. These agents interfere with the biosynthesis of essential substances, either through enzyme inhibition or by incorporation into essential molecules to form false products. They ultimately block the synthesis or functioning of proteins, DNA precursors, or DNA itself, inhibiting cell growth.

A. Folic acid antagonists

1. **Chemistry. Methotrexate**, the primary folic acid antagonist, is an analogue of folic acid that combines irreversibly with the enzyme dihydrofolate reductase (DHF).
2. **Pharmacology**
   a. Inhibition of DHF by methotrexate reduces the production of **tetrahydrofolate** (THF), interfering with the metabolic conversion of deoxyuridine monophosphate (dUMP) to deoxythymidine monophosphate (dTMP).
   b. This deficiency of dTMP results in **inhibited DNA synthesis**.
   c. **Leucovorin** (a reduced form of folic acid) may be given after high-dose methotrexate therapy, to **reduce toxicity to normal cells**. Leucovorin provides intermediary THF, which reestablishes the conversion of dUMP to dTMP.
3. **Therapeutic indications**. Methotrexate may be used for treatment of acute lymphocytic leukemia, choriocarcinoma, mycosis fungoides, osteogenic sarcoma, and cancers of the breast, testis, lung, head, and neck.
4. **Adverse effects**. Toxic reactions to methotrexate are dose-related and may result in anemia, leukopenia, thrombocytopenia, stomatitis, diarrhea, nausea, vomiting, nephrotoxicity, hepatic dysfunction, alopecia, dermatitis, and hyperuricemia.

B. Purine antagonists

1. **Chemistry**. Purine antagonists include **mercaptopurine** (6-MP, Purinethol) and **thioguanine** (6-TG, Lanvis), analogues of the natural purines hypoxanthine and guanine (Fig. 14-4).

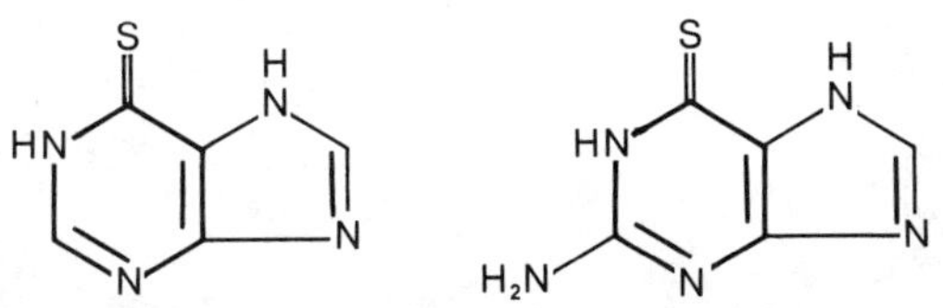

A

B

Figure 14-4. Structural formulas of (*A*) mercaptopurine and (*B*) thioguanine, purine analogue antimetabolites.

2. **Pharmacology**
   a. **Mercaptopurine** interferes with purine synthesis, ultimately interfering with adenine and guanine synthesis or with their incorporation into DNA.
   b. **Thioguanine** appears to be incorporated into DNA synthetic pathways, forming a false DNA code that interferes with the DNA template mechanism.

3. **Therapeutic indications**. Mercaptopurine and thioguanine may be used for treatment of acute lymphocytic, acute granulocytic, and chronic granulocytic leukemias.

4. **Adverse effects**. Major adverse effects of the purine antagonists include leukopenia, thrombocytopenia, anemia, nausea, vomiting, anorexia, jaundice, hepatotoxicity, and hyperuricemia.

C. Pyrimidine antagonists

1. **Chemistry**. Pyrimidine antagonists include **fluorouracil** (5-FU; Fig. 14-5), **floxuridine** (FUDR), and **cytarabine** (ara-C, Cytosar-U).

2. **Pharmacology**
   a. **Fluorouracil** and **floxuridine** compete with deoxyuridine monophosphate (dUMP) for the enzyme thimidylate synthetase, thus inhibiting conversion of dUMP to deoxythymidine monophosphate (dTMP) and ultimately **inhibiting DNA synthesis**.
   b. **Cytarabine**, which differs from natural cytidine by having an arabinose sugar rather than a deoxyribose sugar, competes with cytidine nucleotide and **inhibits the action of DNA polymerase**.

3. **Therapeutic indications**
   a. **Fluorouracil** and **floxuridine** may be of palliative value when used to treat cancers of the breast, stomach, colon, pancreas, ovary, cervix, prostate, urinary bladder, head, and neck.
   b. **Fluorouracil** is also widely used topically for treatment of premalignant skin keratoses and superficial basal-cell cancers.
   c. **Cytarabine** is used for treatment of acute granulocytic and acute lymphocytic leukemias.

4. **Adverse effects**
   a. **Fluorouracil** and **floxuridine** may cause leukopenia, thrombocytopenia, anemia, anorexia, nausea, vomiting, diarrhea, stomatitis, dermatitis, hyperpigmentation, nail changes, alopecia, weakness, and malaise.
   b. **Cytarabine** may cause leukopenia, thrombocytopenia, anemia, megaloblastosis, nausea, vomiting, diarrhea, stomatitis, hepatic dysfunction, hyperuricemia, dermatitis, and fever.

IV. HORMONES

IV. HORMONES. For a complete discussion of the chemistry, pharmacology, major therapeutic uses, and adverse effects of hormones, see Chapter 13. Only the use of hormones for the treatment of neoplastic diseases is discussed here. For the most part, hormones are noncytotoxic.

A. Adrenocorticosteroids

1. Adrenocorticosteroids such as **prednisone** cause direct destruction of lymphocytes and provide **symptomatic relief of the complications of neoplastic disease**.

2. These agents are effective in the treatment of **certain lymphocytic leukemias** and are also widely used as adjuncts with other cytotoxic antineoplastic agents.

B. Estrogens

1. Estrogens such as **diethylstilbestrol** sometimes are used to treat cancers of testosterone-dependent male reproductive tissue, such as **prostatic cancer**. These agents block the effects of androgens, producing chemical castration.

2. These agents also may be used for treatment of **breast cancer in postmenopausal women** for whom surgery and radiotherapy have not been effective.

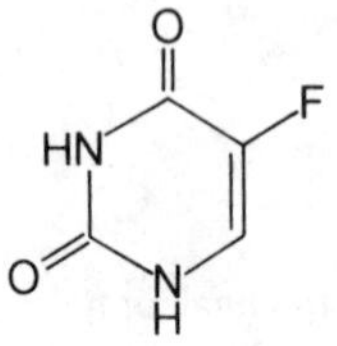

O, F, HN, O, N, H

Figure 14-5. Structural formula of fluorouracil (5-FU), a pyrimidine antagonist.

3. A unique agent, **estramustine** (Emcyt) may be used for treatment of prostatic cancer. A *bis*-2-chloroethylamine derivative of estradiol, this agent is a prodrug that appears to act as a site-specific alkylating agent for estrogen-dependent tissues.

C. **Androgens and anabolic steroids**. Androgens, such as **fluoxymesterone** (Halotestin), and anabolic steroids, such as **nandrolone phenpropionate** (Anabolin), are sometimes used to treat cancers of estrogen-dependent tissues, such as **breast cancer**.

D. **Antihormones**

1. **Tamoxifen** (Nolvadex) acts as an **antiestrogen** by binding to cytoplasmic estrogen receptors and slowing the growth of estrogen-dependent tissues. It is used in the treatment of **breast cancer** in postmenopausal women.
2. **Aminoglutethimide** (Cytadren) acts as an **antiadrenal agent** by interfering with adrenocorticoid synthesis. It is used in the treatment of **adrenal cancer** and **metastatic breast cancer**.

V. ANTIBIOTICS

The antibiotics used in cancer chemotherapy include dactinomycin, daunorubicin, doxorubicin, the bleomycins, plicamycin, and mitomycin.

A. Chemistry

1. These agents are produced by different species of the fungus *Streptomyces*.
2. **Dactinomycin** (also known as actinomycin D), **daunorubicin** (Cerubidine), and **doxorubicin** (Adriamycin) are structurally similar to the tetracyclines.
3. The **bleomycins**, which differ from each other only in their terminal amine moieties, are water-soluble, basic glycopeptides.
4. **Plicamycin** (Mithracin), which was formerly known as mithramycin, is a large structure somewhat similar to dactinomycin.
5. **Mitomycin** (Mutamycin) contains a urethane and a quinone group as well as an aziridine ring, which is essential to its antineoplastic activity.

B. Pharmacology

1. All the antibiotics used in cancer chemotherapy appear to act as **cell-growth inhibitors**.
2. **Dactinomycin**, **daunorubicin**, and **doxorubicin** appear to **bind noncovalently to guanine**, altering the character of the DNA double helix by intercalating with it. This interferes with the transcription of the DNA molecule.
3. **Bleomycin** (Blenoxane) binds to DNA, possibly by intercalation, causing hydrolysis of glycosidic linkages and reductive cleavage of single and double DNA strands. The resulting **fragmentation of the DNA molecule** is sometimes referred to as **nicking**.
4. **Plicamycin** appears to bind to DNA, resulting in an **inhibition of ribonucleic acid (RNA) synthesis**.
5. **Mitomycin** acts as a **bifunctional alkylating agent**, inhibiting DNA synthesis.

C. Therapeutic indications

1. **Dactinomycin** is used to treat Wilms' tumor, rhabdomyosarcoma, testicular cancer, and choriocarcinoma.
2. **Daunorubicin** is used to treat acute granulocytic and acute lymphocytic leukemias.
3. **Doxorubicin** is used to treat sarcomas, Hodgkin's disease, non-Hodgkin's lymphomas, acute leukemias, neuroblastomas, and cancers of the breast, thyroid, lung, stomach, and genitourinary tract.
4. **Bleomycin** is used to treat Hodgkin's disease, non-Hodgkin's lymphomas, and cancers of the head and neck, testis, skin, esophagus, and genitourinary tract.
5. **Plicamycin** is of limited value because of its severe toxicity. It may be used to treat malignant hypercalcemia and testicular cancer.
6. **Mitomycin** is used to treat cancers of the stomach, colon, pancreas, breast, bladder, and cervix.

D. Adverse effects

1. **Dactinomycin** is associated with anemia, leukopenia, thrombocytopenia, anorexia, nausea, vomiting, diarrhea, stomatitis, erythema, desquamation, hyperpigmentation, alopecia, and soft-tissue damage.

2. **Daunorubicin** is associated with bone marrow depression, cardiac toxicity, nausea, vomiting, stomatitis, esophagitis, anorexia, diarrhea, nephrotoxicity, hepatotoxicity, dermatitis, and alopecia.

3. **Doxorubicin** is associated with leukopenia, thrombocytopenia, cardiac toxicity, nausea, vomiting, diarrhea, stomatitis, esophagitis, hyperpigmentation, and alopecia.

4. **Bleomycin** is associated with stomatitis, prolonged anorexia, nausea, vomiting, diarrhea, erythema, vesiculation, desquamation, ulceration, alopecia, pulmonary toxicity, and an acute allergic reaction with profound fever.

5. **Plicamycin** is associated with thrombocytopenia, nausea, vomiting, anorexia, diarrhea, stomatitis, and proteinuria. It is toxic to bone marrow, liver, and kidneys and also produces a severe bleeding syndrome, which may range from epistaxis to generalized hemorrhage.

6. **Mitomycin** is associated with thrombocytopenia, leukopenia, paresthesias, nausea, vomiting, anorexia, stomatitis, dermatitis, fever, malaise, and alopecia.

VI. PLANT PRODUCTS AND DERIVATIVES

A. Vinca alkaloids

1. **Chemistry. Vinblastine** (Velban) and **vincristine** (Oncovin) are alkaloids derived from the periwinkle plant (*Vinca rosea*). They are closely related dimeric compounds.

2. **Pharmacology.** The vinca alkaloids block mitosis by arresting cells in metaphase, thus **inhibiting cell growth.**

3. **Therapeutic indications**
   a. **Vinblastine** is used to treat Hodgkin's disease, non-Hodgkin's lymphomas, and cancers of the breast, testis, and renal cells.
   b. **Vincristine** is used to treat acute lymphoblastic leukemia, neuroblastoma, Wilms' tumor, rhabdomyosarcoma, Hodgkin's disease, and non-Hodgkin's lymphomas.

4. **Adverse effects**
   a. **Vinblastine** is associated with leukopenia, thrombocytopenia, depression, paresthesias, peripheral neuropathy, numbness, loss of deep tendon reflexes, muscle pain and weakness, nausea, vomiting, stomatitis, constipation, ileus, anorexia, abdominal pain, urinary retention, dermatitis, and alopecia.
   b. **Vincristine** is associated with mild anemia and leukopenia, peripheral neuropathy, loss of deep-tendon reflexes, paresthesias, muscle weakness and cramps, ataxia, hoarseness, headache, diplopia, ptosis, constipation, nausea, vomiting, anorexia, stomatitis, urinary retention, and alopecia.

B. Podophyllotoxin derivatives

1. **Chemistry. Etoposide** (VePesid) is a semisynthetic carbohydrate analogue of podophyllotoxin.

2. **Pharmacology.** Etoposide acts by **arresting cell mitosis.**

3. **Therapeutic indications.** This agent is used to treat acute nonlymphocytic leukemia, lymphosarcoma, Hodgkin's disease, testicular cancer, and small-cell lung cancer.

4. **Adverse effects.** Major adverse effects include myelosuppression, leukopenia, thrombocytopenia, nausea, vomiting, headache, fever, and alopecia. Anaphylaxis occurs rarely.

VII. MISCELLANEOUS AGENTS

A. **Hydroxyurea** (Hydrea) appears to inhibit ribonucleotide diphosphate reductase, causing inhibition of nucleotide synthesis. It is used to treat chronic granulocytic leukemia and malignant melanoma.

B. **Procarbazine** (Matulane) appears to cause depolymerization of the DNA molecule, interfering with DNA and RNA synthesis. It is used to treat Hodgkin's disease.

C. **Asparaginase** (Elspar) appears to hydrolyze asparagine, an amino acid commonly found in cancer cells that may be an essential nutrient for them. It is used to treat acute lymphocytic leukemia.

D. **Cisplatin** (Platinol) acts as an alkylating agent to cause both intrastrand and interstrand cross-linking of DNA. It is used to treat neuroblastoma, osteogenic sarcoma, and cancers of the testis, ovary, bladder, head and neck, thyroid, cervix, and endometrium.

STUDY QUESTIONS

Directions: Each question below contains five suggested answers. Choose the **one best** response to each question.

1. Assume that a type of cancer is susceptible to an individual drug. All of the following anticancer combinations are therapeutically rational EXCEPT

A. thiotepa—prednisone
B. cyclophosphamide—6-mercaptopurine
C. doxorubicin—methotrexate
D. melphalan—chlorambucil
E. floxuridine—vinblastine

2. Systemic antifolate therapy has been found to be useful in the treatment of psoriasis. Which of the following agents most likely would be dispensed for this purpose?

A. Cyclophosphamide
B. Vinblastine
C. Bleomycin
D. Methotrexate
E. Carmustine

3. Most of the clinically available anticancer agents have an underlying mechanism of action that acts as

A. cell-growth inhibitors
B. stimulation of natural body defense mechanisms
C. interference with cell wall production
D. inhibition of cancer cell nutrient absorption
E. receptor-site blockade of cancer cell secretions

Directions: Each question below contains three suggested answers of which **one or more** is correct. Choose the answer

A if **I only** is correct
B if **III only** is correct
C if **I and II** are correct
D if **II and III** are correct
E if **I, II, and III** are correct

4. True statements concerning fluorouracil include

I. its chemical structure is a modified pyrimidine that is similar to uracil and thymine
II. bone marrow depression is a common side effect
III. it inhibits the methylation of deoxyuridine monophosphate to form deoxythymidine monophosphate

5. Anticancer agents that act as enzyme inhibitors include

I. doxorubicin
II. methotrexate
III. floxuridine

Directions: The group of questions below consists of lettered choices followed by several numbered items. For each numbered item select the **one** lettered choice with which it is **most** closely associated. Each lettered choice may be used once, more than once, or not at all.

Questions 6–8

For each anticancer agent, select the mechanism of action that most appropriately describes it.

A. Bifunctional alkylating agent
B. Intercalating antibiotic
C. Antimetabolite–antifolate
D. Mitosis-blocking plant alkaloid
E. Antimetabolite–pyrimidine antagonist

6. Cytarabine
7. Vinblastine
8. Doxorubicin

ANSWERS AND EXPLANATIONS

1. The answer is D. (*I B 4; II A 1, 2*) To be therapeutically rational, combinations of anticancer agents should consist of drugs that are individually effective in the type of cancer being treated and should belong to different antineoplastic classes, have different mechanisms of action, or both. Each of the above pairs of drugs includes anticancer agents that belong to different classes and have different mechanisms of action except the melphalan—chlorambucil combination. Both of these agents are bifunctional alkylating agents that act by cross-linking guanine bases in both DNA strands, thus preventing their division and subsequent reproduction of daughter cells.

2. The answer is D. (*I B 2; III A*) An antifolate is an agent that antagonizes the action of folic acid. Methotrexate does this by inhibiting the action of dihydrofolate reductase, thus preventing the reduction of dihydrofolate to tetrahydrofolate. The deficiency of tetrahydrofolate interferes with conversion of deoxyuridine monophosphate to deoxythymidine monophosphate which, in turn, results in inhibited DNA synthesis. Thus, an antifolate acts as a cell-growth inhibitor. Psoriasis is a non-neoplastic disease of the skin but is similar to cancer in that it is characterized by abnormally rapid proliferation of epidermal cells. Methotrexate is indicated only for the treatment of severe, disabling psoriasis that is not adequately responsive to other forms of therapy.

3. The answer is A. (*I B 1, 2, 3*) Cancer cells, unlike most normal cells, continue to reproduce after maturation. Characteristically, this growth is described as uncontrollable. With the possible exception of the hormones (e.g., the adrenocorticoids when used as palliative adjuncts in the treatment of cancers other than certain lymphocytic leukemias), almost all of the approved anticancer drugs act to inhibit or slow down this uncontrollable growth. Another important characteristic of cancer cells is their ability to metastasize.

4. The answer is D (II, III). (*III A 1, C 2*) Methotrexate is an antifolate–antimetabolite that inhibits the action of dihydrofolate reductase. Floxuridine is a pyrimidine antagonist that inhibits the action of thymidylate synthetase. Doxorubicin is an antibiotic that acts by intercalation.

5. The answer is E (all). (*III C; Figure 14-5*) Fluorouracil has a fluoro-group substituted on the 5 position of uracil. Thymine is 5-methyl uracil. Fluorouracil is a cell-growth inhibitor and as such is likely to cause bone marrow depression since it inhibits the growth of normal cells, particularly those that have a high turnover.

6–8. The answers are: 6-E, 7-D, 8-B. (*III C; V B 2; VI A*) Cytarabine is an analogue of the pyrimidine nucleoside, cytosine, in which the ribase sugar moiety has been replaced by arabinose. It is converted to the arabinonucleotide in the body, which then competitively inhibits DNA polymerase and thus blocks DNA synthesis.

Vinblastine is an alkaloid derived from the periwinkle plant (*Vinca rosea*). It and its structurally related homologue vincristine both act as mitotic antagonists by binding to contractile proteins in the mitotic spindle of dividing cells, which leads to inhibition of mitosis. Although the structures and mechanism of action of vinblastine and vincristine are quite similar, the two plant alkaloids are quite different in their therapeutic application and toxicities.

Doxorubicin is an antibiotic. Similar to dactinomycin and daunorubicin, it acts as an intercalating agent. Intercalating agents are substances that bind strongly to DNA by insertion into the space between adjacent base pairs of the double helix and thereby inhibit DNA synthesis and DNA-directed RNA synthesis.

15
Nuclear Pharmacy

Kathryn A. Huntley

I. INTRODUCTION

A. Definitions

1. **Nuclear pharmacy** is the branch of pharmacy that involves the procurement, compounding, dispensing, and quality control of radioactive pharmaceuticals intended for patient and research use.

2. **Radiopharmaceuticals** are agents with proven pharmacologic action that have been made radioactive. Their unstable nuclei disintegrate spontaneously with the emission of nuclear particles or photons.

3. **Half-life**. Radiopharmaceuticals have both a physical and a biologic half-life.
   a. **Physical half-life** refers to the decay rate—the time needed for a radioactive substance to lose 50% of its activity through decay. Each radioisotope has a unique physical half-life.
   b. **Biologic half-life** refers to the time needed for the body to eliminate 50% of the radioactive substance. It is determined by the route of administration and metabolism of the substance.
   c. The combined action of radioactive decay (physical half-life) and elimination (biologic half-life) determine **effective half-life**—the time required for the radioactivity of an administered radioisotope to decrease by 50%.

B. Uses of radiopharmaceuticals. Radiopharmaceuticals are valuable in medical diagnosis and therapy.

1. **Diagnostic uses**. Radiopharmaceuticals serve as tracers that, when introduced into the body, emit radiation that is subsequently detected (e.g., by a scintillation detector) and measured.
   a. For example, to analyze thyroid function, a tracer dose of radioactive iodine (radioiodine) is administered orally; the agent concentrates in the thyroid gland. The thyroid is then scanned to determine radioiodine concentration and location. Greater than normal uptake by the thyroid indicates hyperthyroidism.
   b. Many diagnostic tests using radioactive agents involve radionuclide imaging methods.
   c. In some studies, the radioactivity level of an administered radiopharmaceutical is measured from a serum sample or urine specimen to evaluate organ or tissue function.
   d. Optimally, a radioisotope used in a tracer study is given in the lowest possible dose that permits its accurate detection and measurement.

2. **Therapeutic uses**. Radioisotopes are used as internal or external radiation sources to treat such disorders as hyperthyroidism and cancer.
   a. **Internal radiation source**. A radioisotope administered orally or intravenously or implanted in the target tissue or organ will produce radiation that destroys diseased cells and prevents new tissue growth.
   b. **External radiation source**. Radiation (which can be in the form of x-rays or radioisotopes) may be used for therapy in cancer patients.

C. Criteria for an optimal radiopharmaceutical

1. An agent administered as a radioactive tracer or therapeutic source should have a relatively short half-life.

2. It should emit **gamma particles** (by electron capture or isomeric transition) rather than alpha or beta particles.
   a. Agents emitting alpha and beta particles give the patient a higher radiation dose than those emitting gamma particles, thereby increasing the risk of patient injury.

b. Also, alpha and beta emissions are harder to detect with current methods, making them less desirable in diagnostic studies.

3. The energy of a radiopharmaceutical should range from 30 to 300 kilo electron volts (KeV).

4. Metabolic stability. Radiopharmaceuticals follow first-order kinetics and must be able to localize in the target site before being metabolized.

5. Organ specificity. A radiopharmaceutical should have the capacity to localize readily in the site under study, with a high target-to-nontarget ratio for optimal visualization. Also, it must have sufficient affinity for the target site to permit use of the lowest possible dose.

6. Excretion. The agent must be subject to excretion from the body.

7. Availability. The radiopharmaceutical should be relatively inexpensive and easily produced and obtained.

8. Technetium 99m (^{99m}Tc) currently is the most widely acceptable radioisotope for diagnostic imaging studies.

a. Its half-life is 6 hours.

b. It is eluted in a technetium 99m generator from radioactive decay of molybdenum 99; it is in the form of sodium pertechnetate ($Na^{99m}TcO_4$) with valence + 7 and is easily reduced to valence + 4, for better reaction with prepared components.

c. This agent decays mainly by gamma ray emission, producing gamma rays of 140 KeV, which are ideal for imaging and can be easily shielded, thus safely handled.

II. USE OF RADIOPHARMACEUTICALS FOR ORGAN SYSTEM ANALYSIS

A. Pulmonary system. Radioisotopes commonly are used in **lung perfusion scans**, which help detect acute pulmonary embolism, and **ventilation scans**, which help differentiate pulmonary embolism from chronic obstructive pulmonary disease (COPD).

1. ^{99m}Tc MAA (macro-aggregated albumin)

a. This agent contains spheres of denatured human albumin labeled with ^{99m}Tc.

b. Ninety percent of the particles used must have a diameter of 10 to 90 μm; no diameter can exceed 150 μm.

c. The microspheres are prepared in a suspension for intravenous (IV) administration.

(1) The suspension must be shaken before it is administered.

(2) It should be used no later than 8 hours after preparation.

d. In the **lung perfusion scan**, particles enter the lungs via the pulmonary arteries, then lodge in the precapillary arterioles. Abnormal distribution patterns reflect impaired regional lung perfusion.

e. The lungs clear the particles by enzymatic hydrolysis; half-life with lung clearance is 14 to 15 hours.

f. The recommended dose is 1 to 4 millicuries (mCi) of 60,000 to 120,000 particles.

2. Xenon 133 (^{133}Xe) gas

a. In a **ventilation scan**, this gas may be administered via spirometer or a special breathing apparatus to distribute with respiratory air. With pulmonary embolism, the scan usually is normal; with COPD, it typically shows delayed ventilation and radioactive gas trapping.

b. ^{133}Xe has a half-life of 5.3 days; it decays by beta, gamma, and x-ray emission.

c. Because this gas is highly soluble in oil and grease, stopcocks and fittings on syringes or ventilating machine apparatus should not be lubricated.

d. The usual adult dose is 10 to 15 mCi.

B. Skeletal system

1. General considerations. Nuclear bone scans are particularly valuable for detecting cancer metastases, which appear as areas of increased radionuclide phosphate uptake. Bone scans are more sensitive than x-rays for this purpose because the radionuclide is adsorbed onto the hydroxyapatite bone matrix via chemisorption.

2. ^{99m}Tc methylene diphosphonate (^{99m} Tc medronate; MDP) [Fig. 15-1]

a. Stannous chloride, present in the reaction vial, reduces ^{99m}Tc + 7 to ^{99m}Tc + 4; this substance then complexes with one or more of the phosphate groups.

b. Approximately 50% to 60% of the injected dose distributes throughout the skeleton within 3 hours; the remainder is excreted by the kidneys.

c. The usual dose is 10 to 20 mCi.

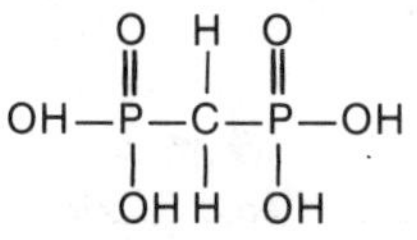

Figure 15-1. Methylene diphosphonate.

C. Hepatobiliary system

1. **General considerations**. Although liver function can be evaluated through various laboratory tests, liver visualization previously proved challenging because the organ is not dense enough to permit useful x-rays. The introduction of **radioactive colloids** has made possible both liver visualization and functional evaluation of reticuloendothelial cells; the use of radiopharmaceutical **reactive dyes** permits visualization of the liver and biliary duct and assessment of hepatocyte function.

2. **^{99m}Tc sulfur colloid (SC)**
   a. This colloidal dispersion contains ^{99m}Tc particles of up to 1 μm in diameter.
   b. In a liver scan, ^{99m}Tc SC is injected intravenously. The radioisotope locates mainly in reticuloendothelial cells of the liver, spleen, and bone marrow, accumulating in tumors and other lesions.
   c. The biologic half-life is 6 hours.
   d. The usual adult dose is 5 to 8 mCi.

3. **Iodine 131 (^{131}I) sodium rose bengal**
   a. A reactive dye, sodium rose bengal is labeled with ^{131}I for use in liver scans.
   b. After IV administration, the substance accumulates in the polygonal cells of the liver.
   c. Normally, it is excreted in the feces via the biliary system. Renal excretion indicates impaired liver function.
   d. ^{131}I decays by gamma and beta emission; its half-life is 8.06 days.
   e. The usual dose is 2 to 3 microcuries (μCi)/kg.

4. **^{99m}Tc disofenin** (Fig. 15-2)
   a. This iminodiacetic acid (IDA) derivative is rapidly extracted from the blood by hepatocytes, then travels to the bile. Because it achieves high biliary concentrations, it has value in gallbladder and bile duct imaging.
   b. ^{99m}Tc disofenin is useful in diagnosing acute cholecystitis and associated cystic duct obstruction. For example, if the agent does not reach the bowel (as shown by a scan), cystic duct obstruction is present.
   c. The agent is excreted in the feces.
   d. The usual dose varies with the patient's serum bilirubin level; it ranges from 2 to 15 mCi.

D. Renal system

Renal system. Radiopharmaceuticals allow both static and dynamic evaluation of the kidneys.

1. **^{99m}Tc gluceptate (glucoheptonic acid)** [Fig. 15-3]
   a. Most valuable in assessment of kidney shape, size, and position, this agent also identifies kidney lesions.
   b. After IV injection, ^{99m}Tc gluceptate concentrates in the renal parenchyma.
   c. The usual adult dose is 10 to 20 mCi.

2. **^{99m}Tc succimer (2,3-dimercaptosuccinic acid; DMSA)** [Fig. 15-4]
   a. Renal scans using this agent can assess the renal parenchyma and distinguish normal renal

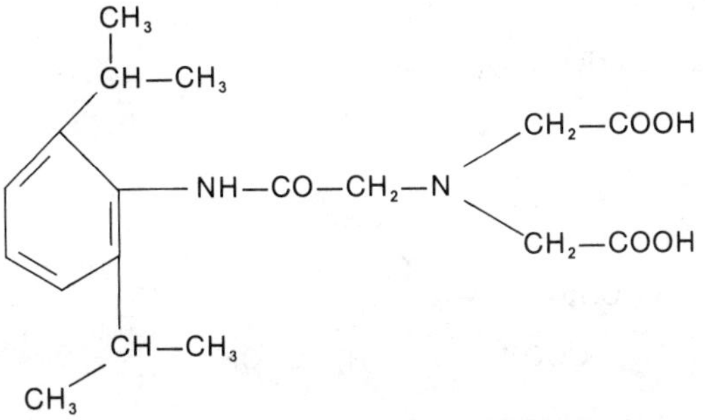

Figure 15-2. Disofenin.

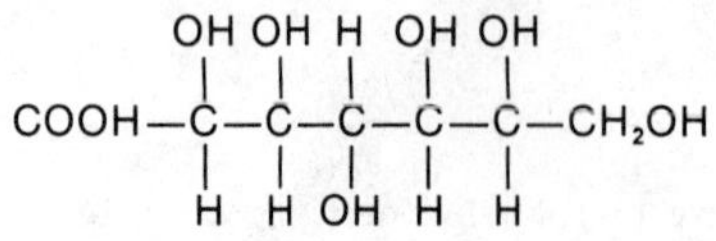

```
      OH OH H  OH OH
      |  |  |  |  |
COOH—C—C—C—C—C—CH2OH
      |  |  |  |  |
      H  H  OH H  H
```

Figure 15-3. Glucoheptonic acid.

anatomic variations from space-occupying lesions. Renal tumors and cysts appear as nonfunctioning renal cortical defects.

b. Results correlate well with relative renal blood flow.

c. ^{99m}Tc DMSA must be used within 30 minutes of preparation.

d. The usual adult dose is 2 to 6 mCi.

3. ^{99m}Tc pentetate (diethylenetriaminepentaacetic acid; DTPA) [Fig. 15-5]

a. Excreted via glomerular filtration, ^{99m}Tc DTPA permits analysis of renal vascular integrity (as in a renal perfusion study). Unperfused regions indicate renal cysts.

b. Rapid sequential views are taken.

c. The usual adult dose is 3 to 5 mCi.

4. ^{131}I orthoiodohippurate sodium (Fig. 15-6)

a. Because this agent is excreted almost entirely by the kidneys (with each kidney excreting about 50%), renal function can be assessed by measuring ^{131}I concentration in each kidney after injection. Inequalities in concentration indicate renal dysfunction (e.g., abnormalities in relative renal blood flow, differential tubular function, and urinary tract patency).

b. The average dose is 3 to 5 μCi/kg; the maximum dose is 350 μCi.

E. Nervous system

1. Brain imaging agents

a. General considerations. Nuclear brain scans serve two main purposes:

(1) To evaluate changes in the blood–brain barrier

(2) To assess cerebral blood flow

b. ^{99m}Tc gluceptate. Discussed in more detail in section II D 1, this is now the agent of choice in tests performed to localize cerebral lesions.

c. $^{99m}TcO_4$

(1) Closely resembling the iodide ion in physiologic behavior, $^{99m}TcO_4$ distributes rapidly in the extracellular fluid, concentrating in the choroid plexus of the brain. (Other concentration sites include the thyroid gland, salivary gland, and stomach.)

(2) It is useful in evaluating cerebral blood flow.

(3) The patient receives 150 to 300 mg of potassium perchlorate 30 to 60 minutes before $^{99m}TcO_4$ is injected, to block uptake in the choroid plexus.

(4) The usual dose is 10 to 20 mCi.

d. ^{123}I iodinated amphetamines (e.g., ^{123}I-iofetamine)

(1) This relatively new class of agents is used in tests that evaluate the brain's white matter, to investigate such conditions as dementia and Alzheimer's disease.

(2) Less active forms of amphetamine, they penetrate the blood–brain barrier but have little or no pharmacologic activity of their own.

(3) Imaging takes place 15 minutes after injection.

(4) The usual dose is 3 to 5 mCi.

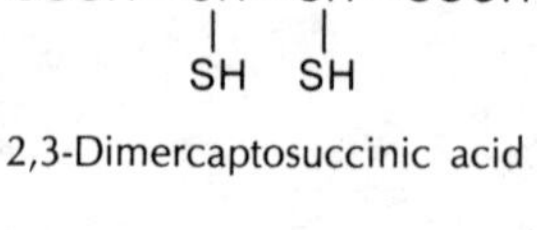

```
COOH—CH—CH—COOH
     |   |
     SH  SH
```

Figure 15-4. 2,3-Dimercaptosuccinic acid (metal chelate).

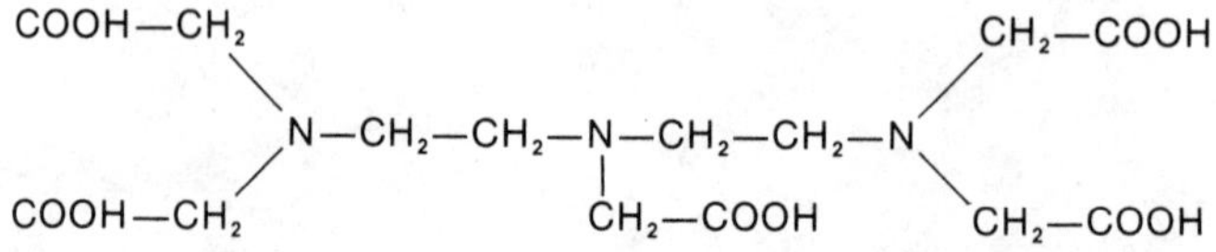

```
COOH—CH2                                  CH2—COOH
        \                                /
         N—CH2—CH2—N—CH2—CH2—N
        /            |           \
COOH—CH2             CH2—COOH     CH2—COOH
```

Figure 15-5. Diethylenetriaminepentaacetic acid.

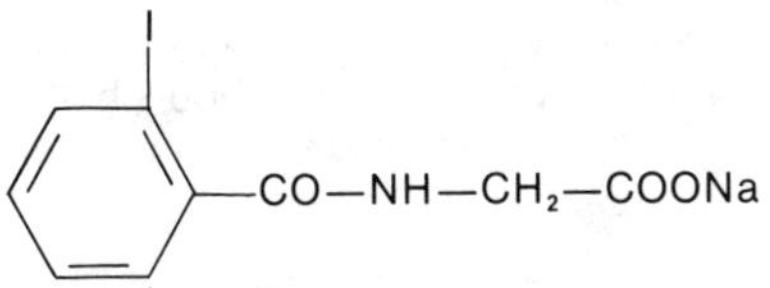

I

—CO—NH—CH$_2$—COONa

Figure 15-6. Iodine 131 orthoiodohippurate sodium.

e. **^{99m}Tc DTPA** (discussed in section II D 3) accumulates in intracranial lesions with excessive neovascularity or when the blood–brain barrier is altered. The dose used for brain scans is 10 to 20 mCi.

2. **Agents used in cerebrospinal fluid (CSF) studies (cisternography).** Indium 111 (^{111}In) DTPA is the preferred agent for CSF dynamic studies, which evaluate the flow of CSF and detect any CSF leakage.
   a. Imaging occurs at approximately 4 hours and 24 hours after administration.
   b. The half-life of ^{111}In is 2.8 days; decay occurs by electron capture.
   c. The dose is 0.5 to 1.4 mCi.

F. Cardiovascular system

1. Nuclear imaging studies of the heart may be static or dynamic.
   a. A **static scan** localizes the site of myocardial infarction and analyzes myocardial perfusion.
   b. A **dynamic study** evaluates cardiac function.
2. **^{99m}Tc pyrophosphate**
   a. This agent is in the same family as the radiopharmaceuticals used in bone scans.
   b. It concentrates in infarcted regions through an unknown mechanism.
   c. Imaging occurs 1 hour and 1½ hours after administration.
   d. The study must be performed within 6 to 10 hours of a myocardial infarction.
   e. The dose is approximately 10 to 15 mCi.
3. **Thallous chloride 201 (^{201}TlCl; thallium 201)**
   a. This agent is used to localize areas of myocardial ischemia and infarction in tests serving as adjuncts to angiography. Mimicking potassium, ^{201}TlCl is taken up by myocardial cells. Diminished or absent uptake signals an ischemic or infarcted area.
   b. To assess for coronary artery disease, ^{201}TlCl is injected as the patient undergoes a stress test (e.g., a treadmill test). An area of reduced myocardial perfusion ("cold spot") that fills in after the patient has rested indicates ischemia rather than an old infarction.
   c. About 4% of the injected dose is extracted by the myocardium within 5 to 15 minutes after injection. It has a half-life of 73 hours, and it decays by electron capture.
   d. The dose is 1 to 2 mCi.

G. Miscellaneous agents

1. **Sodium iodide 123 (Na^{123}I)**
   a. This is the preferred radioisotope in thyroid function studies and imaging studies of the thyroid, liver, brain, and lung.
   b. The radiation dose is lower than that of ^{99m}Tc; also, Na^{123}I has a high target-to-background ratio.
   c. Half-life of ^{123}I is 13.2 hours; decay takes place by emission of 159-KeV gamma rays.
   d. Imaging occurs 24 hours after administration.
   e. The usual adult dose is 100 to 400 μCi.
2. **Gallium citrate 67 (^{67}Ga)** [Fig. 15-7]
   a. This agent helps localize tumors and infections of soft tissue and bone (e.g., lymphomas, hepatoma, bronchiogenic carcinoma).
   b. ^{67}Ga binds to plasma proteins, especially the iron-transport proteins transferrin, lactoferrin, and siderophores.

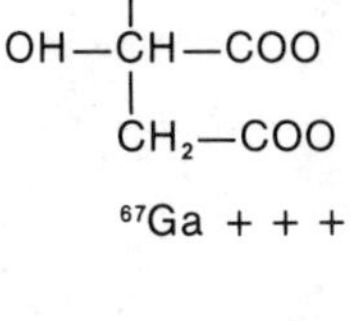

CH$_2$—COO
OH—CH—COO
CH$_2$—COO
^{67}Ga + + +

Figure 15-7. Gallium citrate 67.

c. Because ferric iron may displace some ^{67}Ga from these proteins, ^{67}Ga localization may be inhibited if an excessive dose of ferric iron is administered within 24 hours before the test.
d. The half-life of ^{67}Ga is 78 hours; decay occurs by four different gamma ray emissions ranging from low to high energy.
e. The usual dose is 2 to 10 mCi.

3. **^{111}In oxyquinoline**
   a. This nonpolar lipophilic complex is valuable in the labeling of cellular blood components (such as ^{111}In-labeled leukocytes for the localization of abscesses.)
   b. ^{111}In has a half-life of 2.8 days; decay takes place by electron capture.
   c. The usual dose is 1 mCi.

STUDY QUESTIONS

Directions: Each question below contains five suggested answers. Choose the **one best** response to each question.

1. What type of radioactivity is most often used in radiopharmaceuticals?

A. Gamma rays
B. Alpha particles
C. Beta emissions
D. X-rays
E. Neutrons

2. Which of the following agents is used in diagnostic studies of the biliary system?

A. ^{99m}Tc MDP (^{99m}Tc methylene diphosphonate)
B. ^{99m}Tc DMSA (^{99m}Tc dimercaptosuccinic acid)
C. ^{99m}Tc gluceptate (^{99m}Tc glucoheptonic acid)
D. ^{99m}Tc disofenin
E. ^{99m}Tc MAA (^{99m}Tc macro-aggregated albumin)

3. Which of the following apparatuses has allowed wider use of short-lived radionuclides in locations such as small community hospitals?

A. Cyclotron
B. Nuclear reactor
C. Isotope generator
D. Geiger counter
E. Survey meter

4. What normal function of the liver is used to advantage when a liver scan is performed?

A. Absorption
B. Phagocytosis
C. Adsorption
D. Glomerular filtration
E. Pinocytosis

Directions: Each question below contains three suggested answers of which **one or more** is correct. Choose the answer

A if **I only** is correct
B if **III only** is correct
C if **I and II** are correct
D if **II and III** are correct
E if **I, II, and III** are correct

5. Mrs. Jones, who has chronic bronchial asthma, was sent to the hospital by her physician because she complained of a marked increase in shortness of breath. Her physician is afraid that she may have a pulmonary embolism. Which of the following agents would be used in a differential diagnosis of her shortness of breath?

I. ^{133}Xe (Xenon 133)
II. ^{99m}Tc MAA (^{99m}Tc macro-aggregated albumin)
III. ^{99m}Tc SC (^{99m}Tc sulfur colloid)

6. Monitoring the particle size is important when using which of the following agents?

I. ^{99m}Tc MDP (^{99m}Tc methylene diphosphonate)
II. ^{99m}Tc MAA (^{99m}Tc macro-aggregated albumin)
III. ^{99m}Tc SC (^{99m}Tc sulfur colloid)

Directions: The group of questions below consists of lettered choices followed by several numbered items. For each numbered item select the **one** lettered choice with which it is **most** closely associated. Each lettered choice may be used once, more than once, or not at all.

Questions 7–9

Match the nuclear medicine study with the agent of choice.

A. Sodium iodide 123 ($Na^{123}I$)
B. ^{99m}Tc gluceptate
C. Thallous chloride 201 ($^{201}TlCl$)
D. ^{99m}Tc sulfur colloid (^{99m}Tc SC)
E. Xenon 133 (^{133}Xe)

7. Anatomically viewing the kidney
8. Imaging the thyroid
9. Performing a cardiac stress test

ANSWERS AND EXPLANATIONS

1. The answer is A. (*I B 2 b, C 2, 8 c*) While x-rays from a sealed source are still the most common form of radiation used in medicine and some radioactive isotopes do emit x-rays, radiopharmaceuticals do not make use of x-rays. In nuclear medicine, radioisotopes that emit gamma rays are used most often. Gamma rays are the safest, the most easily shielded, and the most efficiently detected; agents emitting alpha and beta particles must be given in higher doses, thereby increasing the risk of injury to the patient. Neutrons, along with protons, are components of alpha particles.

2. The answer is D. (*II C 4*) Disofenin is an iminodiacetic acid (IDA) derivative. Members of the IDA series are rapidly removed from the blood by liver cells and then concentrate in the bile, a property that is useful for gallbladder and bile duct imaging. When labeled with ^{99m}Tc, medronate (methylene diphosphonate; MDP) is used for bone scans; succimer (dimercaptosuccinic acid; DMSA) and gluceptate (glucoheptonic acid), for kidney studies; and macro-aggregated albumin (MAA), for lung perfusion studies.

3. The answer is C. (*I C 8*) It is best to use an isotope with a short half-life (to minimize the radiation dose received by the patient) when a clinical test requires that a radioisotope be administered internally. The most commonly used radioisotope for diagnostic imaging, technetium 99m(^{99m}Tc), is the "daughter" of molybdenum 99 (^{99}Mo). It is produced by eluting, or "milking," ^{99}Mo in a radioisotope generator, or "radioisotopic cow."

4. The answer is B. (*II C 1*) The liver naturally clears the blood of foreign products by way of its reticuloendothelial cells. These cells engulf the foreign matter, a process known as phagocytosis. If the foreign matter is a radioactive colloid (e.g., ^{99m}Tc sulfur colloid), its cumulation in the reticuloendothelial cells allows both visualization ("scanning") of the liver and functional evaluation of the reticuloendothelial cells.

5. The answer is C (I, II). (*II A, C 2*) Xenon 133 (^{133}Xe) is a gas used to test the patency of the bronchioles in a ventilation scan, and ^{99m}Tc MAA shows the regional pulmonary blood flow in a lung perfusion scan. These studies are useful in distinguishing shortness of breath due to bronchial causes (e.g., asthma) from that due to perfusion abnormalities (e.g., pulmonary embolism), a differential diagnosis that is often a problem without these tests.

6. The answer is D (II, III). (*II A 1, B 2, C 2*) If the particles of ^{99m}Tc MAA are too large, they will block the needed pulmonary blood flow, and pulmonary hypertension could result. If the particles of ^{99m}Tc SC are too large, they will be trapped in the lungs. ^{99m}Tc MDP, used for bone imaging, is a solution and should contain no particles.

7–9. The answers are: 7-B, 8-A, 9-C. (*II D, F 3, G 1*) ^{99m}Tc gluceptate can be used to determine kidney shape, size, and position and to identify kidney lesions. Na^{123}I is the preferred radioisotope in studies of thyroid function and for imaging studies of the thyroid, liver, brain, and lung. ^{201}TlCl is used to localize areas of myocardial ischemia and infarction and to assess for coronary artery disease. It mimics the potassium ion in its myocardial distribution. ^{99m}Tc sulfur colloid is used for liver studies, and xenon 133, a gas, is used for lung ventilation scans.

Part III
Pharmacy Practice

Robert L. McCarthy
Anthony V. Rozzi

16 Interpreting and Dispensing Prescriptions and Medication Orders

Robert L. McCarthy

I. DEFINITIONS

A. Prescriptions are orders for legend products, written by a licensed practitioner who is authorized by statute to prescribe; they are intended for use by patients on an ambulatory basis. Generally, the prescription includes:

1. Patient's name, age, and home address
2. Trade and/or generic name of the legend product
3. Product strength
4. Quantity of medication to be dispensed
5. Directions for compounding (if necessary)
6. Instructions for use
7. Number of refills
8. Prescriber's signature, office address and telephone number, and Drug Enforcement Administration number and/or state controlled substances number

B. Medication orders are orders for legend or nonlegend products that are intended for use by patients on an institutional rather than ambulatory basis. The medication order generally includes:

1. Patient's name, age, and home address
2. Patient identification number and known allergies
3. Prescriber's name and signature
4. Trade or generic name of the legend or nonlegend product
5. Product strength
6. Directions for compounding (if necessary)
7. Instructions for use
8. Any other relevant practitioner instructions regarding patient care (e.g., radiologic procedures, respiratory therapy, diet)

II. INTERPRETING THE PRESCRIPTION OR MEDICATION ORDER.

Upon receipt of a prescription or medication order, the pharmacist should be able to interpret (or determine) the following information:

A. Why the order is indicated, relative to the patient's clinical condition

B. Patient's disease or disorder

C. Terminology used, including apothecary, metric, and English units of measure, and Latin abbreviations

D. Trade or generic name of the product

E. Whether the prescribed product is commercially available or requires extemporaneous compounding

F. What pharmaceutical calculations are necessary to prepare and dispense the prescription

G. Practicality of measuring and administering the prescribed dose [e.g., whether 5.396 ml versus 5.4 ml measured practically by the patient (by rounding off)]

H. Whether the prescription or medication order contains the necessary dispensing information (e.g., route of administration and strength) to allow accurate preparation and dispensing

I. Whether the order contains all the information required by federal and state statutes

III. EVALUATING THE APPROPRIATENESS OF A PRESCRIPTION OR MEDICATION ORDER

A. The pharmacist must evaluate a prescription or medication order to ensure that it is appropriate in light of the following:

1. Patient's disease or disorder

2. Patient's allergies or hypersensitivities

3. Pharmacologic or biologic action of the prescribed product

4. Prescribed administration route

B. Also, the pharmacist should determine whether:

1. Prescribed product might result in a drug–drug or drug–disease interaction

2. Dose and dosage regimen are safe and effective for the patient for whom the product is prescribed

3. Prescribed dosage form will promote optimal safety, therapeutic effectiveness, and patient compliance

4. Quantity of medication to be dispensed is sufficient to allow proper completion of a course of therapy

5. A physical or chemical incompatibility might result (if the product requires extemporaneous compounding)

IV. PROCESSING AND DISPENSING MEDICATIONS. To process and dispense the prescribed product, the pharmacist should follow appropriate guidelines.

A. On the prescription, the pharmacist should record:

1. Prescription number (for initial filling)

2. Date of filling or refilling

3. Quantity dispensed (if different from the quantity prescribed)

4. Lot number and expiration date of the prescribed product (as shown on the manufacturer's container)

5. Pharmacist's initials

6. Any other information required by federal or state statutes

B. The pharmacist must choose the correct product, dose, and dosage form.

C. If the prescription or medication order requires extemporaneous compounding, the pharmacist must properly compound it and prepare it for dispensing.

D. The pharmacist must select the proper packaging and container to ensure product stability and promote patient compliance.

E. Labeling of the prescribed product

1. The pharmacist must include the following information on the prescription product's label:
a. Patient's name
b. Dispensing date
c. Prescription number
d. Directions for use

e. Product's generic and/or trade name
f. Product strength
g. Quantity of medication dispensed
h. Prescriber's name
i. Lot number and expiration date
j. Any other information required by federal or state statutes

2. For a medication order that is dispensed in **unit-dose packages,** the label should clearly identify the patient's name and room number, the product's generic or trade name, product strength, and lot number and expiration date.

F. To ensure proper medication use and storage and compliance with applicable statutes, the pharmacist should affix **auxiliary and/or cautionary labels** as appropriate.

G. The pharmacist should maintain **prescription files and records** in accordance with standards of sound practice and statutory requirements. These records should include a **patient profile system** containing patient demographic information and a complete chronologic record of prescriptions. The patient profile system may be automated (computerized) or manual. (See section VI A for more information on the patient profile system.)

V. COUNSELING PATIENTS AND HEALTH PROFESSIONALS.

The pharmacist's responsibilities include counseling patients and health professionals on the safe and effective use of medication.

A. Counseling patients

1. The pharmacist should advise patients regarding the proper dosage, route of administration, dosing interval or time of administration, and duration of use of prescribed products.

2. Other patient counseling topics may be appropriate as well.
   a. **Special procedures.** As appropriate, the pharmacist may advise patients on how to take the medication (e.g., on an empty stomach or with plenty of water) or may warn patients to avoid alcoholic beverages during drug therapy. Auxiliary labels may be used to reinforce verbal counseling.
   b. **Potential adverse effects.** The pharmacist may warn patients about adverse effects, offer advice on ways to manage or minimize them, and inform patients which adverse effects may warrant consultation with the prescriber or pharmacist.
   c. **Proper storage.** The pharmacist should tell patients how to store products properly to ensure stability.
   d. **Over-the-counter (OTC) products.** The pharmacist should caution patients about the use of OTC products that may interact with the prescribed product.

B. **Counseling nursing personnel.** The pharmacist should advise nurses regarding the indications, contraindications, adverse effects, and usual dosage for medication orders written for patients under their care.

C. **Counseling physicians and other allied health professionals.** To ensure the safe and effective use of prescribed medications, the pharmacist may counsel health professionals on the following topics:

1. Choice of prescription product
2. Proper dosage, dosing intervals, and route of administration
3. Commercially available products and their strengths
4. Potential adverse drug effects
5. Drug interactions
6. Intravenous (IV) incompatibilities
7. Safe handling of chemotherapeutic agents
8. Nutritional support
9. Drug interference with laboratory tests

VI. PATIENT MONITORING.

To determine therapeutic success or failure and to detect any adverse drug effects, drug interactions, drug allergies, and drug toxicity, the pharmacist should establish effective monitoring practices.

A. A comprehensive **patient profile system** is the cornerstone of good patient monitoring. This system permits the pharmacist to detect various problems.

1. **Late refills of maintenance products.** If this problem occurs, the pharmacist should advise the patient about the importance of uninterrupted therapy.
2. **Acute medical conditions for which completion of therapy is essential.** The pharmacist should monitor patients to ensure completion.
3. **Adverse effects or iatrogenic disease** that may have resulted from a prescribed product
4. **OTC (nonlegend) interactions.** The pharmacist must monitor the patient's selection of OTC (nonlegend) products to avoid interactions with prescribed products.
5. **Therapeutic parameters.** To ensure that the prescribed product has safe and effective results, the pharmacist should monitor such parameters as the patient's drug sensitivities, serum drug concentrations, and nutritional status markers.
6. **Duplicate prescribing of medications**
7. **Potential drug misuse or abuse**

B. To prevent potential drug interactions or contraindications, the pharmacist must carefully consult the patient profile when new legend products are added to a patient's regimen.

C. The pharmacist should monitor the patient's clinical condition for evidence of **therapeutic failure** (i.e., drug failure).

D. When **therapeutic intervention** is warranted, the pharmacist must consult with the prescriber promptly.

STUDY QUESTIONS

Directions: Each question below contains five suggested answers. Choose the **one best** response to each question.

1. Medication orders differ from prescriptions in that they

A. are intended for ambulatory use
B. contain only the generic name of the drug
C. may contain nonmedication instructions from the practitioner
D. may be written by a nonlicensed practitioner
E. contain the quantity of medication to be dispensed

2. A prescription label should contain all of the following EXCEPT

A. quantity dispensed
B. lot number
C. patient diagnosis
D. expiration date
E. physician name

3. Auxiliary cautionary labels should be utilized for all of the following purposes EXCEPT

A. to substitute for verbal consultation
B. to ensure proper usage
C. to inform the patient of storage requirements
D. to comply with statutory requirements
E. to warn against the concomitant use of certain drugs or foods

4. A pharmacist must monitor patients receiving medications to detect each of the following problems EXCEPT

A. therapeutic failure
B. adverse reactions
C. drug interactions
D. progression of the disease state
E. noncompliance

ANSWERS AND EXPLANATIONS

1. The answer is C. (*I B*) Medication orders, because they are written for the care of inpatients, often contain laboratory, radiologic, and other nonmedication orders. Both medication orders and prescriptions may contain the trade or generic name of the drug; prescriptions contain the quantity of medication to be dispensed, and neither prescriptions nor medication orders are written by nonlicensed practitioners.

2. The answer is C. (*16 IV E 1*) The quantity of medication dispensed, the lot number and expiration date, and the physician's name should all appear on prescription labels. However, the patient's diagnosis, although listed on the patient's medication profile, is not included on the prescription label.

3. The answer is A. (*IV F; V A 2 a*) Auxiliary cautionary labels are an adjunct to verbal consultation, not a replacement. Appropriate uses for such labels include assurance of proper use, citing storage requirements, compliance with statutory requirements, and warning against food and drug interactions.

4. The answer is D. (*VI*) Pharmacists have the clinical responsibility of monitoring for the therapeutic success or failure of drug therapy and for adverse reactions, drug interactions, and noncompliance. Monitoring patients for progression of their disease state is generally the responsibility of the patient's physician.

17
Hospital Pharmacy Practice

Robert L. McCarthy

I. HISTORICAL PERSPECTIVE. Institutional pharmacy practice has undergone dramatic changes in the last 20 years.

A. During the 1960s, the responsibilities of the hospital pharmacist generally involved supplying medication in bulk to ward stocks and extemporaneously compounding topical ointments, creams, and an occasional sterile ophthalmic preparation.

B. Two major changes in recent decades significantly affected the hospital pharmacist.

1. The unit-dose drug distribution system and pharmacy preparation of intravenous admixtures greatly enhanced the hospital pharmacist's role.

2. The clinical pharmacist emerged as an integral member of the patient care team.

C. These changes thrust hospital pharmacists—who had lagged behind their community counterparts—into leadership positions in the new era of pharmacy practice.

D. Pharmacist involvement in physician rounds and the development of doctor of pharmacy (PharmD) and residency programs further enhanced the stature of the hospital pharmacist.

E. The **American Society of Hospital Pharmacists (ASHP)** has become a leading pharmacy organization in the United States, with a membership and range of activities extending beyond institutional walls.

F. Today, hospital pharmacists are vital players on the health-care team, acting in such important capacities as therapeutic experts, nutritional support unit members, and pharmacokinetic consultants.

II. ADMINISTRATIVE STRUCTURE OF THE HOSPITAL PHARMACY

A. Pharmacy director. Sometimes known as the chief pharmacist or pharmacy manager, the pharmacy director has varied leadership responsibilities.

1. Like all hospital departmental managers, the pharmacy director oversees both personnel and budgetary (fiscal) matters.

2. The director also serves on various hospital committees, typically acting as secretary of the **pharmacy and therapeutics committee.**

3. As a member of the hospital team, the pharmacy director may be involved in community outreach programs (see section III C 4).

4. The pharmacy director sets quality standards for the department, evaluating policies and procedures and implementing changes and innovations as necessary.

B. Associate or assistant director. Depending on department size, the pharmacy may have one or more associate or assistant directors.

1. The associate or assistant director aids the pharmacy director in the operation of the pharmacy.

2. Specific tasks may include overseeing day-to-day pharmacy operations, supervising the sterile products room, and directing pharmacy purchasing.

3. When the pharmacy director is absent, the associate or assistant director assumes managerial responsibility.

C. Staff pharmacists. These employees have daily responsibility for the pharmacy's distributive and clinical duties.

1. **Distributive duties** include:
   a. Physician order review and filling
   b. Unit-dose cart checking
   c. Extemporaneous compounding of ointments, creams, solutions, and intravenous admixtures
   d. Specific assigned tasks, such as purchasing, inventory control, and narcotic distribution and control

2. **Clinical duties** of the staff pharmacist are varied.
   a. **Therapeutic assessment.** In addition to evaluating the appropriateness of prescribed drugs and dosages, the staff pharmacist monitors for drug–drug interactions and adverse drug effects.
   b. The staff pharmacist also advises physicians, participates in physician rounds, and serves on the nutritional support team.
   c. Other clinical duties of the staff pharmacist include pharmacokinetic monitoring, patient discharge counseling, and in-service education.

D. Clinical pharmacists. Because of their specialized education and training, these pharmacists are responsible for providing clinical activities for the hospital pharmacy.

1. Most clinical pharmacists have an advanced degree, such as master of science in clinical pharmacy or PharmD. Some also may have completed a residency or fellowship in a clinical specialty.
2. The clinical pharmacist plays a major role in prescribing, monitoring, and evaluating drug therapy.
3. Depending on departmental organization and hospital size, the clinical pharmacist also may have drug distribution duties.
4. Some clinical pharmacists hold appointments at colleges or schools of pharmacy, serving as preceptors to graduate and undergraduate students.

E. Hospital pharmacy residents. As graduates of pharmacy programs, these staff members have a special interest in hospital practice.

1. Generally, pharmacy residencies are 1-year or 2-year programs offered by hospitals alone or in conjunction with a college or school of pharmacy.
2. Hospital pharmacy residents gain intensive experience in the distributive, clinical, and administrative aspects of institutional practice.
3. Many pharmacy residents go on to graduate school, clinical fellowships, or entry-level hospital pharmacy management positions.
4. The ASHP matches potential pharmacy residents with residency programs to facilitate the selection process for both residency candidates and hospitals.

F. Technicians and other support personnel play an important part in hospital pharmacy operation.

1. Technicians may be pharmacy students fulfilling their internship requirements, or they may be high school graduates.
2. Technicians work under the direct supervision of a pharmacist. In fulfilling their primary duty—helping to carry out the pharmacist's responsibilities—technicians perform the following tasks:
   a. Fill unit-dose carts
   b. Fill floor stock pharmacy supplies
   c. Extemporaneously compound and prepare intravenous admixtures
3. Many hospitals and several schools of pharmacy and community colleges have established 1-year and 2-year technician training programs.
4. The Association of Pharmacy Technicians, a national organization, includes support personnel working in community pharmacies, hospitals, and other settings.

G. Clerical and secretarial support staff. These employees may be involved in pharmacy purchasing and patient billing as well as standard clerical and secretarial duties.

III. RESPONSIBILITIES OF THE HOSPITAL PHARMACY

A. Drug distribution is the primary responsibility of the hospital pharmacy.

1. Recently, drug distribution methods have undergone major changes. For instance, to place pharmacy services closer to patient care areas, many large hospitals have decentralized drug distribution by creating satellite pharmacies and using mobile cart systems.
2. Drug distribution systems fall into two major categories—floor stock and unit-dose systems.
   a. Floor stock drug distribution
   (1) The traditional drug distribution system, the floor stock system, involves a separate pharmacy area in a secured area on each patient care floor.
   (a) Generally, each nursing area has 10 to 100 dosage forms on hand for use by the nursing staff.
   (b) Floor stock may include all or some of the medications carried in the hospital pharmacy.
   (c) In many cases, floor stock consists of a predetermined list of medications, with others sent on request from the nursing staff if they have received physicians' orders for different items.
   (2) Drawbacks
   (a) The floor stock system does not give pharmacists the opportunity to review physicians' orders for accuracy of dosage and scheduling or potential drug interactions. The choice of medication is made by the medicine nurse from floor stock, without the involvement of a dispensing pharmacist.
   (b) Pharmacists have no chance to review the patient's medication profile to monitor drug therapy. They must guess, based on nurses' requests for a resupply, when a particular drug is being used. Modified floor stock systems were developed in an attempt to address the issue of pharmacist review of medication profiles; however, these systems do not deal with the issue of nurse dispensing.
   b. Unit-dose drug distribution system. Developed to reduce medication errors, this system guarantees pharmacist medication review and individual patient dispensing. It has largely replaced the floor stock system.
   (1) The unit-dose system has two main components.
   (a) All physician medication orders are reviewed by a pharmacist before they are dispensed. The pharmacist may review orders directly in the patient care area or may review copies of orders sent to the pharmacy.
   (b) Medications are dispensed as unit-doses or units-of-use, in an individually labeled box or drawer for each patient. Typically, a 24-hour medication supply is sent. For instance, for a patient who is to receive 250 mg of amoxicillin orally three times daily, the pharmacy sends three individually packaged, 250-mg capsules of amoxicillin.
   (2) Advantages. Besides allowing pharmacists to review and dispense all medications, the unit-dose system reduces medication errors and helps cut pharmacy costs (by eliminating floor stock medication supplies).
   (3) Drawbacks. Although the unit-dose system generally is superior to the floor stock system, it has certain flaws.
   (a) Delays may occur in initiating new medication orders.
   (b) Doses may be missed.
   (c) Pharmacy labor costs are higher.
3. **Intravenous admixture programs.** These programs followed closely the implementation of the unit-dose drug distribution system.
   a. Formerly, the nursing staff was responsible for preparing intravenous admixtures.
   b. The responsibility shifted to pharmacists in recognition of their advanced training in this area and the need for sterile preparation areas for intravenous admixtures. These areas contain laminar flow hoods, which eliminate environmental contamination and protect personnel who prepare potentially toxic products (e.g., antineoplastic agents).

B. Clinical functions of the hospital pharmacy

1. **Therapeutic consultation** may be the most important service provided by the hospital pharmacy staff.
   a. Acute-care patients typically receive multiple drug therapy; such complex regimens necessitate the involvement of a pharmacist.
   b. The hospital pharmacist also performs other clinical activities, such as:
   (1) Selecting an antimicrobial therapy regimen or parenteral nutrition formula
   (2) Monitoring the pharmacokinetic aspects of aminogylcoside therapy
   (3) Assessing for drug interactions and adverse effects

2. **Drug information centers,** which are operated by the pharmacies of many large teaching hospitals, field drug-related questions.
   a. Textbooks, journals, and on-line computer information sources serve as the data base.
   b. Health-care professionals both within and outside the hospital may have access to the drug information center.
   c. Some drug information centers act as poison control centers for their geographic region; this requires pharmacist interaction with the public.

3. **Other clinical functions.** Hospital pharmacists participate in in-service and patient education programs. For example, they may give formal lectures to physicians, nurses, and other allied health personnel and may instruct patients about medications upon discharge.

C. Miscellaneous functions of the hospital pharmacy

1. **Purchasing.** This important administrative function has been greatly simplified by advanced technology, such as computer-generated purchase orders and bar codes for ordering.
   a. Generally, a pharmacist or pharmacy technician coordinates pharmacy purchasing.
   b. Pharmaceuticals may be purchased from the manufacturer or a drug wholesaler.
      (1) To reduce drug acquisition costs, the pharmacies of several hospitals may band together to negotiate group contracts with manufacturers.
      (2) A **prime-vendor contract**—in which the pharmacy guarantees that it will purchase a specific dollar amount from the wholesaler—also helps reduce pharmacy costs.
      (3) In return for the guarantee, the wholesaler reduces the mark-up—a practice known as cost plus. For instance, a wholesaler normally charges a mark-up of 8% above the manufacturer's price. Under a cost-plus prime-vendor contract, the wholesaler may use a cost-plus-3% formula, charging only the manufacturer's price plus 3%.

2. **Inventory control**
   a. Hospital pharmacies usually take annual, semi-annual, or quarterly physical inventories.
   b. To maintain the proper inventory, the pharmacy's **turnover rate** must be determined.
      (1) The turnover rate is calculated as follows:

$$\text{Turnover rate} = \frac{\text{Annual purchases (in dollars)}}{\text{Annual inventory (in dollars)}}$$

      (2) A low turnover rate may indicate that inventory is too high.

3. **Committee work**
   a. As discussed in section II A, the pharmacy director typically serves on the **pharmacy and therapeutics committee,** which oversees the use of medications in the hospital.
      (1) Working with the committee chairperson (usually a physician), the pharmacy director sets the committee's agenda. (Other pharmacy staff—for instance, a clinical pharmacist—also may hold committee membership.)
      (2) The committee determines which drugs should be carried on the hospital's formulary; it may also oversee the use of investigational drugs and the handling of hazardous waste.
   b. **Other hospital committees** that may include pharmacy personnel are the pharmacy–nursing committee, infection control committee, human studies committee, and quality assurance committee.

4. **Community relations.** A hospital pharmacist may coordinate community outreach programs such as hypertension and cholesterol screening, poison prevention awareness, and substance abuse prevention programs.

STUDY QUESTIONS

Directions: Each question below contains five suggested answers. Choose the **one best** response to each question.

1. All of the following are considered desirable functions of a contemporary hospital pharmacy EXCEPT

A. clinical consultation services
B. intravenous admixture programs
C. floor stock distribution systems
D. selecting antimicrobial therapy regimens
E. purchasing and inventory control

2. All of the following are advantages of unit-dose drug distribution systems EXCEPT

A. prompt delivery of new medication orders
B. pharmacist review of medication orders
C. a decrease in medication errors
D. reduced pharmacy costs
E. pharmacist dispensing of medications

3. Hospital pharmacy residency programs are governed by the

A. ASCP
B. ASHP
C. APhA
D. ACA
E. NARD

4. Clinical pharmacists often possess which of the following advanced degrees?

A. PD
B. PhD
C. MBA
D. PharmD
E. JD

5. Responsibilities often delegated to hospital pharmacy technicians include

A. counseling of patients being discharged
B. review of physicians' medication orders
C. preparation of intravenous admixtures
D. pharmacokinetic monitoring
E. administration of intravenous admixtures

6. A patient's medication order states that she is to receive "ampicillin 500 mg po q6h." How many doses of ampicillin 250-mg capsules should be placed in the patient's unit-dose drawer daily?

A. 2
B. 4
C. 6
D. 8
E. 10

7. The clinical functions of a hospital pharmacist may include all of the following EXCEPT

A. monitoring drug interactions
B. administration of medications
C. pharmacokinetic consultation
D. participation on a nutritional support team
E. making rounds with physicians

8. Information sources utilized by drug information centers may include all of the following EXCEPT

A. popular literature
B. medical journals
C. textbooks
D. on-line computer information sources
E. pharmacy journals

9. In inventory control, the turnover rate is calculated by which of the following formulas (in dollar amounts)?

A. Annual purchases + annual inventory
B. Annual purchases × annual inventory
C. Annual inventory ÷ annual purchases
D. Annual purchases ÷ annual inventory
E. Annual purchases − annual inventory

ANSWERS AND EXPLANATIONS

1. The answer is C. [*III A 2 a (2), b, B 1 b (1)*] Floor stock drug distribution systems have numerous drawbacks. Therefore, these systems have been replaced largely by unit-dose drug distribution systems in most hospital pharmacies. Clinical consultation services, intravenous admixture programs, providing drug information to hospital staff and to patients, community outreach services, and drug purchasing and inventory control are all important functions of the contemporary hospital pharmacy.

2. The answer is A. (*III A 2 b*) Although unit-dose systems offer numerous advantages, the prompt delivery of new medication orders is not one of them. Traditional floor stock systems, which kept ''mini pharmacy'' supplies of medications in the patient care area, provided much faster access to medications for the initiation of new therapy—at the cost, however, of numerous medication errors and other serious problems.

3. The answer is B. (*II E 4*) The American Society of Hospital Pharmacists (ASHP) matches potential pharmacy residents with residency programs. The ASHP also acts as the accrediting body for hospital pharmacy residencies.

4. The answer is D. (*II D 1*) The Doctor of Pharmacy degree (PharmD), a clinically oriented doctorate, is held by many clinical pharmacists in both institutional and academic settings.

5. The answer is C. (*II F 2*) Counseling patients about medication upon discharge, reviewing physicians' medication orders, and pharmacokinetic monitoring are all functions that must be performed by a pharmacist. The preparation of intravenous admixtures, under the direct supervision of a pharmacist, is an activity often delegated to technicians. The administration of intravenous admixtures is the responsibility of the nursing staff.

6. The answer is D. [*III B 1 b (1) (b)*] Typically, with the unit-dose distribution system, the pharmacy provides a 24-hour medication supply for each patient in an individually labeled unit-dose box or drawer. The patient in the question is to receive 500 mg of ampicillin orally every 6 hours—that is, four times each day. With only 250-mg capsules available, a daily unit-dose supply of eight capsules is necessary.

7. The answer is B. (*I D; III B*) Despite the pharmacist's assumption of numerous clinical functions in recent years, the administration of medications to patients has remained a nursing function.

8. The answer is A. (*III B 2*) Popular literature (e.g., *Time*, *Newsweek*, *People*) is not considered an appropriate information source for a drug information center.

9. The answer is D. (*III C 2*) The annual purchases of a pharmacy (in dollars) divided by the pharmacy's annual inventory (in dollars) will yield the turnover rate. A low turnover rate may indicate that inventory is high.

18
Parapharmaceutics and Medical Devices

Joseph F. Palumbo

I. AMBULATORY AIDS

A. Wheelchairs. Many different types of wheelchairs are available. The patient's disabilities, size, weight, and activities are the main considerations in wheelchair selection.

1. Wheelchairs may be manually or electrically operated.
2. Accessories for wheelchairs include elevated leg rests, removable arm rests, and detachable back rests.

B. Walkers. These lightweight devices, made of metal tubing, have four widely placed legs.

1. They are used by patients who need more support than a cane but have reasonably good arm, hand, and wrist function.
2. The patient holds onto the walker and takes a step, then moves the walker and takes another step.
3. **Types of walkers** include:
   a. Adult adjustable walker
   b. Adult nonadjustable walker
   c. Child's adjustable walker
   d. Folding walker
   e. Reciprocating walker
   f. Wheeled walker
   g. Side walker

C. Canes. These simple ambulatory aids provide balance and transfer weight off a weakened limb.

1. Canes may be wooden or metal.
   a. **Wooden canes** made for males typically are heavier than those made for females. The highest-quality wooden canes are those that have been cut with a hand saw.
   b. **Metal canes** come in adjustable and nonadjustable models and may be monopod or multipod. Good metal canes are those that have been cut with a tubing cutter.
2. **Fitting a cane.** Each cane must be adjusted or cut to fit the individual patient.
   a. To support the arm muscles, the cane should provide about 25° of elbow flexion.
   b. The crease on the inside of the patient's wrist should be level with the top of the hand grip.
   c. The tip of the cane should be 4″ in front of the toes, at approximately a 45° angle.
   d. The cane should be cut about ½″ shorter than the required length to allow for the thickness of the tip.
3. **Using a cane.** In most cases, the patient should carry the cane on the strong side to provide a wide base of support and permit the center of gravity to move forward rather than from side to side.

D. Crutches. These devices generally are used by patients with temporary disabilities (e.g., sprains, fractures).

1. Crutches come in sizes ranging from toddler to large adult.
2. They may be made of wood or aluminum; either type may be fixed or adjustable.
3. Crutch accessories include arm pads, hand grip cushions, and crutch tips.
4. **Types of crutches** include forearm crutch, axillary crutch, quad crutch, and shepherd's crook crutch.

a. The **forearm crutch** (also called Canadian or Lofstrand crutch) supports the wrists and elbows, attaching to the forearm by a collar or cuff. It is used by patients needing crutches on a long-term basis.
b. The **axillary crutch**—the most commonly used crutch—provides more support than the forearm crutch.
c. The **quad crutch** is a forearm crutch with a quadrangular base that is attached to the main shaft with a flexible rubber mount. This design allows the quad feet to maintain constant contact with the ground.
d. The **shepherd's crook crutch,** a type of axillary crutch, resembles a forearm crutch except that the hand grips point to the rear, and axillary rather than forearm support is provided.

5. **Fitting a crutch.** A crutch must be properly measured to prevent "crutch paralysis"— injury to axillary nerves, blood vessels, and lymph nodes.
a. The patient should stand erect, supported by the wall or a chair, for the fitting.
b. The crutch tip should fall 2" next to and 6" in front of the toes.
c. The top rest should fall 2" below the axilla.
d. The hand grips should be set so that the arms form roughly a 30° angle.

II. ORTHOPEDIC BRACES AND SURGICAL FITTINGS

A. These devices are worn by patients with various spinal disorders, including the following:

1. **Kyphosis** (known in lay terms as "hump back" or "hunch back") refers to increased convexity of the curvature of the thoracic spine (as viewed from the side).

2. **Lordosis** (sometimes called "swayback") is an abnormal increase in the curvature of any spinal region.

3. **Scoliosis** is lateral spinal curvature.

B. By limiting patient movement, orthopedic braces and surgical fittings promote proper body alignment.

C. Pharmacists must undergo special training before attempting to fit an orthopedic device.

III. HOSPITAL BEDS AND ACCESSORIES.

Hospital beds may be manually or electrically operated.

A. Most manually operated beds have an adjustable height feature and adjustable head and foot sections.

B. Electrically operated beds can be positioned by the patient while in bed.

C. Bed rails are safety devices that prevent the patient from falling out of bed.

IV. OSTOMY APPLIANCES AND ACCESSORIES

A. **Definitions.** An **ostomy** is a surgical procedure in which portions of the intestinal and/or urinary tract are removed, the remaining ends brought to the abdominal wall, and a stoma (artificial opening) created to allow passage of feces or urine.

B. An **ostomy procedure** is named for its anatomic location.

1. In a **colostomy**, part of the colon is removed. This procedure is done mainly in patients with colon or rectal cancer, lower bowel obstruction, or diverticulitis.
a. The stoma may be located on the ascending, transverse, descending, or sigmoid colon segment.
b. A colostomy may be temporary (as with bowel resection) or permanent (as with removal of the rectum).
c. Stomal discharge may range from liquid or semisolid (as with an ascending colostomy) to solid (as with a sigmoid or descending colostomy).
d. Eventually, the patient can resume normal activities. However, if the lower rectum has been removed, the male patient may be impotent and sterile.

2. In an **ileostomy**, a portion of the ileum is removed. This procedure usually is reserved for patients with severe ulcerative colitis or Crohn's disease.
a. A loop of the proximal ileum is brought to the abdominal wall to create the stoma.
b. Stomal discharge is liquid or semisolid. Because it contains digestive enzymes, it is highly irritating to skin surrounding the stoma.

c. As with a colostomy, the patient eventually can resume normal activities.

3. **Urinary diversion** with stoma creation may be performed in patients undergoing cystectomy.
   a. In an **ileal conduit** (the preferred method), urine is diverted through a loop in the ileum to a stoma on the abdominal surface at the umbilicus. After surgery, the patient wears an external pouch continuously.
   b. Other types of urinary diversion procedures include ureterostomy, nephrostomy, and ileal bladder.

C. **Ostomy appliances.** The selection of an ostomy appliance (the collecting device for stomal discharge) hinges mainly on the type of discharge produced. Other considerations include size of the gasket openings that fit around the stoma, method of attachment to the stoma, and types of activities the patient engages in.

1. **Solid waste appliances** (as for most colostomy patients) are disposable, detachable pouches with a relatively large gasket size. Most are sealed at the bottom.

2. **Semisolid waste appliances** (as for most ileostomy patients) usually are permanent devices attached to the skin either with cement or karaya gum washers to maintain a watertight seal. Instead of being sealed at the bottom, most of these appliances must be folded, then secured with a rubber band or clip; for drainage, the patient removes the rubber band or clip and unfolds the bottom.

3. **Urinary diversion appliances** are permanent rubber pouches that are cemented to the skin. They must be close-fitting and have a leakproof seal.

D. **Ostomy accessories**

1. To ensure a leakproof seal around the stoma, karaya gum washers may be used.

2. Karaya gum powder, used to prepare the skin for ostomy fitting, absorbs moisture and protects the skin from irritation.

3. Foam pads, usually made of nonabsorbent foam rubber, are placed between the appliance faceplate and the skin.

4. Elastic belts are used to attach some ostomy appliances over the stoma.

5. Cement or adhesive disks may be used to affix the ostomy appliance to the skin.

6. Skin barriers (e.g., Stomadhesive) help protect the skin around the stoma from discharge.

7. Protective skin dressings protect the skin when the ostomy appliance is removed.

8. Solvents are used to remove the ostomy appliance.

9. Some colostomy patients may use special irrigating sets instead of pouches.

10. Hypoallergenic tape is used to attach or support the ostomy appliance.

11. Deodorizers help control fecal odor. For local control, a liquid concentrate deodorant can be placed in or an aerosol deodorant sprayed in the pouch. For systemic odor control, the patient may ingest bismuth subgallate, chlorophyll tablets, or charcoal tablets.

E. **Fitting** of an ostomy appliance usually is done by an enterostomal therapist.

F. **Special considerations for ostomy patients**

1. **Irrigation**
   a. To establish regular, conveniently timed bowel evacuation, the patient may administer an enema to the colon via the stoma daily or every few days.
   b. Many ostomates may stop wearing a pouch after a few months, if irrigation has established adequate bowel control. To protect the stoma, the patient places a gauze sponge or stoma cap over it.

2. **Drug therapy**
   a. Ostomates should crush or chew tablets or take oral drugs in liquid form.
   b. Coated or enteric-coated tablets may not dissolve in the intestine after an ostomy.
   c. Antibiotics, sulfa drugs, laxatives, and diuretics may cause problems in ostomates.

V. **URINARY CATHETERS.** These devices allow removal of urine from the bladder in patients who cannot void naturally. A catheter also may be inserted to empty the bladder before surgery or, in special cases, to collect a urine specimen.

A. Most urinary catheters used today are made of soft rubber or plastic. Most are sized by the French scale; the larger the number, the larger the diameter of the catheter.

B. The catheter is inserted through the urethra into the bladder and attached to a urinary leg bag or a bedside collection bag.

C. To avoid injury, the catheter should be inserted only by a physician or specially trained nurse. Sterile technique is crucial to prevent infection.

D. Patients can be trained to insert their own catheters at home.

E. Types of urinary catheters include the indwelling (Foley) and the "Texas" catheter.

1. An **indwelling catheter** is indicated for continuous bladder drainage or when repeated catheterization must be avoided. The catheter's balloon tip, filled with air or a sterile liquid after catheter placement, prevents catheter dislodgment.

2. The **"Texas" catheter**, designed for male patients, is worn externally over the penis and attached to a leg bag.

VI. OTHER SICKROOM SUPPLIES

A. Thermometers. These instruments, which measure body temperature, are essential to medical practice and should be kept in every home.

1. The **standard fever thermometer** has a sealed glass constriction chamber containing liquid mercury.
   a. Responding to temperature changes, the mercury column rises or falls as it expands or contracts.
   b. The mercury column remains at the maximum temperature registered until it is shaken back into the reservoir at the bottom (the constriction chamber acts as a valve check, preventing the mercury from flowing back into the reservoir).
   c. Fever thermometers come in three main types.
      (1) The **oral thermometer** has a slender reservoir and bulb. Usually, it is placed under the tongue and left there for 3 minutes.
      (2) The **rectal thermometer** has a blunt, pear-shaped bulb for added safety and retention. It is inserted into the rectum and left there for 4 minutes. (Rectal temperature normally is 1° higher than oral temperature.)
      (3) The **stubby thermometer** (also called a security thermometer) has a short, stubby bulb. It is used to take oral or rectal temperature in a child or an irrational patient.
   d. If oral or rectal temperature cannot be taken, **axillary temperature** may be taken with any standard fever thermometer. (Axillary temperature is 1° lower than oral temperature.)

2. The **basal thermometer** records temperatures only within 96° to 100° F. Its graduations are in tenths of a degree. Used to estimate the time of ovulation, this thermometer can be placed in the mouth or rectum.

3. **Electronic thermometers** register body temperature quickly and precisely. Heat alters the amount of current running through a resistor; a digital readout then displays body temperature.

4. **Liquid crystal strips,** placed on the skin, calculate core body temperature from surface temperature. These stick-on strips are valuable for continuous temperature monitoring.

5. **Disposable thermometers** are presterilized and intended for single use only. Also available are disposable thermometer covers—thin, sterile plastic sheaths that can be placed over oral thermometers for each temperature measurement, then discarded.

B. Supplies used for heat and cold therapy. For musculoskeletal disorders and certain other conditions, physicians may recommend application of heat or cold to specific body regions.

1. **Heat** may be applied in dry or moist form.
   a. **Dry heat** commonly is recommended to induce vasodilation and leukocytosis, relax muscles and connective tissue, or hasten suppuration. It may be delivered via a hot water bottle or an electric heating pad.
   b. **Moist heat** penetrates more deeply into muscle tissues than dry heat.
      (1) A **moist-heat pack** (hydrocollator) is a bean bag filled with tiny beads; when boiled, the beads form a gelatinous substance that holds its temperature for up to 40 minutes.

(a) The moist-heat pack must be wrapped in several layers of towels before it is placed on the body.

(b) Between uses, the pack should be wrapped in plastic and stored in the refrigerator (or, if a long storage period is anticipated, the freezer).

(2) Other moist-heat devices include electric heating pads with a wettable sponge or cover (e.g., the Thermophore Pad), chemical hot packs, paraffin baths, and poultices.

2. **Cold application** is indicated mainly to decrease circulation to a local area (as for sprains), thereby reducing swelling. Also, severe arthritis may respond better to cold than to heat.
   a. Cold may be delivered via an ice bag, gel pack, or chemical pack.
   b. Cold application is contraindicated in patients with circulatory stasis.

C. Respiratory therapy equipment

1. **Oxygen therapy** may be prescribed to prevent or treat hypoxia in patients with various respiratory or cardiovascular conditions.
   (1) Usually, oxygen is supplied as a compressed gas or liquid or via an oxygen concentrator.
   (2) A registered respiratory therapist should be consulted for information on the correct procedures, cautions, and laws regarding oxygen use.
2. **Vaporizers** generate steam via electricity.
   a. Vaporizers are used in the treatment of colds, the croup, and other upper respiratory ailments.
   b. A pinch of baking soda or borax may be added in soft-water regions to help conduct the current.
   c. Some vaporizers have a chamber or cup for medication, which volatilizes and passes out of the spray.
3. **Humidifiers** deliver a cool mist, adding moisture to dry air. They promote expectoration in patients with tenacious mucus.

STUDY QUESTIONS

Directions: Each question below contains five suggested answers. Choose the **one best** response to each question.

Questions 1 and 2

Mrs. Jackson has come to you for crutches.

1. How far should the top rest be below her axilla?

A. 0.5 inch
B. 1 inch
C. 2 inches
D. 3 inches
E. 4 inches

2. What angle should her arms form when the hand grips are set properly?

A. 10°
B. 30°
C. 45°
D. 60°
E. 90°

Questions 3 and 4

Young Mrs. Jones has a new 3-year-old stepson, who seems to be feverish. In explaining the use of thermometers, you give her the following information.

3. Relative to oral temperature, rectal temperature is

A. 2° lower
B. 1° lower
C. the same
D. 1° higher
E. 2° higher

4. Relative to oral temperature, axillary temperature is

A. 2° lower
B. 1° lower
C. the same
D. 1° higher
E. 2° higher

5. A colostomy or ileostomy might be performed for any of the following diagnoses EXCEPT

A. lower bowel obstruction
B. malignancy of the colon or rectum
C. ulcerative colitis
D. duodenal ulcer
E. Crohn's disease

6. The diameter of urinary catheters is measured by which of the following scales?

A. Luer
B. English
C. French
D. Gauge
E. Metric

ANSWERS AND EXPLANATIONS

1 and 2. The answers are: 1-C, 2-B. (*I D 5*) When a patient is measured for crutches, the top rest should be 2 inches below the axilla, and the hand grips are set so that the arms form about a 30° angle.

3 and 4. The answers are: 3-D, 4-B. (*VI A 1 c*) Relative to oral temperature, rectal temperature is 1° higher, while axillary temperature is one 1° lower. For example, if a patient's oral temperature were 100°, the rectal temperature would be 101° and the axillary temperature would be 99°.

5. The answer is D. (*IV B*) Lower bowel obstruction, malignancy of the colon or rectum, and diverticulitis may all require a colostomy; severe ulcerative colitis and Crohn's disease may require an ileostomy. The treatment of a duodenal ulcer does not include a colostomy or an ileostomy.

6. The answer is C. (*V A*) The French scale is used to measure the diameter of urinary catheters. The Luer scale is used to measure the syringe-tip size on Luer-lok and Luer-slip syringes. The gauge scale is used to measure the outer diameter of needles, and both the English and metric scales are general systems of measurement.

19
Home Health Care

Joseph F. Palumbo
Barbara Schlienz Prosser
Robert A. Smaglia

I. HOME DIAGNOSTIC AIDS

A. Self-care tests or kits, sold in pharmacies for home use, detect specific conditions or measure levels of certain substances for monitoring purposes.

1. These tests have limitations and are intended for use by patients under a physician's care—not for self-diagnosis.
2. Test instructions are written in easily understood language.
3. Many factors can affect the accuracy of home tests; usually, the package lists these factors.
4. Outdated tests can give misleading or inaccurate results.
5. Pharmacists should familiarize themselves with the tests they sell and be prepared to counsel patients on their use.

B. Types of home diagnostic aids

1. **Pregnancy tests.** New types of pregnancy tests come on the market frequently. Purchasers must follow test instructions carefully.
2. **Ovulation tests.** These tests, which help determine when ovulation occurs, are difficult for some women to use—especially those with irregular menstrual cycles.
3. **Acetone, albumin, and bilirubin tests.** Relatively easy to perform, these tests have been available for a long time.
4. **Glucose tests**
   a. **Blood glucose tests** range from lancets for finger pricks to expensive, complex glucose meters.
   b. **Urine glucose tests** include such products as Benedict's solution, tablets, and test strips. Some are used up to four times daily.
5. **Occult blood (stool guaiac) tests** are screening tests for colorectal cancer.
   a. These tests cannot differentiate upper and lower gastrointestinal tract bleeding.
   b. False-positive results may occur.
   c. The patient must avoid certain foods for a prescribed period before these tests are performed.
   d. Patient teaching is essential to ensure successful testing.

II. HOME INFUSION THERAPY

A. Introduction. Since its emergence in the 1960s, the home infusion industry has grown dramatically due to increased health care costs, the development of new drugs, advances in drug delivery, and changes in medical insurance, government legislation and third-party payment policies.

1. The costs of inpatient hospital care have skyrocketed, making home therapy more cost-effective. Studies show that home infusion therapy achieves a cost savings of 50% to 75% over inpatient infusion therapy.
2. New drugs and the development of lightweight ambulatory infusion devices have made home infusion therapy more practical.
3. Third-party payors now recognize and reimburse for most home infusion therapies.

4. The passage of the Catastrophic Illness Act by Congress will offer a broader range of home intravenous (IV) therapies to the medicare population.

B. Types of home infusion therapy

1. **Home nutritional support therapy**
   a. **Parenteral nutrition** fulfills the nutritional requirements of patients via a central or peripheral IV catheter. Typically, the parenteral solution contains amino acids, dextrose, electrolytes, trace minerals, and vitamins. Some patients require concomitant administration of IV lipid suspensions.
   b. **Enteral nutrition** supplies either supplemental or total nutrition via the gastrointestinal tract. The enteral formula may be given by mouth, nasogastric tube or a tube that has been surgically placed in the intestine. Some patients require delivery via an infusion pump.

2. **Home antibiotic therapy.** Administered via a central or peripheral IV line, this therapy necessitates thorough patient teaching to ensure that the patient understands its clinical necessity and the need for close monitoring.

3. **Home analgesic therapy.** This type of therapy permits home pain management in patients who otherwise would require hospitalization. Medication is delivered via a small, patient-controlled analgesic (PCA) pump, which allows the patient to monitor the pain control regimen and make adjustments as necessary.

4. **Home chemotherapy and hydration.** Chemotherapy agents administered in the home are those with minimal side effects. These agents are administered by continuous IV infusion via an ambulatory pump or IV bolus injection or subcutaneously. Home hydration is employed as supportive therapy for the debilitated or terminal patient or as part of a chemotherapy protocol.

5. New infusion therapies now available for home use include the administration of immunoglobulin, heparin, Prolastin, blood products, and chelating agents.

C. Assessing candidates for home infusion therapy. Before patients are approved for home therapy, they must be thoroughly evaluated.

1. The patient, a significant other, or both must be capable of independent functioning and of learning self-administration techniques.

2. The patient's disease must be stable, and no other indication for hospitalization may be present.

3. The patient must be motivated to participate in the home infusion program.

4. The home environment and physical facilities must be appropriate for home therapy.

5. The patient's psychosocial status must be conducive to independent self-care.

6. The patient's venous access must be determined.
   a. A patient who must use a peripheral IV line generally is eligible only for short courses of therapy (lasting a few weeks).
   b. A patient with a central IV line may receive infusion therapy for several months to years.

D. Patient teaching. Patients, significant others, or both must learn the skills needed to administer and monitor home infusion therapy. Patient teaching topics include the following:

1. Infusion techniques

2. Dressing changes (using sterile technique to avoid infection)

3. Mixing of drugs with short-term stability

4. Troubleshooting mechanical problems

5. Monitoring for venous access problems (e.g., infiltration, phlebitis, clotting)

6. Assessing for adverse drug effects

7. Understanding when to obtain emergency medical help (the patient must be instructed to go to a hospital before contacting the home infusion provider)

E. Support personnel. Home infusion therapy requires skilled nursing care, line support, and ancillary supplies.

1. A **patient care coordinator**—usually a nurse—assesses the patient's needs for home nursing

and social services and acts as a liaison between the patient and any agencies involved.

2. A **visiting nurse** provides supplemental nursing services in the home, if necessary.

3. A **patient service representative** manages the patient's inventory and supply deliveries.

4. An **insurance coordinator,** employed by the infusion therapy provider, handles reimbursement matters for the patient.

5. A **durable medical equipment (DME) coordinator** assesses the patient's need for such equipment, coordinates its delivery, and ensures that the patient is properly trained in its use. The DME coordinator acts as a liaison between the patient and DME supplier.

6. A **team of pharmacists** coordinates the patient's drug therapy through regular contact with the nurses, physician, and patient.
   a. The **nutritional support pharmacist** works closely with the nutritional support team to design therapy and monitor the nutritional, metabolic, and fluid needs of the patient receiving home enteral or parenteral nutrition.
   b. The **sterile products pharmacist** oversees the admixture, storage, and safe administration of infusion drugs as well as use of the infusion pump.
   c. The **retail pharmacist** coordinates the patient's oral prescriptions and special needs.

F. **Patient monitoring.** Regular laboratory tests (including drug serum levels) and patient assessment by the visiting nurse help ensure ongoing monitoring. (Home infusion patients cannot be monitored continuously; therefore, they must be educated to assist in monitoring their therapy and to contact the home infusion provider for assistance when needed.)

III. OTHER TYPES OF HOME THERAPY

A. **Home apnea monitoring** may be established for pediatric patients whose apnea has been documented by pneumography or for adults with sleep apnea.

B. **Home phototherapy** may be administered to newborns with hyperbilirubinemia who require an extended course of therapy.

C. **Home respiratory therapy**

1. **Types of therapy**
   a. **Oxygen and nebulizer therapy** commonly are administered at home to patients with asthma or chronic obstructive pulmonary disease (COPD).
   b. **Ventilator therapy** (e.g., intermittent positive-pressure breathing) may be administered to patients who cannot be weaned from a ventilator, such as those with severe COPD, muscular dystrophy, or spinal cord injuries.
   c. **Aerosolized pentamidine therapy** is given prophylactically or therapeutically to patients with *Pneumocystis carinii* pneumonia.

2. Training of hospitalized patients who plan to use certain types of home ventilator therapy may need to begin 6 to 8 weeks before discharge to ensure thorough understanding.

STUDY QUESTIONS

Directions: Each question below contains five suggested answers. Choose the **one best** response to each question.

1. PCA pumps are home care products that are used to administer

A. parenteral nutrition
B. enteral nutrition
C. analgesic medications
D. antibiotics
E. chemotherapy

2. Home phototherapy is used to treat newborns with

A. hyperbilirubinemia
B. azotemia
C. hyperglycemia
D. hypercalcemia
E. hypernatremia

ANSWERS AND EXPLANATIONS

1. The answer is C. (*II B 3*) Patient-controlled analgesia (PCA) pumps are infusion devices that permit pain management at home instead of in the hospital. PCA pumps allow patients to monitor their pain-control regimen and make small adjustments as necessary.

2. The answer is A. (*III B*) Newborn infants with hyperbilirubinemia may require an extended course of phototherapy. Home phototherapy allows the infant to be cared for at home, rather than having to remain in the hospital for a prolonged period.

20 Drug Use In Special Populations

E. Paul Larrat

I. DRUG USE IN PREGNANT PATIENTS. Because virtually any drug a pregnant woman takes can cross the placenta and enter the fetal circulation, drug use in pregnant patients is a source of special concern.

A. Fetal development

1. The effects of drug therapy in pregnancy depend largely on the stage of fetal development. The fetus develops in three distinct stages.
   a. **Blastogenesis.** During this stage (the first 15 to 21 days after fertilization), cleavage and germ layer formation occur. Embryo cells are undifferentiated; increase in embryo size results from general cell proliferation.
   b. **Organogenesis.** From approximately day 21 to day 90 after fertilization, fetal organs and organ systems undergo rapid growth and differentiation.
   c. **Fetogenesis.** This stage, which begins approximately 90 days after fertilization and lasts until birth, is marked mainly by overall fetal growth. All major organ systems now are formed and functioning.
2. The fetus is most vulnerable to the effects of maternal drug therapy during the first and third trimesters of pregnancy.

B. Placental transfer of drugs. A deep red, spongy organ, the placenta serves as the transfer point between the circulatory systems of mother and fetus. (Normally, however, maternal and fetal blood do not mix in the placenta.)

1. The transfer of most nutrients, oxygen, waste products, and other substances occurs via passive diffusion. A few compounds, though, are actively transported across the placental membrane.
2. Formerly, the placenta was thought to guard the fetus from harmful compounds in the maternal circulation. However, the protective characteristics of the placenta are, in fact, limited.
3. **Factors affecting placental drug transfer.** Certain drug properties and placental characteristics can affect the degree of placental drug transfer.
   a. **Molecule size.** Drugs with very large molecules (e.g., heparin) do not cross the placental membrane as readily as those with smaller molecules.
   b. **pH.** The pH gradient between the maternal and fetal circulation and the pH of the drug itself affect the degree of placental transfer. Weakly acidic and weakly basic drugs tend to be rapidly transferred.
   c. **Lipid solubility.** Generally, highly lipid-soluble compounds do not diffuse across the placental membrane as easily as less lipid-soluble compounds.
   d. **Physical characteristics of the placenta.** As pregnancy progresses and the placenta ages, placental drug transfer is less efficient. Also, the presence of placental enzymes and the thickness of the placenta, which change during the course of the pregnancy, may reduce placental transfer.

C. Drugs that cross the placenta may have **embryocidal, teratogenic,** or **fetotoxic effects**.

1. **Embryocidal drug effects**
   a. **Definition.** Embryocidal effects of drugs are those that harm the developing embryo, resulting in termination of pregnancy.
   b. Many drugs, including hormones, antidepressants, angiotensin-converting enzyme (ACE) inhibitors, and certain anti-infectives, administered during blastogenesis are embryocidal.

(1) Because the placenta, which provides some fetal protection, has not yet fully formed by this time, the embryo risks damage from a wide variety of compounds.
(2) The administration of some drugs may result in spontaneous abortion by causing a severe chemical insult to the embryo before cell differentiation.

2. Teratogenic drug effects

a. **Definition.** Teratogenic effects of drugs are those that cause physical defects in the fetus. The risk of teratogenesis is highest during the first trimester, when organs are differentiating.

b. Teratogenesis may lead to physical deformities and mental abnormalities.

c. Because fetal organ systems develop at different times, specific teratogenic effects depend mainly on when the drug was ingested. For instance, the central nervous system (CNS) develops between days 18 and 38 of gestation, whereas the genitals form after day 45. For this reason, a drug taken before day 38 may affect the CNS but probably will not cause genital deformities.

d. The Food and Drug Administration has developed a **classification system** that groups drugs according to the degree of their potential risk during pregnancy.

(1) **Category A.** Controlled studies have not demonstrated a risk to the fetus during the first trimester of pregnancy. The risk of fetal harm from these drugs appears remote.
(2) **Category B.** Animal studies show an adverse drug effect on animal fetuses. However, well-controlled human studies have not revealed similar results.
(3) **Category C.** Although studies show teratogenic risk in animals, no similar human studies are available.
(4) **Category D.** Evidence of human fetal risk exists. However, a threat to the mother's life may warrant use of these drugs despite the potential risks.
(5) **Category X.** Both human and animal studies demonstrate severe harm to the fetus. The risks of these drugs clearly outweigh the benefits.

e. Examples of potentially teratogenic drugs include the following:

(1) **Vitamin A derivatives.** This group, which includes isotretinoin (Accutane), may result in severe human deformities.
(2) **Oral antihyperglycemic agents** (e.g., chlorpropamide, tolbutamide). Whenever possible, these drugs should be replaced with insulin in pregnant women with diabetes mellitus (insulin does not cross the placental membrane). Most toxicity problems associated with diabetic mothers are probably related to high maternal serum glucose levels.
(3) **Warfarin and derivatives.** In some cases, these drugs can be replaced with heparin (which is poorly transferred across the placenta) when anticoagulant therapy is necessary.
(4) **Estrogen and oral contraceptives.** These Category X drugs may cause severe genital tract malformations.
(5) **Other hormonal agents.** Such drugs as thyroid preparations and cortisone may affect the development of fetal endocrine glands.
(6) **Tetracycline.** Mottling of the teeth may occur when this drug is taken after week 18 of gestation. This teratogenic effect does not become evident until later in childhood when tooth eruption occurs.

3. Fetotoxic drug effects

a. **Definition.** Fetotoxic effects of drugs are physiologic effects in the developing fetus. During fetogenesis, these effects are more likely to occur than teratogenic effects.

b. Clinically significant fetotoxic effects include the following:

(1) **CNS depression.** This effect may occur with barbiturates, tranquilizers, antidepressants, and narcotics. Also, analgesics and anesthetics commonly given during labor may cause significant CNS and respiratory depression in newborns.
(2) **Neonatal bleeding.** Maternal ingestion of such agents as nonsteroidal anti-inflammatory drugs (NSAIDs) and certain antidepressant and antianxiety medications may cause serious bleeding in newborns.
(3) **Drug dependence.** Habitual maternal use of barbiturates or narcotics may lead to withdrawal symptoms in the neonate.
(4) **Reduced birth weight.** Pregnant women who smoke cigarettes or consume large amounts of alcohol have an increased risk of delivering an underweight infant.

D. Breast milk transfer of drugs. Most maternal drugs are secreted in at least small quantities into the breast milk of a lactating woman. However, the breast milk concentrations that most drugs achieve are too small to cause a clinical response in the nursing infant.

1. Transfer of drugs through breast milk is governed by many of the same principles affecting placental drug transfer, including:
   a. pH gradient between breast milk and plasma
   b. Degree of drug ionization
   c. Degree of the drug's lipid solubility

2. Drugs that readily enter the breast milk and may adversely affect the infant should be avoided by nursing mothers.
   a. Narcotics, barbiturates, and benzodiazepines, such as diazepam, may have a hypnotic effect on the nursing infant—especially when taken by the mother in large doses. Alcohol consumption may have a similar effect.
   b. Reserpine may cause nasal congestion.
   c. Cascara and danthron may cause diarrhea.
   d. Antithyroid preparations may impair the infant's thyroid function.
   e. Anticholinergic compounds may result in adverse CNS effects in the infant and may reduce lactation in the mother.

II. DRUG THERAPY IN PEDIATRIC PATIENTS

A. General considerations

1. **Age-related characteristics of drug absorption, distribution, metabolism, and excretion** can profoundly influence drug response in pediatric patients.

2. Because the wrong dosage can lead to therapeutic failure or potentially fatal toxicity, special precautions must be taken when calculating pediatric dosages and determining drug regimens.

3. **Prophylactic drugs and biologicals,** often administered to pediatric patients, also must be given with extreme caution to avoid severe side effects.

4. **Therapeutic compliance** poses a challenge in pediatric drug therapy because the patient must rely on others for medication doses.

B. Pharmacokinetics in pediatric patients

1. **Drug absorption**
   a. Reduced production of gastric acid and prolonged gastric emptying time may lead to erratic absorption of oral drugs in neonates. At around 6 months of age values for gastric emptying time approach those of adults. Absorption of aspirin and other acidic drugs and certain other drugs commonly administered to children (e.g., phenobarbital and phenytoin) is also reduced.
   b. The underdeveloped digestive enzyme system of infants and young children may cause impaired absorption of certain oral drugs.
   c. As in the adult patient, absorption of **rectally administered drugs** in pediatric patients is erratic and unpredictable.
   d. **Topical agents** are absorbed faster in children due to the thinner epidermis. Local inflammation (as in diaper rash) may exacerbate percutaneous drug absorption.
   e. **Parenteral drug dosages** must be calculated carefully and drugs administered cautiously because the therapeutic index for such drugs may be quite narrow in pediatric patients.

2. **Drug distribution**
   a. Children have an increased percentage of total body fluids and, in particular, a greater percentage of extracellular fluid compared to adults. As a result, the volume of distribution of water-soluble drugs is greater in pediatric patients.
   b. Because children have less fat in proportion to body mass, lipid-soluble drugs are distributed more slowly in children than in adults.
   c. Children have fewer plasma protein–binding sites than adults.
      (1) As a result, more free drug is available for receptor sites.
      (2) Greater plasma drug concentrations may occur, possibly exacerbating the toxic effects of some drugs.

3. **Drug metabolism.** Until approximately 3 weeks of age, infants have immature metabolic pathways and cannot metabolize full pediatric doses of certain drugs. For example, chloramphenicol may accumulate, leading to **grey baby syndrome** (cardiovascular collapse).

4. **Drug excretion.** Until about age 1 year, infants have a reduced glomerular filtration rate (GFR). Consequently, dosages of drugs excreted mainly via the renal route must be adjusted to avoid accumulation and possible toxicity.

C. Pharmacologic response in pediatric patients

1. The CNS of infants may be especially sensitive to such drugs as narcotics, barbiturates, and antiemetics—possibly due to greater permeability of the blood–brain barrier. This may result in an enhanced CNS response.
2. Some drugs may cause adverse dermatologic effects in pediatric patients. Typically, these effects manifest as an allergic response (e.g., urticaria, edema, or anaphylaxis).
3. Drugs that affect growth and development should be used with extreme caution in pediatric patients. Corticosteroids, for instance, may result in growth suppression.
4. Tetracycline can cause permanent tooth discoloration, enamel defects, and retarded bone growth in children under age 8.
5. Because infants have an erratic temperature-regulating mechanism, they may experience hypothermia with administration of NSAIDs or chlorpromazine, or with topically applied alcohol. Large doses of NSAIDs and sympathomimetics may cause fever.

D. Calculation of pediatric dosages. The child's height, weight, body surface area, and liver and kidney function must be considered when calculating dosages. Established dosages for most commonly used pediatric medications are based on weight.

1. Some existing formulas used for calculating pediatric dosages based on adult dosages are inaccurate. To determine the correct pediatric dosage, current references should be consulted.
2. Pediatric dosages based on body surface area are more accurate than those calculated from adult dosages. This is especially important for drugs with a narrow therapeutic index or with potentially severe side effects. To find a child's body surface area, a **nomogram** is used.

E. Problems of pediatric drug therapy. Poor therapeutic compliance can result from various factors.

1. **Inappropriate dosage form** (e.g., unpalatable or hard-to-swallow medications) can cause a child to resist or refuse doses.
2. **Parents may fail to maintain the proper medication regimen.** Educational efforts aimed at parents may improve compliance.
3. **Spillage or spitting up of oral medications** may cause the child to receive smaller-than-prescribed doses.

III. DRUG USE IN GERIATRIC PATIENTS

A. General considerations

1. The elderly consume more medications than any other age group. Although people over age 65 make up only about 12% of the American population, they consume roughly 25% to 30% of the medications sold in this country.
2. Drug response in elderly patients is affected by age-related changes in physiology and pharmacokinetics.
3. For many reasons, the elderly are more susceptible than younger people to adverse drug reactions.
   a. Many geriatric patients have several illnesses, necessitating multiple medications.
   b. In some cases, more than one physician prescribes medications for an elderly patient. The likelihood of drug-related problems increases when a physician prescribes a medication without knowledge of other medications prescribed for that patient.
   c. The dispensing pharmacist who is not aware of a patient's complete medication regimen is at a disadvantage when counseling this individual.
   d. Many elderly patients receive inadequate medication counseling. Physicians, pharmacists, and other health professionals are often too busy to counsel a patient adequately about the medication regimen. This lack of counseling has been positively correlated with the development of adverse drug reactions and other medication-related problems.
   e. Some elderly patients inappropriately self-medicate.

B. Pharmacokinetics in geriatric patients

1. **Drug absorption.** Age-related changes in the stomach and small intestine may decrease the

absorption rate or cause erratic absorption in elderly patients. (Generally, however, these changes do not affect the **amount** of drug absorbed.)

a. Longer gastric emptying time. In the elderly, many compounds contact the gastric muscosa for longer than normal periods. This may cause several problems.

(1) Interaction with antacids may occur due to the increased chance for binding.

(2) Gastric irritation and ulceration may result from prolonged mucosal contact with ulcerogenic drugs.

(3) Absorption of poorly water-soluble drugs may increase.

(4) Weakly basic drugs (e.g., tricyclic antidepressants, anxiolytics, analgesics, levodopa, anticonvulsants) may have a delayed onset of action.

(5) Incomplete absorption of certain drugs, such as oral antibiotics, antihypertensives, and antiarthritics, may increase the risk of diarrhea.

b. Reduced gastrointestinal motility. Slowed motility in the small intestine may cause erratic absorption of some drugs. The absorption of controlled-release products may be greatly changed.

c. Elevated gastric pH. Reduced gastric acidity may affect the dissolution of weakly acidic drugs, possibly delaying their onset of action.

d. Reduced intestinal blood flow. This may cause delayed or incomplete drug absorption.

2. Drug distribution. Elderly patients have an increased amount of active drug (resulting in a greater risk of adverse reactions) due to several age-related changes in blood and body composition.

a. Decreased plasma albumin level. The albumin portion of plasma proteins diminishes with age. This leads to fewer protein-binding sites and greater levels of unbound active drug. (For this reason, dosages of highly protein-bound drugs should be decreased for elderly patients.)

b. Body composition changes. As a person ages, the percentage of body water and protein falls while the percentage of body fat rises.

(1) Consequently, water-soluble drugs achieve a faster onset of action and a higher blood concentration.

(2) Lipid-soluble drugs, which must be distributed to a greater tissue volume in the elderly, have a slower onset and prolonged duration of action.

3. Drug metabolism. Liver function decreases with age, causing slower drug metabolism and higher plasma levels of active drug (and thus an increased risk of drug toxicity). The following age-related changes affect the hepatic metabolism of drugs.

a. Reduced liver perfusion. Liver metabolism depends greatly on hepatic blood flow. Between ages 25 and 60, blood flow to the liver drops by about 40%.

b. Diminished liver enzyme function. Certain metabolic pathways become less efficient with age, leading to decreased drug metabolism and higher blood levels of active drug.

4. Drug excretion. Age-related reductions in the GFR and kidney perfusion may impair the renal filtration and excretion of drugs. (The GFR may drop as much as 50% between ages 25 and 90.) As a result, many drugs have a longer half-life and may cause toxicity in elderly patients.

a. Drugs that are excreted unchanged in the urine (e.g., digoxin, aminoglycosides, cimetidine, and some cephalosporins) may achieve toxic blood levels due to reduced renal function.

b. Indexes of renal function (e.g., serum creatinine and creatinine clearance levels) may be useful in adjusting drug therapy. (In geriatric patients, creatinine clearance is the more accurate measure of the GFR.)

C. Pharmacologic response in geriatric patients

1. The **site of action** of many drugs may show changes with age, altering the patient's drug response. Typically, an elderly patient has either a heightened or diminished response due to changes in end-organ sensitivity. For example, β-adrenergic receptors may be less responsive to drugs, necessitating an increase in the dosage of such drugs as β-blockers.

2. Major CNS neurotransmitters become depleted as a person ages, leading to enhanced drug effects. Therapy involving antidepressants, barbiturates, antiparkinsonian agents, and benzodiazepines should be monitored for exaggerated effects.

3. The elderly have a greater response to heparin and warfarin due to decreased protein binding and thus are more likely to experience adverse effects from these drugs.

4. Sometimes, behaviors that appear to be related to age or illness actually are undesired responses to medication. For example, confusion or poor interaction with the environment may reflect CNS response to medication rather than dementia.

D. Adjustments in geriatric drug therapy

1. Typically, drug dosages must be adjusted to compensate for the unpredictable drug response in elderly patients.

2. Because some age-related physiologic changes increase the blood level of active drugs while other changes reduce the blood drug level, the net effect of drug therapy in elderly patients is hard to predict. For this reason, drug therapy must be carefully monitored to avoid adverse reactions and inappropriate effects.

E. Problems of geriatric drug therapy. In ambulatory geriatric patients, therapeutic success may hinge on the patient's ability to take medications properly. However, various problems may interfere with patient compliance.

1. **Inappropriate tablet crushing.** Many elderly patients cannot swallow medications whole and crush them instead. When an enteric-coated tablet or controlled-release product is crushed, the drug may become inactivated in the stomach or its initial absorption may be excessive.
2. **Lack of patient teaching.** Elderly patients who do not know the purpose of their drug therapy are nine times more likely than other patients to have medication-related problems, such as adverse drug reactions and noncompliance.
3. **Duplication of medication.** In a surprising number of cases, elderly patients reportedly take two or more concurrent drug products with the same active ingredient. Confusion over brand and generic drug names and prescribing by more than one physician are the main causes of this problem.
4. **Drug swapping.** The elderly are more likely than other patients to swap or share medications with friends and family members.
5. **Underuse and overuse of medications.** An elderly patient may decide to increase or decrease the daily medication dosage, increasing the chance for adverse drug reactions or inadequate blood drug levels.
6. **Reduced sensory acuity.** Because of hearing loss, an elderly patient may not hear medication instructions clearly; impaired vision may lead to the inability to read medication labels.

STUDY QUESTIONS

Directions: Each question below contains five suggested answers. Choose the **one best** response to each question.

1. Placental transfer of a drug is affected by all of the following factors EXCEPT

A. size of the molecule
B. pH of the compound
C. lipid solubility of the compound
D. sex of the fetus
E. physical characteristics of the placenta

2. In the classification system for drug use during pregnancy, category X drugs are compounds for which

A. the possibility of fetal harm is remote
B. animal, but not human, studies have shown adverse effects
C. animal, but not human, studies have shown teratogenic risk
D. both animal and human studies have shown that severe risk to the fetus clearly outweighs the benefits of the drug
E. evidence of human fetal risk exists, but life-threatening situations may necessitate use of the drug despite the risks.

3. Factors that affect the absorption of drugs in the elderly include all of the following EXCEPT

A. lengthened gastric emptying time
B. decreased plasma albumin
C. elevated gastric pH
D. decreased intestinal blood flow
E. decreased gastrointestinal motility

4. Medications that should be avoided by a mother who is breast-feeding include all of the following EXCEPT

A. narcotics
B. barbiturates
C. diazepam
D. alcohol
E. acetaminophen

5. Grey baby syndrome in newborns is associated with the administration of

A. gentamicin
B. penicillin
C. chloramphenicol
D. clindamycin
E. erythromycin

6. All of the following are taken into account when calculating dosage for children EXCEPT

A. height
B. weight
C. hepatic and renal function
D. age
E. body surface area

Directions: The question below contains three suggested answers of which **one or more** is correct. Choose the answer

A if **I only** is correct
B if **III only** is correct
C if **I and II** are correct
D if **II and III** are correct
E if **I, II, and III** are correct

7. Problems encountered in geriatric drug therapy include

I. crushing of enteric-coated tablets
II. underuse of medication
III. overuse of medication

ANSWERS AND EXPLANATIONS

1. The answer is D. (*I B 3*) The placental transfer of a drug from mother to fetus is affected by the size of the drug molecule, the pH of the drug, its lipid solubility, and the physical characteristics of the placenta. The sex of the fetus is irrelevant.

2. The answer is D. (*I C 2 d*) The Food and Drug Administration has developed a classification system to designate the risks of drug use during pregnancy. In this system, category X represents compounds that have demonstrated severe risks to the fetus in both animal and human studies, with the risks clearly outweighing the benefits of the drug.

3. The answer is B. (*III B 1, 2*) Lengthened gastric emptying time, elevated gastric pH, decreased intestinal blood flow, and decreased gastrointestinal motility all may affect drug absorption. Decreases in plasma albumin may alter a drug's distribution but would not affect its absorption.

4. The answer is E. (*I D 2*) Large doses of narcotics, barbiturates, diazepam, and alcohol should be avoided by a mother who is breast-feeding her infant. These medications enter the breast milk and may have a hypnotic effect on the nursing infant. Acetaminophen has not been shown to cause problems in nursing babies.

5. The answer is C. (*II B 3*) The administration of chloramphenicol to newborns may result in drug accumulation and subsequent cardiovascular collapse (grey baby syndrome) due to the immaturity of certain metabolic pathways.

6. The answer is D. (*II D*) When calculating dosage for children, the child's height, weight, body surface area, and renal and hepatic function must be taken into account. Age, although sometimes used, may result in improper dosing due to the variations in body size and level of development found in children of the same age.

7. The answer is E (all). (*III E*) The inappropriate crushing of enteric-coated or controlled-release tablets, drug swapping with friends and family, under- and over-utilization of medication, and duplication of drug products are common problems encountered in geriatric drug therapy. Education about drug therapy may reduce these problems.

21 Nutrition

Robert L. McCarthy

I. GENERAL CONSIDERATIONS

A. Nutritional requirements. To maintain normal physiologic functions, physical activity, growth, and tissue repair, the body needs an ongoing supply of energy from food.

1. **Recommended dietary allowances (RDAs).** The National Academy of Sciences has established recommended dietary allowances for average daily amounts of nutrients that healthy people should consume.
   a. **RDAs** have been established for energy needs, most vitamins, and some minerals. **Safe and adequate intakes** have been established for the remaining vitamins and minerals.
   b. RDAs do not apply to people with such conditions as chronic illness, infection, or metabolic disorders. In these cases, nutrient requirements must be determined on an individual basis.

2. **Metabolism of dietary carbohydrate, fat, and protein** supplies the required energy for body functions.

3. Energy is measured in **kilocalories** (kcal); 1 kcal represents the amount of heat needed to raise the temperature of 1 kg of water by 1°C.
   a. Fat supplies 9 kcal/g.
   b. Carbohydrates and protein supply 4 kcal/g.

4. Fat, carbohydrate, and protein requirements vary greatly depending on age, sex, body size, physical activity, general health, and other factors.
   a. In a healthy person, energy requirements are determined by **basal energy expenditure (BEE)**, **physical activity**, and the **energy used for digestion.**
      (1) **BEE** reflects the amount of energy needed to maintain basic physiologic functions. Measured under special circumstances, BEE is calculated using the Harris-Benedict equations.
         (a) For men:

$$\textbf{BEE} = 66 + (13.7 \times \text{weight in kg}) + (5 \times \text{height in cm}) - (6.8 \times \text{age in years})$$

         (b) For women:

$$\textbf{BEE} = 66.5 + (9.6 \times \text{weight in kg}) + (1.7 \times \text{height in cm}) - (4.7 \times \text{age in years})$$

      (2) Digestion-related energy expenditure (known as the **calorigenic effect of food**) generally equals about 10% of the BEE.
      (3) The amount of energy expended in physical activity depends on the specific activity.
   b. **Disease** and other stressful conditions alter the body's metabolic needs, changing the energy requirements. For example, a postoperative patient may require double the calories normally expended for basal metabolism; a patient with burn injury may need up to triple the calories.

5. **Vitamin and mineral requirements.** See section IV.

B. Nutritional assessment. Nutrition plays an essential—yet sometimes overlooked—role in patient care. Prolonged illness, injury, and the postoperative period may be accompanied by malnutrition, which, in turn, complicates recovery. Early identification of patients who risk malnutrition and early detection of those already suffering from it can help avoid potentially devastating consequences.

1. **Anthropometric measurements** help evaluate nutritional status by estimating body composition. The major anthropometric measurements are **height**, **weight**, **triceps skinfold thickness**, and **midarm circumference.**

a. The patient's body weight is compared to **ideal body weight** relative to body size (height and frame size), as shown in standard reference tables.
b. Triceps skinfold thickness and midarm circumference reflect the patient's protein and fat reserves.

2. **Laboratory tests**
a. **Creatinine-height index** compares urine creatinine excretion with ideal creatinine output according to body size. Malnourished patients commonly have subnormal urine creatinine levels.
b. **Serum albumin and transferrin tests** are used to assess visceral protein stores.
c. **A nitrogen balance study** is used to evaluate protein use.
(1) Nitrogen accounts for approximately 16% of body protein.
(2) Normally, nitrogen intake (in the form of consumed proteins) equals nitrogen output (via the urine, skin, and feces).
(a) Positive nitrogen balance (anabolism) exists when nitrogen intake exceeds nitrogen output, resulting in a protein gain. This occurs during such periods as growth and tissue regeneration (e.g., after surgery or injury).
(b) Negative nitrogen balance (catabolism) indicates that nitrogen output exceeds nitrogen intake, leading to protein loss. If this condition persists, it may result in loss of muscle mass and visceral protein.

II. NUTRITIONAL SUPPORT.

Patients whose nutritional needs cannot be met through standard diets may require parenteral or enteral nutrition therapy.

A. Parenteral nutrition

1. **Indications.** Parenteral nutrition (PN)—also called intravenous (IV) hyperalimentation—is given to malnourished, severely debilitated patients with a nonfunctioning gastrointestinal tract. Examples of such patients include those with Crohn's disease, ulcerative colitis, short bowel syndrome, radiation-induced enteritis, head or neck cancer with esophageal obstruction, severe malabsorption syndrome, enterocutaneous fistulae, severe anorexia nervosa, and congenital malformations of the gastrointestinal tract.

2. **Administration routes**
a. **Peripheral-vein administration** may be used in patients whose clinical status is expected to improve within a few weeks. (The high osmolarity of many peripherally administered solutions usually cannot be tolerated for longer periods.)
b. Central-vein administration is the most common route. An indwelling Broviac or Hickman catheter is placed via the superior vena cava in a large central vein (e.g., the internal jugular, intraclavicular, or supraclavicular vein).

3. **Administration methods.** PN solutions may be administered by **continuous infusion** (the most common method) or **cyclic infusion.**

4. **Types of PN solutions**
a. The composition of PN solutions is designed to approximate the nutrient content of a normal oral diet.
(1) Solutions must contain the three basic caloric sources needed for basal energy (carbohydrate, fat, and protein), as well as electrolytes and vitamins.
(2) PN solutions sometimes are used to deliver IV medications or to treat certain deficiencies (e.g., iron deficiency).
b. **Solution components**
(1) **Amino acids** serve as a source of protein and as a substrate for anabolism.
(a) Unlike earlier PN formulas that used protein hydrolysates, current formulas contain a mixture of essential and nonessential **crystalline amino acids,** which provide 100% bioavailability.
(b) Adult PN patients generally need 1 to 1.5 g/kg/day of protein.
(c) Crystalline amino acid solutions come in concentrations ranging from 3% to 11.4% and are available with or without electrolytes. Examples include Aminosyn, Novamine, Travasol, and FreAmine III.
(2) **Dextrose** (D-glucose) is the main sugar used as a carbohydrate source. It must be given in sufficient amounts to maintain basal energy requirements.
(a) Dextrose is essential to protein synthesis by "sparing" the use of protein as an energy source.
(b) Commercially available dextrose concentrations range from 2.5% to 70%. Concentrations 10% and above are hypertonic and should be infused only through a central vein.

(3) **Fats** (lipids) provide essential fatty acids and additional calories.
  (a) Fats are administered via emulsions **(fat emulsions),** which incorporate a nonaqueous phase into an aqueous phase.
  (b) Prepared from soybean oil, safflower oil, or both, fat emulsions prevent essential fatty acid deficiency and, along with dextrose, provide nonprotein calories.
  (c) Fat emulsions are available commercially in 10% to 20% solutions. Examples include Intralipid, Travamulsion, and Liposyn.
  (d) Until recently, fat emulsions were administered as a separate solution—either through a Y-connector into the main PN line or through a peripheral vein. However, they now can be mixed directly with the amino acid/dextrose formula in a solution called "3-in-1" or "triplex mix."
    (i) **Benefits.** They are easier to administer and require less manipulation of the IV line (resulting in a lower infection risk).
    (ii) **Drawbacks.** These mixtures are difficult to test for clarity, have poor stability, and cannot be filtered. Such problems have led clinicians to question their practical and clinical value.

(4) **Electrolytes** (sodium, potassium, calcium, magnesium, chloride, and phosphate) may be added to the PN solution. Requirements for these substances vary widely. (See Chapter 22 for more information on electrolytes.)

(5) **Vitamins** generally are added to PN solutions in multivitamin preparations. Commercially available multivitamin preparations for PN solutions include Berocca P.N., M.V.I.-12, and M.V.C. 9+3. (See section IV for a detailed discussion of vitamins.)
  (a) Because of stability problems, vitamins are packaged in a two-vial system.
    (i) One vial contains the vitamins A, D, E, B_1, B_2, B_3, B_5, B_6, and C.
    (ii) The second vial contains the vitamins B_{12}, biotin, and folic acid.
  (b) To avoid vitamin degradation by the bisulfite ion in amino acid solutions, multivitamin preparations should be added to the PN solution just before infusion.

(6) **Trace elements** now are included in many solutions, especially those given to patients receiving long-term PN.
  (a) **Zinc, copper, chromium,** and **manganese** were the first trace elements to be added to PN solutions. Many solutions now also include molybdenum, iodine, selenium, cobalt, nickel, and fluorine.
  (b) Each trace element may be added individually or as part of a "cocktail." Commercially available cocktails include T.E.C., Multitrace, and M.T.E.-2 through M.T.E.-7 (the numeral indicates how many trace elements the preparation contains.)
  (c) **Precise requirements** for trace elements have not been determined. However, these substances are known to play an essential role in nutrition and in specific physiologic functions. (See section IV B for more information on trace elements.)

(7) **Insulin** may be added to PN solutions to help the pancreas utilize high-concentration dextrose—especially in centrally administered solutions, which may have final dextrose concentrations of 25% or more.
  (a) Only regular (clear) insulin from animal or human sources should be used.
  (b) Clinicians disagree as to indications for insulin. Some believe it should be added routinely to PN solutions; others advocate insulin addition only if the patient begins to spill sugar into the urine.
  (c) The insulin dosage depends on the patient's specific needs. The proteinaceous nature of insulin sometimes leads to its adsorption onto plastic or glass containers, administration sets and filters. Studies of how much insulin adheres to these surfaces is variable. (Dosage adjustment may be necessary because of this phenomenon.)
  (d) Patients with severe glucose intolerance may require a separate insulin infusion.

(8) **Heparin** may be added to the PN solution to reduce the risk of thrombosis and to maintain catheter patency. Heparin also may increase fat utilization.

(9) **Hydrocortisone** in low doses sometimes is added to peripherally administered PN solutions to reduce the risk of phlebitis from hypertonic formulas.

(10) **Histamine (H_2)-receptor antagonists** (e.g., cimetidine, ranitidine) sometimes are used in PN solutions to prevent gastric stress ulcers—a possible complication of PN.

(11) **Miscellaneous additives** used in special circumstances include antibiotics, albumin, aminophylline, hydrochloric acid, opiates, metoclopramide, cardiac medications, and antineoplastic agents.

c. **Amino acid specialty solutions** are especially formulated for patients with specific disorders.

(1) **Hepatic failure solutions** contain a mixture of essential and nonessential amino acids with a high concentration of branched-chain amino acids (BCAAs: leucine, isoleucine, and valine). This content restores normal BCAA levels, reducing mortality and helping

to improve mental status and electroencephalographic patterns. HepatAmine is a commercially available hepatic failure solution.

(2) **Renal failure solutions** contain only essential amino acids (e.g., histidine, considered essential for uremic patients).

(a) To reduce elevated ammonia levels, **arginine** also may be added.

(b) Hypertonic dextrose solution also is infused to promote protein synthesis and slow rising blood urea nitrogen (BUN) levels; dextrose also helps to maintain the balance of potassium, phosphorus, and magnesium serum levels.

(c) Commercially available renal failure solutions include Aminosyn-RF and Nephramine.

(3) **Stress formulas** contain a mixture of essential and nonessential amino acids, with a high concentration of BCAAs to compensate for BCAAs lost through acute metabolic stress. FreAmine HBC is a commercially available stress formula.

d. Complications of PN solutions parallel those of other parenterally administered solutions (see Chapter 22).

B. Enteral nutrition

1. Indications. Enteral nutrition (EN) is used for patients who cannot ingest adequate nutrients but who have absorptive function in some portion of the gastrointestinal tract. Such patients may include those with inflammatory bowel disease; gastrointestinal or head or neck cancer; acute or chronic pancreatitis; dysphagia; esophageal stricture; and coma.

2. Advantages. Compared to PN, EN causes fewer serious side effects and is less expensive and easier to administer.

3. Administration routes

a. Oral feeding is preferred for patients who can take oral nutrients.

b. Tube feeding is necessary for patients who cannot take food by mouth (e.g., those with drug-induced anorexia or certain neurologic disorders).

(1) Usually, the feeding tube is placed in the stomach via the nose. This is referred to as a nasogastric tube.

(2) In some cases, fluoroscopy or endoscopy is used to place the tube.

(3) Surgical tube placement (tube enterostomy) may be done in patients requiring long-term nutritional support. For instance, a gastrostomy (G) tube is placed directly in the stomach; a jejunostomy (J) tube, directly into the jejunum.

4. Administration methods

a. Continuous administration

(1) This method is indicated when:

(a) EN is initiated.

(b) The patient has not received an enteral feeding for 3 or more days.

(c) The patient is critically ill.

(d) Feedings are delivered directly into the small intestine.

(2) The formula is delivered slowly (50 to 150 ml/hr over 12 to 24 hours).

(3) An **infusion pump** should be used when the delivery rate is less than 150 to 200 ml/hr, when using a smaller tube, and when feeding into the small intestine.

b. Intermittent (bolus) administration

(1) This is the method of choice for ambulatory patients because it does not restrict movement. (However, EN is best initiated with continuous feedings; then, intermittent feedings are introduced gradually.)

(2) Feedings are administered in volumes of 250 to 400 ml, given five to eight times daily.

5. Types of enteral formulas

a. Modular supplements are nutritionally incomplete formulas that provide specific amounts of carbohydrates, proteins, and fats. They are intended as supplements for complete formulas in patients with additional nutritional needs. Commercially available modular formulas include Polycose (glucose polymer), Propac (protein), and Hycal (carbohydrate).

b. Defined formulas

(1) These formulas may be monomeric or polymeric.

(a) **Monomeric formulas** contain amino acids or short peptides and simple carbohydrates.

(b) **Polymeric formulas** contain more complex protein and carbohydrate sources.

(2) Defined formulas come in three basic categories; formulas in any category may be monomeric or polymeric.

(a) **Milk-based formulas** now are used rarely because of low patient tolerance. Examples of these formulas include Sustagen and Sustacal powder and pudding.

(b) **Nutritionally complete, lactose-free formulas,** the most frequently used EN formulas, usually are well-tolerated. Examples include Vital High Nitrogen, Sustacal, Isocal, Osmolite, and Ensure.

(c) **Specialized formulas** are administered to patients with specific disorders.

(i) **Hepatic failure formulas** are high in BCAAs and low in aromatic amino acids (AAA). Hepatic-Aid is an example.

(ii) **Renal failure formulas** (e.g., Amin-Aid) contain only essential amino acids.

(iii) **Stress formulas** (e.g., Stresstein, Traum-Aid) have a high BCAA content and an unrestricted AAA content.

6. Adverse effects and complications

a. Fluid and electrolyte disturbances

(1) EN may cause such problems as dehydration (from osmotic diuresis) and excessive diarrhea.

(2) Tube feeding syndrome may occur. This condition—characterized by dehydration, hypernatremia, hyperchloremia, and azotemia—results from excessive protein intake and inadequate fluid intake.

(3) To prevent dehydration caused by diarrhea and concentrated formula, patients should receive additional water.

(a) After each intermittent feeding or at intervals of 3 to 6 hours during continuous feeding, 25 to 100 ml of water should be given.

(b) The water also rinses the feeding tube and helps prevent clogging.

b. Aspiration pneumonia may occur from gastric reflux and subsequent aspiration of the formula. To prevent regurgitation in a patient using a nasogastric tube, the patient's head should be elevated at a 30° angle for at least 30 minutes after an intermittent feeding and at all times during continuous feeding.

c. Hyperglycemia

d. Diarrhea is the most common adverse effect of EN. The risk of diarrhea can be reduced by modifying the formula's caloric density. For example, if the formula contains 1 to 2 cal/ml (as do most of these high-osmolarity formulas), therapy may be initiated at one-fourth strength (three-fourths water to one-fourth formula), then slowly increased, as tolerated, to one-half strength, three-fourths strength, and full strength.

e. Constipation may result from low residue content of feedings. This problem may warrant the addition of fiber to the formula or the use of laxative medications or enemas.

f. Other gastrointestinal problems (e.g., nausea, abdominal cramps, and distention) also may result.

C. Monitoring nutrition therapy. To ensure therapeutic efficacy of PN or EN and to prevent or detect adverse effects and complications, the following steps should be taken:

1. **Body weight** should be measured daily.

2. **Levels of serum electrolytes, glucose, and creatinine and BUN** should be measured daily until the patient is stable. Then, levels of electrolytes and glucose should be checked twice weekly.

3. **Daily intake** should be documented.

4. The patient's **fluid status** and overall **clinical status** should be followed.

5. The **feeding tube** (with EN) or **catheter** (with PN) should be **inspected** regularly to prevent sepsis and mechanical problems.

III. INFANT FORMULAS

A. General considerations. Although breast-feeding remains the preferred method for meeting the nutritional needs of infants, great strides have been made recently in the development of nutritionally sound infant formulas. Besides traditional milk-based formulas, manufacturers now offer modified formulas using alternate protein sources as well as specialty formulas for infants with specific disorders. Pharmacists can play an important role in advising pediatricians on the most suitable preparations for particular patients.

B. Content of milk and formulas

1. **Human milk** is preferred for most infants. Containing one-third the protein content of cow's milk, human milk also has a lower casein content, a different fat content (monosaturated and medium-chain fatty acids), and a higher percentage of carbohydrates.

2. **Evaporated milk** offers several advantages over whole cow's milk, including convenience, sterility, and better gastrointestinal tolerance. It contains twice the calories of whole milk formulas. However, like unmodified cow's milk, evaporated milk does not supply adequate amounts of vitamins C and E and essential fatty acids.

3. **Skim milk** generally is not recommended for infants less than 1 year old because it does not contain adequate carbohydrate, protein, or fat ratios.

C. **Forms of infant formulas**

1. Infant formulas are available in **concentrated liquid, concentrated powder,** and **ready-to-use liquid.**

2. The concentrated forms must be diluted before use. Standard dilutions are as follows:
   a. Concentrated powder—1 tbsp/60 ml water
   b. Concentrated liquid—equal parts formula and water, to produce a caloric density of 20 kcal/30 ml

D. **Content of standard formulas.** Infant formulas must contain adequate amounts of essential nutrients and must supply calories from carbohydrate, fat, and protein sources. In addition, these formulas must be easily digestible and free from microbial contamination.

1. **Caloric density.** Standard formulas generally contain 67 kcal/100 ml (or 20-30 kcal/oz). Formulas with higher or lower caloric density are considered therapeutic formulas (see section III E).

2. **Osmolality** must be considered. The osmolality of an infant formula should approximate that of human milk (approximately 300 mOsm/kg of water). Hyperosmolar formulas may cause diarrhea and dehydration.

E. **Formulas for term infants**

1. **Milk-based formulas** (e.g., Enfamil, Similac) contain nonfat cow's milk, vegetable oils and lactose or corn syrup as a carbohydrate source. These formulas are available without iron or with added iron. Vitamins and minerals are added by the manufacturer.

2. **Milk-based formulas with added whey proteins** (e.g., SMA Iron-Fortified) contain an increased ratio of whey proteins to casein, approximating the ratio found in human milk. Of high nutritional quality, these formulas result in a relatively low renal solute load (the amount of water-soluble substance that must be removed by the kidneys).

3. **Soy-based formulas** (e.g., Isomil, Nursoy, ProSobee) contain water-soluble soy as a protein source. They are used for infants with suspected or diagnosed milk allergy.

4. **Protein hydrolysate-based formulas** (e.g., Nutramigen, Pregestimil) contain hydrolyzed casein. These formulas are indicated for infants who are sensitive to intact proteins.

5. **Meat-based formulas** have a high protein and fat content, necessitating carbohydrate addition. Gerber's meat-based formula, for instance, derives its protein from beef heart.

F. **Therapeutic formulas** are specialty formulas designed for infants with various disorders or conditions.

1. Soy-based and protein hydrolysate-based formulas (discussed above) are used for infants with milk protein allergy.

2. Formulas containing moderate amounts of medium-chain triglycerides (e.g., Pregestimil, Portagen) are indicated for infants on fat restriction. Conditions requiring fat restriction include cystic fibrosis, short bowel syndrome, and celiac disease.

3. Carbohydrate disorders, due to the lack of an essential carbohydrate enzyme, are sometimes seen in infants with cystic fibrosis, celiac disease, or as a congenital defect. CHO-Free is a formula that may be used in these infants. Soy-based formulas, Nutramigen, or meat-based formulas may be used in infants with galactosemia.

4. Formulas with a high caloric density and low renal solute load are required by infants with congenital heart disease. For example, milk-based formulas with added whey often are given to infants with congestive heart failure.

5. Phenylalanine-restricted formulas (e.g., Lofenalac) are given to infants with phenylketonuria.

6. Formulas with high caloric density are used for low-birth-weight infants because of their need for additional calories and their inability to handle adequate volume. Enfamil Premature Formula was designed specifically for low-birth-weight infants. However, like other high-caloric-density formulas, it may cause an excessive renal solute load.

G. Complications of infant formulas

1. Diarrhea and consequent dehydration may result from milk intolerance or inadequate formula dilution.
2. Hypersensitivity reactions may occur with milk-based formulas.
3. Mechanical obstruction may stem from milk curds in milk-based formulas.
4. Other potential complications include electrolyte imbalance, vitamin and mineral deficiency, anemia, neutropenia, and metabolic alkalosis.

IV. VITAMINS AND MINERALS. To maintain good health, the diet must include adequate amounts of vitamins and minerals. Healthy people who consume a well-balanced diet rarely require vitamin or mineral supplementation. However, chronic illness, infection, pregnancy, unusual diets, and other conditions may lead to vitamin and/or mineral deficiency (or, in rare cases, toxicity). To correct vitamin or mineral deficiencies (which usually involve more than one vitamin or mineral), supplements are given. (In the literature accompanying these supplements, RDAs are shown in ranges only. To determine precise RDAs based on patient weight and age, additional references should be consulted.)

A. Patient counseling

1. When dispensing vitamin and mineral preparations, the pharmacist should inform the patient of those products that contain nearly 100% of the RDA and should warn the patient to stay within RDA guidelines to avoid toxicity from megadose therapy.
2. The pharmacist should advise the patient to take iron supplements and other vitamins and minerals with food to reduce stomach upset and should warn the patient that iron supplements may turn stools black.
3. When dispensing liquid vitamin and mineral preparations, the pharmacist should inform the patient that these products can be added to food or beverages.
4. The pharmacist should tell patients to warn children that vitamins are medicine—not candy.

B. Vitamins. These organic compounds are necessary for various metabolic functions. Vitamins fall into two categories—fat soluble and water soluble.

1. The **fat-soluble vitamins A, D, E, and K** are absorbed along with dietary fat. Because these vitamins are stored in the body when intake exceeds current requirements, toxicities (hypervitaminoses) can occur.
   a. **Vitamin A** is found in fish, eggs, liver, carrots, squash, pumpkin, dark leafy vegetables, and dairy products.
      (1) **Main functions.** Vitamin A aids in body tissue repair and maintenance, infection resistance, visual purple synthesis (for night vision), ribonucleic acid synthesis, and skin hydration. It impedes corneal necrosis and growth retardation and promotes corticosteroid production.
      (2) **Hypervitaminosis A** may stem from chronic excessive vitamin A ingestion. Signs and symptoms include fatigue, malaise, lethargy, rough, dry skin, bone and joint pain, restlessness, night sweats, headache, insomnia, hair loss, brittle nails, peripheral edema, gingivitis, anorexia, weight loss, and liver and spleen enlargement.
      (3) **Hypovitaminosis A** may result from fat malabsorption (e.g., as in cirrhosis of the liver or cystic fibrosis), which causes excessive vitamin A excretion. Clinical manifestations include night blindness, dry skin, tunnel vision, softened tooth enamel, and frequent infections.
      (4) **RDA**
         (a) **Adults**
            (i) **Men:** 5000 international units (IU)
            (ii) **Women:** 4000 IU
         (b) **Infants and children:** 2000 to 3500 IU
      (5) **Supplements** can be given orally or parenterally.
   b. **Vitamin D** is supplied by egg yolks, liver, butter, fatty fish, bone meal, and vitamin D-enriched milk products. Commercially, vitamin D is available as ergocalciferol (vitamin D_2), calcifediol (25-hydroxycholecalciferol), calcitriol (1,25-dihydroxycholecalciferol), and dihydrotachysterol (DHT) and cholecalciferol (vitamin D_3).
      (1) **Main functions.** Vitamin D is important in calcium and phosphorus regulation, myocardial function, blood clotting, and nerve cell maintenance.
      (2) **Hypervitaminosis D,** as from chronic excessive vitamin D ingestion, leads to anorexia, weight loss, nocturia, polyuria, and nausea. In severe cases, soft-tissue calcification, nephrocalcinosis, hypertension, acidosis, and renal failure may occur.

(3) **Hypovitaminosis D** may be caused by renal disease, malabsorption syndrome, lack of sunlight, short bowel syndrome, hypoparathyroidism, or familial hypophosphatemia. Signs and symptoms include rickets (in children) and osteomalacia (in adults).
(4) **RDA**
(a) **Adults:** 200 to 400 IU
(b) **Infants and children:** 400 IU
(5) Supplements may be given orally or by injection.

c. **Vitamin E** is found in vegetable oils, dark green vegetables, milk, eggs, organ meats, nuts, butter, and wheat germ.
(1) **Main functions.** The role of vitamin E has not been precisely determined. However, the vitamin is a known antioxidant and protects cell membranes from peroxidation. Also, it may help retard aging, serve as an anticlotting factor, promote diuresis, and help reduce serum cholesterol.
(2) **Hypervitaminosis E** may result in bleeding, gastrointestinal distress, and poor utilization of vitamins A and K.
(3) **Hypovitaminosis E** is caused by malabsorption and maldigestion disorders, myopathies, neuropathies, and cystic fibrosis. Signs and symptoms include gastrointestinal distress, hair loss, impotence, sterility, muscle wasting, and dry hair.
(4) **RDA**
(a) **Adults**
(i) **Men:** 12 to 15 IU
(ii) **Women:** 12 IU
(b) **Children:** 4 to 10 IU
(5) **Supplements** of vitamin E are given only by the oral route.

d. **Vitamin K** is provided by molasses, green leafy vegetables, yogurt, liver, and safflower oil. In the body, vitamin K is produced by intestinal microorganisms.
(1) **Main functions**
(a) Vitamin K promotes blood clotting.
(b) **Clinical uses.** Vitamin K may be administered to prevent or treat hemorrhage associated with pathologic conditions and adverse drug effects or overdose. In newborns, it is given in low dosages (1 mg) to prevent bleeding.
(2) **Hypervitaminosis K** may lead to hepatomegaly or hemolytic anemia. People with glucose-6-phosphate dehydrogenase deficiency may experience hemolytic reactions even with ordinary doses of vitamin K.
(3) **Hypovitaminosis K** can result from malabsorption syndrome, bowel resection, liver disease, or antibiotic therapy. Clinical findings include diarrhea, bleeding tendency, epistaxis, and miscarriage.
(4) **RDA.** No RDA exists for vitamin K; the requirement probably is very low.
(5) **Supplements** may be administered parenterally or orally.

2. **Water-soluble vitamins** are excreted in the urine when the body contains them in excess; they must be supplied daily by the diet because they are not stored in sufficient amounts.
a. **Vitamin C (ascorbic acid)** is supplied by citrus fruits, leafy vegetables, potatoes, and tomatoes.
(1) **Main functions**
(a) Vitamin C plays a key part in cellular respiration; collagen production; catecholamine synthesis; wound healing; and the metabolism of carnitine, steroids, folinic acid, and tyrosine.
(b) **Clinical uses.** Vitamin C may be given to acidify the urine and enhance the antibacterial activity of methenamine.
(2) **Hypervitaminosis C** results in diarrhea, flatulence, uricosuria, pancreatic damage, and impaired leukocyte bactericidal activity.
(3) **Hypovitaminosis C (scurvy)** occurs from inadequate consumption of vitamin C, as may result from such conditions as alcoholism, advanced age, poverty, or gastrointestinal disease. Signs and symptoms of hypovitaminosis C include bleeding gums, gingivitis, loosened teeth, easy bruising, faulty tooth and bone development, muscle and joint pain, impaired wound healing, anorexia, weakness, hyperkeratotic hair follicles on thighs and buttocks, and hair coiling.
(4) **Test interference.** Vitamin C may cause false-positive results with Clinitest tablets and false-negative results with Tes-Tape and Clinistix.
(5) **RDA**
(a) **Adults:** 50 to 60 mg
(b) **Children:** 45 mg
(c) **Infants:** 35 mg
(6) **Supplements** may be given orally or by injection.

b. Thiamine (vitamin B_1) is found in brown rice, liver, kidney, lean pork, peas, and beans.
- **(1) Main functions.** Thiamine promotes carbohydrate metabolism, circulation, digestion, growth, learning, muscle tone, and neurologic function.
- **(2) Hypovitaminosis B_1 (beriberi)** usually stems from inadequate intake due to unusual diet or overprocessed or overcooked foods. Such conditions as fever, thyrotoxicosis, and alcoholism increase the need for thiamine. Signs and symptoms of hypovitaminosis B_1 include edema, muscle weakness (and later atrophy), and evidence of cardiac insufficiency (e.g., dyspnea, tachycardia). (Wernicke-Korsakoff syndrome, a severe neuropsychiatric thiamine deficiency disorder, sometimes occurs in alcoholics.)
- **(3) RDA**
  - **(a) Adults:** 1.0 to 1.5 mg
  - **(b) Infants and children:** 0.3 to 1.2 mg
- **(4) Supplements** may be administered parenterally or orally.

c. Riboflavin (vitamin B_2) is supplied by milk, eggs, meat, fish, liver, whole grains, leafy green vegetables, and nuts.
- **(1) Main functions.** A coenzyme in tissue respiratory systems, riboflavin promotes antibody and red blood cell formation and energy metabolism.
- (2) Hypovitaminosis B_2 (ariboflavinosis) commonly stems from inadequate milk intake, alcoholism, or a vegetarian diet. Manifestations include corneal vascularization, cheilosis, glossitis, and seborrheic dermatitis.
- **(3) RDA**
  - **(a) Adults:** 1.2 to 1.7 mg
  - **(b) Infants and children:** 0.4 to 1.4 mg
- (4) Supplements may be administered orally.

d. Niacin (vitamin B_3, nicotinic acid, nicotinamide) is provided by whole grains, lean meat, organ meats, peanuts, and seafood. The body also synthesizes niacin, providing approximately half of the RDA.
- **(1) Main functions**
  - (a) Niacin is a component in two enzymes involved in tissue respiration. It promotes circulation, growth, sex hormone production, and pigment metabolism.
  - **(b) Clinical uses.** Niacin is administered in the treatment of hyperlipidemic patients who do not respond to dietary and weight reduction measures.
- **(2) Niacin deficiency (pellagra)** may lead to dermatitis, diarrhea, dementia, stomatitis, depression, and rigidity.
- **(3) RDA**
  - **(a) Adults:** 13 to 19 mg
  - **(b) Children:** 9 to 16 mg
  - **(c) Infants:** 6 to 8 mg
- **(4) Supplements** are available in parenteral and oral forms.

e. Pyridoxine (vitamin B_6) is present in bananas, meats, cereals, lentils, nuts, potatoes, avocados, green leafy vegetables, molasses, and raisins.
- **(1) Main functions.** Pyridoxine is a coenzyme in carbohydrate, protein, and fat metabolism. It promotes antibody formation, digestion, hemoglobin production, and sodium and potassium homeostasis.
- **(2) Pyridoxine deficiency** causes signs and symptoms similar to those occuring from riboflavin and niacin deficiency.
- **(3) Drug interactions**
  - (a) Pyridoxine requirements may increase during administration of isoniazid, cycloserine, penicillamine, hydralazine, and oral contraceptives.
  - (b) Patients with Parkinson's disease who are receiving levodopa should avoid multivitamin preparations containing pyridoxine; this vitamin may cause dopa decarboxylation in peripheral tissues, reducing levodopa's therapeutic efficacy. (Sinemet, containing a levodopa–carbidopa combination, is not affected by concurrent pyridoxine administration.) Multivitamin products without pridoxine are available for such patients.
- **(4) RDA**
  - **(a) Adults:** 1.8 to 2.2 mg
  - **(b) Children:** 0.9 to 1.6 mg
  - **(c) Infants:** 0.3 to 0.6 mg
- **(5) Supplements** are available in tablet or injection form.

f. Cyanocobalamin (vitamin B_{12}) is supplied by beef, fish, eggs, pork, milk products, and organ meats.
- **(1) Main functions.** Cyanocobalamin is essential to myelin and nucleoprotein synthesis, hematopoiesis, cell production, and general growth.

(2) Cyanocobalamin deficiency, usually accompanied by folic acid deficiency, may occur in vegetarians and people lacking intrinsic factor, which is necessary for cyanocobalamin absorption. (Lack of cyanocobalmin results in a condition known as pernicious anemia.) Signs and symptoms of deficiency include glossitis, anemia, fatigue, memory impairment, paresthesias, poor muscle coordination, nervousness, headache, confusion, agitation, hallucinations, and acute psychosis.

(3) **RDA**

(a) **Adults:** 3 μg

(b) **Children:** 2 to 3 μg

(c) **Infants:** 0.5 to 1.5 μg

(4) **Supplements** may be given orally or parenterally.

g. Folic acid (folacin) is provided by eggs, citrus fruits, leafy green vegetables, milk products, organ meat, yeast, seafood, and whole grains.

(1) **Main functions.** Folic acid is required for nucleoprotein synthesis and normal erythropoiesis.

(2) **Folic acid deficiency,** usually resulting from lack of fresh fruits and vegetables, may cause tongue inflammation, diarrhea, fatigue, pallor, digestive problems, irritability, memory lapse, and megaloblastic anemia.

(3) **Drug interactions.** Methotrexate administration results in drug antagonism with folic acid. Leucovorin calcium, the active reduced form of folic acid, is used to diminish the toxicity of this antagonism.

(4) **RDA**

(a) **Adults:** 400 μg

(b) **Children:** 100 to 300 μg

(c) **Infants:** 30 to 45 μg

(5) **Supplements** are available to be given orally or by injection.

h. Pantothenic acid (calcium pantothenate, vitamin B_5) is found in a wide variety of foods, including organ meats, whole grains, fresh vegetables, yeast, and eggs.

(1) **Main functions.** Pantothenic acid is a precursor of coenzyme A, which is crucial to the oxidative metabolism of carbohydrates, gluconeogenesis; fatty acid synthesis and degradation; and synthesis of sterols, steroids, and porphyrin.

(2) **Pantothenic acid deficiency** may lead to diarrhea, hair loss, gastrointestinal and renal problems, muscle cramps, fatigue, premature aging, and respiratory infections.

(3) **RDA**

(a) **Adults:** 4 to 7 mg

(b) **Children:** 3 to 7 mg

(c) **Infants:** 2 to 3 mg

(4) **Supplements** are administered orally.

i. Biotin is a B vitamin found in legumes, organ meats, egg yolks, milk, seafood, and whole grains. Also, it is synthesized by intestinal microorganisms.

(1) **Main functions.** Biotin is involved in carboxylation reactions. It promotes fatty acid production; cell growth; vitamin B utilization; and metabolism of carbohydrate, protein, and fat.

(2) **Biotin deficiency** may stem from overingestion of egg whites (the protein in egg whites prevents biotin absorption) or is found in patients receiving parenteral nutrition without added biotin. Signs and symptoms of deficiency include dry skin, anemia, depression, insomnia, poor appetite, and muscle pain.

(3) **RDA**

(a) **Adults:** 100 to 200 μg

(b) **Children:** 65 to 200 μg

(c) **Infants:** 35 to 50 μg

(4) **Supplements.** Biotin is not available as a single-vitamin supplement; however, it is incorporated into various multivitamin products.

3. Multivitamin preparations

a. Generally, healthy people who consume a well-balanced diet do not need these products. However, others may benefit from a daily multivitamin that supplies nearly 100% of the RDA for each vitamin. Such people include:

(1) Elderly

(2) Adolescents

(3) Infants

(4) Pregnant and lactating women

(5) Impoverished or socially isolated people

(6) Trauma and postoperative patients

(7) Patients with severe infection or severe gastrointestinal disorders or malignancy

(8) Patients with prolonged diarrhea, sprue, obstructive jaundice, or cystic fibrosis

(9) Patients taking oral contraceptives; estrogen; long-term, broad-spectrum antibiotics; isoniazid; or long-term parenteral nutrition

b. Multivitamins containing iron are useful for menstruating women because they replace iron losses during menses. (Dietary iron is only 10% bioavailable and therefore may be inadequate for these women.)

B. Minerals are inorganic substances needed for various physiologic functions and commonly are classified in two groups: trace elements and electrolytes.

1. Trace elements

a. Iron is supplied by red meat, liver, fish, poultry, wheat germ, and eggs.

(1) Main functions. Iron is a component of hemoglobin, myogobin, and several enzymes.

(2) Iron deficiency may stem from dietary insufficiency, malabsorption, pregnancy, lactation, or blood loss. Manifestations of iron deficiency include anemia, pallor, weakness, fatigue, cold sensitivity, constipation, brittle nails, exertional dyspnea, palpitations, and numbness of the extremities. In many cases, however, no symptoms occur and the deficiency is discovered from results of routine blood tests.

(3) RDA

(a) Adults: 10 to 18 mg (menstruating women have a higher requirement)

(b) Infants and children: 10 to 15 mg

(4) Supplements

(a) Oral iron forms include ferrous sulfate, ferrous gluconate, and ferrous fumarate; these forms are available as tablets, capsules, liquid, and sustained-release tablets. The **parenteral form** is iron dextran.

(b) Because all iron salts may cause gastrointestinal distress, they should be taken with food. Constipation and black, tarry stools are common side effects of iron supplements.

b. Iodine is found in seafood, kelp, and iodized salt.

(1) Main functions. Iodine is crucial to the synthesis of thyroxine and triiodothyronine. It plays a part in metabolism, physical and mental development, and energy production.

(2) Iodine deficiency (now extremely rare due to the use of iodized salt) may lead to goiter, cretinism (in infants and children), cold hands and feet, dry hair, irritability, and obesity.

(3) RDA

(a) Adults: 150 μg

(b) Children: 70 to 120 μg

(c) Infants: 40 to 50 μg

(4) Supplements. Iodine may be added to PN formulas.

c. Other trace elements include **zinc, copper, chromium, manganese, molybdenum,** and **selenium.**

(1) Zinc, an enzymatic cofactor, promotes wound healing, taste, smell, skin hydration, and normal growth.

(2) Copper is important in transferring production and in the formation of red and white blood cells (copper deficiency causes anemia).

(3) Chromium helps maintain normal glucose metabolism and nerve cell function.

(4) Manganese is involved in enzyme activation and glycoprotein synthesis.

(5) Molybdenum is a constituent of several enzymes.

(6) Selenium guards cell components against damage during cellular metabolism.

2. Electrolytes. Calcium, phosphate, magnesium, sodium, chloride, and potassium are discussed in Chapter 22.

STUDY QUESTIONS

Directions: Each question below contains five suggested answers. Choose the **one best** response to each question.

1. A nitrogen balance study is used to assess body

A. carbohydrate
B. fat
C. protein
D. insulin
E. glycogen

2. Continuous enteral feeding is the preferred nutritional method for all of the following situations EXCEPT

A. when patients are ambulatory
B. when therapy is initiated
C. when patients are critically ill
D. when feeding into the small intestine is necessary
E. when a patient has not received a feeding for three or more days

3. Which type of insulin must be used when adding insulin to parenteral nutrition solutions?

A. Lente
B. NPH
C. Regular
D. Ultralente
E. Semilente

4. The "tube feeding syndrome" is a combination of

A. dehydration, hypernatremia, hyperkalemia, azotemia
B. dehydration, hypernatremia, hyperchloremia, azotemia
C. hypernatremia, hyperkalemia, hyperchloremia, azotemia
D. dehydration, hypernatremia, hyperkalemia, hyperchloremia
E. hypernatremia, hyperkalemia, hyperchloremia, hypercalcemia

5. Which vitamin may cause false-positive readings with Clinitest tablets and false-negative results with Tes-Tape and Clinistix?

A. Vitamin A
B. Vitamin B
C. Vitamin C
D. Vitamin D
E. Vitamin E

6. Wernicke-Korsakoff syndrome is a severe vitamin deficit seen in some alcoholic patients. Which vitamin is lacking?

A. Vitamin B_1
B. Vitamin B_2
C. Vitamin B_3
D. Vitamin B_6
E. Vitamin B_{12}

7. Compared to cow's milk, human milk contains all of the following EXCEPT

A. a higher protein content
B. a lower casein content
C. monosaturated fatty acids
D. a higher percentage of carbohydrates
E. medium-chain fatty acids

8. All of the following statements about parenteral nutrition are false EXCEPT

A. the nutrition solution is given by subcutaneous infusion
B. a hypertonic dextrose solution is often used
C. lipid concentrations may be high as 30%
D. the final formula is isotonic
E. protein hydrolysates are the preferred source of protein

ANSWERS AND EXPLANATIONS

1. The answer is C. (*I B 2 c*) A nitrogen balance study is used to evaluate a patient's protein use. Approximately 16% of body protein is nitrogen. Therefore, nitrogen intake versus output is often used to determine whether a patient is receiving enough protein to compensate for normal protein catabolism.

2. The answer is A. (*II B 4 b*) Ambulatory patients are usually given enteral nutrition via bolus (intermittent) feedings, because this allows them to conduct their normal daily activities more easily.

3. The answer is C. [*II A 4 b (7)*] Insulin may be added to parenteral nutrition solutions to help the pancreas utilize the high-concentration dextrose present in some of these solutions. Insulin comes in various formulations, and only regular (clear) insulin can be given intravenously. Therefore, only regular insulin from animal or human sources may be added to parenteral nutrition solutions.

4. The answer is B. [*II B 6 a (2)*] The tube feeding syndrome—dehydration, hypernatremia, hyperchloremia, and azotemia—occurs as a result of excessive protein intake and inadequate fluid intake in some patients receiving enteral nutrition therapy.

5. The answer is C. [*IV B 2 a (4)*] Ascorbic acid (vitamin C) is known to interfere chemically with the reliability of Clinitest tablets and Tes-Tape and Clinistix tests.

6. The answer is A. [*IV B 2 b (2)*] Wernicke-Korsakoff syndrome is a severe neurologic disorder characterized by dementia and caused by a lack of thiamine, usually alcohol-related. Therefore, thiamine (vitamin B_1) is often administered orally or parenterally to alcoholic patients to avoid the occurrence of Wernicke-Korsakoff syndrome.

7. The answer is A. (*III B 1*) Human milk has one-third the protein content of cow's milk. Human milk also has a lower casein content; it contains monosaturated fatty acids and medium-chain fatty acids and has a higher percentage of carbohydrates.

8. The answer is B. (*II A 2, 4*) Parenteral nutrition is given intravenously, most often through a large central vein (e.g., the internal jugular). A peripheral vein may be used when parenteral nutrition therapy is expected to be brief. Dextrose concentrations for parenteral nutrition range from 2.5% to 70%; concentrations 10% and above are hypertonic and require central vein administration. Protein hydrolysates were formerly used for parenteral nutrition but have been supplanted by crystalline amino acid solutions. These range in concentration from 3% to 11.4% and provide 100% bioavailability. Lipid concentrations used for parenteral nutrition do not exceed 20%. In addition, the final formula is hypertonic, often necessitating the use of a central line.

22
Sterile Products

Robert L. McCarthy

I. DEFINITIONS

A. **Sterility**, an absolute term, means the absence of living microorganisms.

B. **Sterile products** are pharmaceutical dosage forms that are sterile. Such products include parenteral preparations, irrigating solutions, and ophthalmic preparations. (For information on ophthalmic preparations, see Chapter 27.)

C. **Aseptic technique** refers to the procedures used to maintain the sterility of pharmaceutical dosage forms.

D. **Parenteral preparations** are pharmaceutical dosage forms that are injected through one or more layers of skin. Because the parenteral route bypasses the body's protective barriers, parenteral preparations must be sterile.

E. **Pyrogens** are metabolic by-products of microorganisms or dead microorganisms that cause a pyretic response (i.e., fever) upon injection.

F. The hydrogen ion concentration of a solution, expressed as a logarithm, is referred to as **pH**. It may markedly influence the stability and compatibility of parenteral preparations as discussed in section VI B.

G. **Tonicity** refers to the tone of a solution and is directly related to the osmotic pressure exerted by the solute.

1. **Isotonic solutions** exert the same osmotic pressure as blood or 0.9% sodium chloride solution.

2. **Hypertonic solutions** have a greater osmotic pressure than blood or 0.9% sodium chloride solution. These solutions are administered through a central rather than peripheral vein to avoid the pain caused by red blood cell shrinkage (resulting from water loss).

3. **Hypotonic solutions** have a lower osmotic pressure than blood or 0.9% sodium chloride solution. Because these solutions cause cells to expand, administration may lead to pain and hemolysis.

II. STERILE PRODUCT AREAS: DESIGN AND FUNCTION

A. **Clean rooms.** These areas are specially constructed, filtered, and maintained to prevent environmental contamination of sterile products during the manufacturing process. Clean rooms must meet several requirements:

1. **High-efficiency particulate air (HEPA) filters** are used to cleanse the air entering the room.
   a. HEPA filters remove all airborne particles sized 0.3 μm or larger with an efficiency of 99.97%.
   b. In addition, HEPA-filtered rooms generally are classified as Federal Class 10,000, meaning that they contain no more than 10,000 particles sized 0.5 μm or larger per cubic foot of air.

2. **Positive-pressure air flow** is used to prevent contaminated air from flowing into the clean room. In order to achieve this, the air pressure inside the clean room is greater than the pressure outside the room, so that when a door to the clean room is opened, the air flow is outward.

3. Counters in the clean room are made of stainless steel or other nonporous, easily cleaned material.

4. Walls and floors are free from cracks or crevices and have rounded corners. If walls or floors are painted, epoxy paint is used.

5. As with the HEPA filters used in clean rooms, the air flow moves with a uniform velocity along parallel lines. The velocity of the air flow is 90 (±) 20 feet per minute.

B. Laminar flow hoods. These clean-air work benches are specially designed, like clean rooms, to ensure the aseptic preparation of sterile products. Laminar flow hoods are generally used in conjunction with clean rooms. However, not all pharmacies involved in preparing sterile products have clean rooms; in these instances, laminar flow hoods are vital to ensure aseptic preparation.

1. Requirements

a. Like clean rooms, laminar flow hoods utilize **HEPA filters,** but the hoods use a higher-efficiency air filter than do clean rooms.

b. Hoods are classified as Federal Class 100, meaning that they contain no more than 100 particles sized 0.5 μm or larger per cubic foot of air.

2. Types

a. Horizontal laminar flow hoods were the first hoods used in pharmacies for the preparation of sterile products. Air flow in horizontal hoods moves across the surface of the work area, flowing first through a pre-filter and then through the HEPA filter. The major disadvantage of the horizontal hood is that it offers no protection to the operator. This drawback is especially significant when antineoplastic agents are being prepared.

b. Vertical laminar flow hoods provide two major advantages over horizontal flow hoods.

(1) The air flow is vertical, flowing down on the work space. This air flow pattern protects the operator against potential hazards from the products being prepared.

(2) A portion of the HEPA-filtered air is recirculated a second time through the HEPA filter. The remainder of the filtered air is removed through an exhaust filter. This exhaust may be vented to the outside to protect the operator from chronic, concentrated exposure to hazardous materials.

C. Inspection and certification. Clean rooms and laminar flow hoods are inspected and certified when new, at least every 6 to 12 months thereafter, and, in the case of hoods, when moved to a new location.

1. Inspections are conducted by companies with the sensitive equipment needed for testing procedures and with personnel who are specially trained in these procedures.

2. The **dioctyl phthalate (DOP) smoke test** ensures that no particle larger than 0.3 μm will pass through the HEPA filter. In addition, an **anemometer** is used to determine air flow velocity, and a **particle counter** is used to determine the particle count.

III. STERILIZATION METHODS AND EQUIPMENT.

Sterilization is performed to destroy or remove all microorganisms in or on a product. Sterilization may be achieved through thermal, chemical, radiation, or mechanical methods.

A. Thermal sterilization involves the use of either moist or dry heat.

1. Moist heat sterilization is the most widely used and reliable sterilization method.

a. Microorganisms are destroyed by cellular protein coagulation.

b. The objects to be sterilized are exposed to saturated steam under pressure at a minimum temperature of 121°C for at least 15 minutes.

c. An **autoclave** commonly is used for moist heat sterilization.

d. Because it does not require as high a temperature, moist heat sterilization causes less product damage compared to dry heat sterilization.

2. Dry heat sterilization is appropriate for materials that cannot withstand moist heat sterilization. Objects are subjected to a temperature of at least 160°C for 120 minutes (if higher temperatures can be used, less exposure time is required).

B. Chemical (gas) sterilization is used to sterilize surfaces and porous materials (e.g., surgical dressings) that other sterilization methods may damage.

1. In this method, ethylene oxide is generally used in combination with heat and moisture.

2. Residual gas must be allowed to dissipate after sterilization and before use of the sterile product.

C. **Radiation sterilization** is suitable for the industrial sterilization of contents in sealed packages that cannot be exposed to heat (e.g., prepackaged surgical components and some ophthalmic ointments).

1. This technique involves either electromagnetic or particulate radiation.

2. Accelerated drug decomposition sometimes results.

D. **Mechanical sterilization (filtration)** removes (but does not destroy) microorganisms and clarifies solutions by eliminating particulate matter. For solutions rendered unstable by thermal, chemical, or radiation sterilization, filtration is the preferred method. A depth filter or screen filter may be used.

1. **Depth filters** usually consist of fritted glass or unglazed porcelain—substances that trap particles in channels.

2. **Screen (membrane) filters** are films measuring 1 to 200 μm thick made of cellulose esters, microfilaments, polycarbonate, synthetic polymers, silver, or stainless steel.
   a. A meshwork of millions of microcapillary pores of identical size filter the solution by a process of physical sieving.
   b. Because pores make up 70% to 85% of the surface, screen filters have a higher flow rate than depth filters.
   c. Screen filters come in three basic types.
      (1) **Particulate filters** remove particulates of glass, plastic, rubber, and other contaminants.
         (a) These filters also are used to reduce the risk of phlebitis associated with administration of reconstituted powders; filtration removes any undissolved powder particles that may cause venous inflammation.
         (b) The pore size of standard particulate filters ranges from 0.45 to 5 μm. Consequently, particulate filters cannot be used to filter blood, emulsions (e.g., fat emulsions), or suspensions because these preparations have a larger particle size. (Special filters are available for blood filtration.)
      (2) **Microbial filters**, with a pore size of 0.22 μm or smaller, ensure complete microbial removal or sterilization.
      (3) **Final filters**, which may be either particulate or microbial, are in-line filters used to remove particulates or microorganisms from an intravenous (IV) solution before infusion.

IV. PACKAGING OF PARENTERAL PRODUCTS.

Parenteral preparations and other sterile products must be packaged in a way that maintains product sterility until time of use and prevents contamination of contents during opening.

A. Types of containers

1. **Ampules,** the oldest type of parenteral product containers, are made entirely of glass.
   a. Intended for single use only, ampules are opened by breaking the glass at a score line on the neck.
   b. Because glass particles may become dislodged during ampule opening, the product must be filtered before it is administered.
   c. Their unsuitability for multiple-dose use, the need to filter solutions before use, and other safety considerations have markedly reduced ampule use.

2. **Vials** are glass or plastic containers closed with a rubber stopper and sealed with an aluminum crimp.
   a. Vials have several **advantages** over ampules.
      (1) They can be designed to hold multiple doses (if prepared with a bacteriostatic agent).
      (2) It is easier to remove the product.
      (3) They eliminate the risk of glass particle contamination during opening.
   b. However, vials also have certain **drawbacks.**
      (1) The rubber stopper may become cored.
      (2) Multiple withdrawals (as with multiple-dose vials) may result in microbial contamination.
   c. Some drugs that are unstable in solution are packaged in vials unreconstituted and must be reconstituted with sterile water or sterile sodium chloride for injection before use.
      (1) To accelerate the dissolution rate and permit rapid reconstitution, many powders are lyophilized (freeze-dried).
      (2) Some of these drugs come in vials that contain a double chamber.
         (a) The top chamber, containing sterile water for injection, is separated from the unreconstituted drug by a rubber closure.

(b) To dislodge the inner closure and mix the contents of the compartments, external pressure is applied to the outer rubber closure. This system eliminates the need to enter the vial twice, thereby reducing the risk of microbial contamination.

3. **Prefilled syringes and cartridges** are designed for maximum convenience.
   a. Drugs administered in an emergency (e.g., atropine, epinephrine) are available for immediate injection when packaged in **prefilled syringes** (e.g., Abboject, Bristoject).
   b. **Prefilled cartridges** (e.g., Tubex, Carpuject) are ready-to-use parenteral packages that offer improved sterility and accuracy. They consist of a metal or plastic cartridge holder and a prefilled medication cartridge with a needle attached. The medication is premixed and premeasured.

4. **Infusion solutions** are divided into two categories: **small volume parenterals (SVP)**, those having a volume less than 100 ml; and **large volume parenterals (LVP)**, those having a volume of 100 ml or greater. Infusion solutions are used for the intermittent or continuous infusion of fluids or drugs (see section IX B).

B. **Packaging materials.** Materials used to package parenteral products include glass and plastic polymers.

1. **Glass**, the original parenteral packaging material, has superior clarity, facilitating inspection for particulate matter. Compared to plastic, glass less frequently interacts with the preparation it contains.

2. **Plastic polymers** used for parenteral packaging include polyvinylchloride (PVC) and polyolefin.
   a. PVC is flexible and nonrigid.
   b. Polyolefin is semi-rigid; unlike PVC, it can be stored upright.
   c. Both types of plastic offer several advantages over glass, including unbreakability, easier storage, reduced weight, and improved safety.

V. PARENTERAL ADMINISTRATION ROUTES.

Parenteral preparations may be given by a variety of administration routes.

A. **Subcutaneous administration** refers to injection into the subcutaneous tissue beneath the skin layers—usually of the arm or thigh. Insulin is an example of a subcutaneously administered drug.

B. **Intramuscular administration** means injection into a muscle mass. The mid-deltoid area and gluteus medius are common injection sites.

1. No more than 5 ml of a solution should be injected by this route.

2. Drugs intended for prolonged or delayed absorption (e.g., depo medications such as methylprednisolone) commonly are administered intramuscularly.

C. **IV administration** is the most important and most common parenteral administration route. It allows an immediate therapeutic effect by delivering the drug directly into the circulation. However, this route precludes recall of an inadvertent drug overdose. Antibiotics, cardiac medications, and many other drugs are given intravenously.

D. **Intradermal administration** involves injection into the most superficial skin layer. Because this route can deliver only a limited drug volume, its use generally is restricted to skin tests and certain vaccines.

E. **Intra-arterial administration** is injection directly into an artery. It delivers a high drug concentration to the target site with little dilution by the circulation. Generally, this route is used only for radiopaque materials and some antineoplastic agents.

F. **Intracardiac administration** is injection of a drug directly into the heart.

G. **Hypodermoclysis** refers to injection of large volumes of a solution into subcutaneous tissue to provide a continuous, abundant drug supply. This route occasionally is used for antibiotic administration in children.

H. **Intraspinal administration** refers to injection into the spinal column.

I. **Intra-articular administration** means injection into a joint space.

J. **Intrasynovial administration** refers to injection into the joint fluid.

K. Intrathecal administration is injection into the spinal fluid; it sometimes is used for antibiotics.

VI. PARENTERAL PREPARATIONS

A. IV admixtures. These preparations consist of one or more sterile drug products added to an IV fluid—generally dextrose or sodium chloride solution alone or in combination. IV admixtures are used for drugs intended for continuous infusion and for drugs that may cause irritation or toxicity when given via direct IV injection.

B. IV fluids and electrolytes

1. **Fluids** used in the preparation and administration of parenteral products include sterile water and sodium chloride, dextrose, and Ringer's solutions. These fluids have multiple uses; for example, they serve as vehicles in IV admixtures, provide a means for reconstituting sterile powders, and serve as the basis for correcting body fluid and electrolyte disturbances and for administering parenteral nutrition.
   a. **Dextrose** (D-glucose) solutions are the most frequently used glucose solutions in parenteral preparations.
      (1) Generally, a solution of 5% dextrose in water (D5W) is used as a vehicle in IV admixtures. D5W may also serve as a hydrating solution.
      (2) Because the pH of D5W ranges from 3.5 to 6.5, instability may result if it is combined with an acid-sensitive drug.
      (3) In higher concentrations (e.g., a 10% solution in water), dextrose provides a source of carbohydrates in parenteral nutrition solutions.
      (4) Dextrose solutions should be used cautiously in patients with diabetes mellitus.
   b. **Sodium chloride** usually is given as a 0.9% solution. Because it is isotonic and hence "normal" with blood, this solution is called **normal saline solution** (NSS). (A solution of 0.45% sodium chloride is termed half-normal saline.)
      (1) Sterile sodium chloride for injection—a solution of 0.9% sodium chloride— is used as a vehicle in IV admixtures and for fluid and electrolyte replacement. In smaller volumes, it is suitable for the reconstitution of various medications.
      (2) Bacteriostatic sodium chloride for injection—also a 0.9% solution—is intended solely for multiple reconstitutions. It contains an agent that inhibits bacterial growth (e.g., benzyl alcohol, propylparaben, methylparaben), allowing its use in multiple-dose preparations.
   c. **Waters** are used for reconstitution and for dilution of such IV solutions as dextrose and sodium chloride. Waters suitable for parenteral preparations include sterile water for injection and bacteriostatic water for injection.
   d. **Ringer's solutions**, appropriate for fluid and electrolyte replacement, commonly are administered to postsurgical patients.
      (1) Lactated Ringer's injection (Hartmann's solution, Ringer's lactate solution) contains sodium lactate, sodium chloride, potassium chloride, and calcium chloride. Frequently, it is combined with dextrose (e.g., as dextrose 5%/lactated Ringer's injection).
      (2) Ringer's injection differs from lactated Ringer's injection in that it does not contain sodium lactate and has slightly different concentrations of sodium chloride and calcium chloride. Like lactated Ringer's injection, it may be combined in solution with dextrose.

2. **Electrolyte preparations.** Ions present in both intracellular and extracellular fluid, electrolytes are crucial for various biological processes. Surgical and medical patients who cannot take food by mouth or who need nutritional supplementation require the addition of electrolytes in hydrating solutions or parenteral nutrition solutions.
   a. **Cations** are positively charged electrolytes.
      (1) Sodium is the chief extracellular cation.
         (a) It plays a key role in interstitial osmotic pressure, tissue hydration, acid–base balance, nerve impulse transmission, and muscle contraction.
         (b) Parenteral sodium preparations include sodium chloride, sodium acetate, and sodium phosphate.
      (2) Potassium is the chief intracellular cation.
         (a) It participates in carbohydrate metabolism, protein synthesis, muscle contraction (especially of cardiac muscle), and neuromuscular excitability.
         (b) Parenteral potassium preparations include potassium acetate, potassium chloride, and potassium phosphate.
      (3) Calcium is essential to nerve impulse transmission, muscle contraction, cardiac function, and capillary and cell membrane permeability. Calcium may be given parenterally as calcium chloride, calcium gluconate, or calcium gluceptate.

(4) **Magnesium** plays a vital part in enzyme activities, neuromuscular transmission, and muscle excitability. It is given parenterally as magnesium sulfate.

b. **Anions** are negatively charged electrolytes.

(1) **Chloride** is the major extracellular anion. Along with sodium, it regulates interstitial osmotic pressure. Chloride also helps to control blood pH. Parenteral chloride preparations include calcium chloride, potassium chloride, and sodium chloride.

(2) **Phosphate**, the major intracellular anion, is critical to various enzyme activities. It also influences calcium levels and acts as a buffer to prevent marked changes in acid–base balance. Parenteral phosphate preparations include potassium phosphate and sodium phosphate.

(3) **Acetate** is a bicarbonate precursor that may be used to provide alkali to assist in the preservation of plasma pH. Parenteral acetate preparations include potassium acetate and sodium acetate.

C. **Parenteral antineoplastic agents**. These medications may be toxic to the personnel who prepare and administer them, necessitating special precautions to ensure safety. In addition, patients receiving antineoplastics may experience various problems associated with drug delivery.

1. **Administration methods**. Parenteral antineoplastics may be given by direct IV injection, short-term infusion, or long-term infusion. Some are administered by a nonintravenous route, such as the subcutaneous, intramuscular, intra-arterial, or intrathecal route.

2. **Safe antineoplastic handling guidelines.** All pharmacy and nursing personnel who prepare or administer antineoplastics should receive special training to reduce the risk of injury from exposure to these drugs.

a. A **vertical laminar flow hood** should be used during drug preparation, with exhaust directed to the outside.

b. All syringes and intravenous tubing should have Luer-Lok fittings.

c. Personnel should wear closed-front cuffed surgical gowns and double-layered latex surgeon's gloves.

d. **Negative-pressure technique** should be used during withdrawal of medication from vials.

e. Final dosage adjustment should be made into the vial or ampule, or directly into an absorbent gauze pad.

f. Special care should be taken when intravenous administration sets are primed.

g. Proper procedures should be followed for disposal of materials used in the preparation and administration of antineoplastics.

(1) Needles should not be clipped or recapped.

(2) Preparations should be discarded in containers that are puncture-proof, leak-proof, and properly labeled.

(3) Hazardous waste should be incinerated at a temperature sufficient to destroy organic compounds ($> 1000°C$).

h. After removal of gloves, personnel should wash hands thoroughly.

i. Personnel and equipment involved in the preparation and administration of antineoplastic agents should be monitored routinely.

3. **Patient problems**. Infusion phlebitis and extravasation are the most serious problems that may occur during the administration of parenteral antineoplastics.

a. **Infusion phlebitis** (inflammation of a vein) is characterized by pain, swelling, heat sensation, and redness at the infusion site. Drug dilution and filtration may eliminate or minimize the risk of phlebitis.

b. **Extravasation**—infiltration of a drug into subcutaneous tissues surrounding the vein—is especially harmful when antineoplastics with vesicant properties are administered. Measures must be taken immediately if extravasation occurs. Depending on the drug involved, emergency measures may include stopping the infusion, injecting hydrocortisone or another anti-inflammatory agent directly into the affected area, injecting an antidote (if available), and applying a cold compress (to facilitate a drug–antidote reaction). A warm compress may then be applied to increase the flow of blood, and thus of the vesicant, away from damaged tissue.

VII. IRRIGATING SOLUTIONS.

Although these sterile products are manufactured by the same standards used to process intravenous preparations, they are not intended for infusion into the venous system.

A. **Topical administration**. Irrigating solutions for topical use are packaged in pour bottles so that they can be poured directly onto the involved area. These solutions are intended for such purposes as irrigating wounds, moistening dressings, and cleaning surgical instruments.

B. Infusion of irrigating solutions. This procedure, using an administration set attached to a Foley catheter, is commonly used for many surgical patients. Surgeons performing urologic procedures often use irrigating solutions to perfuse tissues in order to maintain the integrity of the surgical field, remove blood, and provide a clear field of view. To decrease the risk of infection, 1 ml of Neosporin G.U. Irrigant, an antibiotic preparation, is often added to these solutions.

C. Dialysis. Dialysates are irrigating solutions used in the dialysis of patients with such disorders as renal failure, poisoning, and electrolyte disturbances. These products remove waste materials, serum electrolytes, and toxic products from the body.

1. In **peritoneal dialysis**, a hypertonic dialysate is infused directly into the peritoneal cavity via a surgically implanted catheter. Containing dextrose and electrolytes, the dialysate removes harmful substances by osmosis and diffusion. After a specified dwell period, the solution is drained. Antibiotics and heparin may be added to the dialysate.

2. In **hemodialysis**, the patient's blood is transfused through a dialyzing membrane unit that removes the harmful substances from the patient's vascular system. After passing through the dialyzer, the blood reenters the body via a vein.

VIII. NEEDLES AND SYRINGES

A. Hypodermic needles are stainless steel or aluminum devices that penetrate the skin for the purpose of administering or transferring a parenteral product.

1. **Needle gauge** refers to the outside diameter of the needle shaft; the larger the number, the smaller the diameter. Gauges in common use range from 13 (largest diameter) to 27. Subcutaneous injections usually require a 24-gauge or 25-gauge needle; intramuscular injections, a needle gauge between 19 and 22. Needles of 18 gauge to 20 gauge are commonly used for compounding parenterals.

2. **Bevels** are slanting edges cut into needle tips to facilitate injection through tissue or rubber vial closures.
   a. **Regular-bevel needles** are the most commonly used type, suitable for subcutaneous and intramuscular injections and hypodermoclysis.
   b. **Short-bevel needles** are used when only shallow penetration is required (as in IV injections).
   c. **Intradermal-bevel needles** are designed for intradermal injections.

3. **Needle lengths** range from 1/4 to 6 inches. Choice of needle length depends on the desired penetration. For compounding of parenteral preparations, 1 1/2 inch-long needles are commonly used. Intradermal injection necessitates a needle length of 1/4 to 5/8 inch; intracardiac injection, 3 1/2 inches and intravenous infusion, 1 1/4 inches to 2 1/2 inches.

B. Syringes are devices for injecting, withdrawing, or instilling fluids. Originally made of reusable glass, syringes now come primarily in plastic.

1. The **Luer syringe**, the first syringe developed, has a universal needle attachment accommodating all needle sizes.

2. **Syringe volumes** range from 0.3 to 60 ml.

3. Syringes consist of a glass or plastic barrel with a tight-fitting plunger at one end; a small opening at the other end accommodates the head of a needle.
   a. **Calibrations**, which may be in the metric or English system, vary in specificity depending on syringe size; the smaller the syringe, the more specific the scale.
   b. **Insulin syringes** have unit gradations (40 or100 units/ml) rather than volume gradations.

4. **Syringe tips** come in several types.
   a. **Luer-Lok tips** are threaded to ensure that the needle fits tightly in the syringe. Antineoplastic agents should be administered with syringes of this type.
   b. **Luer-Slip tips** are unthreaded. Because they do not lock into place, the needle may become dislodged.
   c. **Eccentric tips,** set off center, allow the needle to remain parallel to the injection site.
   d. **Catheter tips** are used for wound irrigation and administration of enteral feedings. They are not intended for injection.

IX. IV DRUG DELIVERY

A. Injection sites

1. **Peripheral vein injection** is preferred for drugs that do not irritate the veins, for administration

of isotonic solutions, and for patients who require only short-term IV therapy. Generally, the dorsal forearm surface is chosen for venipuncture.

2. **Central vein injection** is preferred for administration of irritating drugs or hypertonic solutions, for patients requiring long-term IV therapy, and when a peripheral line cannot be maintained. Large veins in the thoracic cavity, such as the subclavian, are used.

B. Infusion methods

1. **Continuous drip infusion** is the slow, primary-line infusion of an IV preparation to maintain a therapeutic drug level or provide fluid and electrolyte replacement.
   a. **Flow rates** must be carefully monitored. Generally, these rates are expressed as volume per unit of time (e.g., ml/hr or drops/min).
   b. Such drugs as aminophylline and heparin typically are administered by this method.
2. **Intermittent infusion** allows drug administration at specific intervals (e.g., every 4 hours). Three different techniques may be used.
   a. **Direct (bolus) injection** rapidly delivers small volumes of an undiluted drug. This method is used to:
      (1) Achieve an immediate effect (as in an emergency)
      (2) Administer drugs that cannot be diluted
      (3) Achieve a therapeutic serum drug level quickly
   b. **Additive set infusion**, using a volume-control device, is appropriate for the intermittent delivery of small amounts of IV solutions or diluted medications. The fluid chamber is attached to an independent fluid supply or placed directly under the established primary IV line.
   c. The **piggyback method** is used when a drug cannot be mixed with the primary solution. A special coupling for the primary IV tubing permits infusion of a supplementary solution through the primary system.
      (1) This method eliminates the need for a second venipuncture or further dilution of the supplementary preparation.
      (2) Admixtures in which the vehicle is added to the drug are known as manufacturers' piggybacks.
   d. In some cases, **intermittent infusion injection devices** are used. Also called **scalp-vein, heparin-lock,** or **butterfly infusion sets,** these devices permit intermittent delivery while eliminating the need for multiple venipunctures or prolonged venous access with a continuous infusion.
      (1) To prevent clotting in the cannula, dilute heparin solution or normal saline solution may be added.
      (2) This method is especially suitable for patients who do not require or would be jeopardized by administration of large amounts of IV fluids (e.g., those with congestive heart failure).
      (3) Because intermittent infusion injection devices do not require continuous attachment to an IV bottle or bag and pole, they permit greater patient ambulation.

C. Pumps and controllers

1. These devices are used to administer parenteral infusions when the use of gravity flow alone might lead to inaccurate dosing or risk patient safety. Pumps and controllers are used to administer parenteral nutrition, chemotherapy, cardiac medications, and blood and blood products.
   a. **Pumps** are electronic devices used to deliver IV infusions with accuracy and safety.
      (1) Two types of mechanisms are used in infusion pumps.
         (a) **Piston-cylinder mechanisms** use a piston in a cylinder or a syringe-like apparatus to pump the desired volume of fluid.
         (b) **Peristaltic mechanisms** use external pressure to expel the fluid out of the pumping chamber. Peristaltic pumps may be rotary or linear.
      (2) Pumps, despite their extra costs and the training required by personnel, provide a number of important benefits. They maintain a constant, accurate flow rate; detect infiltrations, occlusions, and air; and may save nursing time.
   b. **Controllers**, unlike pumps, exert no pumping pressure on the IV fluid. Rather, they rely on gravity and control the infusion by counting drops electronically, or they infuse the fluid mechanically and electronically. In comparison to pumps, controllers are less complex, generally are less expensive, contain no moving components, and require less maintenance. They achieve reasonable accuracy and are very useful for uncomplicated infusion therapy.

2. **Types of pumps and controllers**
   a. **Volumetric pumps and controllers** are used for intermittent infusion of medications such as antibiotics and for continuous infusion of IV fluid, parenteral nutrition, anticoagulants, and anti-asthma medications. Examples include IVAC, IMED, and Abbott volumetric devices.
   b. **Syringe pumps** are used to administer intermittent or continuous infusions of medications (e.g., antibiotics and opiates) in concentrated form. Examples of syringe pumps are the Autosyringe and the Harvard Mini Infuser.
   c. **Mobile infusion pumps** are small infusion devices designed for ambulatory and home patients, and are used for administering chemotherapy and opiate medications. Examples include the Cormed and Pancretec pumps.
   d. **Implantable devices** are infusion devices surgically placed under the skin to provide a continuous release of medication, typically an opiate. The reservoir in the pump is refilled by injecting the medication through a latex diaphragm in the pump. An advantage of this type of pump is its alleged lower incidence of infection. The Infusaid pump is an example of this type of device.

D. **IV incompatibilities**. When two or more drugs must be administered through a single IV line or given in a single solution, an undesirable reaction may occur. Although such incompatibilities are relatively rare, their consequences may be significant. A patient who receives a preparation in which an incompatibility has occurred may experience toxicity or an incomplete therapeutic effect.

1. **Types of incompatibilities**
   a. A **physical incompatibility** occurs when a drug combination produces a visible change in the appearance of a solution.
      (1) An example of physical incompatibility is the evolution of carbon dioxide when sodium bicarbonate and hydrochloric acid are admixed.
      (2) Various types of physical incompatibilities may occur:
         (a) **Visible color change or darkening**
         (b) **Precipitate formation**, which may result from the combination of phosphate and calcium
   b. A **chemical incompatibility** reflects the chemical degradation of one or more of the admixed drugs, resulting in toxicity or therapeutic inactivity.
      (1) The degradation is not always visible. Nonvisible chemical incompatibility may be detected only by analytical methods.
      (2) Chemical incompatibility occurs in several varieties.
         (a) **Complexation** is a reaction between products that inactivates them. For example, the combination of calcium and tetracycline leads to formation of a complex that inactivates tetracycline.
         (b) **Oxidation** occurs when one drug loses electrons to the other, resulting in a color change and therapeutic inactivity.
         (c) **Reduction** takes place when one drug gains electrons from the other.
         (d) **Photolysis**—exposure to light—may lead to hydrolysis or oxidation, with resulting discoloration.
   c. A **therapeutic incompatibility** occurs when two or more drugs, IV fluids, or both are combined and the result is a response other than that intended. An example of a therapeutic incompatibility is the reduced bactericidal activity of penicillin G when given after tetracycline. A bacteriostatic agent, tetracycline slows bacterial growth; penicillin, on the other hand, is most effective against rapidly proliferating bacteria. To prevent therapeutic incompatibility in this case, penicillin G should be given before tetracycline.

2. **Factors affecting IV compatibility**
   a. The **pH factor.** Incompatibility is more likely to occur when the components of an IV solution differ significantly in pH. This increased risk is explained by the chemical reaction between an acid and a base, which yields a salt and water; the salt may be an insoluble precipitate.
   b. **Temperature.** Generally, increased storage temperature speeds drug degradation. To preserve drug stability, drugs should be stored in a refrigerator or freezer, as appropriate.
   c. **Degree of dilution.** Generally, the more diluted the drugs are in a solution, the less chance there is for an ion interaction leading to incompatibility.
   d. **Length of time in solution**. The chance for a reaction resulting in incompatibility rises with the length of time that drugs are in contact with each other.
   e. **Order of mixing**. Drugs that are incompatible in combination, such as calcium and phosphate, should not be added consecutively when an IV admixture is being prepared. This keeps these substances from pooling, or forming a layer on the top of the IV fluid, and,

therefore, decreases the chance of an incompatibility. Thorough mixing after each addition is also essential.

3. **Preventing or minimizing incompatibilities.** To reduce the chance for an incompatibility, the following steps should be taken.
   a. Solutions should be administered promptly after they are mixed to minimize the time available for a potential reaction to occur.
   b. Each drug should be mixed thoroughly after it is added to the preparation.
   c. The number of drugs mixed together in an IV solution should be kept to a minimum.
   d. If a prescription calls for unfamiliar drugs or IV fluids, compatibility references should be consulted.

E. **Hazards of parenteral drug therapy.** A wide range of problems can occur with parenteral drug administration.

1. Infusion pump or controller failure may lead to runaway infusion, fluid overload, or incorrect dosages.
2. IV tubing may become kinked, split, or cracked; may produce particulates; may allow contamination; or may interfere with the infusion.
3. Particulate matter may be present in a parenteral product.
4. Glass containers may break, causing injury.
5. Rubber vial closures may interact with the enclosed product.
6. Drug instability may lead to therapeutic ineffectiveness.
7. Incompatibility may result in toxicity or reduced therapeutic effectiveness.
8. Labeling errors may cause administration of an incorrect drug or improper dosage.
9. Phlebitis may result from vein injury or irritation. Generally a minor complication, phlebitis can be minimized or prevented through good IV insertion technique, dilution of irritating drugs, and a decreased infusion rate.
10. Extravasation may occur with administration of drugs with vesicant properties (see section VI C 3 b)
11. Irritation at the injection site can be reduced by varying the injection site and applying a moisturizing lotion to the area.
12. Pain of infusate is most common with peripheral IV administration of a highly concentrated preparation. Switching to central vein infusion and diluting the drug may alleviate the problem.
13. Air embolism, potentially fatal, can result from entry of air into the IV tubing.
14. Drug overdose may be caused by runaway IV infusion, failure of an infusion pump or controller, or nursing or pharmacy errors.
15. Infection, a particular danger with central IV lines, may stem from contamination during IV line insertion or tubing changes. Infection may be local or generalized (septicemia). The infection risk can be minimized by following established protocols for the care of central lines.
16. Allergic reactions may result from hypersensitivity to an IV solution or additive.
17. Central catheter misplacement may lead to air embolism or pneumothorax. To prevent this problem, catheter placement should always be verified radiologically.
18. Preservative toxicity may be a serious complication, especially in children. For example, premature infants receiving parenteral products containing benzyl alcohol may develop a fatal toxic syndrome.
19. Hypothermia, possibly resulting in shock and cardiac arrest, may stem from administration of a cold IV solution. This problem can be prevented by allowing parenteral products to reach room temperature.

X. QUALITY CONTROL AND QUALITY ASSURANCE

A. Definitions

1. **Quality control** is the day-to-day assessment of all operations from the receipt of raw material to the distribution of the finished product, including analytic testing of the finished product.

2. **Quality assurance,** an oversight function, involves the auditing of quality control procedures and systems, with suggestions for changes as needed.

B. **Testing procedures.** Various types of tests are used to ensure that all sterile products are free of microbial contamination, pyrogens, and particulate matter. In addition, ampules are subjected to a leaker test to ensure that the container is completely sealed.

1. **Sterility testing** ensures that the process used to sterilize the product was successful.
   a. The official U.S.P. standard for sterility testing calls for the following:
      (1) A 10% test sample for batches of 20 to 200 units
      (2) A minimum of two test samples for batches of less than 20 units
   b. The **membrane sterilization method** is often used to conduct sterility testing. Test samples are passed through membrane filters; a nutrient medium then is added to promote microbial growth. After an incubation period, microbial growth is determined.

2. **Pyrogen testing** by means of a qualitative fever response test in rabbits and an in vitro limulus test is often difficult to conduct because of lack of facilities. Therefore, people handling sterile products should attempt to avoid problems with pyrogens by purchasing pyrogen-free water and sodium chloride for injection from reputable manufacturers and by using proper handling and storage procedures.

3. **Clarity testing** is used to check sterile products for particulate matter. Before dispensing a parenteral solution, pharmacy personnel should check it for particulates by swirling the solution and then looking at it against both light and dark backgrounds, using a clarity testing lamp or other standard light source.

STUDY QUESTIONS

Directions: Each question below contains five suggested answers. Choose the **one best** response to each question.

1. Parenteral products with an osmotic pressure greater than that of blood or 0.9% sodium chloride are referred to as

A. isotonic solutions
B. hypertonic solutions
C. hypotonic solutions
D. iso-osmotic solutions
E. neutral solutions

2. Sterilization of an ophthalmic solution could be achieved in a community pharmacy by

A. using a 0.45-μm filter
B. using a 0.22-μm filter
C. incorporating the drug in an already sterile vehicle
D. radiation sterilization
E. heat sterilization

3. Which needle has the largest diameter?

A. 25-gauge × 3/4″
B. 24-gauge × 1/2″
C. 22-gauge × 1″
D. 20-gauge × 3/8″
E. 26-gauge × 5/8″

4. Intradermal injection refers to injection into the

A. muscle mass
B. subcutaneous tissue
C. spinal fluid
D. superficial skin layer
E. joint fluid

5. Advantages of the IV route include

A. ease of removal of the dose
B. a depo effect
C. low incidence of phlebitis
D. rapid onset of action
E. a localized effect

6. Which of the following drugs should NOT be prepared in a horizontal laminar flow hood?

A. Aminophylline
B. Dopamine
C. Doxorubicin
D. Nitroglycerin
E. Bretylium tosylate

7. True statements about D5W include all of the following EXCEPT

A. its pH range is 8 to 10
B. it is isotonic
C. it is a 5% solution of D-glucose
D. it should be used with caution in diabetic patients
E. it is often used in IV admixtures

8. As a packaging material for parenteral products, plastic offers all of the following advantages over glass EXCEPT

A. unbreakability
B. improved clarity for visual inspection
C. ease of storage
D. decreased weight
E. safety

9. The central vein may be considered a suitable route for IV administration in which of the following situations?

A. When a nonirritating drug is given
B. When isotonic drugs are given
C. For short-term therapy
D. When venous access is poor
E. For postoperative hydration

10. Procedures for the safe handling of anti-neoplastic agents include all of the following EXCEPT

A. use of Luer-Lok syringe fittings
B. wearing double-layered latex gloves
C. use of positive-pressure technique when medication is being withdrawn from vials
D. wearing closed-front, surgical-type gowns with cuffs
E. not recapping or clipping used needles

11. The formation of an insoluble precipitate as a result of admixing calcium and phosphate is an example of what type of incompatibility?

A. Chemical
B. Physical
C. Pharmacologic
D. Medicinal
E. Therapeutic

12. Parenteral drug products undergo what type of testing to ensure that all microorganisms have been destroyed or removed?

A. Clarity testing
B. Leaker testing
C. Pyrogen testing
D. Sterility testing
E. Solubility testing

ANSWERS AND EXPLANATIONS

1. The answer is B. (*I G*) Hypertonic solutions have an osmotic pressure greater than that of blood (or 0.9% saline), whereas hypotonic solutions have an osmotic pressure less than that of blood, and isotonic or iso-osmotic solutions have an osmotic pressure equal to that of blood.

2. The answer is B. (*III*) The use of a microbial 0.22-μm or smaller filter is necessary to achieve sterilization. The addition of a nonsterile drug to a sterile vehicle will not accomplish this. Radiation sterilization is an industrial technique and is not suitable for use in a community pharmacy. Heat sterilization might degrade the ophthalmic drug, making it unsafe to use.

3. The answer is D. (*VIII A 1*) The gauge size refers to the outer diameter of the needle. The lower the gauge size number, the larger the needle.

4. The answer is D. (*V D*) Intradermal injection refers to parenteral administration into the most superficial layer of skin. This administration route generally is used for certain types of vaccines and skin tests.

5. The answer is D. (*V B, C*) The IV route of drug administration allows for rapid onset of action and, therefore, immediate therapeutic effect. There can be no recall of the administered dose, and phlebitis, or inflammation of a vein, may occur. In addition, a depo effect (i.e., accumulation and storage of the drug for distribution) cannot be achieved by administering a drug intravenously. Delivering a drug by the IV route results in a systemic rather than a localized effect.

6. The answer is C. (*II B 2*) Doxorubicin is an antineoplastic agent and consequently should be prepared only in a vertical laminar flow hood due to the potential hazard of these toxic agents to the operator.

7. The answer is A. (*VI B 1 a*) D5W [dextrose (D-glucose) 5% in water] is acidic, its pH ranges from 3.5 to 6.5, and it is isotonic. It is often used in IV admixtures and should be used with caution in diabetic patients.

8. The answer is B. (*IV B*) As a packaging material for parenteral products, a major disadvantage of plastic is its relative opacity, since visual inspection of the solution for particulate matter or a change in color is an important safety measure.

9. The answer is D. (*IX A*) Nonirritating drugs, isotonic drugs, short-term therapy, and postoperative hydration are best given by peripheral IV administration. Central vein injection is used when access to a peripheral vein is poor, for administration of irritating drugs or hypertonic solutions and for long-term IV therapy.

10. The answer is C. (*VI C 2*) In order to prevent drug aerosolization, a negative-pressure technique (not a positive-pressure technique) should be used when an antineoplastic agent is being withdrawn from a vial. The other precautions mentioned in the question are important safety measures for handling parenteral antineoplastics. All pharmacy and nursing personnel who handle these toxic substances should receive special training.

11. The answer is B. (*IX D 1 a*) Physical incompatibilities occur when two or more products are combined and produce a change in the appearance of the solution, such as the formation of a precipitate.

12. The answer is D. (*X B*) Sterility testing ensures that parenteral products are free from microbial contamination. Pyrogen testing checks products for the presence of pyrogens, clarity testing tests for the presence of particulates, and leaker testing ensures that ampules have been completely sealed during the manufacturing process. Solubility testing may be done to determine the maximum soluble concentration of a drug.

23
Drug Interactions and Adverse Drug Reactions

Anthony V. Rozzi

I. DRUG INTERACTIONS. By maintaining complete patient medication records and supervising drug therapy, pharmacists can play a significant part in preventing or minimizing drug interactions and monitoring the effects of drug therapy for evidence of interactions.

A. Types of drug interactions

1. **Homergic interactions.** These interactions occur when two concurrently administered drugs interact to produce the same quality of effect. **Additive interactions** reflect the cumulative effect of two drugs on the same receptor. Doses of one drug substitute for doses of another in proportion to the relative potency of the drugs. The combined effects are additive linearly.

2. **Heterergic interactions.** These interactions result from concurrent administration of two drugs that cause responses of differing quality. The net response is modified.
   a. **Synergism** occurs when the combined effect of two drugs is greater than the algebraic sum of their individual effects (mathematically expressed as 1 + 1 = 3). For example, exaggerated central nervous system (CNS) effects, analgesia, and respiratory depression may develop when narcotic analgesics are given concurrently with phenothiazines. (Synergism now is considered to be **synonymous with potentiation**; the latter term is rarely used.)
   b. **Antagonism** takes place when the combined effect of two drugs is less than the sum of the drugs acting separately.
      (1) **Chemical antagonism** reflects the interaction of an agonist drug and antagonist drug to form an inactive compound. For example, administration of tetracycline with metal ions (e.g., calcium) results in a poorly absorbed complex (chelate), which prevents tetracycline from reaching optimal blood levels.
      (2) **Competitive antagonism** results when an agonist and antagonist compete for the same receptor sites.
         (a) This type of antagonism usually can be reversed if the agonist is given in a higher concentration.
         (b) An example of competitive antagonism is the interaction between an antihistamine and endogenous histamine, which have an affinity for the same receptor sites.
      (3) **Noncompetitive antagonism** occurs when an antagonist combines with a receptor at a site other than that used by the agonist.
         (a) Because it inactivates the receptor, noncompetitive antagonism is virtually irreversible.
         (b) The interaction between warfarin and vitamin K is an example of noncompetitive antagonism.

B. Mechanisms of drug interactions

1. **Direct interactions.** In some cases, two drugs interact directly—either physically or chemically. The result may be a modified effect of each drug.
   a. Direct drug interactions take place by several mechanisms.
      (1) An **electrostatic interaction** results when certain basic (alkaline) drugs are given concomitantly with certain acidic drugs; the basic compound may inhibit or negate the activity of the acidic agent.
      (2) Certain drugs are **oxidized** when added to some intravenous solutions.
      (3) The combination of tetracycline and a polyvalent cation results in a **chelate**, as described in section I A 2 b (1).
   b. Direct interactions can be avoided by adjusting the drug dosage or schedule.

2. **Alterations in gastrointestinal absorption.** One oral drug can interfere with another's absorption in the gastrointestinal tract by altering any number of variables.

a. **Gastrointestinal motility and gastric emptying rate**
   (1) A drug that increases motility and shortens gastric emptying time may **enhance** the absorption of a subsequent acidic drug (because acidic drugs normally are absorbed from the stomach). In contrast, such a drug may **delay** the absorption of a subsequent basic compound (because basic drugs normally are absorbed from the small intestine).
   (2) A drug that reduces motility and prolongs gastric emptying may reduce the absorption of a subsequent drug (depending on whether the second drug is acidic or basic).

b. **Gastrointestinal flora**. Certain antibiotics may enhance the effects of anticoagulants by altering the gastrointestinal flora and thus interfering with vitamin K synthesis. As a result, anticoagulant efficacy may be altered.

c. **pH of the gastrointestinal tract**. Nonionized drug forms (which are more lipid-soluble) are more readily absorbed than the less lipid-soluble ionized drug forms.
   (1) Acidic drugs (e.g., aspirin) are nonionized in the acidic environment of the stomach; consequently, they are rapidly absorbed. In the alkaline intestinal environment, however, acidic drugs become ionized and thus are absorbed more slowly from the intestine.
   (2) Basic drugs, in contrast, are more readily absorbed from the intestine than from the stomach.
   (3) A drug that alters the pH of the gastrointestinal tract may modify the absorption of a subsequently administered drug.
      (a) For example, antacids raise the pH, possibly inhibiting or delaying the absorption of acidic drugs and enhancing the absorption of basic drugs.
      (b) Changes in gastric pH may cause premature dissolution of certain drugs. For instance, the coating of an enteric-coated tablet may dissolve in the stomach rather than the intestine if taken shortly after an antacid, possibly resulting in gastric irritation and enhanced drug effects.

d. **Complexation**, reflecting chemical antagonism, is discussed in section I A 2 b (1).

e. **Sequestration**. Certain substances can bind with other drugs, preventing their absorption. For instance, cholestyramine resin binds with such drugs as warfarin, thiazides, and cardiac glycosides, inhibiting their absorption.

3. **Alterations of drug distribution**
   a. **Competitive binding.** Two drugs with an affinity for the same plasma protein receptor sites may compete for these sites, resulting in displacement of one drug.
      (1) Displacement increases the free (unbound) level of the displaced drug.
      (2) Competitive binding is most likely to result in an interaction when the displaced drug is at least 90% protein-bound. (See Table 23-1 for examples of highly protein-bound drugs.)
   b. **Reduced plasma protein levels.** A decrease in the serum albumin concentration (i.e., hypoalbuminemia) may reduce overall drug binding and increase free drug levels.
      (1) This increases the risk of drug toxicity.
      (2) Conditions associated with hypoalbuminemia include gastrointestinal, hepatic, and renal disease; cancer; and malnutrition.

4. **Alterations of drug biotransformation.** Drug interactions occurring during biotransformation (metabolism) involve either enzyme induction or enzyme inhibition.
   a. **Enzyme induction.** One drug may enhance the metabolism of another drug—usually by stimulating the production of the hepatic enzymes involved in drug metabolism (e.g., cytochrome P450 microsomal enzymes). An enzyme-including drug may cause faster biotransformation and a decrease in the pharmacologic action of a subsequent drug. Table 23-2 lists some drugs that induce hepatic enzymes.
   b. **Enzyme inhibition.** A drug that inhibits microsomal enzyme production may raise the blood level of a subsequent drug (or its toxic metabolites), causing intensified drug effects and a longer duration of action. For examples of enzyme inhibitors, see Table 23-3.

5. **Alterations of drug excretion**
   a. **Competition for tubular transport between concurrent drugs.** This can block or slow the excretion of the competing drugs. For instance, probenecid competes with penicillin for tubular transport and frequently is given intentionally to prolong penicillin's effects.

Table 23-1. Some Highly Protein-Bound Drugs

Salicylates	Sulfur and sulfonamides
Barbiturates	Clofibrate
Phenylbutazone	Tolbutamide
Phenylpropionic acids	Warfarin

Table 23-2. Some Agents That Induce Microsomal Enzymes

Alcohol	Phenytoin
Chloral hydrate	Chlordiazepoxide
Cortisone	Imipramine
Nicotine	Phenobarbital
Prednisone	Testosterone

b. Changes in urinary pH. Because ionized drugs are more easily excreted than nonionized drugs, a drug that changes the urinary pH may alter the excretion of a subsequent weak-acid or weak-base drug.

(1) A drug that **increases the ionization** of a second drug enhances the second drug's excretion; a drug that **reduces the ionization** of a second drug makes the second drug easier to reabsorb into the bloodstream, thereby prolonging its activity.

(2) For this reason, an acidifying or alkalinizing agent may be given intentionally to prolong the effects of a concurrent drug (e.g., an acidifier administered with methenamine enhances the latter's antibacterial activity). Examples of urinary acidifiers and alkalinizers are shown in Table 23-4.

c. Increased fluid flow. A drug that stimulates the flow of secretory fluids (e.g., perspiration, tears, saliva) may enhance the elimination of drugs that are eliminated via these routes. The interaction, however, is extremely inconsequential.

6. Fluid and electrolyte imbalances. Drugs that affect the pH of body fluids and the concentration of electrolytes can significantly alter the action of concurrent drugs. Potassium-losing diuretics, for instance, may cause hypokalemia, making the heart more sensitive to the effects of digitalis. Consequently, a patient receiving diuretics along with digitalis may experience drug toxicity and cardiac arrhythmias (from hypokalemia). Examples of drugs that may produce fluid and electrolyte disorders include diuretics, ipecac, oncologic agents, and mineral supplements.

C. Drug–food interactions

1. Drug absorption may be modified by the presence of food in the stomach.

a. Foods that alter gastric pH can change the rate and extent of drug absorption by altering the drug's dissolution and ionization.

(1) Drugs with relatively poor dissolution fractions have enhanced absorption when taken with food because food prolongs the gastric emptying time.

(2) The absorption of drugs with relatively good dissolution fractions is inhibited by food.

b. Gastric secretions stimulated by food may enhance or inhibit absorption of certain drugs. Lipid-soluble drugs, for instance, may be better absorbed when given with meals because bile (stimulated by food) helps dissolve these drugs.

Table 23-3. Some Agents That Inhibit Microsomal Enzymes

Allopurinol	Anabolic agents
Oral antidiabetics	Chloramphenicol
Disulfiram	Isoniazid
Metronidazole	Monoamine oxidase inhibitors
Oral anticoagulants	Cimetidine

Table 23-4. Some Urinary Alkalinizers and Acidifiers

Urinary alkalinizers	**Urinary acidifiers**
Acetazolamide	*p*-Aminosalicylate
Diuretics	Ascorbic acid
Potassium citrate	Fatty acids
Sodium acetate	Phenylbutazone
Sodium bicarbonate	Ammonium chloride
Sodium citrate	Calcium chloride
	Sodium acid phosphate
	Fruit juices

c. **Food's buffering effect** can help reduce adverse drug effects (e.g., nausea, abdominal distress, mucosal damage from salicylates).

2. **Effects of food on gastrointestinal motility and drug bioavailability**
   a. **Acidic foods** (e.g., orange juice) reduce gastrointestinal motility and may enhance the degradation of acid-sensitive drugs, such as certain penicillins and erythromycins.
   b. **Alkaline foods** (e.g., effervescent products, milk and dairy products) may inhibit the absorption of weak-acid drugs due to drug ionization and cause the untimely release of long-acting agents. Also milk and diary products chelate with tetracycline, significantly reducing drug absorption.
   c. **Viscous, unchewed foods** decrease gastrointestinal motility and may slow drug absorption.
   d. **Fatty foods** reduce gastrointestinal motility and slow the absorption of drugs with low lipid solubility; however, they enhance the absorption of highly lipid-soluble drugs (e.g., griseofulvin). Also, bile acids, stimulated by ingestion of fatty foods, may cause complexation with certain drugs.
   e. **High-volume, low-viscosity foods** increase gastrointestinal motility, speeding drug absorption.

3. **Effects of drugs on appetite**
   a. Serotonin antagonists and psychotropic agents **stimulate** the appetite.
   b. Antineoplastics and cardiac glycosides **inhibit** the appetite.

4. **Effects of drugs on gastrointestinal motility**
   a. Mineral oil, although a lubricant laxative, **inhibits** gastrointestinal motility.
   b. Stimulant laxatives (e.g., bisacodyl, danthron, senna) **stimulate** gastrointestinal motility.

5. **Effects of drugs on nutritional status**
   a. Neomycin and anticholesteremics (e.g., clofibrate) inhibit the absorption of vitamins, electrolytes, iron, carotenes, and sugar.
   b. Stool softeners (surfactants) interfere with the permeability and absorption of nutrients into cells.
   c. Neomycin, erythromycin, sulfonamides, tetracyclines, penicillins, isoniazid, and chloramphenicol reduce folic acid utilization, decrease vitamin K synthesis, and impair absorption of vitamin B_{12}, calcium, and magnesium.
   d. Methotrexate, fluorouracil, phenytoin, and phenobarbital inhibit the absorption of folic acid, vitamin B_{12}, fats, and electrolytes.
   e. Alcohol increases the excretion of magnesium and blocks the tubular reabsorption of vitamin B_{12} and folic acid.
   f. All diuretics except those that spare potassium increase electrolyte excretion and interfere with carbohydrate metabolism.
   g. Isoniazid and hydralazine impede absorption and utilization of vitamin B_6.
   h. Mineral oil reduces the absorption of fat-soluble vitamins.

II. ADVERSE DRUG REACTIONS.

As defined by the Food and Drug Administration, an adverse drug reaction is "any response to a drug which is noxious and unintended and which occurs at doses used in man for prophylaxis, diagnosis or therapy." (This definition excludes untoward effects resulting from medication errors, inadequate doses, bioavailability problems, drug abuse, noncompliance, and poisoning.)

A. General considerations

1. Adverse reactions are extremely individualized and unpredictable because of physiologic variations among patients.

2. Not all adverse reactions result from a drug's active ingredient. Some stem from impurities, preservatives, vehicles, degradation products, additives, or metabolites.

3. The incidence of adverse reactions is approximately 6% to 15% of all drug administrations in clinical settings.

4. **No universal classification system** for adverse reactions exists. The various systems that have been used include the following:
   a. **Probability.** Older systems classify adverse reactions as **definite**, **probable**, **possible**, or **remote**.
   b. **Body system**. Adverse reactions may be identified by the body system they affect (e.g., hepatic, renal, and cardiac reactions).
   c. **Underlying mechanism**. Adverse reactions may be classified as **immunologic** or **nonimmunologic** (idiosyncratic).

B. Immunologic adverse reactions

1. These reactions are **characterized by an antigen–antibody reaction**.
   a. Upon first exposure to the agent, no apparent reaction occurs. However, signs and symptoms appear subsequently—usually within a few days after drug therapy begins.
   b. Effects of an immunologic reaction do not resemble the drug's pharmacologic effects and usually also occur at doses below the therapeutic range.
   c. Involving only a small patient population, immunologic reactions cause a limited number of allergy-related syndromes.
   d. **The Boston Collaborative Drug Surveillance Program**, conducted in the mid-1970s, found that the agents most often responsible for adverse drug reactions include penicillins, sulfa antibiotics, corticotropin, erythromycin, and blood products.

2. **Types of hypersensitivity reactions**. These adverse reactions fall into four categories based on the underlying immunologic mechanism.
   a. **Type I: Immediate hypersensitivity reactions, or anaphylaxis**
      (1) This type of reaction has several stages.
         (a) **Initial sensitization** (antibody formation) occurs on first exposure to a specific drug. No signs and symptoms appear at this time, however.
         (b) During the **inductive phase** that follows, immunoglobulin E (IgE) antibodies are produced; these antibodies circulate and affix to the surface of mast cells throughout the body.
         (c) The antigenic drug becomes bound to IgE antibodies on mast cells on subsequent exposure.
         (d) This triggers **degranulation of mast cells**, which then release large amounts of mediators, such as histamine and slow-reacting substance of anaphylaxis (SRS-A).
         (e) **Histamine release** causes peripheral vasodilation and increased vascular permeability, leading to local vascular congestion and edema. Bronchiolar smooth muscle constriction also typically occurs. Signs and symptoms appear immediately after parenteral administration or up to 6 hours after oral administration.
      (2) Drugs that may cause type I hypersensitivity reactions include penicillins, iron dextrans, and certain biologic products [e.g., antisera, red blood cells (RBCs)].
   b. **Type II: Cytotoxic hypersensitivity reactions**
      (1) These reactions occur when IgM or IgG antibodies react with antigen on the cell surface, resulting in cell destruction from phagocytosis or cell lysis.
      (2) Usually, activation of the complement system is involved, leading to the destruction of RBCs or specific target cells.
      (3) Three groups of type II hypersensitivity reactions have been identified.
         (a) **Hapten-induced hemolysis** occurs when drug molecules that are too small to act as antigens bind to cellular proteins to produce larger complexes. The immune system then recognizes and destroys the complexes.
         (b) **"Innocent bystander" reactions** take place when a drug induces antibodies and subsequent formation of antigen–antibody complexes that circulate and coat RBCs. The complexes and the RBCs are then destroyed by the immune system via complement activation. Examples of drugs that can induce this reaction include isoniazid, chlorpromazine, rifampin, and insulin. The RBC here is an innocent bystander.
         (c) **Autoimmune hemolysis** develops when an antibody to a drug has cross-sensitivity to endogenous proteins, such as RBCs. Methyldopa, for example, can induce this reaction.
   c. **Type III: Immune complex reactions**
      (1) In these reactions, antigen–antibody complexes circulate and lodge in smaller blood vessels (typically including those of the kidneys) or other target tissues.
      (2) These intravascular complexes activate the complement system, leading to an inflammatory reaction that results in tissue destruction.
      (3) **Serum sickness** is an example of an immune complex disease in which complex deposition in the vascular system produces vasculitis. Characteristic lesions develop in the glomerular walls, leading to destruction of glomerular tissue. Hematuria and proteinuria may occur from increased permeability of the glomerular basement membrane.
         (a) Penicillin is the leading cause of serum sickness.
         (b) Other causative agents include cephalosporins, sulfonamides, and streptomycin.
      (4) In **Arthus' reaction**, another type III hypersensitivity disorder, cellular inflammation and necrosis occur at the site of antigen injection in a previously sensitized person. Antibody precipitation and complement activation lead to an acute localized vasculitis.
      (5) **Systemic lupus erythematosus-like** drug reactions probably reflect type III hypersensitivity.

d. Type IV: Cellular (delayed) hypersensitivity reactions. In these T-cell dependent reactions, interaction between antigens and cytotoxic T lymphocytes causes release of lymphokines, which then attract monocytes, neutrophils, and basophils. An inflammatory response destroys the foreign matter.

(1) Type IV hypersensitivity reactions commonly develop on the skin (as in contact dermatitis).

(2) Other examples of this type of hypersensitivity include the reaction to the tuberculin skin test, transplant or graft rejection, and reactions to such substances as ethylenediamine (found in aminophylline), parabens, neomycin, and para-aminobenzoic acid (PABA).

C. Drug toxicity

1. Renal toxicity. The kidney is especially sensitive to the effects of drugs—perhaps to a greater degree than any other organ. Drugs may cause serious and, in some cases, irreversible kidney damage.

a. The structure and function of the kidney account for its vulnerability.

(1) The kidney is among the most highly perfused organs, receiving roughly 25% of the cardiac output. Consequently, it is exposed to high concentrations of toxins.

(2) Drugs and their carrier proteins uncouple at the tubule (a drug that is innocuous when bound may be toxic when free).

(3) Changes in urinary pH affect the solubility of many of the compounds that reach the kidneys for excretion; in some cases, precipitation occurs.

(4) The kidney's large endothelial surface makes it especially vulnerable to deposition of antibody–antigen complexes, which may trigger a type III hypersensitivity reaction.

b. Nephrotoxic mechanisms

(1) Drugs that can result in **direct glomerular or tubular damage** include aminoglycosides, cephalosporins, and polymyxins (in doses greater than 3 mg/kg).

(2) **Defects in tubular function** may result from the following drugs.

(a) Lithium, methoxyflurane, and sulfonylureas can cause nephrogenic diabetes insipidus by inhibiting the action of antidiuretic hormone (ADH) at the renal tubule.

(b) Outdated and degraded tetracycline can lead to Fanconi syndrome, which is characterized by tubular dysfunction.

(3) **Acute interstitial nephritis** may result from a type III hypersensitivity reaction caused by methicillin, nafcillin, ampicillin, rifampin, phenytoin, and thiazides.

(4) **Chronic interstitial nephritis** is characterized by changes in the biochemical defense system that protects renal cells from oxidative damage. Abuse of over-the-counter (OTC) analgesics (e.g., aspirin, acetominophen) can lead to analgesic nephropathy—a form of chronic interstitial nephritis. This disorder may occur with administration of large doses of analgesics over a prolonged period (e.g., 2 g to 4 g daily for more than 5 years).

(5) **Obstructive nephropathy** can develop by several mechanisms.

(a) Sulfonamides and certain other drugs may precipitate in the kidney, leading to formation of crystals, stones, or both.

(b) Drugs that cause increased uric acid excretion can result in uric acid crystallization in various renal areas. Causative agents include allopurinol, probenecid, methotrexate, and sulfinpyrazone.

(c) Such drugs as methysergide may cause ureter constriction and subsequent renal ischemia.

2. Hepatotoxicity. Drugs can damage the liver either by an intrinsic property or through an idiopathic mechanism.

a. Intrinsic hepatotoxicity occurs with compounds whose chemical structure promotes liver injury.

(1) **Direct intrinsic hepatotoxicity** results when a substance directly destroys hepatocytes. Carbon tetrachloride, arsenic, and acetaminophen (in excessive doses) are examples of direct hepatotoxins.

(2) **Indirect intrinsic hepatotoxicity** occurs when a drug interferes with the metabolic or secretory processes of hepatocytes. Oral contraceptives and anabolic steroids can impede hepatocyte metabolism; tetracycline and ethanol can disrupt hepatocyte secretion.

b. Idiopathic hepatotoxic reactions are unpredictable and vary from patient to patient. They may involve host hypersensitivity or interference with liver enzyme activity.

(1) **Autoimmune reactions**, similar to type III hypersensitivity, present as hepatocellular hepatitis. Phenothiazines, methyldopa, and hydantoins are examples of causative agents.

(2) A drug that interferes with liver enzyme activity may cause rapid accumulation of toxic

metabolites and subsequent cellular damage when the reaction has a rapid onset. With slow onset, active drug accumulates; if the drug is potentially toxic, cellular damage will occur (as with halothane).

3. Hematologic toxicity

a. General considerations. Hematotoxicity reflects drug interference with hematopoiesis, resulting in abnormalities in blood cell components or their numbers. (See Figure 23–1 for a representation of normal hematopoiesis.)

(1) Some drugs affect the bone marrow, thereby disrupting all formed elements of the blood. Other drugs may interfere with only a particular type of blood component.

(2) Most hematotoxic effects disappear with drug withdrawal.

b. Anemia is characterized by RBC abnormalities.

(1) Aplastic anemia develops when a drug suppresses or destroys bone marrow stem cells, causing deficiencies of all formed elements of the blood. Benzene derivatives, insecticides, and chloramphenicol are some of the compounds that can cause asplastic anemia.

(2) Megaloblastic anemia stems from impaired synthesis of deoxyribonucleic acid (DNA) by RBCs, resulting in slow cell division and production of large, immature, dysfunctional RBCs.

(3) Hemolytic anemia, characterized by premature RBC destruction, may be induced by two different drug-related mechanisms.

(a) Certain **oxidant drugs** (e.g., antimalarials, sulfonamides, nitrofurantoin) interfere with RBCs in patients with glucose-6-phosphate dehydrogenase (G6PD) deficiency.

(b) A drug-induced **immune hemolytic anemia** results from certain antigen–antibody reactions. For example, with penicillin administration, IgG antibodies may react with the RBC–penicillin complex, resulting in hemolysis.

c. Leukopenia results when a drug or disorder reduces the white blood cell (WBC) level.

(1) Agranulocytosis is a severe reduction in the number of granulocytes (basophils, eosinophils, and neutrophils).

(a) This disorder may stem from a type II hypersensitivity mechanism (as with sulfonamides, sulfonylureas, and phenylbutazone).

(b) Bone marrow suppression at the myeloblast level also may cause agranulocytosis. Such drugs as antineoplastics, zidovudine, and phenylbutazone may induce this form of agranulocytosis.

(2) Neutropenia is characterized by a decreased neutrophil level. Such causative agents include the oncologic drugs.

(3) Signs and symptoms of leukopenia include fever, sore throat, chills, rash, and secondary infections.

d. Thrombocytopenia, an abnormal reduction in the platelet level, may occur if a drug or disorder increases platelet destruction or decreases platelet production. (See Table 23-5 for a list of drugs that can induce thrombocytopenia.)

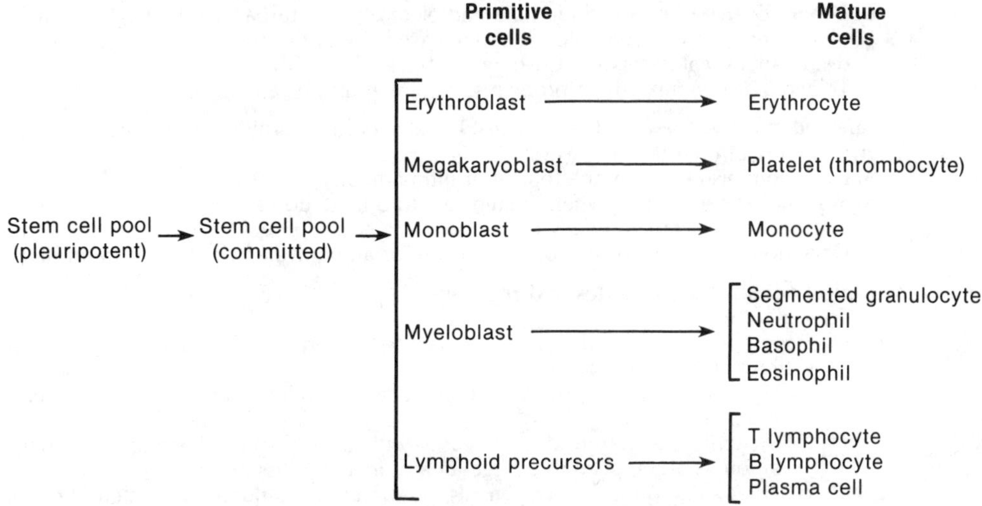

Figure 23-1. Simplified diagram of hematopoiesis.

Table 23-5. Drugs That Suppress Platelet Function

Aminosalicylic acid	Indomethacin
Amitriptyline	Naproxen
Chlorpromazine	Nitrofurantoin
Diphenhydramine	Nortriptyline
Dipyridamole	Papaverine
Fenoprofen	Promethazine
Ibuprofen	Tolmetin
Imipramine	

D. Corticosteroid therapy and toxicity

1. Highly potent hormones, corticosteroids have multiple physiologic functions and pharmacologic effects.
   a. **Cell stabilization**. Corticosteroids polymerize hyaluronic acid, which stabilizes cell and lysosomal membranes; prevent intracellular swelling and the release of proteolytic enzymes; and reduce capillary membrane permeability.
   b. **Anti-collagen activity**. Corticosteroids minimize the formation and deposition of collagen and fibrous tissue.
   c. **Vasoconstriction**. When applied topically, corticosteroids promote vasoconstriction of the cutaneous microcirculation.
   d. **Mitosis inhibition**. Corticosteroids inhibit epidermal cell mitosis.
   e. **Vitamin D antagonism**. Corticosteroids antagonize the effects of vitamin D on calcium absorption from the intestine, thereby helping to regulate serum calcium.
   f. **Lymphocytolysis**. Corticosteroids reduce lymphatic tissue mass and cause redistribution of circulating lymphocytes.
   g. **Anti-inflammatory effects**. Corticosteroids suppress the inflammatory response caused by antigen–antibody reactions; inhibit macrophage accumulation at sites of potential inflammatory immune reactions; and promote monocytopenia, lymphocytopenia, and eosinopenia.
   h. **Thrombocyte protection**. Corticosteroids guard thrombocytes from autolysis and phagocytosis.
   i. **Positive inotropic effect**. By increasing myocardial contractile force, corticosteroids can enhance cardiac output.

2. **Adverse effects of corticosteroids**. Because they profoundly alter the body's metabolism and immune responses, corticosteroids can cause a wide range of adverse effects.
   a. **Prolonged, high-dose corticosteroid therapy causes suppression of the hypothalamic-pituitary-adrenal (HPA) axis** through a negative feedback mechanism. Drug withdrawal must be tapered gradually to permit the HPA axis to recover; abrupt withdrawal may lead to adrenal insufficiency—a life-threatening emergency—as well as acute exacerbation of the original disorder.
   b. **Other adverse effects** include fluid and electrolyte disturbances, hyperglycemia, glycosuria, osteoporosis, peptic ulcers, an increased risk of infection, myopathy, psychological disturbances, cataracts, and Cushing's habitus.
   c. To avoid or minimize these problems, therapy must be carefully planned and monitored.

3. **Safe and effective therapeutic regimens**. Usually, corticosteroids are safe and effective when given in any of the following ways:
   a. Local administration (by the topical or intra-articular route)
   b. Systemic administration when limited to 1 to 3 large doses
   c. Alternate-day or tapered daily regimens
   d. Daily doses of 40 mg or less of prednisone (or an equivalent) for a maximum of 10 days

4. **Typical administration routes and regimens**
   a. **Topical administration**
      (1) Depending on the underlying skin disorder, a corticosteroid may be applied with or without an occlusive dressing.
         (a) When an occlusive dressing is used, local anti-inflammatory effects may increase as much as 100-fold.
         (b) Systemic absorption also increases with an occlusive dressing and when large amounts are applied to a large area of inflamed tissue.
      (2) When applied to the face or genitals, position 9 alpha-fluorocorticosteroid derivatives may cause rebound pustulation and/or rosacea on withdrawal. For use on these areas, hydrocortisone products are recommended instead.

b. **Inhalation therapy.** For maintenance therapy of asthma, beclomethasone is given in the form of oral inhalation powder, in a dosage of 50 μg/puff.
   (1) This drug acts locally. No HPA suppression or significant adverse systemic effects occur.
   (2) Oral *Candida* and *Aspergillus* infections are common side effects of inhalation corticosteroid therapy.
   (3) Alternate-day oral therapy (15 mg or less of prednisone or an equivalent) may be replaced with beclomethasone inhalation therapy.

c. **Tapered oral therapy.** Usually lasting 5 to 12 days, oral therapy is used in the treatment of acute, self-limiting inflammatory conditions. To assure natural HPA function, the dosage must be decreased by 10% daily; most decreasing doses may exceed the equivalent of 7.5 mg prednisone.

d. **Alternate-day regimen**
   (1) Used as maintenance therapy for chronic inflammatory conditions, this regimen minimizes HPA suppression and reduces the untoward metabolic effects associated with long-term corticosteroid therapy. Alternate-day doses allow partial recovery of the HPA system between doses.
      (a) Alternate-day therapy is not suitable for initial therapy, treatment of an acute condition, or administration of long-acting corticosteroids.
      (b) A single dose of prednisone (40 mg or less) is given every other morning.
      (c) Corticosteroids have a half-life of 24 to 36 hours and a duration of action of approximately 2 days. Consequently, because HPA suppression may persist for up to 36 hours, some HPA function occurs on the days when no doses are received.
   (2) **Dosages**. Methylprednisone and triamcinolone are each administered in a dosage of 8 to 32 mg every other day; prednisolone and prednisone, each in a dosage of 20 to 80 mg every other day.

e. **Daily regimen**
   (1) The total daily dosage is taken in the morning, when natural adrenal hormone secretions peak.
   (2) If the dose must be divided, two-thirds of the total daily dose is given in the morning; the other third is divided among the remaining scheduled doses.

f. **Basic dosing protocol**
   (1) The corticosteroid is given in three or four divided doses for 7 to 10 days.
   (2) The total daily dose is given every morning for 7 to 10 days.
   (3) At least twice the total daily dose is given every other morning for an indefinite period. (The patient may receive up to four times the daily dose every other day before HPA suppression equals that occurring with daily therapy.)
   (4) Doses are given more frequently during symptom exacerbation. For example, three or four daily doses are given for several days or a tapered regimen lasting 5 to 10 days is used.

5. **Withdrawal of prolonged, systemic corticosteroid therapy**. When HPA suppression is proven or assumed, the drug must be tapered gradually to avoid adrenal insufficiency and acute exacerbation of the preexisting condition.

a. **HPA suppression**
   (1) Suppression is **assumed** after continuous therapy or an increasing daily dosage equivalent to 7.5 mg or more of prednisone for 7 or more consecutive days.
   (2) Suppression is a direct result of corticosteroid therapy, depending on posology, duration of therapy, time of day of administration, biologic half-life, and preexisting HPA condition.
   (3) **Recovery time after full HPA suppression**. Restoration of basal secretion (20 to 30) mg/day of hydrocortisone) may take up to 9 months; restoration of stress-induced surge secretion (200 to 300 mg/day of hydrocortisone) may take up to 1 year.

b. **Signs and symptoms of adrenal insufficiency**. Abrupt corticosteroid withdrawal or acute stress during corticosteroid therapy may lead to adrenal insufficiency, manifested by fatigue, arthralgia, dizziness, lethargy, depression, syncope, orthostatic hypotension, dyspnea, anorexia, and evidence of hypoglycemia.
   (1) **Acute adrenal insufficiency** in a patient receiving corticosteroids may result from major surgery or serious illness or infection as well as from abrupt drug withdrawal. To treat the insufficiency, 200 to 400 mg of Solu-Cortef are given intravenously in 1000 ml of normal saline solution, or 100 to 400 mg of Solu-Cortef may be given by intravenous push or bolus with supplemental sodium chloride for the acute situation.
   (2) **Subacute adrenal insufficiency** in a patient receiving corticosteroids may stem from minor surgical procedures (e.g., dental work, endoscopy) and disorders such as otitis media, *Streptococcus* pharyngitis, colds, and influenza. To treat this problem, 50 mg of

hydrocortisone or 10 to 15 mg of prednisone are given in twice-daily oral doses for 3 to 5 days.

(3) A patient receiving corticosteroids should wear a medical identification bracelet and carry a prefilled syringe containing 4 mg of Decadron injection in case of an emergency.

c. Dosage reduction schedule

(1) With hydrocortisone, the daily dosage is reduced by 10% every 1 to 2 weeks until symptoms are controlled by 20 mg/day. (Generally, with prednisone, the daily dosage may be decreased by 1.0 to 2.5 mg every 2 weeks.)

(2) Then, the daily dosage is reduced by 2.5 mg every week until the patient is receiving 10 mg daily.

(3) Levels of plasma hydrocortisone and urinary 17-hydroxysteroids are measured on the mornings when no doses are taken to assess HPA function.

(4) During stressful situations or symptom exacerbation, the daily corticosteroid dosage should be increased until symptoms disappear once more.

STUDY QUESTIONS

Directions: Each question below contains three suggested answers of which **one or more** is correct. Choose the answer

- **A** if **I only** is correct
- **B** if **III only** is correct
- **C** if **I and II** are correct
- **D** if **II and III** are correct
- **E** if **I, II, and III** are correct

1. According to the Food and Drug Administration, adverse drug reactions are defined as untoward effects resulting from

   I. therapeutic dosages
   II. bioavailability problems
   III. medication errors

2. Type II (cytotoxic) hypersensitivity reactions can be identified as

   I. hapten-induced
   II. "innocent bystander" reactions
   III. Arthus' reaction

ANSWERS AND EXPLANATIONS

1. The answer is A (I). (*II A*) Adverse drug reactions, as defined by the Food and Drug Administration, are limited to those occurring at normal therapeutic, prophylactic, or diagnostic dosages, and they are considered to be unpredictable and unpreventable. These adverse reactions can be classified generally as immunologic or idiosyncratic.

Many effects do not fit in this definition. The majority are due to drug overuse and misuse, errors in medication prescribing and administration, and lack of patient compliance. Differences in bioavailability between brands of drugs also can cause a variety of effects and contribute to toxicity or lack of therapeutic effect.

2. The answer is C (I, II). [*II B 2 b (3), c (4)*] Hypersensitivity reactions are categorized into four types: type I, immediate hypersensitivity reactions; type II, cytotoxic hypersensitivity reactions; type III, immune complex reactions; type IV, cellular (delayed hypersensitivity) reactions. These types do not necessarily occur independently.

Hapten-induced hypersensitivity can be classified as type II. Haptens are partial antigens and can cause an immune response only when combined with tissue- or serum-derived carrier proteins to produce larger complexes, which the immune system recognizes as foreign and then attacks.

''Innocent bystander'' reactions also are classified as type II. Drugs can induce allergic and autoallergic responses against red blood cells (RBCs). The drug induces antibodies and the formation of antigen–antibody complexes, which coat the RBCs (the ''innocent bystander'').

Arthus' reaction is a type IV hypersensitivity reaction, which occurs with inflammation and necrosis at the site of antigen injection in and around walls of small blood vessels, usually in the skin.

24
OTC Products: Enteral Drugs

Robert L. McCarthy
Anthony V. Rozzi

I. ORAL HYGIENE PRODUCTS

A. Preparations for common oral sores

1. Definitions

a. Cold sores (sometimes called **fever blisters**) are small vesicles on an erythematous base, caused by the **herpes simplex virus.**

(1) In many cases, the lesions recur periodically—usually at the same site. Factors that may precipitate recurrences include colds, influenza, exposure to sunlight, and stress.

(2) Although highly contagious, cold sores are self-limiting. (However, secondary bacterial infection is possible.)

b. Canker sores (aphthous stomatitis) are recurrent, painful, ulcerous lesions. Although their cause remains unknown, hypersensitivity to *Streptococcus* organisms is suspected. Some researchers also suspect a hereditary predisposition and believe that the lesions may be exacerbated by stress.

2. Treatment goals. With both cold sores and canker sores, the goal of treatment is to promote lesion healing and alleviate discomfort.

3. Products for cold sores

a. Emollients (e.g., Orabase) are effective moisturizers.

b. Topical local anesthetics can be used for analgesia.

c. Topical antibiotic ointments or creams can be applied if signs of secondary bacterial infection appear.

d. Other OTC products used to treat cold sores include Orajel, Anbesol, Tanac, and Blistex. To prevent sunlight-induced cold sores, a sunscreen containing para-aminobenzoic acid (PABA) can be applied before exposure to the sun.

4. Products for canker sores

a. Emollients, local anesthetics, and oral analgesics are the mainstays of therapy.

b. OTC products used for canker sores include Orajel, Kank-A, Tanac, and Orabase with Benzocaine.

B. Halitosis preparations

1. General considerations

a. Definition. Halitosis (fetor oris) is an offensive odor of the oral cavity.

b. Causes. Halitosis may stem from such factors as poor oral hygiene (as from food particles embedded in the teeth or plaque-coated tongue) and disease (e.g., tuberculosis, purulent lung infection, bronchiectasis, sinusitis, tonsillitis, rhinitis, and severe hyperglycemia). Drugs associated with halitosis include rifampin, dimethyl sulfoxide 50% (DMSO), and alcohol.

2. General therapeutic principles

a. When halitosis stems from poor oral hygiene, thorough toothbrushing, flossing, and the use of mouthwash are helpful.

b. Halitosis secondary to an underlying disease necessitates treatment of the disease.

3. Products. Mouthwashes may contain antiseptics (e.g., phenol, cetylpyridinium chloride); anesthetics (e.g., eugenol, clove oil); and astringents (e.g., zinc chloride).

II. ANTACID PRODUCTS

A. General considerations

1. **Uses.** Physicians may recommend or prescribe antacids for the symptomatic relief of peptic ulcer, gastritis, gastric hyperacidity, and hiatal hernia. However, many people take antacids inappropriately for a wide range of symptoms.

2. **Definitions**
   a. **Peptic ulcer** is an ulcerative lesion of the upper gastrointestinal mucous membrane, resulting from exposure to gastric acid and pepsin.
   b. **Gastritis** is an inflammation of the gastric mucosa caused by underlying disease (e.g., peptic ulcer), chronic aspirin or alcohol ingestion, or toxins.
   c. **Gastric hyperacidity** is excessive secretion of gastric juice, which may lead to mucosal irritation and peptic ulcer.
   d. **Hiatal hernia** is the protrusion of a portion of the stomach through the esophageal hiatus into the chest.

B. Treatment goal.

Antacid therapy is directed at decreasing the concentration and total load of gastric acid.

C. Products (Table 24-1)

1. **Absorbable (systemic) antacids**
   a. **Definition.** Absorbable antacids are soluble, readily absorbed, and capable of changing the pH of extracellular fluid.
   b. **Examples of absorbable antacids**
      (1) **Sodium bicarbonate.** Widely used as an antacid, this compound immediately neutralizes hydrochloric acid (HCl) in the stomach.
      (2) **Calcium carbonate.** A very potent and fast-acting antacid, calcium carbonate is highly soluble and available for systemic absorption.
   c. **Problems associated with absorbable antacids**
      (1) Systemic alkalosis may occur.
      (2) **Milk alkali syndrome** may develop if absorbable antacids are taken with milk. In this

Table 24-1. Some Common OTC Antacid Products

Sodium bicarbonate products
Alka-Seltzer
Bell/ans
Calcium carbonate products
Amitone
Chooz
Titralac
Tums
Aluminum hydroxide products
ALterna GEL
Amphojel
Magnesium hydroxide product
Milk of Magnesia
Magaldrate product
Riopan
Bismuth salt product
Pepto-Bismol
Magnesium and aluminum products
Aludrox
Gelusil
Maalox
Mylanta
WinGel

syndrome, excess calcium is absorbed, leading to hypercalcemia, alkalosis, nephrocalcinosis, and azotemia.

(3) With sodium bicarbonate, excess drug rapidly leaves the stomach and is absorbed from the gastrointestinal tract. The liberated CO_2 then causes gastric distention, posing a risk to people who have gastric ulcers approaching the perforation stage.

(4) Sodium absorption (which may result from sodium-containing antacids) may be dangerous to people with congestive heart failure (CHF) or hypertension.

(5) **Hyperacidity rebound** may occur after the antacid has increased gastric pH. Antral secretion of gastrin persists even after pH returns to a level that normally terminates secretion. Rebound is a particular problem with calcium carbonate.

2. Nonabsorbable (nonsystemic) antacids

a. Definition. Nonsystemic antacids are those that form insoluble compounds in the intestine. Because these compounds are not significantly absorbed, they lack systemic effects.

b. Magnesium-containing antacids

(1) Magnesium hydroxide. This compound is nearly insoluble. The hydroxide reacts with HCl to form magnesium chloride, as demonstrated by the following equation:

$$Mg(OH)_2 + HCl = MgCl_2 + H_2O$$

(a) Some of the magnesium hydroxide that does not react with gastric HCl at the time of administration remains in the stomach, reacting with subsequently secreted acid.

(b) Consequently, magnesium hydroxide has a longer duration of action than sodium bicarbonate or calcium carbonate, and its neutralizing action is nearly as prompt and complete.

(c) Precautions

(i) The salt ($MgCl_2$) is absorbable and exerts a cathartic effect, possibly resulting in neurologic, neuromuscular, or cardiovascular impairment.

(ii) Magnesium hydroxide is contraindicated in patients with renal insufficiency.

(2) Magnesium trisilicate

(a) This compound reacts with gastric acid as shown in the following equation:

$$Mg_2Si_3O_8 \cdot nH_2O + 4H^+ = 2Mg^{++} + 3SiO_8 + (n + 2)H_2O$$

(b) In this slow reaction, hydrated silicon dioxide formed in the stomach passes into the intestinal tract, where its fate is unclear.

(c) The double magnesium salts in the intestine may cause diarrhea, even at normal adequate doses.

(3) Magnesium carbonate. This compound is similar to magnesium hydroxide, except that CO_2 is liberated during its neutralization.

c. Aluminum-containing antacids. Aluminum hydroxide neutralizes HCl in the stomach, with no hydroxyl ions formed and liberated, as shown by the following equation:

$$Al(OH)_3 + HCl = AlCl_3 + H_2O$$

(1) Its onset is relatively slow.

(2) Precautions

(a) Constipation may occur.

(b) Hypophosphatemia may develop with prolonged use.

d. Combination antacids. Many antacid products contain both magnesium and aluminum.

(1) Magaldrate (e.g., Riopan) is a complex of hydroxymagnesium aluminates.

(a) Combining slow-acting aluminum hydroxide with fast-acting hydroxymagnesium, magaldrate results in a sustained, even action.

(b) The constipating effect of aluminum hydroxide counteracts the laxative effect of magnesium hydroxide.

(c) Magaldrate contains very little sodium and thus can be taken safely by people on sodium-restricted diets.

(d) Precaution. With prolonged use, hypermagnesemia and hypophosphatemia may occur.

(2) Other combination antacid products contain varying amounts of aluminum hydroxide and magnesium hydroxide.

e. Additional antacid ingredients

(1) Simethicone is an inert silicon polymer with a surfactant action that produces an antiflatulent effect.

(2) Oxethazaine is a local anesthetic that has a topical anesthetic effect on the gastric mucosa.

(3) Alginic acid reacts with saliva to form a nonsoluble complex that floats atop the gastric contents, minimizing reflux into the esophagus.

D. Dosages. The buffering and acid-neutralizing capacities of an antacid product must be considered when determining the appropriate dosage. Typical antacid regimens are as follows:

1. For acute symptoms, an aluminum, magnesium, or combination antacid is given in a dosage of 30 ml every 2 hours until symptoms abate. Then, 30 ml is given 1 to 3 hours after meals and at bedtime.

2. For treatment of a duodenal ulcer, 80 mEq of buffering capacity is required, regardless of the type of antacid used.

E. Drug interactions

1. Antacids may alter the absorption rate or renal elimination of some concurrently administered drugs. Examples are as follows:
   a. Magnesium trisilicate slows phenothiazine absorption.
   b. Antacids increase levodopa absorption.
   c. Antacids reduce the absorption of oral digoxin; doses should be scheduled as far as possible from digoxin doses.

2. Antacids may destroy the coating of an enteric-coated tablet, leading to premature drug dissolution in the stomach.

3. Some antacids form complexes (chelate) with certain drugs, decreasing the amount of drug absorbed. For example, sodium bicarbonate, as well as magnesium, aluminum, and calcium salts, forms complexes with tetracycline.

III. ANTIEMETICS AND EMETICS

A. General considerations

1. **Definitions**
   a. **Nausea** refers to the sensation that one is about to vomit.
   b. **Vomiting** is the forceful expulsion of gastric contents through the mouth.

2. **Mechanism.** Vomiting is coordinated by the vomiting center in the medulla.
   a. Stimuli from the peripheral nervous system and within the central nervous system act on the vomiting center via modulation of the **chemoreceptor trigger zone (CTZ)**. The gastrointestinal tract and labyrinth apparatus also may directly stimulate the vomiting center.
   b. Responding to these impulses, the vomiting center stimulates the abdominal muscles, stomach, and esophagus to induce vomiting.

3. **Factors associated with vomiting**
   a. **Blood-borne emetic substances** (e.g., cancer chemotherapeutic agents) or **medical conditions** (e.g., pregnancy, administration of radiation therapy, uremia, electrolyte or endocrine disturbances) can lead to vomiting.
   b. Afferent stimulation also may trigger vomiting. Such stimulation arises from tactile pharyngeal impulses, labyrinth disturbances, increased intracranial pressure, pain, visceral distention, and psychological factors.

B. Products

1. **Antiemetics** are used to treat nausea and vomiting. Some of the most effective antiemetics, such as anticholinergics (e.g., scopolamine) and phenothiazines (e.g., prochlorperazine) are legend drugs. OTC antiemetics have limited value.
   a. **Antihistamines** act by reducing afferent stimulation. Cyclizine, meclizine, and dimenhydrinate are used to treat motion sickness. (These drugs are contraindicated in pregnant women.)
   b. **Phosphorated carbohydrate solution** presumably reduces gastric muscle contraction. However, its antiemetic effectiveness has not been proven.
      (1) The solution is a mixture of levulose (fructose), dextrose (glucose), and phosphoric acid.
      (2) Emetrol and Especol are OTC products containing phosphorated carbohydrate solution.

2. **Emetics** are agents that induce vomiting.
   a. These drugs are valuable in the treatment of poisoning.
   b. **Syrup of ipecac** induces vomiting both by stimulating the CTZ and by directly irritating the gastric mucosa.
      (1) **Adult dosage.** Adults receive 15 to 30 ml, followed by three to four glasses of water. A dose (15 ml) may be repeated in 20 minutes if vomiting has not occurred.

(2) **Pediatric dosage**
   (a) Children less than 1 year of age receive 5 to 10 ml, followed by one-half to one glass of water. The use of syrup of ipecac in children less than 6 months of age is controversial.
   (b) Children greater than 1 year and up to 12 years of age receive 15 ml, followed by one to two glasses of water.

IV. LAXATIVES

A. General considerations

1. **Definition. Constipation** is the difficult or infrequent passage of stools. (Frequency of bowel movements varies widely among individuals; normal frequency ranges from three times per day to three times per week.)

2. **Etiology.** The causes of constipation are wide-ranging and include both organic and functional conditions.
   a. **Organic causes** include intestinal obstruction, tumors, diverticulitis, inflammatory bowel disease, anal fissures, endocrine abnormalities (e.g., hypothyroidism), and metabolic disorders (e.g., hypokalemia, hyperglycemia).
   b. **Functional causes** include the following:
      (1) Failure to respond to the urge to defecate
      (2) Lack of regular, unhurried bowel habits
      (3) Low-fiber diet
      (4) Lack of exercise
      (5) Prolonged use of such drugs as narcotics, muscle relaxants, adrenergic agents, antacids containing aluminum or calcium salts, antidepressants, and antihypertensives.

B. Products

1. **Stimulant laxatives.** These agents presumably act directly on the colon to increase peristalsis.
   a. **Anthraquinones**
      (1) **Cascara sagrada** generally produces a bowel movement in 8 to 12 hours.
         (a) Liquid forms (which are more reliable than solid forms) should be taken with food or milk.
         (b) The usual adult dosage is 300 to 1000 mg.
         (c) OTC products containing cascara include Fletcher's Castoria, Cascara Sagrada, Senna, Senna I, and Senna II.
      (2) **Danthron** has actions and properties similar to those of cascara sagrada. OTC products containing danthron include Doxidan and Dorban.
      (3) **Aloe**, another stimulant laxative, is no longer recommended.
   b. **Diphenylmethane derivatives**
      (1) **Phenolphthalein** acts within 6 hours.
         (a) As much as 15% of this drug is absorbed; the remainder is excreted in the feces.
         (b) The usual adult dosage is 30 to 270 mg.
         (c) OTC products containing phenolphthalein include Feen-A-Mint, Ex-Lax, and Phenolax.
      (2) **Bisacodyl** acts on the entire colon, causing powerful contractions.
         (a) With rectal administration, bisacodyl may be effective within 1 hour; with oral administration, within 6 hours. (The oral tablet is enteric-coated and should not be chewed, crushed, or taken with hot liquids or alkalinizing agents.)
         (b) Dulcolax is an OTC product containing bisacodyl.
   c. **Castor oil** acts in the small intestine.
      (1) Pancreatic lipases hydrolyze castor oil to glycerol and ricinoleic acid, which stimulate peristalsis.
      (2) Because of its strong cathartic effect, castor oil is not recommended as a first-line agent for the treatment of constipation.
   d. **Precautions**
      (1) **Anthraquinones** may appear in secretions, including breast milk, and may color the urine pale yellow to reddish brown.
      (2) **Phenolphthalein**
         (a) This agent may color the urine and feces pink.
         (b) In susceptible people, this agent may cause an allergic reaction (e.g., skin rash).
         (c) Phenolphthalein is contraindicated in pregnant women.

2. **Bulk-forming laxatives.** These agents absorb intestinal water and swell, increasing the bulk

and moisture content of the stool to promote peristalsis. They act in both the small and large intestines.

a. The slowest but safest laxatives, bulk-forming laxatives cause few adverse effects and minimal systemic effects.

b. Natural bulk-forming laxatives include bran, karaya gum, psyllium seeds (Metamucil, Konsyl) and alginates.

c. Semisynthetic bulk-forming laxatives include methylcellulose and carboxymethylcellulose.

d. Precautions

(1) Certain bulk-forming laxative products contain sugar and may be harmful to diabetics.

(2) Some of these products also contain significant amounts of sodium and should not be used by people on sodium-restricted diets.

(3) Bulk-forming laxatives may impair the absorption of nutrients and concurrent drugs.

(4) For people with dysphagia, these laxatives may be hard to swallow.

3. Emollient laxatives. These surfactant agents soften the stool, facilitating its passage.

a. Mechanism of action. Emollients are wetting agents that increase the wetting efficiency of intestinal water by formation of an oil-in-water emulsion.

(1) By facilitating the admixture of fatty substances and fecal mass, they lower surface tension, thereby promoting a softer mass.

(2) Emollient laxatives are recommended for the treatment of hard stools—especially in people who must avoid straining at stool.

(3) These agents do not inhibit nutrient absorption.

b. Docusate, an **ionic emollient**, is available in three salt forms [calcium (Surfak), potassium (Dialose, Diocto-K), and sodium (Colace, Doxinate)].

c. Poloxamers are **nonionic emollients** whose properties resemble those of docusate.

d. Precaution. Emollient laxatives may increase the absorption of concurrent drugs.

4. Saline and osmotic laxatives

a. Saline laxatives include various magnesium and sodium salts and other tartrates, sulfates, and phosphates. Compounds contained in OTC saline laxatives include magnesium hydroxide (Milk of Magnesia), magnesium citrate (Citroma), magnesium sulfate (Epsom Salts), sodium phosphate (Fleet Phosphosoda), disodium phosphate, and monosodium phosphate.

b. Osmotic laxatives include lactulose (Chronulac) and glycerin (Fleet Babylax).

c. Mechanism of action

(1) Saline laxatives cause osmosis by attracting water into the intestinal lumen.

(a) As intestinal fluid accumulates, distention occurs, facilitating peristalsis.

(b) These laxatives also promote release of cholecystokinin-pancreozymin, a hormone that causes accumulation of fluid and electrolytes in the small intestine.

(2) Osmotic laxatives

(a) Glycerin (administered in suppository or enema form) draws water into the feces, softening the stool and lubricating it to promote its passage. The suppository form also may stimulate rectal contractions.

(b) Lactulose has an osmotic effect in the colon; the resulting fluid accumulation encourages peristalsis.

d. Precautions

(1) Absorption of ions may occur, possibly causing systemic toxicity in patients with renal impairment or CHF.

(2) Adequate fluid intake must be ensured to prevent dehydration from hypertonic saline laxatives.

5. Lubricant laxatives. These agents increase water retention in the stool, softening the fecal mass and promoting its passage.

a. Mineral oil and the emulsion of mineral oil and magnesium hydroxide (Haley's M-O) are examples of OTC lubricant laxatives.

b. Precautions

(1) Lubricant laxatives interfere with the absorption of vitamins A, D, and K and such minerals as calcium and phosphate.

(2) These substances may reduce prothrombin time.

(3) Prolonged oral administration of large amounts of mineral oil may lead to systemic absorption that causes hepatic changes.

(4) Lipid pneumonitis may occur with extensive use (especially in children and elderly or debilitated people).

(5) Contact dermatitis may develop with prolonged use.

V. ANTIDIARRHEALS

A. General considerations

1. **Definition. Diarrhea** is the abnormally frequent passage of loose stools having an increased weight (above 150 to 300 g/day) and increased water content (60% to 90%).
   a. Although increased stool weight usually indicates diarrhea, some colonic diseases cause **small-volume diarrhea**, characterized by frequent passage of blood, mucus, or pus.
   b. In diarrhea, excess water that normally is reabsorbed from the intestine is passed via the stool.

2. **Classification.** Diarrhea may be classified by mechanism or etiology.
   a. **Classification by mechanism**
      (1) **Osmotic diarrhea** results when excess water-soluble substances cause osmotic retention of intraluminal water.
         (a) Ingestion of large meals or osmotically active substances (e.g., sorbitol, glycerin, and other polyhydric alcohols) can lead to osmotic diarrhea.
         (b) Dumping syndrome and disaccharidase deficiency are other possible causes.
      (2) **Secretory diarrhea** occurs when damage or inflammation causes the intestinal mucosa to secrete, rather than absorb, water and electrolytes.
         (a) Bacterial toxins (e.g., cholera organisms), infection (as with *Shigella* or *Salmonella* organisms), and inflammatory bowel disease may induce secretory diarrhea.
         (b) Other causes include certain drugs (e.g., prostaglandins) and tumors that secrete activating hormones.
      (3) **Altered intestinal transit**
         (a) Diarrhea may occur if the exposure time between intestinal chyme and the absorbing surface of the gastrointestinal tract is reduced. Shortened exposure time may result from bowel or gastric resection, pyloric sphincter surgery, vagotomy, and use of certain drugs.
         (b) Prolonged exposure between chyme and the absorbing surface may promote diarrhea by allowing fecal bacteria to proliferate in the small intestine. Causes of prolonged exposure include scleroderma, strictured bowel segments, and antibiotic administration.
      (4) **Exudative diarrhea**, characterized by abnormal mucosal permeability, leads to intestinal loss of blood, serum proteins, and mucus. This, in turn, increases fecal bulk and fluid content.
   b. **Classification by etiology**
      (1) **Infection**. Common infectious pathogens include *Escherichia coli*, *Shigella*, *Salmonella*, and *Staphylococcus aureus* organisms.
         (a) *E. coli* and *S. aureus* cause diarrhea via an enterotoxin.
         (b) *Shigella* and *Salmonella* organisms invade mucosal epithelial cells, producing a dysentery-like syndrome characterized by fever and frequent passage of small-volume stools that may contain blood and pus.
         (c) *E. coli* frequently causes **traveler's diarrhea** ("turista"), in which ingestion of contaminated food or water leads to extensive changes in the intestinal bacterial flora. This syndrome has a sudden onset and is characterized by loose stools, nausea, vomiting, and cramps.
         (d) In **infantile diarrhea,** caused by a viral infection, vomiting, low-grade fever, and watery diarrhea occur, possibly leading to severe dehydration.
         (e) **Protozoal diarrhea** stems from infection by *Giardia lamblia* or *Entamoeba histolytica* organisms. In this type of infection, explosive watery diarrhea and severe cramps have a sudden onset.
      (2) **Drug-induced diarrhea**
         (a) Antibiotics promote diarrhea by causing mild intestinal irritation, alteration of the intestinal microbial flora, and increased intestinal motility.
         (b) Other drugs associated with diarrhea include antineoplastics, digitalis, laxatives, colchicine, quinidine, and guanethidine.
      (3) **Malabsorption syndromes** (e.g., celiac sprue, short bowel syndrome states, diverticula) can lead to diarrhea.
      (4) **Food-induced diarrhea** most commonly results from food allergy, fatty or spicy foods, milk intolerance, high-fiber foods, or foods containing polyhydric alcohol (e.g., molasses).
      (5) Other causes of diarrhea include psychological factors, pancreatic disease (e.g., diabetes mellitus), pelvic disease, hyperthyroidism, and malnutrition.

B. General therapeutic measures

1. Foods are withheld for 12 to 24 hours. However, clear, lukewarm fluids may be given, especially if the patient has acute watery diarrhea.
2. When the patient can tolerate them, soft foods (e.g., gelatin) are permitted in small portions.
3. If the patient is dehydrated, Pedialyte or Lytren may be given.
4. The World Health Organization has established guidelines for fluid and electrolyte replacement in severe diarrhea.
   a. Ingredients include:
      (1) Glucose: 20 g
      (2) Sodium chloride: 90 mEq
      (3) Sodium bicarbonate: 30 mEq
      (4) Potassium chloride: 20 mEq
      (5) Water: as needed to make 1 L
   b. Products containing these ingredients include Pedialyte and Dicrolyte (available in the United Kingdom).

C. Products

1. **Opiates** exert a direct musculotropic effect, inhibiting propulsive intestinal movement. This reduces hyperperistalsis and slows passage of the intestinal contents, leading to reabsorption of intestinal water and electrolytes. OTC opiate products include Donnagel-PG and paregoric.
2. **Adsorbents** are chemically inert powders that adsorb bacteria, toxins, and gases. They are not systemically absorbed.
   a. **Activated attapulgite**, a naturally occurring aluminum magnesium silicate, is considered to be safe and effective in the treatment of diarrhea.
      (1) It is available in both suspension and tablet form (Rheaban, Diar-Aid).
      (2) **Dosages**
         (a) Adults receive 1200 mg after each bowel movement. Total daily dosage should not exceed 8400 mg.
         (b) Children aged 6 to 12 years receive half the adult dosage; children aged 3 to 6 years receive one-fourth the adult dosage.
   b. **Bismuth salts** (bismuth subnitrate, subgallate, and subsalicylate) are considered safe and effective in the prophylaxis and treatment of traveler's diarrhea. (Bismuth subsalicylate also inhibits prostaglandin synthesis, relieving cramp-induced pain.)
   c. **Kaolin** is a natural hydrated aluminum silicate whose effectiveness remains unproven.
      (1) It may adsorb drugs such as lincomycin and digoxin.
      (2) Combined with pectin (a polyuronic polymer of purified carbohydrate extracted from citrus fruits or apple pomace), kaolin is available as Kaopectate and Donnagel-MB.
   d. **Activated charcoal** is a powder residue from the distillation of various organic materials. Although valuable as an antidote for various oral drugs, its effectiveness as an antidiarrheal is questionable.
   e. **Polycarbophil** absorbs free fecal water, reducing stool fluidity. It is considered to be safe and effective.
      (1) A **stool normalizer**, it can be used to treat constipation as well as diarrhea.
      (2) **Dosages**
         (a) Adults may take 4 to 6 g/day (eight 500-mg tablets).
         (b) Children aged 6 to 12 years receive 1.5 g/day; children aged 3 to 6 years receive 1 g/day.
3. **Anticholinergics** (e.g., atropine, hyoscyamine) are contained in such combination products as Donnagel Suspension and Donnagel-PG. Although these agents reduce intestinal spasms, their value as antidiarrheals is unproven.
4. **Lactobacillus preparations** have yet to be proven effective in the treatment of diarrhea. These agents replace the normal flora and fauna of the intestinal tract.

VI. HEMORRHOID PREPARATIONS

A. General considerations

1. **Definition.** Hemorrhoids are vascular masses in the anal canal.
2. **Classification**
   a. **Internal hemorrhoids** are varicose dilatations of the superior hemorrhoidal plexus. Bulging into the rectum above the dentate line, they are covered with mucous membrane.

b. External hemorrhoids are varicose dilatations of the inferior hemorrhoidal plexus that originate below the dentate line and protrude outside the anal sphincter.

3. **Signs and symptoms** of hemorrhoids include rectal bleeding, inflammation, irritation, itching, burning, swelling, and pain.

4. **Predisposing and precipitating factors** include hereditary predisposition, prolonged sitting or standing, straining at stool, a low-fiber diet, inadequate fluid intake, constipation, diarrhea, pregnancy, anal infection, and rectal cancer.

B. General therapeutic measures

1. After each bowel movement, the perianal area should be cleansed with hygienic wipes to alleviate itching, burning, and pain.

2. Warm compresses, analgesic ointments, and sitz baths also help relieve discomfort.

3. In some cases, hemorrhoids must be ligated, excised, or sclerosed by injection.

C. Products. OTC hemorrhoid preparations include ointments, creams, suppositories, aerosol foams, lotions, solutions, and perianal wipes and pads. Ingredients contained in these products may include the following:

1. **Corticosteroids.** These agents reduce swelling and inflammation. Most corticosteroids used to treat hemorrhoids require a prescription. However, Dermolate Anal-Itch cream, containing 0.5% hydrocortisone, is available OTC.

2. **Local anesthetics.** These agents, which relieve pain, burning, and itching, are available in such products as Medicone rectal ointment, Americaine ointment, Anusol ointment, and ProctoFoam aerosol foam.

3. **Vasoconstrictors.** Ephedrine, epinephrine, phenylephrine, and other vasoconstrictive agents reduce swelling and congestion of anorectal tissue. Pazo and Wyanoids hemorrhoidal suppositories contain vasoconstrictors.

4. **Astringents.** Witch hazel, zinc oxide, and other astringents alleviate anorectal irritation and inflammation. Products containing astringents include Tucks pads and Preparation H cleansing pads.

5. Other ingredients found in OTC hemorrhoid preparations include antiseptics, emollients, counterirritants, keratolytics, and wound-healing agents.

STUDY QUESTIONS

Directions: Each question below contains five suggested answers. Choose the **one best** response to each question.

1. Which of the following drugs is available over-the-counter for the treatment of nausea and vomiting?

A. Dimenhydrinate
B. Perphenazine
C. Prochlorperazine
D. Scopolamine
E. Danthron

2. All of the following statements about cold sores are true EXCEPT

A. they may recur periodically
B. they are not contagious
C. they tend to be self-limiting
D. they may produce a secondary bacterial infection
E. emollients are helpful in treatment

3. Predisposing causes of hemorrhoids include all of the following EXCEPT

A. prolonged standing
B. heredity
C. high-fiber diet
D. inadequate fluid intake
E. diarrhea

Directions: Each question below contains three suggested answers of which **one or more** is correct. Choose the answer

A if **I only** is correct
B if **III only** is correct
C if **I and II** are correct
D if **II and III** are correct
E if **I, II, and III** are correct

4. Treatment of halitosis may include

I. good toothbrushing and flossing
II. the use of mouthwashes
III. treatment of the causative disease process

5. Nonprescription products used in the treatment of hemorrhoids include

I. corticosteroids
II. local anesthetics
III. vasoconstrictors

6. True statements about polycarbophil include which of the following?

I. It is a bulk-forming laxative
II. It can be used in constipation
III. It can be used in diarrhea

7. Aluminum-containing antacids have the disadvantage of causing

I. constipation
II. phosphate binding
III. diarrhea

ANSWERS AND EXPLANATIONS

1. The answer is A. (*III B 1* a) Perphenazine, prochlorperazine, and scopolamine are all used in the treatment of nausea and vomiting, but they are all legend drugs. Of the drugs listed in the question, only dimenhydrinate is available OTC. Other OTC products for this use are cyclizine and meclizine. All three OTC antiemetics are contraindicated in pregnant women. Danthron is a stimulant laxative, not an antiemetic.

2. The answer is B. (*I A 1* a, *3* a, c) Cold sores (fever blisters) are caused by the herpes simplex virus and are highly contagious. Although each episode is self-limiting, cold sores tend to recur periodically. Factors that precipitate recurrences include upper respiratory tract infections, exposure to sunlight, and stress. In treatment, emollients and local anesthetics help to relieve discomfort. A topical antibiotic may be applied if secondary bacterial infection occurs. A sunscreen preparation may help to prevent sunlight-induced recurrences.

3. The answer is C. (*VI A 4*) A low-fiber diet, not a high-fiber diet, may predispose a patient to hemorrhoids. Other predisposing factors, besides those listed in the question, are straining at stool, constipation, prolonged sitting, pregnancy, anal infection, and rectal cancer.

4. The answer is E (all). (*I B 2*) When poor oral hygiene causes halitosis, good toothbrushing, flossing, and the use of mouthwashes are all helpful measures. If an underlying disease process is the cause, its treatment may result in effective treatment of the halitosis.

5. The answer is E (all). (*VI C*) Corticosteroids, local anesthetics, and vasoconstrictors are only three of the many types of ingredients contained in various OTC products available for the treatment of hemorrhoids. The wide variety of medications available, and their varied formulations, reflect the vexatious nature of this common malady.

6. The answer is D (II, III). (*V C 2* e) Polycarbophil is considered to be a stool normalizer that regulates the amount of water in the gut. It absorbs free fecal water, reducing stool fluidity in diarrhea and softening the stool mass in constipation.

7. The answer is C (I, II). (*II C 2* c) Aluminum, having an ionic charge of three, will repel water and have a constipating effect. Aluminum will also combine with circulating phosphates to decrease free phosphates. With prolonged use, this can cause hypophosphatemia, which depletes the calcium in bones. However, hypophosphatemia is unlikely to develop if the diet is normal, since dietary phosphorus levels parallel the dietary protein levels.

25 OTC Products: Cough, Cold, and Allergy Drugs

Robert L. McCarthy
Anthony V. Rozzi

I. ANTITUSSIVES

A. General considerations. Antitussives are cough inhibitors that decrease the frequency of cough. They are used when frequent coughing causes marked fatigue—especially when the cough is dry and nonproductive.

B. Centrally acting antitussives. These agents act either by depressing the medullary cough center or by suppressing sensory nerve receptors in the respiratory tract.

1. **Narcotic antitussive. Codeine** is the standard of centrally acting narcotic antitussives. At antitussive doses, it rarely leads to dependency and is considered to be safe and effective.
   a. Codeine is available OTC only in some states (it is sold alone and in combination in Puerto Rico).
   b. **Dosages**
      (1) Adults receive 15 mg three times daily.
      (2) Children receive 1.0 to 1.5 mg/kg/day in four divided doses.
   c. **Precautions**
      (1) Codeine may cause drowsiness, sedation, nausea, and constipation.
      (2) This agent is contraindicated in increased intracranial pressure and should be used cautiously in chronic obstructive pulmonary disease, head injury, hepatic or renal disease, or a history of drug dependency.

2. **Nonnarcotic antitussives**
   a. **Dextromethorphan**. A dextro-isomer of levorphanol, this agent has no analgesic activity and does not lead to dependency. Many clinicians believe it is equipotent to codeine.
      (1) **Dosages**
         (a) Adults receive 10 to 20 mg every 4 hours.
         (b) Children ages 6 to 12 years receive 5 to 10 mg every 4 hours.
         (c) Children ages 2 to 5 years receive 2.5 to 5.0 mg every 4 hours.
      (2) **Precautions**
         (a) Dextromethorphan may cause drowsiness and gastrointestinal distress.
         (b) With large doses, bizarre behavior may occur—especially in children.
   b. **Noscapine**. This opium alkaloid, related to papaverine, is used to manage cough—especially in asthma and emphysema. However, its effectiveness has not been proven conclusively.
      (1) The actions of noscapine are dose-dependent.
      (2) At usual dosages, it does not affect respiration.
      (3) Noscapine has no addictive potential.
      (4) **Dosages**
         (a) Adults receive 15 to 30 mg every 4 to 6 hours.
         (b) Children ages 6 to 12 years receive 7.5 to 15.0 mg every 4 to 6 hours.
         (c) Children ages 2 to 5 years receive 3.75 to 7.50 mg every 4 to 6 hours.
   c. **Diphenhydramine**. This agent has both antitussive and antihistamine properties. Its antitussive effect results from direct medullary action.
      (1) **Dosages**
         (a) Adults receive 25 mg every 4 hours.
         (b) Children ages 6 to 12 years receive 12.5 mg every 4 hours.
         (c) Children ages 2 to 5 years receive 6.25 mg every 4 hours.
      (2) **Precautions**
         (a) Diphenhydramine may cause sedation and anticholinergic effects.
         (b) This drug should be used cautiously in patients who have acute asthma, narrow-angle glaucoma, or a history of seizures.

C. Peripherally acting antitussives. These agents act on the bronchioles and other smooth muscle of the respiratory tract to reduce irritation and inflammation, thereby decreasing cough-inducing medullary stimulation. **Demulcents** are peripherally-acting antitussives whose protective action helps reduce irritation and prevent dehydration. Demulcents are produced in the form of lozenges, gargles, and pastilles.

1. **Demulcent antibiotic products** may contain such ingredients as pyridium, cetylpyridium, and hexylresorcinol. However, these agents are considered to be only possibly effective.

2. **Demulcent anesthetic products** generally are effective for short periods, although their value is controversial. The ingredients in these products include benzocaine (5% to 20%), phenol (0.5% to 1.5%), and benzyl alcohol (10%).

II. EXPECTORANTS. These agents may enhance the production of respiratory tract fluids to help reduce the viscosity of thick, tenacious secretions. They are used primarily in colds and chronic pulmonary disorders. However, the value of traditional expectorants has been challenged.

A. Ammonium chloride presumably loosens secretions by reflex stimulation of bronchial mucous glands via gastric mucosal irritation.

1. **Dosage**. Adults typically receive 250 to 500 mg every 2 to 4 hours.

2. **Precautions**
   a. This agent is contraindicated in renal, hepatic, or chronic heart disease.
   b. Ammonium chloride sometimes is used as a urine acidifier and thus may alter the excretion of concurrent drugs.
   c. Acidosis may occur.

B. Guaifenesin. This agent acts by reflex gastric stimulation. However, it has questionable clinical value.

1. **Dosages**
   a. Adults receive 100 to 200 mg every 2 to 4 hours.
   b. Children receive 12 mg/kg/day in six divided doses.

2. **Precaution**. With large doses, guaifenesin may cause nausea and vomiting.

C. Ipecac. This agent (which also is used as an emetic) increases the flow of respiratory tract secretions via gastric irritation.

1. **Dosages**
   a. Ipecac is administered to adults three to four times daily in a dosage of 0.5 to 1.0 ml.
   b. It is administered to children three to four times daily in a dosage of 0.25 to 0.5 ml.

2. **Precautions**. Emetine and cephaeline, chief alkaloids of ipecac, are highly toxic. Consequently, ipecac is not recommended for children under age 6.

D. Terpin hydrate. This volatile oil derivative is thought to act by directly stimulating secretory glands in the lower respiratory tract, reducing the production and viscosity of secretions.

1. **Dosage**. Adults receive 5 to 10 ml every 4 to 6 hours.

2. **Precaution**. This agent has a high alcoholic content and should not be given in large doses.

III. DECONGESTANTS. These agents are sympathomimetic vasoconstrictors that reduce nasal congestion and permit freer nasal air passage. They are used in colds, allergy, rhinitis, and sinusitus.

A. Topical decongestants include various sympathomimetic amines, which cause local sympathetic nerve fiber stimulation. They vary in onset, duration of action, and intensity of effect.

1. **Short-acting topical decongestants**
   a. **Ephedrine sulfate** is available in concentrations ranging from 0.5% to 1.0%.
      (1) Peak levels occur approximately 1 hour after administration.
      (2) **Dosage**. Three or four drops are applied to the nasal mucosa every 4 hours, as needed. (Ephedrine is not recommended for children under age 6.)
      (3) **Precaution**. Tachycardia may occur.
   b. **Phenylephrine hydrochloride** (e.g., Neo-Synephrine) is available in concentrations of 0.25% to 1.00%.
      (1) **Dosage**. Two to three drops or sprays are applied every 4 hours, as needed.
      (2) **Precaution**. Nasal irritation, tachycardia, and palpitations may occur.

c. **Naphazoline** (e.g., Privine) is more potent than phenylephrine. It is available in concentrations ranging from 0.05% to 0.10%.
   (1) **Dosage**. Two sprays or drops are applied to the nasal mucosa every 3 to 6 hours.
   (2) **Precautions**
      (a) In children, systemic side effects may occur with prolonged or excessive use.
      (b) This agent can cause central nervous system (CNS) depression.

2. **Long-acting topical decongestants**
   a. **Oxymetazoline hydrochloride** (e.g., Afrin, Duration) has effects lasting up to 12 hours. It is available in concentrations of 0.025% to 0.050%.
      (1) This agent is administered twice daily for up to 3 days.
      (2) **Precaution**. Severe rebound nasal congestion may result from prolonged or excessive use.
   b. **Xylometazoline hydrochloride** (e.g., Sine-Off, Long-Acting Neo-Synephrine) also has a duration of about 12 hours.
      (1) **Dosage**. Two or three drops or two sprays of 0.1% solution are applied to the nasal mucosa every 8 to 10 hours.
      (2) **Precaution**. Excessive or prolonged used may lead to rebound nasal congestion or irritation.

B. **Oral decongestants**. These agents cause generalized vasoconstriction. Usually, their effects are longer-lasting but less intense than those of topical decongestants. Also, they cause more pronounced adverse effects (e.g., nervousness, insomnia) than do topical agents.

1. **Phenylephrine hydrochloride** is considered to be safe and effective. The adult dosage is 10 mg every 4 hours. Children ages 6 to 12 years receive 5 mg every 4 hours; children ages 2 to 5 years receive 2.5 mg every 4 hours.

2. **Phenylpropanolamine hydrochloride** causes fewer CNS effects than do other sympathomimetic amines.
   a. **Dosages**
      (1) Adults receive 25 mg every 4 hours.
      (2) Children ages 6 to 12 years receive 12.5 mg every 4 hours.
      (3) Children under age 6 may receive 6.25 mg every 4 hours. However, phenylpropanolamine is not recommended for this age group.
   b. **Precautions**. Nausea, dizziness, nervousness, headache, and insomnia may occur.

3. **Pseudoephedrine** (e.g., Sudafed) has a relatively short duration of action. It produces fewer adverse effects than do other oral decongestants.
   a. **Dosages**
      (1) Adults receive 60 mg every 6 to 8 hours.
      (2) Children ages 6 to 12 receive 30 mg every 6 to 8 hours.
      (3) Children ages 2 to 5 years receive 15 mg every 6 hours. However, the use of pseudoephedrine in this age group is questionable.
   b. **Precaution**. Nervousness and palpitations may occur.

IV. ANTIHISTAMINES

A. General considerations

1. Antihistamines are antagonizing agents that compete for receptor sites with natural **histamine,** a biogenic amine present in most body cells and tissues.
   a. When most cells lyse (in response to a necrotic process, inflammation, or an antigen–antibody response), they release histamine. This triggers generalized and localized vasodilation, with edema and increased capillary permeability.
   b. Nasal vasodilation results in swollen nasal turbinates, reducing nasal air passage. This leads to congestion and runny nose.

2. **Classification**. Antihistamines used in cold and allergy remedies are pharmacologically classified as $histamine_1$ antagonists. Those used in OTC preparations are further classified by chemical structure, as ethanolamines, ethylenediamines, or alkylamines.

B. **Ethanolamines**. The most sedating antihistamines, these agents include **diphenhydramine** (discussed in section I B 2 c), **doxylamine**, and **phentoloxamine**.

C. **Ethylenediamines**. Less sedating than ethanolamines, these agents probably also are less effective. They include **pyrilamine** and **thonzylamine**.

D. Alkylamines. These highly effective agents are less sedating than ethanolamines and ethylenediamines. They include **brompheniramine** and **chlorpheniramine**.

E. Precautions. Antihistamines can lead to a wide range of adverse effects that may severely limit their use.

1. **Hepatic enzyme induction**. Because antihistamines induce the microsomal enzyme system and facilitate their own destruction, they become less effective with continued use. This commonly necessitates a change of antihistamine product.

2. **Anticholinergic effects**. These annoying but common side effects usually are manageable and do not warrant drug discontinuation. They include dry mouth, urinary retention, and blurred vision.

3. **CNS depression**. Drowsiness is a common side effect with all antihistamines and may be exacerbated (via synergism) by concurrent use of another CNS depressant.

4. **Paradoxical effects**. Antihistamines sometimes cause CNS stimulation instead of drowsiness. Flushing, hyperactivity, anorexia, and palpitations also may occur. Paradoxical effects are most common in children.

STUDY QUESTIONS

Directions: Each question below contains five suggested answers. Choose the **one best** response to each question.

1. Oxymetazoline acts as a nasal decongestant by

A. causing a local anesthetic action
B. blocking at the synaptic ganglia
C. constricting blood vessels by local sympathetic nerve fiber stimulation
D. dilating blood vessels by local sympathetic nerve fiber inhibition
E. blocking muscarinic receptors

2. Antihistamines are used in OTC cold preparations for their

A. histamine-blocking action
B. anticholinergic effects
C. sympathomimetic effects
D. vasodilating effects
E. microsomal enzyme-inducing effects

3. All of the following are considered centrally acting antitussives EXCEPT

A. noscapine
B. dextromethorphan
C. codeine
D. benzocaine
E. diphenhydramine

Directions: Each question below contains three suggested answers of which **one or more** is correct. Choose the answer

A if **I only** is correct
B if **III only** is correct
C if **I and II** are correct
D if **II and III** are correct
E if **I, II, and III** are correct

4. Phenylpropanolamine is used in which of the following types of OTC products?

I. Analgesics
II. Appetite suppressants
III. Decongestants

5. Long-acting topical nasal decongestants share which of the following properties?

I. They are sympathomimetic agents
II. They are likely to produce rebound congestion with prolonged use
III. Their effects last for more than 24 hours

6. The expectorant terpin hydrate has which of the following properties?

I. It acts by direct bronchial stimulation
II. It decreases mucus production
III. It decreases mucus viscosity

ANSWERS AND EXPLANATIONS

1. The answer is C. (*III A*) Oxymetazoline is a long-acting sympathomimetic, which produces vasoconstriction by α-adrenergic stimulation. Because it is a long-acting decongestant, twice daily administration is sufficient.

2. The answer is A. (*IV A, E*) In OTC cold and allergy formulations, antihistamines are used because they compete for receptor sites with histamine, the natural biogenic amine that causes nasal vasodilation, congestion, and edema in response to cold viruses and allergens. Drowsiness, a natural side effect of antihistamines is useful in the induction of sleep. The anticholinergic effects of antihistamine are annoying and unwanted side effects (e.g., dry mouth, blurred vision). Decongestants, not antihistamines, are used in cold and allergy products for their sympathomimetic effects. A vasodilating effect would be undesirable in a cold or allergy remedy. The induction of hepatic microsomal enzymes is an unwanted side effect of antihistamines.

3. The answer is D. (*I B 1, 2; C 2; Chapter 26 IV B 2*) Benzocaine is a topically acting anesthetic, reducing the peripheral cough reflex and throat irritation. Codeine is a centrally acting narcotic antitussive with a very low risk of dependency. Dextromethorphan and diphenhydramine are nonnarcotic centrally acting antitussives. Noscapine, although an opium alkaloid, is also considered a nonnarcotic centrally acting antitussive because, except for its antitussive effect, it has no other significant CNS effects in the therapeutic dosage range.

4. The answer is D (II, III). (*III B 2; Chapter 26 IV B 1*) Phenylpropanolamine produces its decongestant effects by direct peripheral vasopressor activity. This causes vasoconstriction in the nasal turbinates, allowing more air space for incoming and outgoing air. Phenylpropanolamine is also used as an appetite suppressant, but its effectiveness for this use is questionable. Phenylpropanolamine has no analgesic properties.

5. The answer is C (I, II). (*III A 2*) The effects of long-acting topical nasal decongestants last for about 12 hours. Excessive or prolonged use of any of these products can lead to rebound nasal congestion, and so they should not be used for more than 3 days.

6. The answer is E (all). (*II D*) Terpin hydrate, a volatile oil derivative, acts by stimulating the secretory glands in the bronchi, thereby reducing the production and viscosity of mucous secretions.

26
OTC Products: Centrally Acting Drugs

Robert L. McCarthy
Anthony V. Rozzi

I. ANALGESICS AND ANTIPYRETICS

A. General considerations. OTC analgesics and antipyretics alleviate mild to moderate pain (caused by stimulation of slow pain fibers), relieve inflammation, and reduce fever. Indications typically include headache, neuralgia, myalgia, arthralgia, and generalized inflammatory conditions (e.g., bursitis). [Migraine pain is **not** appropriately treated by OTC analgesics.]

1. **Pathogenesis of pain**
   a. An intense stimulus (e.g., tissue injury) triggers pain receptors to send pain impulses over afferent nerve fibers to the central nervous system (CNS).
   b. Awareness of pain takes place in the thalamus; pain recognition and localization occur in the cortex.
2. **Etiology of pain**. Pain results from injury, disease, or, in some cases, psychogenic sources. (Psychogenic pain commonly stems from chronic muscle tension, a minor somatic sensation, or an imaginary complaint and may contribute to pain arising from other factors.)
3. **Analgesic action**. OTC analgesics inhibit (either centrally, peripherally, or both) the biosynthesis of **prostaglandins**, substances involved in the development of pain and inflammation.

B. Products

1. **Salicylates** (e.g., aspirin, salsalate)
   a. **Therapeutic uses**. Salicylates are used to relieve pain and inflammation and to reduce fever.
   b. **Mechanism of action**
      (1) **Analgesic and anti-inflammatory actions**. Salicylates form an interacting false substrate (eicosatetraenoic acid) that interferes with cyclooxygenase, an enzyme responsible for the production of prostaglandins (Fig. 26-1). This action is both central and peripheral.
      (2) **Antipyretic action**. Salicylates inhibit prostaglandin formation in the hypothalamus, which is responsible for heat conservation and other thermoregulatory mechanisms. Thus, salicylates reduce fever by augmenting heat loss rather than by altering heat production.
   c. **Dosages and administration forms**
      (1) For mild to moderate pain (especially of somatic origin), 325 to 650 mg of a salicylate usually is sufficient initially; then 325 to 650 mg are administered three times daily.
      (2) Chronic inflammatory conditions typically warrant a dosage of 650 to 1200 mg administered twice daily.
      (3) Rheumatoid inflammatory conditions may call for administration of up to 4 g/day in adults.
      (4) Children's dosages are based on the age of the child (e.g., infants and children up to 2 years of age should be given 80 to 100 mg two to three times a day; children ages 2 to 4 years should be given 160 mg every 4 hours).
      (5) Choline salicylate is available in liquid form, and magnesium salicylate is available in tablets. The salts are available in combination in tablets and liquid form.
   d. **Precautions**
      (1) Salicylates inhibit platelet aggregation by blocking prostaglandin synthesis, which may lead to increased bleeding time.
      (2) In low dosages, salicylates may increase uric acid levels; in high dosages, they may cause uricosuria.
      (3) Salicylates inhibit biosynthesis of gastric prostaglandins and thus may cause gastrointestinal irritation (including bleeding and ulceration).

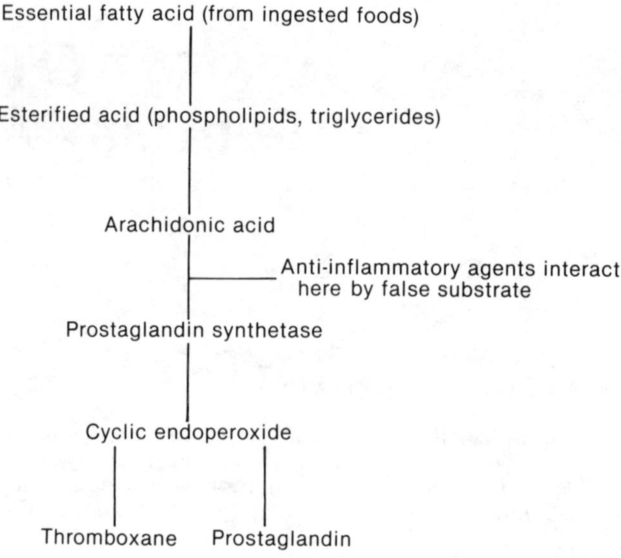

Figure 26-1. Prostaglandin biosythesis.

(4) Salicylate hypersensitivity may occur; most commonly, this manifests as bronchoconstriction.

(5) Salicylate toxicity may range from mild to severe. Mild toxicity causes such signs and symptoms as headache, tinnitus, nausea, vomiting, and sweating. With more serious toxicity, acidosis, hemorrhage, and encephalopathy may develop.

(6) Papillary necrosis may arise from reduced renal blood flow and drug acetylation in the kidney.

(7) **Drug interactions**. Salicylates bind extensively and firmly with plasma proteins and thus may displace less highly bound drugs, such as oral anticoagulants and oral antidiabetic agents.

2. **Para-aminophenols** (i.e., acetaminophen—phenacetin is no longer available OTC due to its undersirable adverse effects)
   a. **Therapeutic uses**. These agents are used as valuable alternatives to salicylates in people with peptic ulcer or other contraindications for salicylates. However, although para-aminophenols are effective analgesics and antipyretics, they have little value in reducing inflammation.
   b. **Mechanism of action**. Para-aminophenols reduce pain and fever by interfering with prostaglandin synthesis in a way similar to salicylates. However, because their action is confined to the CNS, they lack an anti-inflammatory effect.
   c. **Dosages** for para-aminophenols are similar to those for salicylates.
   d. **Precautions**
      (1) These agents may cause direct **hepatocellular toxicity** by saturation of hepatic enzymes.
         (a) Overdoses above 100 mg/kg suggest **possible** hepatocellular damage. This dose level warrants removal of gastric contents.
         (b) Overdoses above 150 mg/kg indicate **probable** hepatocellular damage. In this case, 140 mg/kg of acetylcysteine (Mucomyst) should be administered every 4 hours initially, then 70 mg/kg every 4 hours for 17 doses.
      (2) Para-aminophenols induce hepatic enzymes, accelerating hepatic metabolism of susceptible drugs.
      (3) Para-aminophenols may cause papillary necrosis in the same way as occurs with salicylates.

3. **Phenylpropionic acids** (e.g., ibuprofen)
   a. **Therapeutic uses**. These agents have analgesic, antipyretic, and anti-inflammatory activity. Due to higher patient tolerance, they may be preferred over salicylates. Ibuprofen is the only OTC phenylpropionic acid.
   b. **Mechanism of action**. Phenylpropionic acids are potent prostaglandin inhibitors, acting both centrally and peripherally.

c. **Dosages**. Ibuprofen is available OTC at 200-mg strength. For mild to moderate pain, the usual dosage is 200 to 400 mg taken three or four times daily.

d. **Precautions**

(1) Ibuprofen may cause gastrointestinal distress, including epigastric pain and nausea. It must be used cautiously in patients with peptic ulcer.

(2) Less common adverse effects include visual disturbances, skin rash, headache, edema, and thrombocytopenia.

(3) Cross-sensitivity with aspirin may occur.

(4) Like salicylates and para-aminophenols, phenylpropionic acids may cause papillary necrosis.

II. SLEEP AIDS

A. General considerations

1. **Definition. Insomnia** refers to the inability to fall asleep or remain asleep throughout the night. At least half of all people experience insomnia at some time. Usually, it is transient and self-limiting.

2. **Common causes** of insomnia include situational stress and anxiety, pain or other physical discomfort, changes in daily routine, increasing age, depression, endocrine abnormalities, sleep apnea, nocturnal myoclonus, conditions with nocturnal exacerbation, and drug use. **Chronic insomnia** may signal a serious disease.

B. Products

1. **Antihistamines**. Many OTC sleep aids contain antihistamines—mainly of the ethanolamine class—for their sedative effects. For example, Nytol contains **diphenhydramine**, Unisom contains **doxylamine**, and Quiet World contains **pyrilamine**.

a. **Dosages**. Usually, administration of 25 mg of diphenhydramine, doxylamine, or pyrilamine produces sedation adequate to induce sleep.

b. **Precautions**

(1) Antihistamines may cause such adverse effects as ataxia, dizziness, tinnitus, blurred vision, dry mouth and throat, and paradoxical CNS stimulation (rare).

(2) Gastrointestinal problems (e.g., nausea, vomiting, diarrhea) sometimes occur but are rarest with the ethanolamines (a fact that contributes to their popularity as sleep aids).

2. **L-Tryptophan**. This agent is thought to reduce latency (i.e., the time it takes to fall asleep), increase sleep time, and reduce the number of nocturnal awakenings. However, it is not presently approved as a sleep aid.

3. **Other ingredients in sleep aids. Analgesics** may be added to sleep aids to reduce any pain that may be interfering with sleep. Examples of sleep aids containing analgesics include Sominex-2 Pain Relief (with acetaminophen) and Quiet World (with aspirin and acetaminophen).

III. STIMULANTS

A. **Therapeutic uses.** Stimulants improve mental alertness, reduce the urge to sleep, and elevate the mood. **Caffeine** is the only approved OTC stimulant. OTC products containing caffeine include No Doz, Vivarin, and Dexitac.

B. **Mechanism of action**. A methylated xanthine derivative, caffeine produces stimulant activity in both the CNS (medulla and cortex) and the periphery; its peripheral actions enhance the force of skeletal muscle contractions and reduce muscle fatigue.

C. **Dosages**. OTC caffeine products contain 100 to 250 mg of caffeine in either immediate- or sustained-release form.

D. Precautions

1. **Caffeinism** may occur when caffeine intake exceeds 1 g/day (the equivalent of about 10 cups of coffee). Signs and symptoms of this syndrome include anxiety, muscle twitching, agitation, restlessness, and irritability.

2. **Caffeine overdose** may cause convulsions, vomiting, delirium, sensory disturbances, tachycardia, and gastrointestinal pain.

3. Caffeine is mildly habit-forming.

IV. APPETITE SUPPRESSANTS

A. General considerations

1. **Definition. Obesity** is an abnormal increase in subcutaneous fat cells; a body weight of 20% or more above ideal weight generally indicates obesity.

2. **Causes**. Obesity may result from physiologic, genetic, environmental, or psychological factors (in many cases, it stems from a combination of these).

3. **Therapeutic approaches to obesity**. The most successful weight-reduction regimens incorporate appetite control with planned physical activity and participation in a support group.

4. **Appetite control**. Researchers believe appetite is regulated by the extent of glucose utilization by cells called **glucostats**.
   a. When glucose utilization by glucostats is low, a feedback signal from the **satiety center** (located in the hypothalamus) reduces inhibitory messages to the **appetite center** (also in the hypothalamus). This action stimulates the appetite.
   b. High glucose utilization by glucostats decreases the appetite.

B. Products

1. **Phenylpropanolamine hydrochloride** is a sympathomimetic amine chemically related to amphetamines. Because it has strong peripheral adrenergic effects and weak central stimulant action, this agent is classified as an indirect adrenergic. However, its effectiveness as an appetite suppressant is questionable. OTC products containing phenylpropanolamine include Dexatrim, Unitrol, and Acutrim.
   a. **Dosages.** Immediate-release products contain 25 mg or 37.5 mg of phenylpropanolamine; sustained-release products contain 50 mg or 75 mg.
   b. **Precautions**
      (1) This agent may cause nervousness, tremor, restlessness, insomnia, headache, nausea, and increased blood pressure.
      (2) **Drug interactions**
         (a) Phenylpropanolamine may produce additive CNS and peripheral stimulation when taken with other stimulatory drugs (e.g., caffeine).
         (b) Phenylpropanolamine is contraindicated in patients taking monoamine oxidase (MAO) inhibitors.

2. **Benzocaine**. An insoluble local anesthetic, benzocaine has a direct anesthetic effect on the gastrointestinal mucosa, possibly suppressing appetite by reducing taste sensitivity. However, its value as an appetite suppressant is controversial.
   a. Benzocaine is contained in OTC products such as Ayds and Slim-Line.
   b. **Precaution**. Rare cases of cyanotic reactions and methemoglobinemia have been reported.

STUDY QUESTIONS

Directions: Each question below contains five suggested answers. Choose the **one best** response to each question.

1. Symptoms and signs of "caffeinism" may include all of the following EXCEPT

A. anxiety
B. muscle twitching
C. agitation
D. restlessness
E. cough

2. Besides salicylates, the two classes of drugs that are used as OTC analgesics are

A. phenylpropionates and para-aminophenols
B. phenylpropionates and ethanolamines
C. para-aminophenols and phenylmercurics
D. para-aminophenols and ethanolamines
E. ethanolamines and alkylamines

3. Tinnitus, headache, nausea, and sweating are symptoms of

A. aspirin hypersensitivity
B. acetaminophen toxicity
C. ibuprofen toxicity
D. salicylate toxicity
E. acetaminophen hypersensitivity

4. Acetylcysteine is used to treat overdoses of

A. Benadryl
B. Ayds
C. aspirin
D. No Doz
E. acetaminophen

Directions: Each question below contains three suggested answers of which **one or more** is correct. Choose the answer

A if **I only** is correct
B if **III only** is correct
C if **I and II** are correct
D if **II and III** are correct
E if **I, II, and III** are correct

5. Phenylpropanolamine is contained in which of the following OTC appetite suppressants?

I. Ayds
II. Dexatrim
III. Unitrol

6. Which of the following drugs might be present in an OTC sleep aid product?

I. Diphenhydramine
II. Doxylamine
III. Phenylpropanolamine

7. Para-aminophenol derivatives are useful for

I. treating arthritic pain
II. reducing fever
III. treating headache

8. Side effects of ibuprofen include which of the following?

I. Hepatotoxicity
II. Acidosis
III. Papillary necrosis

ANSWERS AND EXPLANATIONS

1. The answer is E. (*III D 1, 2*) Anxiety, muscle twitching, agitation, and restlessness may all be symptoms of "caffeinism," a syndrome that can occur with excessive caffeine intake (more than 1 g/day—the equivalent of about 10 cups of coffee). Caffeine has a relaxing, not irritating, effect on bronchial smooth muscle.

2. The answer is A. (*I B 2, 3*) The three chemical classes of drugs with analgesic effects that are available in OTC products are salicylates (e.g., aspirin), para-aminophenols (e.g., acetaminophen), and phenylpropionic acids (e.g., ibuprofen). Ethanolamines (e.g., doxylamine) and alkylamines (e.g., chlorpheniramine) are antihistamines, while phenylmercurics are little-used topical antiseptics.

3. The answer is D. [*I B 1 d (5)*] Salicylate toxicity (salicylism) will produce all of the symptoms listed in the question. It is important to recognize that these symptoms are not due to aspirin hypersensitivity, which is manifested most often as bronchoconstriction. Toxic doses of acetaminophen can cause severe liver damage; early symptoms include nausea, vomiting, diarrhea, and sweating, but not tinnitus. Hypersensitivity to acetaminophen is uncommon. Ibuprofen can cause gastrointestinal disturbances.

4. The answer is E. [*I B 2 d (1) (b)*] Acetylcysteine (Mucomyst) is used to treat acetaminophen toxicity; early administration is important. Acetylcysteine presumably acts by increasing the glutathione levels in the liver. Conjugation with glutathione is an important hepatic mechanism for inactivating drugs, and an overdose of acetaminophen rapidly depletes the liver's supply of glutathione.

5. The answer is D (II, III). (*IV B 1*) Dexatrim, Unitrol, and Acutrim all contain phenylpropanolamine, an adrenergic amine that can cause CNS and peripheral stimulation (nervousness, insomnia, increased blood pressure). Ayds and Slim-Line contain benzocaine, a local anesthetic, as an appetite suppressant. The value of either phenylpropanolamine or benzocaine as appetite suppressants is questionable.

6. The answer is C (I, II). (*II B 1*) Diphenhydramine and doxylamine are both antihistamines and are present in several OTC sleep aid products. The sedative effect of antihistamines—an unwanted side effect with allergy and cold remedies—is put to use in these sleep aid products. Phenylpropanolamine is a sympathomimetic amine. It is used in some OTC products for its decongestant properties, and in others for its putative anorexiant properties.

7. The answer is D (II, III). (*I B 2*) Para-aminophenols (e.g., acetaminophen) are effective antipyretics and analgesics but do not reduce inflammation. Therefore, they would not be the best choice for treating arthritic pain, since arthritis is an inflammatory disorder. The phenylpropionates (e.g., ibuprofen), like the salicylates (e.g., aspirin), are anti-inflammatory as well as analgesic and antipyretic.

8. The answer is B (III). (*I B 3 d*) Ibuprofen, a para-aminophenol, can cause necrosis of the renal papillae with long-term use of the drug. This unwanted effect can also occur with the other classes of OTC analgesics, namely the salicylates and the para-aminophenols. Hepatotoxity is a potential toxic effect of para-aminophenols; acidosis can occur with salicylate toxicity.

27
OTC Products: Otic and Ophthalmic Drugs

Robert L. McCarthy
Anthony V. Rozzi

I. OTIC DRUGS

A. General considerations

1. **Auditory apparatus**. The ear has three parts—external ear, middle ear, and internal ear.
   a. The **external ear** consists of three major structures.
      (1) The **auricle** (pinna) is an appendage attached to the side of the head, under the ear canal.
      (2) The **external acoustic meatus** (ear canal) is a tube running from the auricle into the temporal bone. About ¼″ long, it protects the middle ear and internal ear.
      (3) The **tympanic membrane** (eardrum), stretching across the inner end of the auditory canal, reacts to sound waves.
   b. The **middle ear** (tympanic cavity), located in the temporal bone, contains the **auditory ossicles** (malleus, incus, and stapes) and the **eustachian (auditory) tube.**
      (1) Sound waves entering from the external ear move the malleus, causing it to vibrate. This vibration moves the incus and, in turn, the stapes, triggering fluid conduction of sound waves.
      (2) The eustachian tube links the middle ear with the nasopharynx.
         (a) Equalizing middle ear pressure with atmospheric pressure, the eustachian tube also serves as a route for infections to reach the middle ear.
         (b) In children, the eustachian tube is very narrow and nearly horizontal, increasing the chance for middle ear infection.
   c. The **internal ear** contains the **bony labyrinth** and the **membranous labyrinth** (located within the bony labyrinth).
      (1) The three parts of the bony labyrinth are the **vestible**, **cochlea**, and **bony semicircular canals**.
      (2) The membranous labyrinth contains the **utricle**, **saccule**, **cochlear duct**, and **membranous semicircular canals**.
      (3) The internal ear contains **receptors** for the senses of hearing and equilibrium.

2. **Ear disorders**
   a. **External ear disorders**
      (1) **External otitis** (also known as swimmer's ear) usually stems from bacterial or fungal infection.
         (a) Penetration of contaminated water or mechanical trauma (as from a foreign object, dust, or other irritant) can set the stage for acute external otitis.
         (b) Psoriasis and seborrhea sometimes lead to chronic external otitis.
      (2) **Auricular disorders** include dermatologic problems, trauma (e.g., hematoma), cellulitis, and boils.
      (3) **Cerumen impaction** may follow attempts to clean the ear.
      (4) **Foreign bodies in the ear** are most common in children.
   b. **Middle ear disorders**
      (1) **Otitis media** is an inflammation or infection of the middle ear.
         (a) **Serous (secretory) otitis media** refers to transudation of sterile serous fluid. It is caused by an obstruction and resulting buildup of negative pressure in the middle ear. Serous otitis media may be acute or chronic.
         (b) **Suppurative otitis media** generally develops from bacterial infection and usually follows an upper respiratory infection; pathogens enter the middle ear via the eustachian tube. Like serous otitis media, suppurative otitis media may be acute or chronic.
      (2) **Mastoiditis**, usually a complication of otitis media, is a bacterial infection of mastoid air cells. Pus accumulates under pressure in the middle ear cavity, leading to necrosis of adjacent tissue and spread of infection into mastoid cells.

(3) **Tympanic membrane perforation** follows an impact injury or severe acoustic trauma.

c. **Internal ear disorders**

(1) **Labyrinthitis** is an inflammation of the labyrinth. This disorder may cause severe, incapacitating vertigo. Viral labyrinthitis commonly stems from upper respiratory tract infection.

(2) Other internal ear disorders include sensory hearing loss, motion sickness, and Ménière's disease.

B. Agents used in otic drugs

1. **Acetic acid** is an anti-infective agent administered as a sterile solution in water. With a pH of 2.9 to 3.3, it has value against organisms that commonly cause external otitis (such organisms cannot grow at low pH).
   a. Acetic acid also has anti-inflammatory and antipruritic action.
   b. For otic use, it is available as a 2% to 5% solution.
2. **Aluminum acetate solution** (Burow's solution) fights infection by reducing the pH of the external ear canal. It also acts as an astringent.
3. **Antipyrine** is an anti-inflammatory and anesthetic agent used to treat the congestive and serous stages of acute otitis media.
   a. Typically, antipyrine is prepared as a 5.4% solution with 1.4% benzocaine (Auralgan).
   b. It also can be used to facilitate removal of cerumen, a brown or yellowish wax secreted by sweat glands in the auricle.
4. **Boric acid**, with very weak anti-infective properties, is therapeutic for external ear canal infections. It is contraindicated in children under 12 years old.
5. **Camphor** is a mild topical antipruritic and analgesic agent with soothing and counterirritant properties. Although it does not relieve inflammation, it induces reflex local vasoconstriction, which has a mild decongestant effect.
6. **Carbamide peroxide** is a ceruminolytic that softens impacted cerumen for irrigation.
7. **Glycerin** is an emollient that softens ear wax and retains moisture.
8. **Menthol**, like camphor, is a counterirritant that provides mild analgesia.
9. **Olive oil**, which is used as an ingredient in over-the-counter (OTC) otic agents, has lubricant and emollient properties that help soften cerumen.
10. **Phenol**, an anti-infective, is not commonly found in otic preparations.

II. OPHTHALMIC DRUGS

A. General considerations

1. **Visual system**

a. The **orbit**, which houses the eyeball, is a skull recess formed by nine bones.

b. The **eye** has three layers.

(1) The **sclera** is the dense, fibrous, protective outer layer.

(a) The **cornea**, which refracts light waves, is the transparent, convex, anterior portion of the eyeball that is continuous with the sclera. Consisting of five layers, the cornea is bathed by aqueous humor.

(b) The **Schlemm's canal** lies at the scleral–corneal junction.

(2) The **choroid**, or middle layer, is highly vascular and heavily pigmented.

(a) The **ciliary body** lies in the anterior portion of the choroid.

(b) The **iris** contains circular and radial smooth muscle fibers. At its center is the **pupil**, a circular opening that responds to changes in light and other stimuli.

(3) The **retina** is the eye's innermost layer.

(a) Containing three layers of neurons, the retina receives light waves from all portions of the eye.

(b) **Visual receptors** called **rods** and **cones** are stimulated by light waves passing through the retina.

(i) Distributed throughout the retina, **rods** respond to low levels of light and detect moving objects.

(ii) **Cones**, concentrated in the **fovea centralis** (a depression in the center of the retina), are specialized for response to bright lights and fine detail.

c. **Accessory structures**

(1) The **eyelids** (palpebrae) consist of skin and muscle; connective tissue forms a ridge at the lid's free edge. Eyelids protect the eyes and help distribute tears.

(2) The **conjunctiva** is a mucous membrane that lines the eyelid and continues over the surface of the eyeball.

(3) The **lacrimal apparatus** consists of tear-secreting structures—the lacrimal glands, lacrimal ducts, lacrimal sacs, and nasolacrimal ducts.

2. Eye disorders

a. Injuries to the eye include lacerations, lid contusions ("black eye"), globe trauma, anterior chamber hemorrhage, eyelid burns, and chemical burns of the cornea and conjunctiva.

b. Lacrimal and eyelid disorders include blepharitis, orbital cellulitis, dacryocystitis, stye, chalazion, and hypoproduction and hyperproduction of tears.

c. Conjunctival disorders include conjunctivitis and trachoma.

d. Corneal problems include keratitis, keratopathy, corneal ulcer, and keratoconus.

e. Uveal tract disorders include uveitis.

f. Retinal and lens disorders include cataract, vascular retinopathies, retinal detachment, and retinitis pigmentosa.

g. Other ocular problems include glaucoma, papilledema, optic atrophy, nystagmus, strabismus, and ophthalmoplegia.

B. Agents used in ophthalmic drugs

1. General considerations. All ophthalmic preparations are sterile products formulated and packaged for instillation into the eye. OTC ophthalmic preparations are intended for use in the following disorders:

a. Insufficient tears (as in keratoconjunctivitis sicca)

b. Corneal edema

c. Eye inflammation and irritation (as from loose foreign matter in the eye and allergic conjunctivitis)

2. Medicinal agents

a. Antipruritic agents include **antipyrine** (0.1% to 0.4%), **camphor**, and **menthol** (which are also counterirritants).

b. Anti-infectives include **boric acid**, a bacteriostatic agent used as an irrigating solution (2%) or an ointment (5% or 10%) [e.g., Blinx, Collyrium].

c. Astringents include **zinc sulfate**, which produces an astringent action on the conjunctiva. Administered as a 0.2% solution, it relieves ocular congestion and irritation.

d. Decongestants and **vasoconstrictors** relieve itching and redness due to ocular inflammation and irritation.

(1) Agents include **naphazoline hydrochloride**, **phenylephrine hydrochloride**, and **tetrahydrozoline hydrochloride**. **Naphazoline**, **phenylephrine**, and **tetrahydrozoline** have a local adrenergic action on conjunctival blood vessels, producing vasoconstriction.

(a) Naphazoline is instilled as a 0.012%, 0.1%, or 0.02% solution (e.g., Clear Eyes, Vasoclear).

(b) Phenylephrine is administered as a 0.12% or 0.25% solution (e.g., Prefrin, Isopto Frin).

(c) Tetrahydrozoline is used in a concentration of 0.05% (e.g., Clear and Bright, Visine).

(2) These agents tend to oxidize, turning pink and then brown.

(3) **Precaution**. Decongestants and vasoconstrictors are contraindicated in people with glaucoma or heart disease.

3. Nontherapeutic substances

a. Tonicity adjusters used in OTC ophthalmic preparations include dextrose, glycerin, potassium chloride, propylene glycol 1%, dextran 40, dextran 70, and sodium chloride.

b. Antioxidants and stabilizers include edetic acid and the sodium salts of bisulfite, metabisulfite, and thiosulfate.

c. Buffers. The ideal pH for ophthalmic preparations is equivalent to that of tears—7.4. However, this pH is hard to achieve because most active ingredients in such products are weak bases, which are most stable at an acidic pH. Consequently, pH generally is adjusted to maintain product stability. Commonly used buffering agents include boric acid, potassium bicarbonate, potassium borate, potassium carbonate, sodium acetate, sodium bicarbonate, sodium borate, and sodium carbonate.

d. Nonionic wetting agents, which increase spreadability by reducing surface tension, include polysorbate 80, polysorbate 120, and tyloxapol.

e. Preservatives include benzalkonium chloride, benzethonium chloride, thimerosal, and parabens. Another preservative—chlorobutanol—is used only in products that are not packaged in plastic.

f. Viscosity-enhancing agents help lengthen time of contact between the eye and the ophthalmic preparation. These agents include dextran 40, dextran 70, celluloses such as hydroxyethylcellulose, gylcerin, polyethylene glycol, and polyvinyl alcohol.

III. CONTACT LENS CARE PRODUCTS

A. General considerations

1. **Definition.** A **contact lens** is a molded plastic device shaped to fit over the cornea.
2. **Uses.** Generally, contact lenses are used to correct refraction, thereby improving visual acuity, and to improve a person's cosmetic appearance. However, they also have value in the treatment of several serious pathologic disorders (e.g., bullous keratopathy). When used therapeutically, contact lenses act as bandages, protecting the corneal epithelium and allowing medication to reach the eye.
3. **Types of contact lenses**
   a. **Rigid (hard) hydrophobic lenses** are made from polymerized esters of acrylic acid, such as polymethylmethacrylate (PMMA). Some may contain Lucite or Plexiglas.
      (1) Because these lenses do not assume the shape of the cornea, they are particularly well-suited for patients who have an irregularly shaped cornea.
      (2) Rigid hydrophobic lenses have a low water content and negligible gas (oxygen) permeability.
      (3) Initially, eye discomfort (foreign body sensation) and irritation occur, possibly reducing wearing time. With continued use, however, these early complaints usually abate.
      (4) These lenses must be cleaned regularly and may be easily scratched or damaged.
   b. **Rigid gas-permeable lenses** (also called extended-wear lenses) are relatively new lenses intended for extended or continuous wear.
      (1) Prolonged wearing time is possible because oxygen can easily penetrate the lens and reach the cornea.
      (2) These lenses are made of silicone acrylate, cellulose acetate butyrate, or polystyrene.
   c. **Soft (flexible) lenses** are hydrophilic, swelling to assume the corneal shape when hydrated.
      (1) Soft lenses are made of soft hydroxyl or lactam moieties of acrylate (hydroxyethylmethacrylate).
      (2) They require very little adaptation time.
      (3) However, they do not refract light as well as hard lenses and thus cannot completely correct certain refractive abnormalities. Also, they are contraindicated in people with an irregularly shaped cornea.
4. **Contraindications**. Contact lenses are contraindicated in anyone with one of the following conditions:
   a. Dust-filled environments
   b. Inadequate blink reflex
   c. Hypoproduction of tears
5. **Cautions.** The following conditions call for cautious use of contact lenses:
   a. Epilepsy
   b. Diabetes mellitus
   c. Arthritis
   d. Fluid-retention pathologies
   e. Pregnancy

B. Contact lens care products.
Each type of contact lens calls for specific care products.

1. **Rigid lens care products**
   a. **Storage and soaking solutions** remove lens debris, prevent microbial growth, and provide hydration. Typically, these solutions contain benzalkonium chloride.
   b. **Wetting solutions** provide a hydrophilic coating and usually include a viscosity-imparting agent, a surfactant, and a preservative. Ingredients in these solutions include polyvinyl alcohol and methylcellulose derivatives.
   c. **Cleaning solutions and gels** contain surfactants that remove debris from the lens surface.
   d. **Adjunctive solutions** (e.g., artificial tears) are applied directly into the eye while the contact lens is in place to hydrate the lens and prolong wearing time.
2. **Rigid gas-permeable lens care products** include surfactant cleaner and a chemical disinfectant for storage.
3. **Soft lens care products**
   a. **Chemical disinfection systems**—alternatives to thermal (heat) disinfection—may involve

two solutions (one for disinfection, the other for rinsing) or a single solution for both rinsing and storage.

b. **Surfactant cleaning solutions** are used for daily removal of lens debris before chemical disinfection.

c. **Rinsing and storage solutions** are used in conjunction with heat disinfection for lens rinsing and storage.

d. **Enzymatic cleaners,** used weekly, remove deposits from the lens surface.

STUDY QUESTIONS

Directions: Each question below contains five suggested answers. Choose the **one best** response to each question.

1. Which of the following substances is used in ophthalmic products to increase the time that the active drug remains in contact with the eye?

A. Hydroxyethylcellulose
B. Sodium borate
C. Sodium chloride
D. Benzalkonium chloride
E. Antipyrine

2. Which of the following conditions could a pharmacist treat with an OTC product?

A. Black eye
B. Glaucoma
C. Hypolacrimation
D. Papilledema
E. Blepharitis

3. Tyloxapol is used in ophthalmic preparations as

A. an anti-infective
B. a viscosity enhancer
C. a tonicity adjuster
D. a wetting agent
E. a preservative

Directions: Each question below contains three suggested answers of which **one or more** is correct. Choose the answer

A if **I only** is correct
B if **III only** is correct
C if **I and II** are correct
D if **II and III** are correct
E if **I, II, and III** are correct

4. Which of the following contact lenses were designed specifically for extended wear?

I. Hard hydrophobic lenses
II. Soft hydrophilic lenses
III. Rigid, gas-permeable lenses

5. Burow's solution is used in OTC preparations as

I. an astringent
II. an anti-infective
III. a tonicity adjuster

ANSWERS AND EXPLANATIONS

1. The answer is A. (*II B 3 f*) Hydroxyethylcellulose possesses high viscosity and surface tension. It will retain medicaments in the eye and increase the contact time between the preparation and the eye. Sodium borate is used in ophthalmic preparations as a buffer; sodium chloride, to adjust tonicity; benzalkonium chloride, as a preservative; and antipyrine, as an antipruritic.

2. The answer is C. (*II A 2, B 1*) Hypolacrimation (insufficient tears) is the only condition listed in the question that can be treated with over-the-counter (OTC) products (artificial tears). A black eye can represent a serious condition, with tissue damage and ocular mechanical damage, and the patient should be referred to a physician. Glaucoma and papilledema (swelling of the optic nerve) are also serious conditions requiring treatment by a physician, with prescription products. Blepharitis (inflammation of the eyelids, often with crusting) may be due to infection or allergy and also calls for referral to a physician.

3. The answer is D. (*II B 3 d*) Tyloxapol and similar surfactants reduce surface tension. They are added to ophthalmic preparations to increase the wettability of the preparation.

4. The answer is B (III). (*III A 3*) Rigid, gas-permeable lenses allow oxygen to penetrate the lens and reach the cornea, which allows for extended wear.

5. The answer is C (I, II). (*I B 2*) Burow's solution is an aluminum acetate solution. It is a powerful astringent and an adequate anti-infective agent. It is not a tonicity adjuster and, in fact, may alter the isotonicity of an ophthalmic preparation.

28
OTC Products: Skin Care, External Drugs, and Contraceptives

Robert L. McCarthy
Anthony V. Rozzi

I. DRY SKIN PRODUCTS

A. General considerations

1. Integumentary system

a. The **skin** has three primary layers.

(1) The **epidermis** is the outermost, superficial layer.

(a) The **stratum corneum**, the top epidermal stratum, is made up of dead cells converted to **keratin**, an insoluble protein that flakes off.

(b) The **malpighian** layer, beneath the stratum corneum, consists of four sublayers.

(2) The **dermis** (also called corium) is the skin's middle layer. It consists of loose connective tissue interwoven with blood and lymphatic vessels, nerves, glands, and hair follicles.

(3) Subcutaneous tissue is the deepest skin layer. Composed mainly of fat, it also contains blood and lymphatic vessels, hair follicle roots, secretory parts of sweat glands, and sensory nerve endings.

b. Epidermal appendages include the nails, glands, and hair.

(1) Nails are composed of epidermal cells that have been converted to hard keratin. They protect the ends of the fingers and toes.

(2) Hair, found over most of the body, originates at the hair follicle. Melanocytes in the hair bulb determine hair color.

(3) Glands

(a) Sebaceous glands are distributed throughout the body (except for the palms and soles). They secrete **sebum**, a substance containing fat, cellular debris, and keratin. Sebum lubricates the hair and skin.

(b) Apocrine glands, found mostly in the axillae, genital area, and mammary areas, secrete sweat with a strong odor ("body odor").

(c) Eccrine glands ("sweat glands"), located throughout the skin except for the ears and lips, produce perspiration that helps regulate body temperature.

2. Dry skin

a. Definition. Dry skin (xerosis) refers to lack of moisture or sebum in the stratum corneum. This condition, characterized by flaking, scaling, and itching, may be acute or chronic. It is most common in winter.

b. Etiology. Dry skin results from inadequate moisture retention in the stratum corneum, as caused by any of the following factors:

(1) Increasing age. As skin ages, it produces less sebum.

(2) Low humidity. Decreased relative and ambient humidity cause the skin to lose water and become dry and hardened.

(3) Skin disorders. Inherited skin disorders (e.g., ichthyosis) or acquired skin disorders (e.g., psoriasis, contact dermatitis, scleroderma) can impair the skin's ability to retain moisture.

(4) Overexposure to sunlight. This can cause skin proteins to keratinize (cross-link), resulting in skin hardening and reduced moisture retention.

(5) Excessive cleansing or bathing. Overexposure to water can bring on dry skin.

c. Treatment goal. The moisture level of the stratum corneum must be increased to improve skin permeability and restore elasticity.

B. Agents used in OTC dry skin products

1. Lubricants. These agents reduce frictional heat, preventing further moisture loss via frictional heat and perspiration. They have a general soothing effect.

2. **Moisturizing agents**. These agents raise the moisture level or increase the relative moisture content of the stratum corneum. They are classified as either humectants or occlusive agents.
   a. **Humectants** promote moisture retention through a hygroscopic action. (The stratum corneum contains natural hygroscopic factors.) Humectants include **glycerin, urea,** and **polyethylene glycols.**
   b. **Occlusive agents** produce an airtight seal over the skin, increasing perspiration and enhancing moisture content. Highly effective in the treatment of dry skin, such agents include **petrolatum** and **zinc oxide paste**. (Occlusive dressings, such as plastic wrap, may be used with certain agents to increase drug absorption.)

3. **Chemical keratinous compounds** soften keratin within the skin. Some of these agents act by disrupting the natural keratinizing process; others are keratolytic, promoting softening and dissolution of the stratum corneum; a few act by altering keratin structure. By allowing moisture to pass into keratinized skin protein for storage, keratinous compounds increase the moisture content of the stratum corneum.
   a. **Urea**, available OTC in concentrations of 10% to 30%, improves the skin's moisture-binding capacity. At high concentrations, it is proteolytic and may cause irritation and burning. Examples include Aquacare and Carmol 20 Cream.
   b. **Lactic acid** increases skin hydration by controlling the rate of keratinization. Markedly hygroscopic, it is a chief element in the skin's natural hygroscopic factor. It is available OTC in concentrations of 2% to 5%. Examples include Lowila Cake and LactiCare.
   c. **Allantoin** relieves dry skin by disrupting keratin structure. Although less effective than urea, it can be used as a protectant because it desensitizes many skin-sensitizing drugs. OTC products may contain allantoin in concentrations of 0.5% to 2%. Examples include Alphosyl, Psorex, and Tegrin.

4. **Hydrocortisone**. This agent, available OTC in a concentration of 0.5%, reduces inflammatory response that accompanies dry skin conditions (inflammation and keratinization have mutually exacerbating effects). Although hydrocortisone does not directly increase skin hydration, it does inhibit skin dehydration.

5. **Nonkeratinized proteins**. These hydrolyzed collagens of low molecular weight (proteins with 10 to 300 amino acids and a molecular weight of 1000) have excellent moisture-binding capacity and directly promote skin hydration. Due to lack of FDA categorization, however, these agents generally are considered cosmetic rather than therapeutic. They may impart a more youthful look to the skin.

II. ACNE PRODUCTS

A. General considerations

1. **Definition. Acne vulgaris** is a common, chronic inflammatory disease of the sebaceous glands, characterized by such lesions as comedones, pustules, papules, and cysts. Usually beginning at puberty, when androgens stimulate sebum production, acne may continue throughout the period of sex hormone activity. Affected areas typically include the face, upper arms, chest, and back.

2. **Etiology**. The precise cause of acne is unknown.
   a. **Factors associated with acne development** include increased sebum production, androgen secretion, bacteria, and keratinization of the follicular wall, leading to blockage and entrapment of sebum and cellular debris.
   b. Other factors associated with acne development include:
      (1) Genetic predisposition
      (2) Overgrowth of the acne bacillus (*Propionibacterium acnes*) on the skin
      (3) Hypersensitivity to sebaceous gland stimulation
      (4) Use of such drugs as iodine, lithium, corticosteroids, halogens, and anticonvulsants
      (5) Contact with tars, oils, and chlorinated hydrocarbons
      (6) Use of oil-based cosmetics
      (7) Stress
      (8) Poor hygiene
      (9) Ingestion of chocolate, colas, and dairy products
      (10) Mechanical factors (e.g., rubbing or stretching of the skin, friction pressure from shirt collars)

3. **Pathogenesis**
   a. The earliest acne lesion is a **microcomedo**—an invisible, noninflamed plug resulting from obstruction of sebaceous glands with sebum and keratin debris.

b. A **comedo** may then develop.

(1) A **closed comedo (whitehead)** occurs in a closed excretory duct; its opening is covered with epidermis, preventing oxidation and drainage.

(2) An **open comedo (blackhead)** is a widely dilated hair follicle filled with dark, horny material that forms a plug. Oxidation of pigment granules causes the dark color.

c. The comedo blocks the flow of sebum to the skin surface. Bacterial lipases then break down triglycerides in sebum. This triggers release of free fatty acids, which irritate the follicular wall, causing inflammation.

d. Inflammation leads to the development of erythematous papules, pustules, or cysts.

(1) Papules are solid, raised, inflamed lesions.

(2) Pustules are papules containing pus.

(3) Cysts are closed, highly inflamed sacs containing fluid or semisolid material.

e. Eventually, most pustules and cysts open, drain, and heal. Deep papules and cysts may leave permanent scars.

4. General therapeutic principles. Treatment aims to reduce inflammation by promoting drainage of sebaceous glands, avoiding rupture of acne lesions, and restricting bacterial growth.

a. Excess sebum is removed from the skin by gently washing the affected area several times daily.

b. Exacerbating cosmetics, drugs, and foods are eliminated.

c. In some cases, a systemic antibiotic (e.g., tetracycline) or a keratolytic (e.g., isotretinoin, tretinoin) is prescribed.

d. Topical OTC acne products may be used to reduce the occurrence of acne lesions, relieve symptoms, and minimize scarring.

B. Agents used in OTC acne products

1. Benzoyl peroxide. One of the most popular and effective acne agents, benzoyl peroxide has antibacterial and comedolytic activity. It is contained in topical liquids, soaps, lotions, creams, and gels that are sold under various trade names (e.g., Fostex, Oxy, Benoxyl, Propa PH, Dry and Clear).

2. Sulfur preparations are antibacterial and keratolytic. They are available in concentrations of 2% to 10% in various creams, lotions, gels, and cleansers.

3. Other keratolytics in OTC acne products include **salicylic acid** (3% to 6%) and **resorcinol** (1% to 2%). These agents are available in creams, gels, lotions, and cleansers.

4. Astringents include **zinc oxide** and **zinc sulfate**. Like keratolytics, they are available in various forms.

III. SUNSCREEN AND SUNTAN PRODUCTS

A. General considerations

1. Definition. Sunburn is an acute reaction caused by overexposure or hypersensitivity of the skin to sunlight or another actinic source.

2. Etiology. Sunburn and suntan result from exposure to ultraviolet (UV) light rays of 290 to 320 nm (referred to as UV-B light). Generalized erythemic reactions peak 6 to 20 hours after exposure.

a. Factors affecting exposure to sunlight

(1) Time of day. In temperate zones, the greatest exposure to harmful light rays occurs between 10 A.M. and 2 P.M.

(2) Season. In northern temperate zones, sunburn is less likely to occur in winter. In summer, an initial exposure of more than 30 minutes at midday can cause sunburn.

(3) Altitude. Sunburn is more likely to occur at high altitudes.

(4) Environmental factors. Snow, sand, and water increase exposure to sunlight by reflecting light rays. However, direct sunlight—although not necessary to sunburn—greatly reduces the amount of UV exposure needed to produce a burn.

b. Predisposing factors. People with fair skin and light hair or with hypersensitivity to sunlight are at greater risk for developing sunburn.

3. Other reactions to sunlight exposure

a. Actinic keratosis may occur after many years of excessive exposure to sunlight. Typically arising during middle age or later, this disorder manifests as a sharply demarcated, roughened or hardened growth, which may be flat or raised.

b. Cancer. Chronic overexposure to sunlight may lead to squamous cell carcinoma, basal cell carcinoma, or, less commonly, malignant melanoma.

c. Phototoxic contact dermatitis. This reaction, which resembles sunburn, may arise where skin has been exposed to sunlight after contact with a photosensitizing substance. Among the most common offending substances are oil of bergamot and coal-tar derivatives.

d. Phototoxicity reactions. These unusual reactions stem from use of certain drugs or from such disorders as albinism or porphyria.

(1) In **drug-related phototoxicity**, sunlight reacts with the drug to produce a toxic drug form. Photosensitizing drugs include thiazides, tetracyclines, sulfonamides, oral hypoglycemic agents, and phenothiazines.

(2) Within a few minutes of exposure to the sun, an exaggerated sunburn-like response develops.

(3) The intensity of drug-related phototoxicity is probably dose-related.

e. Photoallergy. In this delayed hypersensitivity reaction, a person who has been previously sensitized to a particular drug may develop eczema or an exudative or papulovesicular reaction after exposure to light.

(1) Sunlight chemically alters the drug in the skin, changing it to an active antigen.

(2) Usually, the reaction occurs after an incubation period of 24 to 48 hours of combined drug and sunlight exposure.

(3) Photoallergy is not dose-dependent.

B. OTC sunscreen products. These products help prevent sunburn and/or promote gradual tanning. Applied properly, they block the most harmful UV rays while permitting penetration of less damaging rays that allow tanning.

1. Classification. Based on how much UV light they allow to penetrate the skin, sunscreen products fall into three categories.

a. Sunburn preventive agents. These products absorb at least 95% of UV light in the 290 to 320-nm range.

b. Suntan agents. Absorbing 85% of UV light within 290 to 320 nm, these products permit tanning in some people but may allow sunburn in those with greater susceptibility (e.g., fair-skinned people).

c. Opaque sunblocks. These agents reflect, or scatter, all UV light from 290 to 770 nm, preventing or minimizing sunburn and suntan.

2. Sun protection factor (SPF). Most sunscreen products display a numerical SPF that reflects how effectively the product prevents sunburn in the average person.

a. SPF is determined from a formula that uses the minimal erythema dose (MED)—the amount of solar energy needed to produce minimally perceptible skin redness.

b. The SPF of a specific product equals the MED in skin protected with the product, divided by the MED in unprotected skin.

$$\text{SPF} = \frac{\text{MED in protected skin}}{\text{MED in unprotected skin}}$$

c. The higher a product's SPF, the more protection it offers. For example, a sunscreen with SPF 15 allows the user to stay in the sun fifteen times longer without burning, compared to unprotected exposure. A product with SPF 3 allows safe exposure lasting only three times as long as unprotected exposure.

3. Application of sunscreen products

a. Because a sunscreen takes roughly 30 minutes to bind on the skin, it should be applied at least that long before exposure to the sun.

b. The sunscreen should be applied to all areas of anticipated exposure.

c. After prolonged swimming or excessive perspiration, the sunscreen should be reapplied.

d. Precaution. Some people are sensitive to sunscreen agents.

4. Agents used in OTC sunscreen products

a. Chemical sunscreens. These agents reduce the risk of sunburn by absorbing harmful UV rays from incident sunlight and transmitting only less damaging wavelengths.

(1) Aminobenzoic acid (para-aminobenzoic acid, PABA). Considered to be a very effective chemical sunscreen agent, PABA protects against sunburn when prepared as a 5% solution in 70% ethanol. It has an extremely low incidence of hypersensitivity and other adverse reactions.

(2) PABA esters [glyceryl PABA, padimate A (amyldimethyl PABA), padimate O (octyl dimethyl PABA)]. Although these agents are as effective as PABA, they cause more adverse reactions.

(3) Benzophenones, sulisobenzone, dioxybenzone, and so forth. Because they absorb the broadest spectrum of UV light (250 to 400 nm), these agents protect against the phototoxic and photosensitive effects of drugs as well as against sunburn.

(4) **Cinnamic acid, homosalate (homomenthyl salicylate), and digalloyl trioleate**. Introduced before the PABA series, these agents have a weak absorptive ratio and are a poor choice for people who need photosensitivity protection.

b. Physical sunscreens. Acting as a physical barrier, these agents deflect or scatter UV light in the 200 to 700-nm range.

(1) The three major physical sunscreen agents are **red veterinary petrolatum (RVP), titanium dioxide**, and **zinc oxide.**

(2) Although unsuitable for people who wish to get a tan, physical sunscreens offer excellent protection against sunburn and photosensitivity.

(3) These agents are opaque and therefore less cosmetically acceptable than chemical sunscreens. Usually, they are applied over limited areas (e.g., the nose and lips).

IV. FOOT CARE PRODUCTS

A. Corn, callus, and wart products

1. General considerations

a. Corn

(1) **Definition**. A **corn** is a painful hyperkeratotic mass, usually found over a toe joint (most commonly, on the fifth toe), or between the toes.

(2) **Etiology**. Corns typically result from irritation by ill-fitting shoes.

(3) **Classification**

(a) **Hard corns**—usually caused by an underlying bony prominence—are raised, shiny areas on the toe surface.

(b) **Soft corns** typically appear as hyperkeratotic regions in the web between the fourth and fifth toes. Accumulated perspiration makes these corns appear soft.

b. Callus

(1) **Definition**. A **callus** is a circumscribed region of hyperkeratosis at locations of repeated trauma (e.g., friction or pressure). Unlike a corn, a callus usually lacks a central core. The typical callus is yellow and slightly raised, with a more extensive hyperkeratotic region than that of a corn. It is usually painless.

(2) **Etiology**. A callus commonly stems from loose shoes, an orthopedic problem, or walking barefoot.

c. Wart

(1) **Definition**. A **wart (verruca)** is an intraepidermal skin tumor with a horny surface. Most common in children, a wart may resolve spontaneously (although this sometimes takes years.)

(2) **Etiology.** Warts are caused by the human papillomavirus, which may be transmitted by direct contact or autoinoculation.

(a) Immunologic susceptibility is involved.

(b) Public showers and swimming pools are typical transmission sites.

(3) **Classification**

(a) **Common warts (verrucae vulgaris)** are sharply demarcated tumors with a diameter of 2 to 10 mm.

(i) They may be yellow, light gray, brown, or brownish-black.

(ii) Most frequently, common warts arise at sites subjected to repeated trauma (e.g., the hands or fingers).

(iii) A **plantar wart** is a type of common wart that forms on the sole of the foot. It may be extremely painful due to pressure from walking.

(iv) **Periungual** and **subungual warts** are common warts that form around and beneath the nail beds.

(b) **Venereal warts (condyloma acuminata)** are small, soft, moist, pink or red lesions that grow rapidly. Usually developing in clusters resembling cauliflower heads, these warts may be sexually transmitted.

(c) **Filiform warts** are thin, long projections that typically arise on the face and neck.

(d) **Flat warts** are slight elevations that form in clusters of up to several hundred. They may have a linear distribution, reflecting their spread via scratching. They are most common in children.

d. Treatment goals

(1) For **corns and calluses**, treatment aims to correct the underlying cause—for instance, by avoiding walking barefoot or by wearing orthopedic shoes. OTC products may provide palliative relief.

(2) For **warts**, treatment is directed at removing the lesions and relieving pain, using

topical agents or surgical excision. However, in many cases, warts do not respond to treatment or recur after seemingly successful treatment.

2. **Agents used in OTC corn, callus, and wart products.** Keratolytics, emollients, and local anesthetics are the major agents in these products.
   a. **Salicylic acid**. This keratolytic is the most common active ingredient in corn, callus, and wart products. At concentrations of 10% to 40%, it is contained in plasters, flexible collodions, and occlusive ointments (e.g., Freezone, Compound W, and Off-Ezy).
   b. **Glacial acetic acid and lactic acid**. These corrosive agents help remove corns, calluses, and warts.
   c. **Collodions** commonly serve as vehicles for keratolytics because they form an adherent flexible or rigid film that prevents moisture evaporation and helps the active ingredient penetrate the affected area. Compound W and Off-Ezy are examples of products containing collodions.
   d. **Castor oil**, an emollient, is an ingredient in some corn and callus products. It may also be used alone.
   e. **Local anesthetics** impart analgesia to corn and callus products. Agents used include **diperodon**, **benzocaine**, **menthol**, and **camphor.**
   f. **Zinc chloride**, an astringent and caustic, is available in several products.
   g. **Calcium pantothenate** stimulates epithelialization and relieves itching. It is the active ingredient in Vergo Cream.

B. Athlete's foot products

1. **General considerations**
   a. **Definition. Athlete's foot (tinea pedis)** is a common fungal infection of the foot, characterized by itchy, scaly lesions between the toes that later may affect the plantar surface of the arch. Vesicles and bullae may develop during acute exacerbations.
   b. **Etiology**. Athlete's foot stems from infection by *Trichophyton mentagrophytes*, *T. rubrum*, or *Epidermophyton floccosum*. Transmission usually occurs by walking barefoot in locker rooms or hotel bathrooms.

2. **Agents used in OTC athlete's foot products**. Antifungals, keratolytics, astringents, and anti-inflammatory agents are the major agents in these products.
   a. **Carbol-fuchsin solution (Castellani's paint)** is an antifungal agent that also acts as a local anesthetic and astringent.
   b. **Tolnaftate**, also an antifungal, is used for both treatment and prophylaxis of athlete's foot. Most effective against the dry, scaly form of the disease, tolnaftate is available in such OTC products as Aftate and Tinactin.
   c. **Organic fatty acids**, such as **sodium caprylate** and **sodium propionate**, are antifungal agents contained in Deso-Creme, and Verdefam.
   d. **Triacetin** (glyceryl triacetate) exerts an antifungal action by reducing the pH of the affected area when hydrolysis of triacetin by fungal enzymes causes release of acetic acid. Triacetin is an ingredient in Enzactin and Fungacetin.
   e. **Undecylenic acid** and **zinc undecylenate** are antifungal agents used in the treatment of mild athlete's foot. (Zinc undecylenate also has astringent properties.) These compounds are contained in various OTC products, including Desenex and Ting.
   f. **Calcium undecylenate** resembles zinc undecylenate, having mild astringent as well as antifungal properties. It is found in Caldesene and Cruex.
   g. **Phenolic compounds and derivatives**, such as **phenol**, **resorcinol**, and **chloroxylenol**, are antifungal and keratolytic agents.
   h. **Salicylic acid**, a keratolytic, is contained in some OTC products. It is found in Blis-to-sol.
   i. **Quaternary ammonium compounds**, such as **benzethonium chloride** and **methylbenzethonium chloride**, have detergent and antiseptic properties.
   j. **Quinoline derivatives** exert antifungal activity.
   k. **Aluminum acetate (Burow's solution)** and **aluminum chloride** have astringent properties that help reduce inflammation. In higher concentrations, they also are antibacterial.

V. ANTIPARASITIC PRODUCTS

A. General considerations

1. **Pediculosis**
   a. **Definition. Pediculosis** refers to infestation by lice of the family Pediculidae, which feed on human blood and lay their eggs (nits) in body hairs or clothing.
   b. **Classification**
      (1) **Pediculosis capitis (head lice)** is infestation of the scalp or, occasionally, the eyebrows, eyelashes, or beard.

(a) Most common in children, this disease is often transmitted through poor personal hygiene and overcrowded conditions.
(b) Severe itching and scalp excoriation are typical manifestations.
(c) Nits, attached to hair shafts, are visible on inspection.

(2) **Pediculosis corporis (body lice)** is infestation of the body.
(a) Nits typically live in seams of clothing worn next to the skin (e.g., underwear).
(b) Body lice can spread through bedsheets and shared clothing, especially in overcrowded areas.
(c) Signs and symptoms include itching, red papules (typically on the shoulders or trunk), and, in later stages, rashes or wheals.

(3) **Pediculosis pubis (pubic lice)** is infestation of the pubic hairs or, less commonly, other sites such as body hair and axillary hair.
(a) The disease is transmitted venereally and by contact with infested bedsheets, towels, or clothing.
(b) Anogenital itching and skin irritation develop and small blue-gray spots may arise on the thighs.
(c) Nits attach to the skin at the base of the hair. Their relatively large size makes them fairly easy to detect.

2. Scabies

a. Definition. Scabies is infestation by the parasite *Sarcoptes scabiei* (itch mite).
(1) The mite burrows into the stratum corneum, where the female deposits eggs. Within a few days, larvae hatch and gather around hair follicles.
(2) Characteristic scabies lesions result from a sensitivity reaction. These itchy, erythematous nodules typically become excoriated from scratching.
(3) Common lesion sites include finger webs, the flexor surface of the wrist and elbows, axillary folds, nipples in females, and genitals in males.

b. Etiology. Scabies is transmitted venereally or by skin contact with an infested person.

3. Other parasites that may infest human beings include mange mites (animal scabies), bedbugs, ticks, and chiggers.

B. General therapeutic measures

1. Pediculosis

a. Lindane (gamma benzene hexachloride, GBH) or **benzyl benzoate**—both prescription drugs—are applied daily for two days. Benzyl benzoate comes in lotion form; lindane is available as a shampoo, cream, ointment, or lotion.
b. Clothes and bedding should be laundered, ironed, or dry-cleaned.
c. Other contaminated objects (e.g., combs) should be boiled or otherwise decontaminated.
d. Benzyl benzoate or lindane may be reapplied in 1 week.

2. Scabies

a. After bathing with soap and water, lindane or benzyl benzoate is applied over the entire body from the neck down and left on for 24 hours. It may be reapplied in 1 week.
b. Bedding and clothing should be laundered or dry-cleaned and other objects decontaminated as appropriate.

C. OTC pediculicides and scabicides. As mentioned above, the preferred agents—lindane and benzyl benzoate—are available by prescription only. The OTC agents described below are considered second-line drugs.

1. Pyrethrins (e.g., A-200 Pyrinate, Pyrinyl, Rid) are extracted from chrysanthemum flowers.

a. Mechanism of action. Pyrethrins stimulate the parasitic nervous system by competitively inhibiting cationic conductances, thereby blocking nerve impulse transmission. This, in turn, paralyzes and kills the parasite.

b. Precautions
(1) Water-based pyrethrins are less toxic (but also less effective) than kerosene-based pyrethrins. Nonetheless, they should not be applied to the face, mucous membranes, or orifices.
(2) Because of their greater toxicity, kerosene-based pyrethrins are best suited for application on contaminated objects rather than on human skin.

2. Piperonyl butoxide. This agent inhibits the hydrolytic enzymes that metabolize pyrethrins and is effective when used in conjunction with pyrethrins (potentiation results). It is available in concentrations of 1.65% to 4%.

VI. CONTRACEPTIVES

A. General considerations

1. **Definition. Contraception** refers to prevention of conception—that is, of ovum fertilization by a spermatozoon.

2. **Contraceptive methods** include medications, devices, and techniques that prevent or alter a process involved in conception.
   a. **Mechanical barrier methods** prevent sperm from entering the cervix or uterus; **spermicides** kill or immobilize sperm before they can reach the uterus. Many vaginal OTC contraceptives act by both mechanisms.
   b. Other contraceptive methods work by preventing follicular development, altering ovum transport, preventing nidation (embryonic implantation into the endometrium), or eliminating unprotected intercourse during ovulation (as with basal body temperature calculation).

B. OTC contraceptive products

1. **Condom**. A sheath made of rubber or animal membrane, the condom is a barrier device that traps semen, preventing it from contacting the vagina.
   a. Besides protecting against pregnancy, condoms also help prevent transmission of some sexually transmitted diseases (STDs).
   b. For maximum protection, the condom should be placed on the penis as soon as erection occurs and worn throughout coitus. As soon as possible after ejaculation, the penis should be withdrawn from the vagina with the rim of the condom held firmly to prevent leakage of semen.
   c. Rubber condoms offer greater protection against STDs. However, they dull sensations somewhat and may cause an allergic reaction in some people. Condoms made of animal membranes are thinner. Consequently, they offer greater sensitivity (by allowing transmission of body heat) but provide less protection against pregnancy and STDs.
   d. Condoms are available in a wide variety of colors. Some come with special features, such as ribbing, a reservoir tip (which helps prevent bursting), and spermicidal coating.

2. **Vaginal contraceptives**. Except for the condom, all OTC contraceptives are vaginal spermicidal agents.
   a. **Spermicidal creams and jellies**. Inserted into the vagina with an applicator, these agents melt or spread over vaginal surfaces, immobilizing sperm.
      (1) When used with a diaphragm, these products provide highly effective contraception.
      (2) Creams, which offer more lubrication than jellies, are considered more effective because they fill the vaginal canal more effectively. However, jellies are water-soluble and thus easier to remove if accidentally spilled.
      (3) Creams and jellies should be inserted 10 to 30 minutes before intercourse and must remain in the vagina for 6 to 8 hours afterward. Each subsequent act of intercourse necessitates an additional application.
   b. **Aerosol foams**. These agents, inserted via applicator, are highly effective because they completely fill the vagina and cover the cervical os.
   c. **Vaginal suppositories**. Upon contact with vaginal fluids, these products produce a foam that acts as a spermicidal barrier.
      (1) Inserted about 10 minutes before coitus, each suppository remains effective for 1 hour.
      (2) If intercourse is delayed for more than 1 hour after suppository insertion or if intercourse is repeated, a new suppository must be inserted.
   d. **Vaginal sponge**. A relatively new device, the vaginal sponge is made of polyurethane impregnated with spermicide. Acting as a barrier, the sponge releases the spermicide and absorbs vaginal fluids.
      (1) To activate the spermicide, the sponge must be moistened with water before insertion.
      (2) The sponge may be inserted up to 24 hours before intercourse and should not be removed for at least 6 hours after the last act of intercourse. Intercourse can be repeated for up to 24 hours after insertion without the need for a new sponge or additional spermicidal agents.

3. **Spermicidal agents**
   a. **Nonionic surfactants. Menfegol, nonoxynol 9,** and **octoxynol 9** are category I spermicides: They act directly on the lipid layer that protects the sperm surface, immobilizing the sperm.
   b. Other agents, such as **phenylmercuric acetate** and **phenylmercuric nitrate**, are category II agents: They kill sperm directly by producing a hostile environment by altering vaginal pH.

STUDY QUESTIONS

Directions: Each question below contains five suggested answers. Choose the **one best** response to each question.

1. Urea is used to treat dry skin because it is

A. a humectant
B. a mild soap
C. an occlusive agent
D. an anti-inflammatory agent
E. a demulcent

2. An example of a sunblocking agent would be

A. cinnamic acid
B. padimate A
C. homosalate
D. titanium dioxide
E. sweet oil

3. Tinea pedis is commonly known as

A. athlete's foot
B. corns
C. calluses
D. warts
E. blackheads

4. Tolnaftate is used in the treatment of athlete's foot because it is

A. anti-inflammatory
B. antifungal
C. astringent
D. keratolytic
E. antibacterial

Directions: Each question below contains three suggested answers of which **one or more** is correct. Choose the answer

A if **I only** is correct
B if **III only** is correct
C if **I and II** are correct
D if **II and III** are correct
E if **I, II, and III** are correct

5. Benzoyl peroxide is the active ingredient in which of the following skin care products?

I. Fostex
II. Dry and Clear
III. Propa PH

6. Which of the following substances might be used as an occlusive agent?

I. Polyethylene glycol
II. Petrolatum
III. Zinc oxide

7. True statements about piperonyl butoxide include which of the following?

I. It is a natural pediculicide
II. It is useful in mange control
III. It inhibits pyrethrin metabolism

8. True statments about the vaginal sponge include which of the following?

I. It acts as a physical barrier to sperm
II. It is impregnated with a nonionic spermicide
III. It may be inserted up to 24 hours prior to intercourse

ANSWERS AND EXPLANATIONS

1. The answer is A. (*I B 2 a*) Humectants such as urea will keep the skin moist by drawing water into the area. At high concentrations, urea is also proteolytic, and may cause irritation and burning. In OTC products for treating dry skin, urea is used at a concentration of 10% to 30%.

2. The answer is D. (*III B 1 c, 4 b*) Titanium dioxide is the only complete sunblocking agent listed in the question. Its solid particles deflect ultraviolet light rays, offering excellent protection.

3. The answer is A. (*IV B 1 a*) Tinea pedis, or athlete's foot, is a common fungal infection of the foot. A wide variety of OTC products are marketed for the treatment of athlete's foot; these may contain antifungal agents, keratolytics, astringents, or anti-inflammatory agents, either alone or in combination.

4. The answer is B. (*IV B 2 b*) Tolnaftate is an antifungal agent that is used to treat athlete's foot, a common condition caused by fungi. Tolnaftate is useful not only therapeutically but also prophylactically.

5. The answer is E (all). (*II B 1*) Fostex, Dry and Clear, and Propa PH all contain benzoyl peroxide, a popular and effective anti-acne agent used for its antibacterial and comedolytic effects.

6. The answer is D (II, III). (*I B 2 b*) Occlusive agents produce an airtight seal over the skin, increasing perspiration and thereby enhancing the skin's moisture content. Such agents include petrolatum and zinc oxide. Lassar's paste is a mixture containing zinc oxide and white petrolatum. When applied it will produce an effective occlusive covering for the treatment of dry skin.

7. The answer is B (III). (*V C 2*) Piperonyl butoxide is used in conjunction with pyrethrins in the treatment of pediculosis (lice) and scabies. Piperonyl butoxide inhibits the parasite's natural ability to metabolize pyrethrins and therefore enhances the pesticidal effects of pyrethins.

8. The answer is E (all). (*VI B 2 d*) The vaginal sponge (Today's Sponge) is a relatively new contraceptive device. Made of polyurethane and impregnated with a nonionic surfactant spermicide, the vaginal sponge serves both as a physical barrier and as a spermicidal agent. It may be inserted as early as 24 hours before intercourse, and intercourse may be repeated during that time period without the need for a new sponge or additional spermicide.

Part IV
Clinical Pharmacy and Therapeutics

Alan H. Mutnick
Paul F. Souney

29
Therapeutic Drug Monitoring

Lyndon D. Braun

I. THERAPEUTIC DRUG MONITORING

A. Basic pharmacokinetic terms and principles

1. **Bioavailability** is the fraction of an administered dose that reaches the systemic circulation.
2. **Volume of distribution** is the amount of drug in the body relative to the concentration of drug in the blood (or plasma).

$$V_d = D/C_p$$

where V_d is the apparent volume of distribution, D is the drug dose, and C_p is the plasma concentration of the drug.
3. **Clearance** is the volume of blood (or plasma) that can be completely cleared of a drug per unit of time (units = volume/time).
4. **Half-life** is the time required for the drug concentration in the blood (or plasma) to be reduced 50% (provided no drug absorption occurs during the decline). Half-life is also a measure of the time required for the drug concentration in the blood (or plasma) to reach steady-state concentration with a new dosing regimen.
5. **Steady-state concentration** is the drug concentration at which the body is in equilibrium (i.e., the rate of drug availability equals drug elimination).
6. **Loading dose**. The amount of drug that must be administered to bring the drug concentration in the blood (or plasma) into the therapeutic range rapidly when initiating therapy or increasing the dosing rate after inadequate therapy.
7. **Maintenance dose** is the amount of drug that must be administered to maintain steady-state concentration.
8. **Dosing interval**. The amount of time between consecutive doses of a regularly administered drug. This is usually a multiple of 24 hours or a number that is easily divided into 24 hours.
9. **Trough or minimum concentration** is the lowest concentration of a drug within a dosing interval. This typically is reached at the end of the dosing interval, immediately before the next dose administration.
10. **Peak or maximum concentration** is the highest drug concentration within a dosing interval. This usually is reached within 2 hours of dose administration but depends on the route of administration.

B. Drug criteria for therapeutic drug monitoring

1. Serum drug concentration and the concentration at the receptor site must be in equilibrium..
2. Intensity and duration of the pharmacodynamic effect (efficacy and toxicity) must be correlated with the timing of the sampling and drug concentration at the receptor site.

C. Benefits of therapeutic drug monitoring

1. At initiation of drug therapy, when rapid and effective treatment is needed (as in antibiotic therapy or anticonvulsant therapy), drug monitoring helps determine the proper dose and dosing rate quickly.
2. During maintenance therapy in stable, chronically ill patients (such as those requiring antiarrhythmic therapy or antimanic therapy), drug monitoring can help determine the best possible dosage regimen, one that provides therapeutic outcome while avoiding toxicity.

3. When interacting drugs are added to or removed from a dosage regimen, monitoring can help maintain optimal therapy.

4. Patients with altered physiologic and pharmacokinetic parameters may benefit from therapeutic drug monitoring.
   a. **Impaired renal function**
      (1) Dosage modification may be necessary, depending on the extent of renal impairment and the amount of drug normally excreted unchanged in the urine.
      (2) Renal function normally declines with increasing age; therefore, middle-aged and older patients, in addition to patients with nephrotoxicity or acute or chronic renal failure, may require therapeutic monitoring.
      (3) Usually creatinine clearance is used to estimate renal function. The Cockroft and Galt equation is:

$$\frac{(140-\text{age})(\text{kg of body weight})}{(72)(\text{serum creatinine in mg/dl})}\ (0.85 \text{ for females}) = \text{ml/min}$$

   b. **Impaired hepatic function**
      (1) Dosage modification may be necessary, depending on the:
         (a) Extent of hepatic impairment (often difficult to determine)
         (b) Amount of drug normally metabolized
         (c) Contribution of metabolites to therapeutic efficacy or toxicity
      (2) Impaired hepatic albumin production may necessitate a dosage change for drugs that are highly protein-bound.
      (3) Unlike renal function tests, liver function tests measure the presence of hepatic injury, not the extent of hepatic function.
   c. **Congestive heart failure** can impair absorption, distribution, and elimination of many drugs.
   d. Disease states and other changes that affect **protein binding** are discussed in section I F 4.

D. Routes of drug administration

1. **Intravenous (IV).** This route delivers 100% of the drug directly into the circulation (bioavailability = 100%).
   a. **Bolus.** The entire dose is administered rapidly, producing high plasma concentration and (usually) the most rapid effect. Injection volume is unlimited.
   b. **Infusion.** The drug is administered at a constant rate. At steady state, the rate of drug administration is equal to the rate of drug elimination. Plasma concentration is 50% of the way from starting concentration to steady-state concentration after 1 half-life; 75% after 2 half-lives; 90% after 3.3 half-lives. Injection volume is unlimited.

2. **Subcutaneous (SC).** The drug is injected into subcutaneous tissue (bioavailability ≤ 100%).
   a. Entry of the drug into circulation is slower than through IV administration and is limited by drug solubility, drug lipophilicity, and subcutaneous circulation.
   b. The peak effect is generally much less than with IV administration; however, the duration of effect is generally longer than with IV administration, owing to slower release into the circulation.
   c. The maximum injection volume is approximately 1 ml.

3. **Intramuscular (IM).** The drug is administered into muscle tissue (usually deep muscle, such as gluteus or deltoid) [bioavailability ≤ 100%].
   a. Entry of the drug into the circulation is slower than with IV administration and is limited by drug solubility, drug lipophilicity, and muscular circulation.
   b. The peak effect is generally much less than with IV administration; however, the duration of effect is generally longer than with IV administration, owing to slower release into the circulation.
   c. Administration into a depot site of a minimally soluble drug or vehicle can produce therapeutic levels of some drugs for up to 2 to 4 weeks.
   d. The maximum injection volume is approximately 2 to 5 ml.

4. **Intradermal (ID).** The drug is injected into dermal tissue. This route is generally used for local effect (e.g., allergy testing) and only rarely, if ever, for systemic effects, due to poor distribution into the systemic circulation. The maximum injection volume is approximately 1 ml.

5. **Oral (PO).** The drug is swallowed (bioavailability ≤ 100%). Entry of the drug into the circulation is slower than with IV administration and limited by many factors, detailed in section I E.
   a. **First-pass effect.** Orally administered drugs must pass through portal circulation and the liver before entering systemic circulation. This reduces the bioavailability of many drugs because they are significantly metabolized before reaching the bloodstream. Some drugs need to be administered in much larger doses orally than intravenously (e.g., propranolol requires an oral dose 20 to 40 times larger than its IV dose).

b. Metabolic activation. Some drugs are activated on passage through the liver before entering the systemic circulation. Drugs that are administered in inactive form (e.g., chlorazepate, sulindac) must be metabolically altered to a physiologically active and available form. This type of drug would have a much smaller effect if administered intravenously since only a small fraction of the systemic circulation passes through the liver. This contrasts to gastrointestinal absorption, in which virtually all of the portal circulation passes through the liver.

6. **Sublingual (SL)**. The drug is administered by placement under the tongue (bioavailability is ≤ 100% but often greater than with oral administration). Advantages of this administration route include rapid absorption, due to the vascularity of sublingual tissues, and a large extent of bioavailability, because sublingual circulation passes directly into the systemic circulation rather than into portal circulation. The usual sublingual form is a tablet, but some agents are commercially available in a spray.

7. **Rectal (PR)**. The drug is administered rectally, usually in suppository form, but otherwise as a liquid (bioavailability ≤ 100%). Absorption is slow, erratic, and often incomplete. Bioavailability may be greater than with oral administration because only one (the superior hemorrhoidal vein) of the three rectal veins empties into the portal circulation.

8. **Vaginal (PV)**. The drug is administered vaginally, as a suppository, tablet, cream, or foam. Drug effects are usually local, but systemic absorption does occur through vaginal mucosa. Systemic effects are usually side effects, rather than the desired therapeutic end.

9. **Topical**. The drug is applied to the skin and absorbed into systemic circulation after passing through all five layers of stratum corneum (the outermost epidermis).
   a. Bioavailability is variable and depends on thickness of the skin surface, circulation in the local area, drug lipophilicity, and skin condition (see section I E 4).
   b. Advantages of topical drug administration include a long duration of action and the ability to remove (wipe off) the dosage form once it has been administered.
   c. Absorption is generally slower than with most other routes of administration.

10. **Inhalation**. The drug is inhaled into the lungs, where the site of action may be local (e.g., beclomethasone) or systemic (e.g., enflurane and other inhalation anesthetics).
    a. Absorption is generally rapid, due to the vascular nature of the pulmonary capillary system, but it also depends on drug lipophilicity, droplet or particle size, pulmonary function, and respiratory status.
    b. Most systemic inhaled drugs are generally short-acting (minutes to hours) and may be eliminated by the lungs. Locally acting inhaled drugs generally have longer durations of action and may last from 2 to 12 hours or more.

11. **Buccal**. The drug is absorbed through the oral mucosa, usually placed between cheek and gum. Absorption is usually rapid, and bioavailability is similar to that of sublingual administration (see section I D 6).

12. **Intranasal**. The drug is inhaled nasally and then absorbed through the nasal mucosa. Onset is generally rapid, but bioavailability can be variable and dependent on the condition of nasal membranes. Drugs may be administered for a local (e.g., phenylephrine) or systemic (e.g., desmopressin) effect. The duration of action may be from minutes to hours, depending on the drug.

13. **Ophthalmic (OU, OS, OD)**. The drug is administered onto the conjunctiva. The effect is usually local, with systemic side effects occasionally occurring. Absorption into the central nervous system (CNS) is sometimes a problem because of the proximity of the eyes to the brain and the lipophilic nature of ophthalmically active medications.

14. **Otic (AU, AS)**. The drug is administered into the auditory canal, usually for local results such as an anti-inflammatory or anti-infective effect.

E. Absorption

1. **Dissolution**. Drugs administered in solid dosage forms must be dissolved so that they can be absorbed across membranes. Determinants of dissolution are particle size, coating or protective layer (e.g., tablets), and drug solubility. Some tablets owe their sustained-release properties to slow dissolution. Most highly bioavailable oral dosage forms are readily soluble in gastric juices.

2. **Membrane transport**. Drug molecules must cross the membrane of absorption to enter the systemic circulation. Most drugs cross the membrane by simple diffusion, which depends on the lipophilicity of the drug molecule (highly lipophilic drugs cross the membrane more rapidly and more easily) and the drug concentration gradient existing across the membrane

(a larger gradient causes faster transport). Some drugs (e.g., vitamins) are carried across the absorption membrane by enzymes; such carrier-mediated transport may be passive or active and can move drugs against a concentration gradient as well as down the gradient.

3. **Blood flow to the absorbing organ**. Rapid and extensive blood flow to the organ or membrane of absorption facilitates rapid and complete absorption of the drug. Greater blood flow can help reduce the drug concentration on the systemic side of the absorption membrane and thereby increase the concentration gradient across which the drug molecule is absorbed. Greater blood flow also facilitates more rapid drug entry into the systemic circulation, enabling the drug to exert its effect at the intended site of action.

4. **Skin condition**. This is a concern only for topically administered medications. Highly vascular skin (e.g., on the scrotum or eyelid), broken skin (e.g., burned or eczematous), or hydrated skin leads to a more rapid and complete systemic absorption of topically applied drugs. Thick and highly keratinized skin areas (e.g., calluses, soles of feet) are poor sites for systemic drug absorption because the thickened stratum corneum retards the passage of drug molecules. Drugs applied to such sites should be intended for local effects only, not systemic.

5. **pH-Dependence**. Some drugs (e.g., weak acids and weak bases) carry a molecular charge at different pHs. Weak bases become positively charged at low pH, such as that in the stomach. Charged molecules cannot cross the lipid membrane of the skin easily. Such molecules can be absorbed only when they are uncharged, as occurs lower in the gastrointestinal tract, where the pH is higher. Weak acids are more easily absorbed in acidic environments, where they are uncharged.

6. **Bioavailability**. Some drugs are incompletely absorbed from the administration site. Oral drugs are most commonly mentioned, but intramuscular, topical, and rectal administration sites are also common sites where incomplete absorption occurs. For example, some sustained-release tablets may pass through the gastrointestinal tract and leave the body without their enteric coatings dissolving or they may retain some active drug in their wax matrices. In addition to the first-pass effect discussed in section I D 5 a, incomplete absorption is the other leading cause of low bioavailability.

7. **Compliance**. If drugs are not actually taken in prescribed amounts or at planned intervals, plasma levels will be subtherapeutic. Therapeutic drug monitoring is sometimes used to monitor the compliance of patients.

8. **Food coadministration**. Many oral agents will be incompletely absorbed if they are taken with food. Food can increase the gastric pH and hinder the dissolution of some medications. Also, certain foods contain specific products that interfere with absorption. Although higher plasma levels are usually achieved with most drugs (particularly antibiotics) when taken on an empty stomach, many drugs can still achieve therapeutic concentrations if taken with food. Tetracycline, however, may chelate calcium ions if taken with dairy products and will form a complex that cannot be absorbed.

F. **Distribution**. The distribution of drugs to various body tissues and compartments is affected by many factors, such as body composition and binding propensities. Measuring drug concentrations (most commonly in plasma) helps assess drug distribution, a key element in therapeutic effect. Plasma concentrations may or may not reflect drug concentration at the site of action or the site of toxicity.

1. **Concept of therapeutic concentration and therapeutic index**
   a. For many drugs, the drug concentration at which most patients begin to experience **therapeutic effects** (the minimum effective concentration) is known. Similarly, the concentration at which **toxic effects** are seen (the maximum effective concentration) is also known for many drugs. These concentrations are generally used as the upper and lower limits of the therapeutic concentration range or window. The science of clinical pharmacokinetics is concerned with designing dosage regimens to keep a drug concentration in a specific patient within the therapeutic window.
   b. The **therapeutic index** of a drug is the ratio of the maximum effective concentration to the minimum effective concentration. If the therapeutic index is small, the patient is more likely to experience toxicity or ineffective therapy. If the therapeutic index is large, the therapeutic window is usually larger, and it is easier to achieve an effective, nontoxic dosage regimen.

2. **Tissue binding**. Some drugs are bound to extravascular tissues, such as muscle or fat. Such drugs have low concentrations in the plasma compartment and a large apparent volume of distribution. Some drugs preferentially distribute to specific body tissues, depending on blood flow, pH conditions, and the lipophilicity of the tissue. Other drugs remain largely in the

plasma compartment, have an apparent small volume of distribution, and produce higher plasma concentrations for any given dose of drug.

3. **Body composition**. The composition of the body—which can change with certain disease states and will change with age—can be an important consideration for the distribution of certain drugs. The examples of obesity and edema are discussed here, but similar principles are true for other abnormal physiologic conditions.
   a. **Obesity**. Apparent volume of distribution is usually based on patient weight.
      (1) In addition to increased adipose tissue, obese patients have excess fluid in comparison to lean body mass.
      (2) Some drugs preferentially leave the plasma in **favor** of **adipose tissue**; thus plasma concentration for these drugs is lower and has a larger volume of distribution in obese patients.
      (3) Drugs that have a **low solubility in fat** remain in the plasma and produce higher plasma concentrations. In obese patients, therefore, their volume of distribution is smaller (per weight unit) than in thinner patients. Doses for drugs that distribute poorly to adipose tissue (e.g., aminoglycosides) are usually based on a patient's lean body weight, rather than total body weight. This consideration can be important because the relative proportion of adipose and lean tissue mass changes with age, with fat composing a larger percentage of the body weight with increasing age.
   b. **Edema**. Some hydrophilic drugs (e.g., lithium, aminoglycosides) remain largely in the plasma compartment. Patients with edema or ascites may distribute a large percentage of such drugs into the extra body fluid rather than into the target tissue (e.g., infected muscle tissue). If doses of such drugs are based on patient weight, their plasma concentration will be lower (because of the large plasma compartment) and the observed concentration may be subtherapeutic.

4. **Protein binding**
   a. **Free and bound concentrations**. Many drugs are bound to plasma proteins. In the plasma, these drugs exist in a state of equilibrium, with some of the drug free (unbound) and some bound to proteins. Drug plus protein is referred to as a **drug–protein complex**.
      (1) Only the free drug can cross membranes to enter body tissues, and only the free drug can interact with receptors to produce therapeutic or toxic effects.
      (2) Clinical laboratories generally report total plasma drug concentrations (free plus bound drug). For most patients and most drugs, this report provides sufficient information, because standard therapeutic concentrations reflect such factors as drug affinity for protein and free drug concentrations. Special circumstances exist, however, in which data on total drug concentrations prove insufficient or misleading. Information about the free drug concentration in a blood sample is obtainable for some drugs (notably, phenytoin), but the test is expensive, difficult to perform, and not always available.
   b. **Displacement**. Drugs are generally considered highly protein-bound when over 90% of the total drug in plasma is protein-bound. These drugs can sometimes be displaced by other substances that bind the same protein. In such instances, the second drug "pushes" the first drug off the protein. This causes the first drug to have a much higher free concentration while the total concentration remains unchanged.
      (1) **Example**. If a patient has been stabilized on aspirin (which binds albumin) and then begins taking phenylbutazone (which also binds albumin), the phenylbutazone may displace some salicylic acid and increase the free salicylate concentration. This previously stable patient may now experience some symptoms of salicylate toxicity due to an increased plasma concentration of free salicylate, despite an apparently normal reported salicylic acid (free plus bound) concentration. Eventually the higher free salicylic acid concentration will cause more salicylic acid to be excreted and a new equilibrium (steady state) will be reached.
      (2) **Albumin**
         (a) The main plasma and drug-binding protein, albumin, is an abundant protein that occurs in a concentration of 120 g/3 L (0.6 mmol) in the plasma.
         (b) Most drugs bound to albumin are acidic, including those listed in Table 29-1; some of them are also capable of displacing drugs bound to albumin.
         (c) For a drug to be an effective displacer, it must occupy a large number of binding sites on albumin (i.e., it must accumulate to high concentrations or be given in large doses).
         (d) Drugs such as aspirin, phenylbutazone, and sulfa drugs are the most common albumin displacers. Other substances, such as bilirubin, may bind albumin and may be displaced. For example, sulfa drugs will displace albumin-bound bilirubin, which can cause free bilirubin to increase to toxic concentrations. Because kernicterus can result, sulfa drugs should not be administered to neonates.

Table 29-1. Some Drugs That Bind to Albumin

Clofibrate	Salicylic acid
Ethacrynic acid	Sulfa drugs
Flufenamic acid	Sulfinpyrazone
Oxyphenbutazone	Warfarin
Phenylbutazone	

(e) Albumin levels may also be altered by certain disease states, listed in Table 29-2. Increases in albumin concentration decrease the free concentration of drugs that bind to albumin; conversely, decreases in albumin concentration increase the free concentration of albumin-binding drugs.

(3) Alpha$_1$-acid glycoprotein (AAG)

(a) After albumin, AAG is the second most important drug-binding plasma protein. AAG occurs in much smaller concentrations [2 to 4 mg/L (0.01 to 0.02 mmol)] than albumin and primarily binds basic drugs, listed in Table 29-3.

(b) Circumstances affecting AAG concentrations are listed in Table 29-4.

(c) The same basic protein-binding principles as discussed for albumin hold true for AAG. Conditions that increase AAG concentrations decrease free concentrations of drugs that bind AAG; those that decrease AAG increase free drug concentrations. One notable exception, however, is that few drugs are nearly totally bound to AAG, as some are to albumin. AAG exists in much smaller concentrations in the blood and is, therefore, unlikely to bind most of a drug, unless that drug is given in very small doses.

(d) Drug binding to AAG is not as likely to be as clinically significant as drug–albumin binding.

5. **Sample timing**. Objectives of monitoring include assessing a drug in its steady state and anticipating drug clearance (particularly for toxic agents); thus, sampling should take into account approximate distribution time and the half-life of the drug.

a. Distribution. The rate and pattern of distribution vary widely among drugs and require estimation when considering a monitoring plan.

(1) For example, certain drugs, such as aminoglycosides, reside in the plasma compartment prior to distribution to target tissues. This initial residence may last up to about 30 minutes for an aminoglycoside. Therefore, drawing a plasma aminoglycoside sample within 30 minutes of administration should be avoided as it would misrepresent the true plasma concentration. The concentration would appear to be too high because the drug would not have had a chance to distribute into the tissues.

(2) The probable location of receptor sites for specific drugs is important for sample planning. Digoxin, for example, exerts its therapeutic and toxic effects through receptor sites that seem to reside in the tissue compartments of the heart. Thus, concentrations only become relevant after the drug has had a chance to redistribute from the plasma to the tissue compartment (about 6 hours for digoxin). Samples should not be drawn within 6 to 8 hours after administration of an IV dose of digoxin (longer for an oral dose).

b. Half-lives. When a change in administration rate is being considered, the patient should

Table 29-2. Conditions That May Change Plasma Albumin Concentrations

Decrease Plasma Albumin	Increase Plasma Albumin
Acute infection	Benign tumor
Bone fractures	Gynecologic disorders
Burns	Myalgia
Cystic fibrosis	Schizophrenia
Inflammatory disease	
Liver disease	
Malnutrition	
Myocardial infarction	
Neoplastic disease	
Nephrotic syndrome	
Pregnancy	
Renal disease	
Surgical procedures	

Table 29-3. Some Drugs That Bind to Alpha$_1$-Acid Glycoprotein

Amitriptyline	Lidocaine
Chlorpromazine	Meperidine
Dipyridamole	Nortriptyline
Disopyramide	Propranolol
Erythromycin	Quinidine
Imipramine	

be at or near steady state when the sample is taken for evaluation. Steady state is usually achieved after the passage of four half-lives, with constant dosage.

(1) If the sample is taken too soon—before steady state has been reached—and the infusion rate is raised based on the results of the premature sample, the patient will begin to accumulate drug from the new infusion while continuing to accumulate drug from the initial dose.

(2) Anticipating clearance of toxic agents may require sampling after only two half-lives in order to gauge the rate of progress toward steady state while it is still possible to exert control, as in reducing the dosage rate.

G. Elimination

1. Metabolism. The liver is the site of metabolism for most drugs, but other organs and tissues (e.g., the lungs, kidneys, and intestines) may also metabolize drugs. Lipophilic drugs, for example, require chemical modification (e.g., acetylation, conjugation, and so forth) by the liver to render them more water-soluble and thus more readily removable by renal filtration.

a. Extraction ratio

(1) Drugs that are extensively metabolized during a single pass through the liver are said to have a high extraction ratio (i.e., the proportion of extracted drug to total drug that entered the liver is high). If a significant proportion of the drug has been extracted (rendered inactive) before entering systemic circulation—the **first-pass effect** (see section I D 5 a)—then the amount of active drug left to produce the desired effect is significantly reduced.

(2) The difference in extraction ratios among drugs accounts for the difference in magnitude of the first-pass effect from drug to drug.

(3) Oral agents traverse the liver before entering systemic circulation. If a drug is administered orally and has a high extraction ratio (e.g., propranolol), then most of the drug will be eliminated before reaching systemic circulation. Therefore, the effective dose for such a drug given orally may be much higher than for the same drug administered intravenously.

b. Hepatic blood flow changes

(1) Changes in hepatic blood flow affect the rate at which the liver is presented with a drug. Since the liver effectively processes drugs as they arrive, a change in presentation rate changes the rate at which drugs with a high extraction ratio are metabolized. (Most low-extraction-ratio drugs are affected only minimally or not at all by changes in hepatic flow rate.)

(2) Some drugs [e.g., most histamine$_2$ (H_2) antagonists] reduce hepatic blood flow and thus require close monitoring of plasma drug concentrations if administered to a patient already receiving a high-extraction-ratio drug (e.g., theophylline, propranolol, or lidocaine).

c. Changes in enzyme activity

(1) Metabolic enzyme activity, rather than hepatic blood flow, determines the **removal rate of low-extraction-ratio drugs**.

Table 29-4. Circumstances That May Change Plasma AAG* Concentrations

Decrease Plasma AAG	Increase Plasma AAG
Nephrotic syndrome	Burns
	Chronic pain
	Inflammatory disease (e.g., Crohn's disease, rheumatoid arthritis)
	Myocardial infarction
	Neoplastic disease
	Surgical procedures
	Trauma, injury

*AAG = Alpha$_1$-acid glycoprotein.

(2) Drugs and other substances can affect this activity, enhancing or inhibiting it by altering the amount of enzymes or influencing their function.

(a) **Induction of enzyme metabolism**

(i) Phenobarbital, for example, can stimulate hepatic enzymes to speed metabolism and change the effect of the other drugs metabolized by the liver. Thus, a patient who has been stabilized on rifampin (a low-extraction–ratio drug) may experience subtherapeutic rifampin concentrations once phenobarbital is added to the regimen.

(ii) Smoking can also increase enzyme activity. For example, the theophylline clearance rate is higher in smokers than in nonsmokers.

(b) **Inhibition of enzyme metabolism** may allow drug concentrations to build to toxic levels. For example, less theophylline can be removed if cimetidine is added to the regimen, because cimetidine inhibits cytochrome P-450 (a key element of the oxidative enzyme system).

d. Metabolites. Many metabolites are inactive and are simply removed by the kidneys. In some circumstances, however, drug metabolites must be considered in therapeutic drug monitoring. Like their parent drugs, metabolites may contribute both therapeutic and toxic effects.

(1) **Efficacy**. Some metabolites actually contribute to the therapeutic effectiveness of a drug. For instance, *N*-acetylprocainamide has antiarrhythmic properties that contribute to the effectiveness of procainamide, the parent drug. Other drugs with metabolites that enhance their therapeutic effectiveness include primidone, diazepam, flurazepam, and imipramine.

(2) **Toxicity**. Some metabolites may be more toxic than the parent drug. An example of a toxic metabolite is normeperidine, which is produced from meperidine. In most patients, normeperidine is quickly removed, but in patients with impaired renal function, it may build up to toxic levels and produce seizures. Other drugs with toxic metabolites include ethanol and acetaminophen.

(3) **Prodrugs**. Some drugs are inactive when they are administered and must be "activated" (usually by the metabolic process) to be effective. Examples of prodrugs include sulindac, clorazepate, and aspirin.

(4) **Assay interference**. Drug metabolites may be misinterpreted by the clinical laboratory for active drugs. Most clinical laboratories and commercially available assays can distinguish between parent drugs and metabolites, but mistakes have occurred. This can be particularly relevant if a patient has impaired renal function and metabolites have built up to significant levels. If necessary, plasma concentrations for drug metabolites, such as *N*-acetylprocainamide or desipramine, can be obtained from the clinical laboratory.

2. Excretion

a. Urinary excretion. Most drugs are removed by the kidneys, either as unchanged drug or as a metabolite; therefore, renal function greatly influences drug concentration and thus figures prominently in adjustments of drug regimens.

(1) **Renal function** is usually estimated using the Cockroft and Galt equation [see section I C 4 a (3)]. Generally, all aspects of renal function are assumed to rise or fall together; thus, filtration, secretion, and reabsorption are considered impaired to the same degree in a patient with renal failure. However, the effect of an individual drug may rely more heavily on one of these three aspects. The individual processes are discussed in section II.

(2) **Dose adjustment**. Many nomograms have been developed to help determine dosage adjustments (amount or frequency) in given circumstances. Generally, the greater the degree of renal impairment and the larger the fraction of drug excreted unchanged, the greater the dosage adjustment necessary to maintain drug concentration in the plasma within the therapeutic range.

b. Biliary and fecal excretion

(1) Some drugs undergo biliary excretion and enterohepatic recycling. These drugs may be eliminated in the feces, even though they were administered intravenously. For some drugs, this may be an important consideration. A patient who has taken an overdose of theophylline, for example, may be saved if activated charcoal is administered. The charcoal will work, even if the theophylline was not administered orally, because it will adsorb the theophylline on contact in the gastrointestinal tract, promote gastrointestinal trapping of the theophylline, and hasten its elimination.

(2) Biliary elimination usually only becomes a consideration if a patient has impaired biliary function, because some drugs may accumulate.

c. Other routes. Several other minor routes of drug elimination exist; however, these are insignificant for purposes of therapeutic drug monitoring.

(1) Some volatile anesthetics (e.g., halothane) are eliminated primarily on exhalation.

(2) A few drugs are eliminated through perspiration, saliva, tears, and breast milk.

II. PHARMACOKINETIC DRUG INTERACTIONS.

Coadministration of drugs can enhance, inhibit, or negate the effect each drug should achieve when administered alone. These interactions can occur when one drug alters, opposes, or potentiates the basic pharmacokinetics of the drug, according to the general principles outlined in section I.

A. Absorption

1. Rate

a. The rate of absorption can be **decreased** by administration of drugs that decrease local blood flow (as for topically administered drugs) or that slow stomach emptying (as for orally administered drugs). For example, in the coadministration of propantheline and acetaminophen, propantheline slows stomach emptying; therefore, acetaminophen will be absorbed more slowly.

b. Conversely, the absorption rate **increases** if a drug that speeds stomach emptying is coadministered. For example, metoclopramide, which speeds stomach emptying, increases the absorption rate of coadministered oral acetaminophen.

2. Extent. Coadministration can affect drug availability.

a. Increased bioavailability of digoxin, for example, can be achieved through oral coadministration of digoxin and propantheline. The propantheline slows stomach emptying and improves the availability of the slow-dissolving digoxin tablets.

b. Decreased absorption (bioavailability) results from coadministration in many instances. Coadministration of heavy metal ions and tetracyclines results in the formation of nonabsorbable complexes; kaolin-pectin adsorbs coadministered digoxin and results in less digoxin absorption.

c. Only un-ionized molecules can cross lipid absorption membranes. For this reason, drugs that alter the **ionic status** of other drug molecules can affect their absorption. For example, ketoconazole is only absorbed from an acidic stomach; coadministration of antacids will greatly impair ketoconazole absorption.

B. Volume of distribution.

Changes in protein binding (see section I F 4) are generally the cause of altered volumes of distribution. For example, the volume of distribution increases for salicylic acid when phenylbutazone is coadministered.

C. Clearance

1. Metabolic clearance. Several factors can influence metabolic clearance (see section I G 1).

a. For high-extraction–ratio drugs, metabolism can be **inhibited** by coadministration of a drug that reduces hepatic blood flow. For example, coadministration of lidocaine and cimetidine inhibits elimination of lidocaine (a high-extraction–ratio drug) and may produce higher-than-expected lidocaine concentrations.

b. Metabolic clearance may be **increased** for a low-extraction–ratio drug by coadministration of an enzyme inducer. For example, warfarin (a low-extraction–ratio drug) metabolism is increased when phenobarbital is also administered. If a patient has been stabilized on warfarin and phenobarbital is introduced, close monitoring is required to help maintain the appropriate anticoagulant status.

2. Renal clearance. Drugs eliminated by glomerular filtration are only affected by drugs that modify renal function, a pharmacodynamic interaction (e.g., nephrotoxic cisplatin impairs renal elimination of gentamicin). Secretion and reabsorption are more subject to pharmacokinetic interactions.

a. Secretion. Some drugs, such as penicillins, are actively secreted. Coadministration of a drug that competes for secretion, such as probenecid, can inhibit the secretion of penicillin and result in sustained blood levels of penicillin. This is sometimes used to clinical advantage to improve therapeutic outcome in patients with a history of poor compliance.

b. Reabsorption. Drugs that are filtered or secreted and then reabsorbed can also be subject to drug interactions.

(1) If a drug becomes ionized in the renal tubule due to a change in pH, it is impossible for it to be reabsorbed, because only un-ionized molecules can cross biologic membranes. For example, ammonium chloride decreases urinary pH. Amphetamine becomes positively charged at the lower pH and cannot be reabsorbed. More amphetamine is thus eliminated.

(2) Urine acidification or alkalinization is often used to advantage in cases of overdoses and poisonings.

STUDY QUESTIONS

Directions: The question below contains five suggested answers. Choose the **one best** response to the question.

1. All of the following are true statements about intramuscular (IM) drug administration EXCEPT

A. entry of the drug into the circulation is affected by the drug's degree of lipophilicity
B. peak effect is generally less than with intravenous (IV) administration
C. bioavailability equals 100%
D. maximum injection volume is 2 to 5 ml
E. drug effects generally last longer than with IV administration

Directions: Each question below contains three suggested answers of which **one or more** is correct. Choose the answer

A if **I only** is correct
B if **III only** is correct
C if **I and II** are correct
D if **II and III** are correct
E if **I, II, and III** are correct

2. True statements about protein binding include which of the following?

I. Only bound drug can interact with receptors to produce therapeutic or toxic effects
II. Drugs are considered highly protein bound when over 90% of the total drug in plasma is protein-bound
III. Albumin is the main plasma protein that binds drugs

3. Which of the following patients should have therapeutic drug monitoring?

I. An 80-year-old man with congestive heart failure
II. A 6-year-old boy with kidney disease
III. A 3-month-old girl with acute gastroenteritis

4. Conditions that may decrease plasma albumin include

I. malnutrition
II. pregnancy
III. myalgia

ANSWERS AND EXPLANATIONS

1. The answer is C. (*I D 3*) With intramuscular (IM) administration, bioavailability will not always be 100%. Only intravenous (IV) administration consistently provides 100% bioavailability. The other statements listed in the question are correct. The entry of an intramuscularly injected drug into the circulation is limited by the drug's solubility and lipophilicity, and by the blood supply in the muscle. Because an IM drug enters the blood more slowly and gradually than an IV drug, the peak effect of an IM drug is not as great, but its duration of action is generally longer than with IV administration. Not more than 2 to 5 ml should be injected into any one IM site.

2. The answer is D (II, III). (*I F 4*) Only free drug can interact with receptors to produce a therapeutic (or toxic) effect. A drug that is bound to plasma protein cannot cross membranes to enter body tissues and cannot interact with receptors to produce an effect. Albumin, one of the major proteins of blood plasma, is the main plasma protein that binds drugs. The second most important drug-binding plasma protein is alpha$_1$-acid glycoprotein (AAG). Albumin binds acidic drugs; AAG binds basic drugs.

3. The answer is E (all). (*I C 1, 4*) Patients who need rapidly effective treatment, and patients with altered physiologic and pharmacokinetic parameters, would benefit from therapeutic drug monitoring. Also, extremes of age affect drug absorption, distribution, metabolism, and excretion, so that elderly patients and very young patients require special care in dosage determinations. Congestive heart failure can impair absorption, distribution, and elimination of many drugs. Impaired renal function often requires dosage modification. Acute gastroenteritis in an infant can rapidly cause dehydration and electrolyte imbalance, and therefore calls for rapid, effective treatment and close monitoring.

4. The answer is C (I, II). (*Table 29-2*) Albumin levels may be altered by a variety of disease states. Infections, malnutrition, myocardial infarction, and renal disease are among the numerous diseases that can lower the plasma albumin levels. Pregnancy can also cause a decrease in plasma albumin. Conditions that may increase plasma albumin levels include myalgia and some gynecologic disorders. A decrease in plasma albumin would increase the free concentration of a drug that binds to albumin, and thus would increase the effects of the drug. Conversely, an increase in plasma albumin would lower the concentration of free drug and thus would reduce its effects.

30
Common Clinical Laboratory Tests

Larry N. Swanson

I. GENERAL PRINCIPLES

A. Monitoring drug therapy

1. **Laboratory test results** are monitored by pharmacists to:
   a. **Assess the therapeutic and adverse effects of a drug** (e.g., monitoring the serum uric acid level after allopurinol is administered or checking for elevated liver function test values after administration of isoniazid)
   b. **Determine the proper drug dose** (e.g., assessment of the serum creatinine value before use of a renally excreted drug)
   c. **Assess the need for additional or alternate drug therapy** (e.g., assessment of white blood cell [WBC] count after penicillin is administered)
   d. **Prevent test misinterpretation resulting from drug interference** (e.g., determination of a false positive for a urine glucose test after cephalosporin administration)
2. These tests can be **very expensive** and should be requested only when a definite need exists.

B. Definition of normal values

1. Laboratory test results are defined as **normal within a predetermined range of values** and as **abnormal outside that range.**
   a. However, **normal limits may be defined somewhat arbitrarily**, and values outside that range may not necessarily indicate disease or the need for treatment (e.g., asymptomatic hyperuricemia).
   b. Many factors (e.g., age, sex, time since last meal, and others) must be taken into account when evaluating test results.
   c. Normal values also **vary among institutions** and may depend on the method used to perform the test.
2. **Laboratory error** may also affect test results.
   a. Common sources of laboratory error include spoiled specimens, incomplete specimens, specimens taken at the wrong time, faulty reagents, technical errors, incorrect procedures, and failure to take diet or medication into account.
   b. Laboratory error must always be considered when **test results do not correlate with expected results for a given patient**. If necessary, the test should be repeated.
3. During hospital admission (or routine physical examination), a **battery of tests** is usually given to augment the history and physical examination. Tests may include an electrocardiogram (ECG), a chest x-ray, a sequential multiple analyzer (SMA) profile, electrolyte tests, a hemogram, and urinalysis.

II. HEMATOLOGIC TESTS.
Blood contains three types of formed elements: red blood cells (RBCs), WBCs, and platelets (Fig. 30-1).

A. Red blood cells (erythrocytes)

1. The **RBC count** reports the number of RBCs found in a cubic millimeter (mm^3) of whole blood.
   a. This test provides an **indirect estimate of the blood's hemoglobin content**.
   b. **Normal values** are 4.5 to 6.0 million/mm^3 of blood for males; 4.0 to 5.5 million/mm^3 for females.

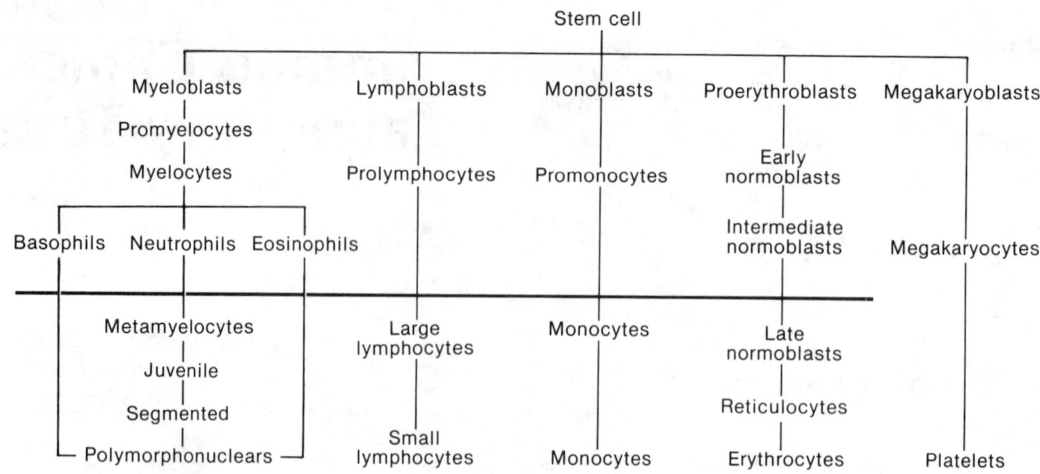

Figure 30-1. Derivation of blood elements from stem cells. Cells located below the *horizontal line* are found in normal peripheral blood, with the exception of the late normoblasts.

2. The **hematocrit (Hct)** or **packed cell volume (PCV)** measures the percentage by volume of packed RBCs in a whole blood sample after centrifugation.
   a. The Hct value is usually **three times the hemoglobin value** (see section II A 3) and is given as a **percent**.
   b. A **low Hct** indicates such conditions as anemia or overhydration; a **high Hct**, such conditions as polycythemia or dehydration.
3. The **hemoglobin (Hgb) test** measures the grams of hemoglobin contained in 1 dl of whole blood and provides an estimate of the oxygen-carrying capacity of the RBCs.
   a. **Normal values** range from 14 to 18 g/dl for males and from 12 to 16 g/dl for females.
   b. The Hgb value depends on the **number of RBCs** and the **amount of Hgb in each RBC**.
   c. A **low Hgb value** indicates anemia.
4. **RBC indices** (also known as **Wintrobe indices**) provide important information regarding RBC size, Hgb concentration, and Hgb weight. They are used primarily to categorize anemias, although they may be affected by average cell measurements.
   a. **Mean corpuscular volume (MCV)** is the ratio of the Hct to the RBC count:

$$\frac{\text{Hct (\%)} \times 10}{\text{RBC count (in millions)}} = \text{MCV}$$

      (1) The MCV value essentially assesses average RBC size and reflects any **anisocytosis** (variation in RBC size).
      (2) A **low MCV** indicates **microcytic** (undersized) **RBCs**, as occurs in iron deficiency. A **high MCV** indicates **macrocytic** (oversized) **RBCs**, as occurs in a vitamin B_{12} or folic acid deficiency.
      (3) The **normal range** for MCV is 90 ± 10.

   b. **Mean corpuscular hemoglobin (MCH)** assesses the amount of Hgb in an average RBC.
      (1) MCH is defined as:

$$\frac{\text{Hgb} \times 10}{\text{RBC count (in millions)}} = \text{MCH}$$

      (2) The **normal range** for MCH is 30 ± 4.

   c. **Mean corpuscular hemoglobin concentration (MCHC)** represents the average concentration of Hgb in an average RBC, defined as:

$$\frac{\text{Hgb} \times 100}{\text{Hct}} = \text{MCHC}$$

      (1) The **normal range** for MCHC is 34 ± 3.
      (2) A **low MCHC** indicates **hypochromia** (pale RBCs resulting from decreased Hgb content), as occurs in iron deficiency.

d. A peripheral blood smear can provide most of the information obtained through RBC indices. Observations of a smear may show variation in RBC shape (**poikilocytosis**), as might occur in sickle cell anemia, or it may show a variation in RBC size (**anisocytosis**), as might occur in a mixed anemia (folic acid and iron deficiency).

5. The **reticulocyte count** provides a measure of immature RBCs (reticulocytes), which contain remnants of nuclear material (reticulum). Normal RBCs circulate in the blood for about 1 to 2 days in this form. Hence, this test provides an index of bone marrow production of mature RBCs.

a. Reticulocytes normally comprise 0.5% to 1.5% of the total RBC count, or 25,000 to 75,000/mm³.

b. An **increased count** occurs with such conditions as hemolytic anemia, acute blood loss, and response to the treatment of a factor deficiency (e.g., an iron, vitamin B_{12}, or folate deficiency). **Polychromasia** (the tendency to stain with acidic or basic dyes), noted on a peripheral smear laboratory report, usually indicates increased reticulocytes.

c. A **decreased count** occurs with such conditions as drug-induced aplastic anemia.

d. In some cases, a **corrected reticulocyte count** may be used, calculated as:

$$\text{\% of observed reticulocytes} \times \frac{\text{Hct}}{45} = \text{corrected reticulocyte count}$$

6. The **erythrocyte sedimentation rate (ESR)** measures the rate of RBC settling of whole, uncoagulated blood over time, and primarily reflects plasma composition. Most of the sedimentation effect results from alterations in plasma proteins.

a. Normal ESR rates (Westergren method) range from 0 to 15 mm/hr for males and from 0 to 20 mm/hr for females.

b. The ESR value increases with acute or chronic infection, tissue necrosis or infarction, well-established malignancy, and rheumatoid collagen diseases.

c. The ESR has two main uses:

(1) For following the clinical course of a disease

(2) For demonstrating the presence of occult organic disease

d. The ESR can also be used to differentiate conditions with similar symptomatology (e.g., angina pectoris [no change in ESR value] as opposed to a myocardial infarction [increase in ESR value]).

B. White blood cells (leukocytes)

1. The **WBC count** reports the number of WBCs in a cubic millimeter of whole blood.

a. The **normal range** is 5000 to 10,000 WBCs/mm³.

b. An **increased WBC count** (leukocytosis) usually signals infection; it may also result from leukemia or from tissue necrosis. It is most often seen with bacterial infection; viral infections tend to cause normal counts or even leukopenia.

c. A **decreased WBC count** (leukopenia) indicates bone marrow depression, which may result from viral infection or from toxic reactions to substances such as antineoplastic agents.

2. The **WBC differential** evaluates the distribution and morphology of the five major types of WBCs—the **granulocytes** (**neutrophils, basophils,** and **eosinophils**) and the **nongranulocytes** (**lymphocytes** and **monocytes**). A certain percentage of each type comprises the total WBC count (Table 30-1).

a. Neutrophils may be mature (**polymorphonuclear leukocytes**, also known as PMNs, "polys," segmented neutrophils, or "segs") or immature ("**bands**" or "stabs").

(1) Neutrophils, which **phagocytize and degrade many types of particles**, serve as the body's first line of defense when tissue is damaged or foreign material gains entry. They congregate at sites in response to a specific stimulus, through a process known as **chemotaxis**.

Table 30-1. Normal Percentage Values for White Blood Cell Differential

Cell Type	Normal Percentage Value
Polymorphonuclear leukocytes	50%–70%
Bands	3%–5%
Lymphocytes	20%–40%
Monocytes	0%–7%
Eosinophils	0%–5%
Basophils	0%–1%

(2) In response to an appropriate stimulus, the **total neutrophil count rises** (neutrophilic leukocytosis), often with an increase in the percentage of immature cells (a "**shift to the left**").

(3) **Neutrophilic leukocytosis with a shift to the left** may represent a severe local bacterial infection or a systemic bacterial infection, such as pneumonia (Table 30-2).

(a) **Certain viruses** (e.g., chicken pox and herpes zoster); some **rickettsial diseases** (e.g., Rocky Mountain spotted fever); some **fungi**; and **stress** (e.g., physical exercise, acute hemorrhage or hemolysis, and acute emotional stress) may also cause this response.

(b) Other causes include **inflammatory diseases** (e.g., acute rheumatic fever, rheumatoid arthritis, acute gout); **hypersensitivity reactions to drugs**; **tissue necrosis** (e.g., from myocardial infarction, burns, and certain cancers); **metabolic disorders** (e.g., uremia and diabetic ketoacidosis); **myelogenous leukemia**; and **use of certain drugs** (e.g., epinephrine and lithium).

(4) **Neutropenia** (a decrease in the number of neutrophils) may occur with an **overwhelming infection of any type** (bone marrow is unable to keep up with the demand). It may also occur with **certain viral infections** (e.g., mumps and measles) and with **idiosyncratic drug reactions**.

b. **Basophils** stain deeply with blue basic dye. Their function in the circulation is not clearly understood; in the tissues they are referred to as **mast cells**.

(1) **Basophilia** (an increased number of basophils) may occur with chronic myelogenous leukemia as well as other conditions.

(2) A decrease in basophils is generally not apparent because of the small numbers of these cells in the blood.

c. **Eosinophils** stain deep red with acid dye and are classically associated with immune reactions. **Eosinophilia** (increased number of eosinophils) may occur with such conditions as **acute allergic reactions** (e.g., asthma, hay fever, and drug allergy) and **parasitic infestations** (e.g., trichinosis and amebiasis).

d. **Lymphocytes** play a dominant role in immunologic activity and appear to produce antibodies. They are classified as B lymphocytes or T lymphocytes; T lymphocytes are further divided into helper-inducer cells (T_4 cells) and suppressor cells (T_8 cells).

(1) **Lymphocytosis** (an increased number of lymphocytes) usually accompanies a normal or decreased total WBC count and is most commonly caused by **viral infection**.

(2) **Lymphopenia** (a decreased number of lymphocytes) may result from **severe debilitating illness, immunodeficiency**, or the **AIDS virus**, which has a propensity to attack T_4 cells.

(3) **Atypical lymphocytes** (T lymphocytes in a state of immune activation) are classically associated with **infectious mononucleosis**.

e. **Monocytes** are phagocytic cells. **Monocytosis** (an increased number of monocytes) may occur with **tuberculosis, subacute bacterial endocarditis, monocytic leukemia**, and during the recovery phase of some **acute infections**.

C. Platelets (thrombocytes)

1. Platelets, the smallest formed elements in the blood, are involved in **blood clotting** and are vital to the formation of a hemostatic plug after vascular injury.

Table 30-2. Examples of Changes in Total White Blood Cell Count and White Blood Cell Differential in Response to Bacterial Infection

	White Blood Cell Count	
Cell Type	**Normal**	**With Bacterial Infection**
Total white blood cells	8000 (100%)	15,500 (100%)
Neutrophils		
Polymorphonuclear leukocytes	60%	82%
Bands	3%	6%
Lymphocytes	30%	10%
Monocytes	4%	1%
Eosinophils	2%	1%
Basophils	1%	0%

2. The **normal range** for a platelet count is 150,000 to 300,000/mm³.

3. **Thrombocytopenia** (a decreased platelet count) can occur with a variety of conditions, such as idiopathic thrombocytopenic purpura or, occasionally, from such drugs as quinidine and sulfonamides.

4. Thrombocytopenia is considered **moderate** when the count is less than 100,000/mm³; **severe** when the count is less than 50,000/mm³.

III. COMMON SERUM ENZYME TESTS.

Small amounts of enzymes (catalysts) circulate in the blood at all times and are released into the blood in larger quantities when tissue damage occurs. Thus, serum enzyme levels can be used to **aid diagnosis of certain diseases**.

A. Creatine phosphokinase (CPK)

1. CPK, also known as **creatine kinase** (CK), is found only in heart muscle, skeletal muscle, and brain tissue.

2. CPK levels are used primarily to **aid in the diagnosis of acute myocardial** (Fig. 30-2) **or skeletal muscle damage**. However, vigorous exercise, a fall, or deep intramuscular injections can cause significant elevations in CPK levels.

3. The **isoenzymes** of CPK (**CPK-MM**, found in skeletal muscle; **CPK-BB**, found in brain tissue; and **CPK-MB**, found in heart muscle) can be used to differentiate the source of damage.
   a. Normally serum CPK levels are virtually all the **CPK-MM isoenzyme**.
   b. Increases in **CPK-MB** levels provide a sensitive indicator of myocardial necrosis.

B. Lactic acid dehydrogenase (LDH or LD)

1. LDH catalyzes the interconversion of lactate and pyruvate and represents a group of enzymes present in almost all metabolizing cells.

2. Five individual **isoenzymes** make up the total LDH serum level.
   a. **LDH_1** and **LDH_2** appear primarily in the heart.
   b. **LDH_3** appears primarily in the lungs.
   c. **LDH_4** and **LDH_5** appear primarily in the liver and in skeletal muscles.

3. The **distribution pattern** of LDH isoenzymes aids in diagnosing myocardial infarction, hepatic disease, and lung disease.

C. Alkaline phosphatase (ALP)

1. ALP is produced primarily in the **liver** and in **bones**.

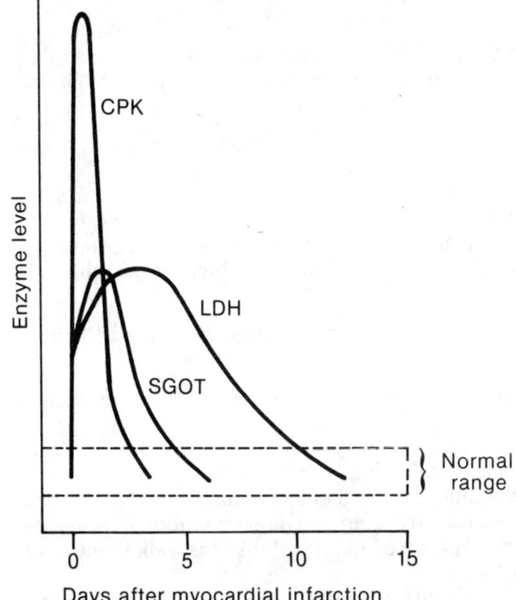

Figure 30-2. The graph shows the elevation of serum creatine phosphokinase (CPK), lactic dehydrogenase (LDH), and serum glutamic-oxaloacetic transaminase (SGOT) levels following a myocardial infarction.

2. Serum ALP levels are **particularly sensitive to partial or mild biliary obstruction**—either extrahepatic (e.g., caused by a stone in the bile duct) or intrahepatic, which causes levels to rise.

3. **Increased osteoblastic activity** (as occurs in Paget's disease, hyperparathyroidism, osteomalacia, and others) also increases serum ALP levels.

D. Serum glutamic-oxaloacetic transaminase (SGOT)

1. SGOT, also known as **aspartate aminotransferase** (AST), is found in a number of organs, primarily in heart and liver tissues and, to a lesser extent, in skeletal muscle, kidney tissue, and pancreatic tissue.

2. **Damage to the heart** (e.g., from **myocardial infarction**; see Fig. 30-2) results in elevated SGOT levels about 8 hours after the injury.
   a. Levels are **elevated markedly** with **acute hepatitis**; they are **elevated mildly** with **cirrhosis** and **fatty liver**.
   b. Levels are also **elevated** with **passive congestion of the liver** (as occurs in congestive heart failure).

E. Serum glutamic-pyruvic transaminase (SGPT)

1. SGPT, also known as **alanine aminotransferase** (ALT), is found primarily in the liver, with lesser amounts in the heart, skeletal muscles, and kidney.

2. Although SGPT values are **relatively specific for liver cell damage**, SGPT is **less sensitive than SGOT**, and more extensive or severe liver damage is necessary before abnormally elevated levels are produced.

3. SGPT also **rises less consistently and less markedly than SGOT** following an **acute myocardial infarction**.

IV. LIVER FUNCTION TESTS

A. Liver enzymes

1. Levels of certain **enzymes** (e.g., LDH, ALP, SGOT, and SGPT) **rise with liver dysfunction**, as discussed in section III.

2. These **enzyme tests indicate only that the liver has been damaged**—they do not assess the liver's ability to function.

3. **Other tests** provide indications of liver dysfunction.

B. Serum bilirubin

1. Bilirubin, a breakdown product of Hgb, is the **predominant pigment in bile**. Effective bilirubin conjugation and excretion depends on **hepatobiliary function** and on the rate of RBC turnover.

2. Serum bilirubin levels are reported as **total bilirubin** (conjugated and unconjugated) and as **direct bilirubin** (conjugated only).
   a. Bilirubin is released by Hgb breakdown and is bound to albumin as water-insoluble **unconjugated bilirubin** (indirect bilirubin), which is not filtered by the glomerulus.
   b. Unconjugated bilirubin travels to the liver, where it is separated from albumin, conjugated with a diglucuronide, and then actively secreted into the bile as **conjugated bilirubin** (direct bilirubin), which is filtered by the glomerulus (Fig. 30-3).

3. The **normal range** of **total serum bilirubin** is 0.3 to 1.3 mg/dl; of **direct bilirubin**, 0.1 to 0.4 mg/dl.

4. An **increase** in serum bilirubin results in **jaundice**, from bilirubin deposition in the tissues. There are three major causes of increased serum bilirubin.
   a. **Hemolysis** increases total bilirubin; direct bilirubin (conjugated) is usually normal or slightly elevated. Urine color is normal, and no bilirubin is found in the urine.
   b. **Biliary obstruction**, which may be intrahepatic (as with a chlorpromazine reaction) or extrahepatic (as with a biliary stone) increases total bilirubin and direct bilirubin; intrahepatic cholestasis (e.g., from chlorpromazine) may increase indirect bilirubin as well. Urine color is dark, and bilirubin is present in the urine.
   c. **Liver cell necrosis**, as occurs in viral hepatitis, may cause an increase in both direct bilirubin (because inflammation causes some bile sinusoid blockage) and indirect bilirubin

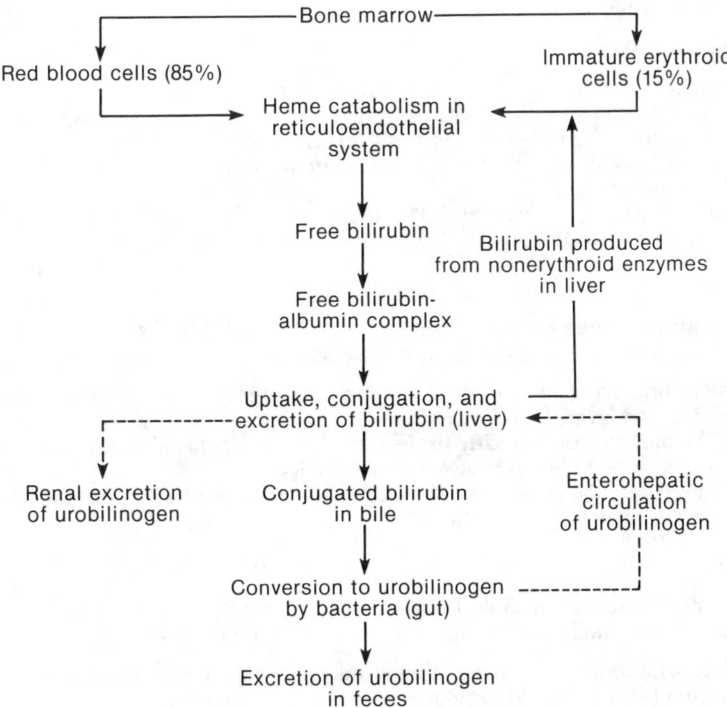

Figure 30-3. Schematic representation of bilirubin metabolism.

(because the liver's ability to conjugate is altered). Urine color is dark, and bilirubin is present in the urine.

C. Serum proteins

1. The **primary serum proteins** measured are albumin and the globulins (alpha, beta, and gamma).
   a. **Albumin** maintains serum osmotic pressure and serves as a transport agent. Because it is primarily manufactured by the liver, liver disease can decrease albumin levels.
   b. **Globulins** function as transport agents and play a role in certain immunologic mechanisms. A decrease in albumin levels usually results in a compensatory increase in globulin production.

2. The **normal range for total serum protein levels** is 6.0 to 8.0 g/dl.

V. URINALYSIS. Standard urinalysis provides basic information regarding renal function, urinary tract disease, and presence of certain systemic diseases. Components of a standard urinalysis include appearance, pH, specific gravity, protein level, glucose level, ketone level, and microscopic examination.

A. Appearance

1. Normal urine is **clear** and ranges in color from **pale yellow to deep gold**.

2. **Changes in color** can result from drugs, diet, or disease.
   a. A red color may indicate, among other things, the presence of blood or phenolphthalein (a laxative).
   b. A brownish-yellow color may indicate the presence of conjugated bilirubin.
   c. Other shades of red, orange, or brown may be caused by ingestion of various drugs.

B. pH

1. **Normal pH** ranges from 4.5 to 9 but is typically **acid** (around 6).

2. An **alkaline pH** may indicate such conditions as alkalosis, a *Proteus* infection, or acetazolamide use. It may also reflect changes caused by leaving the urine sample at room temperature.

C. Specific gravity

1. The **normal range** for specific gravity is 1.003 to 1.035; it is usually between 1.010 and 1.025.
2. Specific gravity is influenced by the number and nature of **solute particles** in the urine.
   a. An **elevated** specific gravity may occur with such conditions as diabetes mellitus (excess glucose in the urine) or nephrosis (excess protein in the urine).
   b. A **decreased** specific gravity may occur with diabetes insipidus, which decreases urine concentration.
   c. A specific gravity **fixed at 1.010** (the same as plasma) occurs when the kidneys lose their power to concentrate or dilute.

D. Protein

1. The **normal value** for urine protein is 50 to 80 mg/24 hr, as the glomerular membrane prevents most protein molecules in the blood from entering the urine.
2. **Proteinuria** occurs with many conditions (e.g., renal disease, bladder infection, venous congestion, and fever).
   a. The presence of a **specific protein** can help to identify a specific disease state (e.g., Bence Jones protein may indicate multiple myeloma).
   b. Most often, the protein in urine is **albumin**. Albuminuria may indicate abnormal glomerular permeability.

E. Glucose

1. The normal **renal threshold** for glucose is a blood glucose level of about 180 mg/dl; glucose **does not normally appear in urine** as detected by popular testing methods.
2. **Glycosuria** usually indicates diabetes mellitus. There are certain less common causes (e.g., a lowered renal threshold for glucose).

F. Ketones

1. Ketones **do not normally appear in urine**. They are excreted when the body has utilized available glucose stores and begins to metabolize fat stores.
2. The **three ketone bodies** are betahydroxybutyric acid (80%), acetoacetic acid (about 20%), and acetone (a small percentage). Some commercial tests (e.g., Ames products) measure only acetoacetic acid, but usually all three are excreted in parallel proportions.
3. **Ketonuria** usually indicates uncontrolled diabetes mellitus, but it may also occur with starvation and with zero- or low-carbohydrate diets.

G. Microscopic examination

1. Microscopic examination of centrifuged urine sediment normally reveals 0 to 1 RBC, 0 to 4 WBCs, and only an occasional cast per high-power field.
2. **Hematuria** (presence of RBCs) may indicate such conditions as trauma, a tumor, or a systemic bleeding disorder. In women, a significant number of **squamous cells** suggests vaginal contamination (menstruation).
3. **Casts** (protein conglomerations outlining the shape of the renal tubules in which they were formed) may or may not be significant. Excessive numbers of certain types of casts indicate renal disease.
4. **Crystals**, which are pH-dependent, may occur normally in acid or alkaline urine. **Uric acid crystals** may form in acid urine; **phosphate crystals** may form in alkaline urine.
5. **Bacteria** do not normally appear in urine. The finding of 20 or more bacteria per high-power field may indicate a urinary tract infection; smaller values may indicate urethral contamination.

VI. COMMON RENAL FUNCTION TESTS

A. Introduction

1. Assessment of **blood urea nitrogen** (BUN) and **serum creatinine** helps determine kidney function.
   a. These tests primarily evaluate glomerular function by assessing the **glomerular filtration rate** (GFR).

b. In many **renal diseases**, urea and creatinine accumulate in the blood because they are not excreted properly.
c. These tests also aid in determining **drug dosage** for drugs excreted through the kidneys.

2. Excessive retention of nitrogenous waste products (BUN and creatinine) in the blood is termed **azotemia**.
   a. **Renal azotemia** results from renal disease, such as glomerulonephritis and chronic pyelonephritis.
   b. **Prerenal azotemia** results from such conditions as severe dehydration, hemorrhagic shock, and excessive protein intake.
   c. **Postrenal azotemia** results from such conditions as ureteral or urethral stones or tumors and prostatic obstructions.

3. The clinical syndrome resulting from decreased renal function and azotemia is called **uremia**.

4. **Clearance** (a theoretical concept defined as the volume of plasma from which a measured amount of substance can be completely eliminated, or cleared, into the urine per unit time) can be used to estimate glomerular function.

5. Renal function **decreases with age**, which must be taken into account when interpreting test values.

B. Blood urea nitrogen (BUN)

1. **Urea**, the end product of protein metabolism, is produced only in the liver. From there, it travels through the blood and is excreted by the kidneys.

2. Urea is **filtered at the glomerulus**, where the tubules reabsorb approximately 40%. Thus, under normal conditions, **urea clearance** is about 60% of the true GFR.

3. **Normal values** for BUN range from 10 to 20 mg/dl.
   a. BUN levels may be **low** with **significant liver disease**.
   b. **Elevated BUN levels** may indicate **renal disease**. However, factors other than glomerular function (e.g., protein intake, reduced renal blood flow, and blood in the gastrointestinal tract) readily affect BUN levels, making interpretation of results difficult.

C. Serum creatinine

1. **Creatinine**, the metabolic breakdown product of muscle creatine phosphate, has a relatively constant level of daily production. Blood levels vary little in a given individual.

2. Creatinine is **excreted** by glomerular filtration and tubular secretion. Creatinine clearance parallels the GFR within a range of ± 10%.

3. This test is a **more sensitive indicator of renal damage than BUN levels** because renal impairment is almost the only cause of serum creatinine elevation.

4. **Normal values** for serum creatinine range from 0.6 to 1.2 mg/dl.
   a. Values vary with the **amount of muscle mass**—a value of 1.2 mg/dl in a muscular athlete may represent normal renal function, whereas this same value in a small, sedentary person with little muscle mass may indicate significant renal impairment.
   b. Generally, the **serum creatinine value doubles with each 50% decrease in GFR**. For example, if a patient's normal serum creatinine is 1 mg/dl, 1 mg/dl represents 100% renal function, 2 mg/dl represents 50% function, and 4 mg/dl represents 25% function.

D. Creatinine clearance

1. Creatinine clearance, which represents the **rate at which creatinine is removed from the blood by the kidneys**, roughly approximates the GFR.
   a. The value is given in units of **ml/min**, representing the volume of blood (in milliliters) cleared of creatinine by the kidney per minute.
   b. **Normal values for men** range from 75 to 125 ml/min.

2. Calculation requires knowledge of **urinary creatinine excretion** (usually over 24 hours) and concurrent **serum creatinine levels**. Creatinine clearance is **calculated** as follows:

$$Cl_{CR} = \frac{C_U V}{C_{CR}}$$

Here, Cl_{CR} is the creatinine clearance in ml/min, C_U is the concentration of creatinine in the urine, V is the urine volume (in ml/min of urine formed over the collection period), and C_{CR} is the serum creatinine concentration.

3. As an example, suppose serum creatinine concentration is 1 mg/dl, and 1440 ml of urine were collected in 24 hours (1440 min) for a urine volume of 1 ml/min. The urine contains 100 mg/dl of creatinine. Creatinine clearance is calculated as:

$$\frac{100 \text{ mg/dl} \times 1 \text{ ml/min}}{1 \text{ mg/dl}} = 100 \text{ ml/min}$$

4. Incomplete bladder emptying and other problems may interfere with obtaining an accurate timed urine specimen. Thus, **estimations of creatinine** may be necessary. These estimations require only a serum creatinine value.
   a. One estimation uses the method of **Cockcroft and Gault**, which is based on body weight, age, and gender.
   b. This formula provides an **estimated value**, calculated for **males** as:

$$Cl_{CR} = \frac{(140 - \text{age in years})\ (\text{body weight in kg})}{72\ (C_{CR} \text{ in mg/dl})}$$

   Again, Cl_{CR} is the creatinine clearance in ml/min, and C_{CR} is the serum creatinine concentration.
   c. For **females**, use 0.85 of the value calculated for males.

VII. AUTOANALYZER METHODS

A. Multiple laboratory assessments of blood can be performed by automated electronic systems, such as the **sequential multiple analyzer (SMA)**. These devices perform a battery of blood tests that screen for the presence of disease.

B. An example is the SMA-12 panel of tests, which may include total protein, albumin, calcium, phosphorus, cholesterol, glucose, BUN, creatinine, uric acid, total bilirubin, ALP, and SGOT levels.

STUDY QUESTIONS

Directions: Each question below contains five suggested answers. Choose the **one best** response to each question.

1. Hematologic testing of a patient with AIDS is most likely to show which of the following abnormalities?

A. Basophilia
B. Eosinophilia
C. Lymphopenia
D. Reticulocytosis
E. Agranulocytosis

2. Hematologic studies are most likely to show a low reticulocyte count in a patient with

A. aplastic anemia secondary to cancer chemotherapy
B. acute hemolytic anemia secondary to quinidine treatment
C. severe bleeding secondary to an automobile accident
D. iron deficiency anemia, 1 week after treatment with ferrous sulfate
E. megaloblastic anemia of folate deficiency, 1 week after treatment with folic acid

3. All of the following findings on a routine urinalysis would be considered normal EXCEPT

A. pH: 6.5
B. glucose: negative
C. ketones: negative
D. WBC: 3 per high-power field, no casts
E. RBC: 5 per high-power field

4. M.T. is a 12-year-old black male being treated for otitis media with cefaclor (Ceclor). On the seventh day of therapy, he "spikes" a fever and develops an urticarial rash on his trunk. Which of the following laboratory tests could best help confirm the physician's suspicion of a hypersensitivity (allergic) reaction?

A. Complete blood count and differential
B. Serum hemoglobin and reticulocyte count
C. Liver function test profile
D. LDH isoenzyme profile
E. RBC count and serum bilirubin

5. An elevated hematocrit is a likely finding in all of the following individuals EXCEPT

A. a man who has just returned from a 3-week skiing trip in the Colorado Rockies
B. a woman who has polycythemia vera
C. a hospitalized patient who mistakenly received 5 L of IV dextrose 5% in water over the last 24 hours
D. a man who has been rescued from the Arizona desert after spending 4 days without water
E. a woman who has chronic obstructive pulmonary disease

6. T.O. is a 29-year-old white male who is seen in the emergency room of Carney Hospital. His WBC count is 14,200 with 80% "polys." All of the following conditions could normally produce these laboratory findings EXCEPT

A. a localized bacterial infection on the tip of the index finger
B. acute bacterial pneumonia caused by *Streptococcus pneumoniae*
C. heart attack
D. a gunshot wound to the abdomen, with a loss of 2 pints of blood
E. an attack of gout

7. S.M. is a 52-year-old male construction worker who drinks "fairly heavily" when he gets off work at night. He is seen in the emergency room in Suburban General Hospital with, among other abnormal laboratory results, an elevated CPK level. All of the following circumstances could explain this elevation EXCEPT

A. he fell against the bumper of his car in a drunken stupor and bruised his right side
B. he is showing evidence of some liver damage due to the heavy alcohol intake
C. he has experienced a heart attack
D. he received an intramuscular injection a few hours before the blood sample was drawn
E. he pulled a muscle that day in lifting a heavy concrete slab

8. A 45-year-old male patient with jaundice has spillage of bilirubin into his urine. All of the following statements could apply to this patient EXCEPT

A. his total bilirubin is elevated
B. his direct bilirubin is increased
C. he may have viral hepatitis
D. he may have hemolytic anemia
E. he may have cholestatic hepatitis

Questions 9–11

Use the following information in answering questions 9 through 11.

J.G. is a 70-year-old black male weighing 154 lb who complains of chronic tiredness. Several laboratory tests were performed with the following results:

BUN: 15 mg/dl
SGOT: within normal limits
WBC: 7500/mm^3
RBC: 4.0 million/mm^3
HCT: 29%
Hgb: 9.0 g/dl

9. J.G.'s mean corpuscular hemoglobin concentration (MCHC) is

A. 27.5
B. 28.9
C. 31.0
D. 33.5
E. 35.4

10. J.G.'s mean corpuscular volume (MCV) is

A. 61.3
B. 72.5
C. 77.5
D. 90.2
E. 93.5

11. From the data provided above and from the calculations in questions 9 and 10, J.G. is best described as

A. normal except for a slightly elevated BUN
B. having normochromic, microcytic anemia
C. having sickle cell anemia
D. having hypochromic, normocytic anemia
E. having folic acid deficiency

Directions: Each question below contains three suggested answers of which **one or more** is correct. Choose the answer

A if **I only** is correct
B if **III only** is correct
C if **I and II** are correct
D if **II and III** are correct
E if **I, II, and III** are correct

12. Factors likely to cause an increase in the blood urea nitrogen (BUN) level include

I. intramuscular injection of diazepam (Valium)
II. severe liver disease
III. chronic kidney disease

13. A patient who undergoes serum enzyme testing is found to have an elevated serum glutamic-oxaloacetic transaminase (SGOT) level. Possible underlying causes of this abnormality include

I. methyldopa-induced hepatitis
II. congestive heart failure
III. pneumonia

14. Serum enzyme tests that may aid in the diagnosis of myocardial infarction include

I. alkaline phosphatase
II. CPK
III. LDH

ANSWERS AND EXPLANATIONS

1. The answer is C. [*II B 2 d (2)*] Valuable diagnostic information can be obtained through quantitative and qualitative testing of the cells of the blood. A finding of lymphopenia (i.e., decreased number of lymphocytes) suggests a severe attack on the immune system or some underlying immunodeficiency. The AIDS virus attacks the T_4 population of lymphocytes, thus leading to lymphopenia.

2. The answer is A. (*II A 5*) The reticulocyte count measures the amount of circulating immature red blood cells (RBCs), which provides information about bone marrow function. A low reticulocyte count is a likely finding in a patient with aplastic anemia—a disorder characterized by a deficiency of all cellular elements of the blood due to a lack of hematopoietic stem cells in bone marrow. A variety of drugs (e.g., those used in anticancer therapy) and other agents produce marrow aplasia. A high reticulocyte count would likely be found in a patient with hemolytic anemia or acute blood loss or in a patient who has been treated for an iron, vitamin B_{12}, or folate deficiency.

3. The answer is E. (*V B, E–G*) Microscopic examination of the urine sediment normally shows fewer than 1 red blood cell (RBC) and from 0 to 5 white blood cells (WBCs) per high-power field. Other normal findings on urinalysis include an acid pH (i.e., around 6) and an absence of glucose and ketones.

4. The answer is A. (*II B 2 c*) An allergic drug reaction will usually produce an increase in the eosinophil count (eosinophilia). This could be determined by ordering a white blood cell (WBC) differential.

5. The answer is C. (*II A 2 b*) Overhydration with an excess infusion of dextrose 5% in water will produce a low hematocrit. The other situations will result in elevations of the hematocrit.

6. The answer is A. (*II B 2 a*) The patient has leukocytosis with an elevated neutrophil count (neutrophilia). A localized infection will not normally result in an increase in the total leukocyte count or neutrophil count. The other situations given in the question can produce a neutrophilic leukocytosis.

7. The answer is B. (*III A*) Because creatine phosphokinase (CPK) is not present in the liver, alcoholic liver damage would not result in an elevation of this enzyme. CPK is present primarily in cardiac and skeletal muscle. The other situations described in the question could all result in the release of increased amounts of CPK into the bloodstream.

8. The answer is D. (*IV B*) The patient with jaundice (deposition of bilirubin in the skin) will usually have an increase in the total bilirubin serum level. Spillage of bilirubin into the urine requires an elevated direct bilirubin, which is likely with viral hepatitis or cholestatic hepatitis. In hemolytic anemia, direct bilirubin is not usually increased, and therefore there would be no spillage of bilirubin into the urine.

9. The answer is C. (*II A 4 c*) The mean corpuscular hemoglobin concentration (MCHC) is calculated as follows:

$$\text{MCHC} = \frac{\text{Hgb} \times 100}{\text{Hct}} = \frac{9 \times 100}{29} = 31.0$$

10. The answer is B. (*II A 4 a*) The mean corpuscular volume (MCV) is calculated as follows:

$$\text{MCV} = \frac{\text{HCT (\%)} \times 10}{\text{RBC count (in millions)}} = \frac{29 \times 10}{4} = 72.5$$

11. The answer is B. (*II A 4; VI B 3*) The patient J.G. is anemic, since his hemoglobin (Hgb) is 9 (normal, 14–18). The anemia is normochromic, since the patient's MCHC of 31 is normal (normal range, 31–37), but the anemia is microcytic, since the patient's MCV is 72.5 (normal, 80–100). The patient's blood urea nitrogen (BUN), 15 mg/dl, is within the normal range of 10 to 20 mg/dl.

12. The answer is B (III). (*VI B 3*) Chronic kidney disease can cause an increase in the blood urea nitrogen (BUN) level; a heavy protein diet and bleeding into the gastrointestinal tract are other factors that can produce this finding. Severe liver disease can prevent the formation of urea and, therefore, is likely to cause a decrease in the BUN level. Although an intramuscular injection of diazepam (Valium) may cause an increase in the serum creatine phosphokinase (CPK) or serum glutamic-oxaloacetic transaminase (SGOT) level, it would have no effect on the BUN.

13. The answer is C (I, II). (*III D*) A lung infection, such as pneumonia, normally would not cause an increase in the release of serum glutamic-oxaloacetic transaminase (SGOT), an enzyme primarily found in the liver and heart. In acute hepatitis, a marked elevation of SGOT is a likely finding. SGOT levels also can be elevated with passive congestion of the liver, as occurs in congestive heart failure.

14. The answer is D (II, III). (*III A, B, C*) Usually, the creatine phosphokinase (CPK), serum glutamic-pyruvic transaminase (SGPT), serum glutamic-oxaloacetic transaminase (SGOT), and lactic acid dehydrogenase (LDH) enzyme levels are elevated after a myocardial infarction. Alkaline phosphase is not present in cardiac tissue and therefore would not be useful in diagnosis of a myocardial infarction.

31
Ischemic Heart Disease

Barbara Szymusiak-Mutnick

I. INTRODUCTION

A. Definition. Ischemic heart disease (IHD) is a condition in which there is an insufficient supply of oxygen to the myocardium (cardiac tissue) so that oxygen demand exceeds the oxygen supply.

B. Manifestations

1. **Angina pectoris**, an episodic, reversible oxygen insufficiency, is the most common form of IHD (see section II).
2. **Acute myocardial infarction** occurs with a severe, prolonged deprivation of oxygen to a portion of the myocardium, resulting in irreversible myocardial tissue necrosis (see section III).
3. **Sudden death.** Myocardial ischemia or infarction can trigger the abrupt onset of ventricular fibrillation (the most disorganized arrhythmia), which can stop cardiac output. Without immediate intervention—such as a precordial thump, cardiopulmonary resuscitation, or defibrillation countershock—the result is death. Episodic recurrences of ventricular fibrillation, sudden "death," and resuscitation are known as **sudden death syndrome**.

C. Etiology. The processes, singly or in combination, that produce IHD include: decreased blood flow to the myocardium, increased oxygen demand, and decreased oxygenation of the blood.

1. **Decreased blood flow** (Coronary blood flow is illustrated in Figure 31-1.)
   a. **Atherosclerosis**, with or without coronary thrombosis, is the most common cause of IHD. In this condition, the coronary arteries are progressively narrowed by smooth muscle cell proliferation and the accumulation of lipid deposits (plaque) along the inner lining (intima) of the arteries.
   b. **Coronary artery spasm**, a sustained contraction of one or more coronary arteries, can occur spontaneously or be induced by irritation (e.g., by coronary catheter or intimal hemorrhage), exposure to the cold, or ergot-derivative drugs. These spasms can cause Prinzmetal's angina and even myocardial infarction.
   c. **Traumatic injury**, whether blunt or penetrating, can interfere with myocardial blood supply (e.g., the impact of a steering wheel on the chest causing a myocardial contusion, in which the capillaries hemorrhage).
   d. **Embolic events**, even in otherwise normal coronary vessels, can abruptly restrict the oxygen supply to the myocardium.
2. **Increased oxygen demand** can occur, for example, with exertion (as in exercise or shoveling snow) and emotional stress, which increases sympathetic stimulation and thus heart rate. Some factors affecting cardiac workload, and therefore myocardial oxygen supply and demand, are listed in Table 31-1.
   a. Under normal circumstances, almost all of the oxygen is removed (during diastole) from the arterial blood as it passes through the heart. Thus, little remains to be extracted if oxygen demand increases. To increase the coronary oxygen supply, the blood flow has to increase. The normal response mechanism is for the blood vessels, particularly the coronary arteries, to dilate, increasing the flow.
   b. The two phases of systole (contraction and ejection) strongly influence oxygen demand.
      (1) The **contractile (inotropic) state** of the heart influences the amount of oxygen it requires to perform.
      (2) As systolic wall tension increases, influenced by **left ventricular volume** and **systolic pressure**, oxygen demand increases.
      (3) Lengthening of **ejection time** (the duration of systolic wall tension per cardiac cycle) also increases oxygen demand.
      (4) Changes in **heart rate** influence oxygen consumption by changing the ejection time.

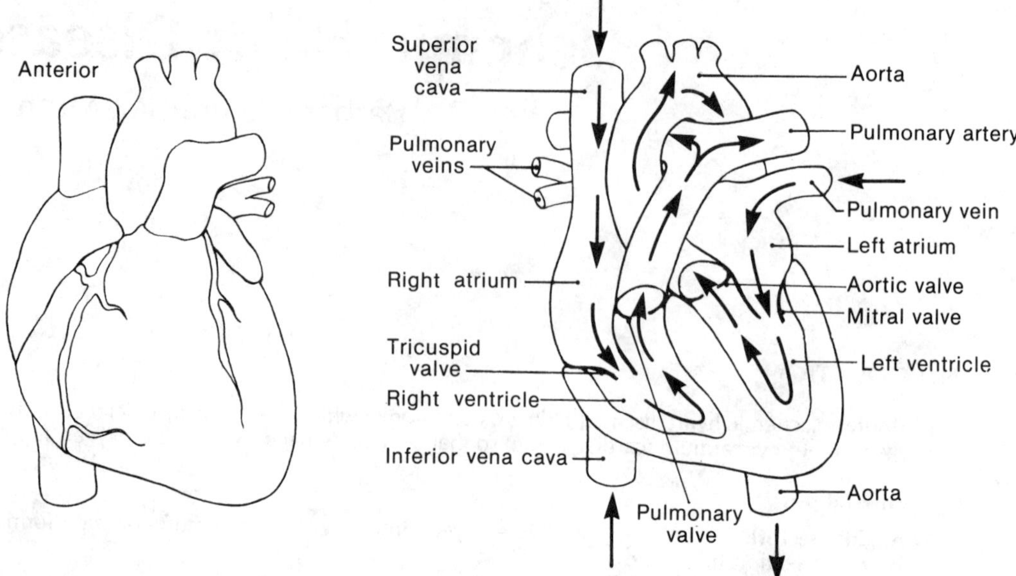

Figure 31-1. Oxygen and other nutrients are borne to the myocardium through the two major coronary arteries (the left and right) and their tributaries. The hemodynamic consequences of ischemic heart disease (IHD) depend on which of the coronary vessels is involved and what part of the myocardium that vessel supplies.

3. **Reduced blood oxygenation**. The oxygen-carrying capacity of the blood may be reduced, as occurs in various anemias.

D. **Risk factors** for IHD appear in Table 31-2.

E. **General therapeutic considerations**. As most IHD occurs secondary to atherosclerosis (a long-term, cumulative process), medical efforts focus on reducing risk factors through individual patient education and media campaigns. Once manifestations occur, treatment addresses their variables.

II. ANGINA PECTORIS

A. **Definition**. This term is applied to varying forms of **transient chest discomfort** that are attributable to insufficient myocardial oxygen.

B. **Common etiologies**. Atherosclerotic lesions producing a narrowing of the coronary arteries is the major cause of angina. However, tachycardia, anemia, hyperthyroidism, hypotension, and arterial hypoxemia are all capable of causing an oxygen imbalance.

C. **Types**

1. **Stable (classic) angina**

a. In this most common form, exertion, emotional stress, or a heavy meal usually precipitates chest discomfort relieved by rest, nitroglycerin, or both.

Table 31-1. Some Factors Affecting Cardiac Parameters That Control Myocardial Oxygen Demand

Factors	Heart Rate	Blood Pressure	Ejection Time	Ventricular Volume	Inotropic Effect
Exercise	Increase	Increase	Decrease	Increase or decrease	Increase
Cold	Increase	Increase	n/a	n/a	n/a
Smoking	Increase	Increase	Increase	n/a	Increase
Nitroglycerin	Increase	Decrease	Decrease	Decrease	Increase
β-Blockers	Decrease	Decrease	Increase	Increase	Decrease

Table 31-2. Risk Factors for Ischemic Heart Disease

Hyperlipidemia
Excess serum cholesterol
Increased ratio of low-density lipoproteins to high-density lipoproteins
Excess triglycerides
Hypertension
Smoking
Diabetes mellitus
Obesity
Family history of ischemic heart disease
Sedentary life-style
Chronic stress or type A personality (aggressive, ambitious, chronically impatient, competitive)
Age and sex (prevalence is higher among men than among premenopausal women and increases for both sexes with age)
Oral contraceptive use
Gout

b. Characteristically, the discomfort builds to a peak and then subsides without residual sensation. If related to physical exertion, the discomfort usually subsides quickly (in 3 to 5 minutes) with rest; if precipitated by emotional stress, the episode tends to last longer (about 10 minutes).

2. Unstable angina

a. Angina is considered unstable and requires further evaluation if a patient experiences:

(1) New-onset angina

(2) Pattern changes—an increase in intensity, duration, or frequency

(3) Occurrences at rest for the first time

(4) Decrease in response to rest or nitroglycerin

b. Progressive unstable angina may signal incipient myocardial infarction and should be reported to the physician promptly.

3. Angina decubitus (nocturnal angina)

a. This angina occurs in the recumbent position and is not specifically related to either rest or exertion.

b. Increased ventricular volume causing increased oxygen needs produces this angina, which may indicate cardiac decompensation.

c. Diuretics alone or in combination are effective in reducing left ventricular volume and may aid the patient.

d. Nitrates such as nitroglycerin, by reducing preload and improving left ventricular dysfunction, may relieve the paroxysmal nocturnal dyspnea associated with angina decubitus.

4. Prinzmetal's angina (vasospastic or variant angina)

a. Coronary artery spasm, reducing blood flow, precipitates this angina.

b. It usually occurs at rest—pain may disrupt sleep—rather than with exertion or emotional stress.

c. Characteristically, an electrocardiogram (ECG) taken during an attack reveals a transient ST-segment elevation.

d. Calcium-channel blockers are most effective for this form of angina, rather than β-blockers. Nitroglycerin may not provide relief, depending on the cause of the vasospasm.

D. Characteristic patient complaints. Patient descriptions of angina include squeezing pressure, sharp pain, burning, aching, bursting, and indigestion-like discomfort. These sensations commonly radiate or move to the arms, legs, neck, shoulders, and back.

E. Physical examination

1. Physical examination is usually not revealing, especially between attacks.

2. The patient's history, risk factors, and full description of attacks—precipitation pattern, intensity, duration, relieving factors—usually prove diagnostic.

F. Diagnostic test results

1. The **ECG** is normal in 50% to 70% of patients at rest and who are asymptomatic. During chest pain, the ST segment will usually be depressed, except in Prinzmetal's angina (see section II C 4 c).

2. **Stress testing (exercise ECG)** aids diagnosis in the patient who has a normal resting ECG. ST-segment depression of more than 1 mm is fairly indicative of vascular abnormality, but the degree of positivity is most indicative of the degree of abnormality.

3. **Coronary arteriography and cardiac catheterization** are most specific and sensitive but are also invasive, expensive, and bear a slight risk (the mortality rate is about 1% to 2%), so they are rarely used just to confirm suspected angina.

G. Treatment goals

1. **To reduce risk of sudden death**

2. **To prevent myocardial infarction**

3. **To increase myocardial oxygen supply or reduce oxygen demand**

4. **To reduce discomfort and anxiety** associated with angina attack

5. **To remove or reduce risk factors**
   a. Hyperlipidemia should be reduced through diet, drugs, or both, with serum monitoring and feedback to the patient at regular intervals.
      (1) Cholesterol-lowering drugs such as cholestyramine (Questran), clofibrate (Atromid-S), colestipol (Colestid), niacin, probucol (Lorelco), gemfibrozil (Lopid), and lovastatin (Mevacor) have not yet shown significant lowering of the overall mortality rates when compared to diet and placebo.
      (2) Despite the controversies, these agents have been used in an attempt to reduce the incidence of nonfatal myocardial infarction.
   b. Hypertension should be controlled.
   c. Smoking should be stopped, unless increasing anxiety offsets the benefits.
   d. Obesity should be reduced through diet and an appropriate exercise program.

H. Therapeutic agents

1. **Nitrates, nitroglycerin**
   a. **Mechanism of action**
      (1) The primary value of nitrates is venous dilation, which reduces left ventricular volume (preload) and myocardial wall tension, decreasing oxygen requirements.
      (2) They may also reduce arteriolar resistance, helping to reduce afterload, both of which decrease myocardial oxygen demand.
      (3) By reducing pressure in cardiac tissues, nitrates also facilitate collateral circulation, which increases blood distribution to ischemic areas.
   b. **Indications**
      (1) Acute attacks of angina pectoris can be managed using sublingual, transmucosal (spray or buccal tablets), or intravenous (IV) delivery.
      (2) Indications include prevention of anticipated attacks using tablets (oral or buccal) or transdermal paste or patches. Sublingual nitrates can be used prior to eating, sexual activity, or a known stress-producing event.
   c. **Choice of preparation** should be based on onset of action, duration of action, and patient compliance and preference, because all nitrates have the same mechanism.
   d. **Precautions and monitoring effects**
      (1) To maximize therapeutic effect, patients should thoroughly understand the use of their specific dosage forms (e.g., sublingual tablets or transdermal patches or pastes).
      (2) Blood pressure and heart rate should be monitored because all nitrates can increase heart rate while lowering blood pressure.
      (3) Preload reduction can be assessed through reduction of pulmonary symptoms such as shortness of breath, paroxysmal nocturnal dyspnea, or dyspnea.
      (4) **Nitrate-induced headaches** are the most common side effect.
         (a) The patient should be warned of the nature, suddenness, and potential strength of this effect to minimize the anxiety that might otherwise occur.
         (b) Compliance can be enhanced if the patient understands that the effect is transient and that the reaction will probably disappear with continued therapy.
         (c) Acetaminophen ingested 15 to 30 minutes before nitrate administration may prevent the headache.
   e. **Effective therapy** should result in a reduction in the number of anginal attacks without inducing significant adverse effects (such as postural hypotension or hypoxia). If maximal doses are reached and the patient still experiences attacks, additional agents should be administered.

2. **β-Adrenergic blockers**
   a. **Mechanism of action**. β-Blockers **reduce oxygen demands**, both at rest and during exertion, by decreasing the heart rate and myocardial contractility, which also decreases arterial blood pressure.
   b. **Indications**. These agents reduce the frequency and severity of exertional angina that is not controlled by nitrates.
   c. **Precautions and monitoring effects**
      (1) Doses should be increased until anginal episodes have been reduced or until unacceptable side effects occur.
      (2) β-Blockers should be avoided in **Prinzmetal's angina** (caused by coronary vasospasm) because they increase coronary resistance.
      (3) **Asthma** is a relative contraindication because all β-blockers increase airway resistance and have the potential to induce bronchospasm in susceptible patients.
      (4) **Diabetic patients** and others predisposed to **hypoglycemia** should be warned that β-blockers mask tachycardia, which is a key sign of developing hypoglycemia.
      (5) Patients should be monitored for **excessive negative inotropic effects**. Findings such as fatigue, shortness of breath, edema, and paroxysmal nocturnal dyspnea may signal developing cardiac compensation, which will also increase the metabolic demands of the heart.
      (6) Sudden cessation of β-blocker therapy may trigger a **withdrawal syndrome** that can exacerbate anginal attacks, especially in patients with coronary artery disease, or cause myocardial infarction.
   d. **Individual agents**. All β-blockers are likely to be equally effective for stable (exertional) angina. For further review of β-adrenergic blockers, see Chapter 36, section III B 7 a.

3. **Calcium-channel blockers**
   a. **Mechanism of action**. Two actions are most pertinent to the treatment of angina.
      (1) These agents prevent and reverse coronary spasm by inhibiting calcium influx into vascular smooth muscle and myocardial muscle. This results in increased blood flow, which enhances myocardial oxygen supply.
      (2) Calcium-channel blockers decrease total peripheral vascular resistance through dilation of peripheral arterioles and reduce myocardial contractility, resulting in decreased oxygen demand.
   b. **Indications**
      (1) Calcium blockers are used in **stable (exertional) angina** that is not controlled by nitrates and β-blockers and in patients for whom β-blocker therapy is inadvisable. Combination therapy—with nitrates, β-blockers, or both—may be most effective.
      (2) These agents are particularly valuable in the treatment of **Prinzmetal's angina**, alone or with a nitrate.
   c. **Individual agents**
      (1) **Verapamil and diltiazem**
         (a) These drugs produce **negative inotropic effects**, and patients must be monitored closely for signs of developing cardiac decompensation—fatigue, shortness of breath, edema, and paroxysmal nocturnal dyspnea. When coadministered with β-blockers or other agents also having a negative inotropic effect (e.g., disopyramide, quinidine, procainamide, flecainide), the negative effects are additive.
         (b) Patients should be monitored for signs of developing bradyarrhythmias and heart block because these agents have **strong negative chronotropic effects**.
      (2) **Nifedipine**
         (a) This calcium-channel blocker does not seem to have a strongly negative inotropic effect; therefore, it is preferred for combination therapy with agents that do.
         (b) Because nifedipine increases the heart rate somewhat, it can produce **tachycardia**, which would increase oxygen demand. Coadministration of a β-blocker should prevent reflex tachycardia.
         (c) Its potent peripheral dilatory effects can decrease coronary perfusion and produce excessive hypotension, which can **aggravate myocardial ischemia**.
         (d) **Dizziness**, **lightheadedness**, and **lower extremity edema** are the most common adverse effects, but these tend to disappear with time or dose adjustment.

III. MYOCARDIAL INFARCTION

A. **Definition**. In myocardial infarction, a portion of the cardiac muscle suffers a severe and prolonged restriction of oxygenated coronary blood. This results in cellular ischemia, tissue injury, and tissue necrosis. Because myocardial tissue dies, a myocardial infarction, unlike angina pectoris, is irreversible.

B. Signs and symptoms

1. The foremost characteristic of a myocardial infarction is **persistent, severe chest pain or pressure**, commonly described as crushing, squeezing, or heavy (likened to having an elephant sitting on the chest). The pain generally begins in the chest and, like angina, may radiate to the left arm, the abdomen, back, neck, jaw, or teeth. The onset of pain generally occurs at rest or with normal daily activities; it is not commonly associated with exertion.

2. Unlike an angina attack, sensations associated with a myocardial infarction usually persist—longer than 15 minutes—and are unrelieved by nitroglycerin.

3. **Other common patient complaints** include a sense of impending doom, sweating, nausea, vomiting, and difficulty breathing.

4. **Observable findings** include extreme anxiety; restless, agitated behavior; and ashen pallor.

5. Some patients, particularly diabetics or the elderly, may experience only mild or indigestion-like pain or a **clinically silent myocardial infarction**, which may only manifest in worsening congestive heart failure, loss of consciousness, a sudden drop in blood pressure, or a lethal arrhythmia.

C. Diagnostic test results. Because a myocardial infarction is a life-threatening emergency, diagnosis is presumed—and treatment is instituted—based on patient complaints and the results of an immediate 12-lead ECG. Laboratory tests and further diagnostic tests can rule out or provide confirmation of a myocardial infarction and help identify the locale and extent of myocardial damage.

1. **Serial 12-lead ECG**. Abnormalities may be absent or inconclusive during the first few hours after a myocardial infarction and may not aid diagnosis in about 15% of the cases. When present, characteristic findings show progressive changes.
   a. First, ST-segment elevation (injury current) appears in the leads reflecting the injured area.
   b. Then T waves invert (reflecting ischemia), and Q waves develop (indicating necrosis).
   c. Unequivocal diagnosis can only be made in the presence of all three abnormalities. However, the manifestations depend on the area of injury. For example, in subendocardial infarction, only ST-segment depression may appear.
   d. Arrhythmias commonly appear after the acute event.

2. **Chest x-ray findings** are commonly normal unless congestive heart failure is developing, indicated by cardiomegaly, pulmonary vascular congestion, or pleural effusion.

3. **Myocardial scanning**, with technetium 99, for example, is useful in confirming or localizing damage; a "hot spot" on the film indicates the area of uptake by damaged tissue.

D. Cardiac enzyme studies. Changes in some of the laboratory values do not appear until between 6 and 24 hours after the myocardial infarction (Table 31-3).

E. Treatment goals

1. **To relieve chest pain and anxiety**

2. **To reduce cardiac workload and stabilize cardiac rhythm**

3. **To reduce myocardial infarction** by limiting the area affected and preserving pump function

4. **To prevent or arrest complications**, such as lethal arrhythmias, congestive heart failure, or sudden death

Table 31-3. Serum Cardiac Enzyme Values in Myocardial Infarction

Test	Approximate Post-Myocardial Infarction Appearance Time	Comments
CPK (creatine phosphokinase)	6 hours	MB isoenzyme elevation is particularly telling as it derives almost exclusively in the myocardium
SGOT (serum glutamic-oxaloacetic transaminase)	6–12 hours	Activity peaks in 24–48 hours; returns to normal in 3–5 days
LDH (lactic dehydrogenase)	24 hours	LDH_1 exceeds LDH_2
WBC (white blood cells)	24 hours	A count of 12,000–15,000/μl indicates necrosis

F. Therapeutic agents. Intramuscular drug administration in myocardial infarction therapy can invalidate the results of cardiac enzyme studies; therefore, this route should be avoided.

1. Nitrates, nitroglycerin

a. These agents may help relieve pain, especially if coronary spasm produced the myocardial infarction. Also, regardless of the cause, the pain of a myocardial infarction can trigger the release of catecholamines, which can produce a coronary spasm.

b. The nitrates decrease oxygen demand and facilitate coronary blood flow, as detailed in section II H 1 a.

2. Morphine

a. The drug of choice for myocardial infarction pain and anxiety, morphine also causes venous pooling and reduces preload, cardiac workload, and oxygen consumption.

b. Precautions and monitoring effects

(1) Because morphine increases peripheral vasodilation and decreases peripheral resistance, it can produce **orthostatic hypotension and fainting**.

(2) Patients should be monitored for **hypotension** and signs of **respiratory depression**.

(3) Morphine has a vagomimetic effect that can produce **bradyarrhythmias**. If ECG monitoring reveals excess bradycardia, it should be reversed by the administration of atropine (0.5 to 1 mg).

(4) Nausea and vomiting may occur, especially with initial doses, and patients must be protected against **aspiration of stomach contents**.

(5) Severe **constipation** is a potential problem with ongoing morphine administration. The patient may use a **Valsalva maneuver** while straining at the stool, which can produce a bradycardia or overload the cardiac system and trigger cardiac arrest. Docusate (100 mg twice daily) has proven a useful prophylactic.

3. Oxygen

a. Current advanced cardiac life support recommendations require the institution of oxygen therapy in any patient who is suffering from chest pain and who may be ischemic.

b. Continuing hypoxia rapidly increases myocardial damage, so increasing the oxygen content of the blood and thus improving oxygenation of the myocardium is a top priority.

4. Lidocaine

a. Lidocaine is administered as a prophylactic against ventricular arrhythmias.

b. This antiarrhythmic has a rapid effect and is highly controllable because its effects diminish rapidly once the infusion is withdrawn.

c. Precautions and monitoring effects

(1) Only lidocaine preparations without sympathomimetic amines or other vasoconstrictors should be used in myocardial infarction. Other forms can cause lethal arrhythmias and are therefore contraindicated.

(2) Coadministration of a β-blocker diminishes the metabolism of lidocaine and may result in lidocaine toxicity. At the first signs of toxicity (e.g., dizziness, somnolence, confusion, paresthesias, or convulsions), the lidocaine should be withdrawn.

(3) The risk of lidocaine toxicity increases with an increased rate of infusion.

5. Thrombolytic agents

a. Indications

(1) Suspected myocardial infarction with chest pain of less than 6 hours duration

(2) ST-segment elevation unresponsive to nitroglycerin

b. Intracoronary or IV administration of **streptokinase** or **urokinase** may restore blood flow in an occluded artery if administered within about 6 hours of the beginning of an attack.

(1) They promote thrombus dissolution, usually within about 30 minutes, by triggering the activation of endogenous plasminogen to plasmin, which hydrolyzes fibrin.

(2) These agents put the patient at risk for intramyocardial and systemic hemorrhage.

c. Heparin and oral anticoagulants should be administered as a follow-up to thrombolytic therapy. Long-term (1–3 years) β-blocker therapy should also be considered.

d. It is hoped that **tissue-type plasminogen activator (t-TPA)**, recently released, will provide the desired therapeutic effects with fewer and less serious adverse effects.

6. β-Adrenergic blockers

a. If administered early in the acute phase, β-blockers, usually propranolol, may help reduce the potential zone of infarction, decrease oxygen demands, and decrease cardiac workload.

b. β-Blocker therapy has also been shown to reduce significantly post–myocardial infarction mortality due to sudden cardiac death.

c. Precautions and monitoring effects (see section II H 2 c).

G. **Complications**. Myocardial infarction potentiates many complications; the most common of these include:

1. **Lethal arrhythmias**. Arrhythmias refractory to lidocaine may respond to amiodarone, bretylium, or tocainide.

2. **Congestive heart failure**. (See Chapter 34 for a more detailed discussion.)
   a. Left ventricular failure causes pulmonary congestion. **Diuretics**, especially furosemide, help reduce the congestion.
   b. **Digitalis glycosides** have a positive inotropic effect, which improves myocardial contractility, helping to compensate for myocardial damage.

3. **Cardiogenic shock**
   a. In this life-threatening complication, cardiac output is decreased and pulmonary artery and pulmonary capillary wedge pressures are increased. This typically occurs when the area of infarction exceeds 40% of muscle mass and compensatory mechanisms only strain the already compromised myocardium.
   b. Vasopressors, such as norepinephrine, epinephrine, and dopamine (high doses) enhance blood pressure through α-receptor stimulation and may be indicated.
   c. Inotropic drugs, such as epinephrine, dopamine (middle doses), dobutamine, isoproterenol, and digitalis glycosides, are rapidly acting agents used to increase myocardial contractility and improve cardiac output.
   d. Vasodilators, such as nitroprusside and nitroglycerin, help reduce preload by lowering pulmonary capillary wedge pressure through venous dilation while reducing afterload by decreasing resistance to left ventricular ejection.
   e. Additional treatment may include invasive procedures such as intra-aortic balloon pumping.

STUDY QUESTIONS

Directions: Each question below contains five suggested answers. Choose the **one best** response to each question.

1. Exertion-induced angina, which is relieved by rest, nitroglycerin, or both, is referred to as

A. Prinzmetal's angina
B. unstable angina
C. classic angina
D. variant angina
E. preinfarction angina

2. All of the following factors have been shown to increase myocardial oxygen demand EXCEPT

A. exercise
B. smoking
C. cold temperatures
D. isoproterenol
E. propranolol

3. Which of the following agents used in Prinzmetal's angina has spasmolytic actions, which increase coronary blood supply?

A. Nitroglycerin
B. Nifedipine
C. Timolol
D. Isosorbide dinitrate
E. Propranolol

4. What adverse drug effect must be monitored in the angina pectoris patient who is receiving propranolol plus diltiazem?

A. Decreased cardiac output
B. Decreased heart rate
C. Increased heart rate
D. Decreased cardiac output and decreased heart rate
E. Decreased cardiac output and increased heart rate

5. Which of the following choices represents maximal medical therapy for treating angina pectoris?

A. Diltiazem, verapamil, nitroglycerin
B. Atenolol, isoproterenol, diltiazem
C. Verapamil, nifedipine, propranolol
D. Isosorbide, atenolol, diltiazem
E. Nitroglycerin, isosorbide, atenolol

6. The term ischemic heart disease (IHD) is used to designate all of the following conditions EXCEPT

A. angina pectoris
B. sudden cardiac death
C. congestive heart disease
D. arrhythmias
E. myocardial infarction

7. The development of ischemic pain occurs when the demands for oxygen exceed the supply. All of the following choices determine oxygen demand EXCEPT

A. contractile state of the heart
B. myocardial ejection time
C. left ventricular volume
D. right atrial pressure
E. systolic pressure

8. The use of morphine in the myocardial infarction patient centers around three distinct pharmacologic properties. Which of the following choices includes these properties?

A. Relief of pain, relief of anxiety, and increased oxygen supply
B. Relief of anxiety, afterload reduction, increased preload
C. Relief of anxiety, preload reduction, and relief of pain
D. Vagomimetic effect, relief of anxiety, respiratory depression
E. Bradycardia, preload reduction, and increased afterload

9. Although all of the evidence has yet to be accumulated, it seems appropriate to suggest that one group of antianginals has been shown to be effective post–myocardial infarction for the prevention of sudden death. Which of the following agents represents this group of antianginals?

A. Isosorbide dinitrate
B. Metoprolol
C. Nifedipine
D. Streptokinase
E. Heparin

ANSWERS AND EXPLANATIONS

1. The answer is C. (*II B 1 a*) Classic, or stable, angina refers to the syndrome in which physical activity or emotional excess causes chest discomfort, which may spread to the arms, legs, neck, and so forth. This type of angina is relieved promptly (within 1 to 10 minutes) with rest, nitroglycerin, or both.

2. The answer is E. (*I C 2; Table 31-1*)) Due to the β-adrenergic blocking effects of propranolol (decreased heart rate, decreased blood pressure, and decreased inotropic effect), there is a net decrease in myocardial oxygen demand. This is directly opposite of the effects seen with the β-agonist isoproterenol. Exercise, cigarette smoking, and exposure to cold temperatures have all been shown to increase myocardial oxygen demand.

3. The answer is B. [*II C 4, H 3 c (2)*] Due to the calcium-channel blocking properties of nifedipine, primarily coronary dilation and spasmolytic effects, there is proven benefit of this agent in treatment of Prinzmetal's angina, a syndrome believed due more to a spastic event rather than to a fixed coronary occlusion.

4. The answer is D. (*II H 2, 3*) As propranolol (a β-adrenergic blocker) and diltiazem (a calcium-channel blocker) both reduce heart rate (a negative chronotropic effect) and reduce cardiac contractility (negative inotropic effect), patients receiving both drugs must be monitored for signs of decompensation (reduced cardiac output) and brady arrhythmias.

5. The answer is D. [*II H 3 b (1)*] The use of a nitrate (isosorbide) in conjunction with a β-adrenergic blocker (atenolol) and a calcium-channel blocker (diltiazem) represents the maximal medical regimen that presently could be used in a nonresponsive angina patient. Venous dilation and coronary dilation due to nitrates reduces oxygen demand while increasing oxygen supply, respectively. The addition of diltiazem further reduces oxygen demand by decreasing heartrate and cardiac contractility. The use of a β-blocker such as atenolol reduces oxygen demand even more, resulting in a total net reduction in myocardial oxygen demand.

6. The answer is C. (*I B*) Ischemic heart disease (IHD) is a clinical condition that exists, when there is a lack of oxygen to the heart. This may be due to increased demands of or decreased supplies to the heart. Angina pectoris, sudden cardiac death due to toxic ventricular arrhythmias, and myocardial infarction represent the various conditions associated with IHD.

7. The answer is D. (*I C 2*) As with most muscles in the body, the contractile force of the heart dictates the amount of oxygen that the heart needs to perform. Consequently, as contractility decreases, the oxygen needs of the heart increase. As contractility continues to decrease, the volume of fluid in the left ventricle increases due to poor muscle performance and increasing tension within the ventricle, resulting in additional oxygen requirements. As the amount of tension within the ventricle increases per cardiac cycle, there is again an added requirement for oxygen by the heart muscle.

8. The answer is C. (*III F 2*) Venous dilation (preload reduction) along with relief of pain and anxiety make morphine a very helpful agent in the myocardial infarction patient. In the clinical situation, pain and anxiety in the myocardial infarction patient represent an added stress, which only increases myocardial oxygen demands further, thus adding potential insult to the already compromised myocardium. Venous dilation would help in reducing venous return to the heart and, therefore, reduce oxygen demands placed on the myocardium. Both of these physiologic responses aid in reestablishing the balance between myocardial oxygen supply and demand.

9. The answer is B. (*III F 6*) As a β-adrenergic blocker, metoprolol and other β-blockers have been shown to reduce the incidence of sudden death after a myocardial infarction. Studies are currently underway using calcium-channel blockers like nifedipine to determine if there are beneficial effects resulting from their use as well.

32
Cardiac Arrhythmias

Alan H. Mutnick

I. GENERAL CONSIDERATIONS

A. Definition. Cardiac arrhythmias are deviations from the normal heartbeat pattern. They include **abnormalities of impulse formation**, such as heart rate, rhythm, or site of impulse origin; and **conduction disturbances**, which disrupt the normal sequence of atrial and ventricular activation.

B. Electrophysiology

1. **Conduction system**
   - a. The conduction system of the heart initiates two electrical sequences that cause the heart chambers to fill with blood and contract.
     - (1) **Impulse formation**, the first sequence, takes place when an electrical impulse is generated automatically.
     - (2) **Impulse transmission**, the second sequence, occurs once the impulse has been generated, signalling the heart to contract.
   - b. The conduction system consists of four main structures composed of tissue that can generate or conduct electrical impulses.
     - (1) The **sinoatrial (SA) node**, in the wall of the right atrium, contains cells that spontaneously initiate an action potential. Serving as the heart's main pacemaker, the SA node initiates 60 to 100 beats/minute.
       - **(a)** Impulses generated by the SA node trigger atrial contraction.
       - **(b)** Impulses travel through internodal tracts—the anterior tract, middle (Wenckebach) tract, posterior (Thorel's) tract, and anterior interatrial tract (Bachmann's bundles) [Fig. 32-1].
     - (2) At the **atrioventricular (AV) node**, situated in the lower interatrial septum, the impulses are delayed briefly to permit completion of atrial contraction before ventricular contraction begins.
     - (3) At the **bundle of His**—muscle fibers arising from the AV junction—impulses travel along the left and right bundle branches, located on either side of the intraventricular septum.
     - (4) The impulses reach the **Purkinje fibers**, a diffuse network extending from the bundle branches and ending in the ventricular endocardial surfaces. Ventricular contraction then occurs.
   - c. The AV junction, bundle of His, and Purkinje fibers are **latent pacemakers**; they contain cells capable of generating impulses. However, these regions have a slower firing rate than the SA node. Consequently, the SA node predominates except when it is depressed or injured (which is known as overdrive suppression).

2. **Myocardial action potential**. Before cardiac contraction can take place, cardiac cells must depolarize and repolarize.
   - a. Depolarization and repolarization result from changes in the electrical potential across the cell membrane, caused by the exchange of sodium and potassium ions.
   - b. The **action potential**, which reflects this electrical activity, has five phases (Fig. 32-2).
     - (1) **Phase 0 (rapid depolarization)**. This takes place as sodium ions enter the cell through fast channels; the cell membrane's electrical charge changes from negative to positive.
     - (2) **Phase 1 (early rapid repolarization)**. As fast sodium channels close and potassium ions leave the cell, the cell rapidly repolarizes—returns to resting potential.
     - (3) **Phase 2 (plateau)**. Calcium ions enter the cell through slow channels while potassium ions exit. As the cell membrane's electrical activity temporarily stabilizes, the action potential reaches a plateau (represented by the notch at the beginning of this phase in Fig. 32-2).

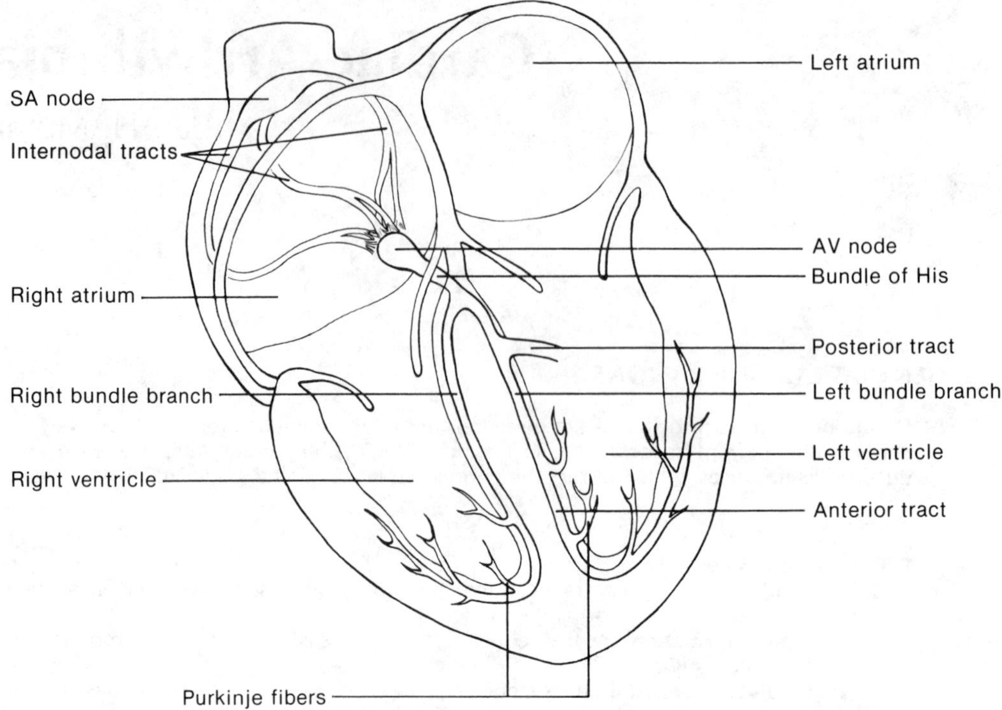

Figure 32-1. Electrical pathways of the heart. *SA* = sinoatrial; *AV* = atrioventricular.

(4) **Phase 3 (final rapid repolarization).** Potassium ions are pumped out of the cell as the cell rapidly completes repolarization and resumes its initial negativity.

(5) **Phase 4 (slow depolarization)**. The cell returns to its resting state, with potassium ions inside the cell and sodium and calcium ions outside.

c. During depolarization/repolarization, a cell's ability to initiate an action potential varies.

(1) The cell cannot respond to any stimulus during the **absolute refractory period** (beginning during phase 1 and ending at the start of phase 3).

(2) A cell's ability to respond to stimuli increases as repolarization continues. During the **relative refractory period**, occurring during phase 3, the cell can respond to a strong stimulus.

(3) When the cell has been completely repolarized, it can again respond fully to stimuli.

d. Cells in different cardiac regions depolarize at various speeds, depending on whether fast or slow channels predominate.

(1) **Sodium** flows through **fast channels**; **calcium**, through **slow channels**.

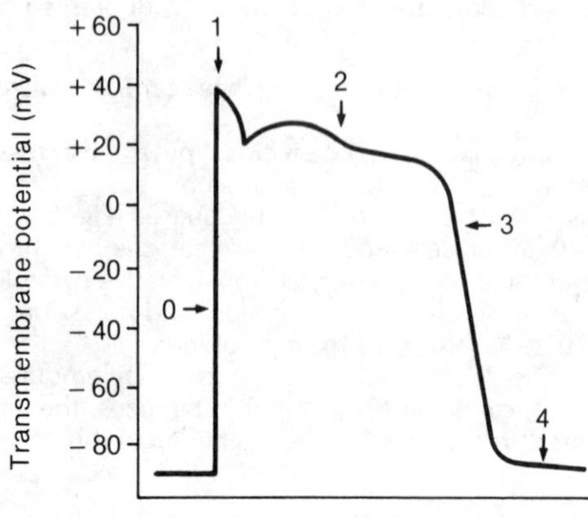

Figure 32-2. Myocardial action potential curve. This curve represents ventricular depolarization/repolarization. *0* = phase 0 (rapid depolarization); *1* = phase 1 (early rapid repolarization); *2* = phase 2 (plateau); *3* = phase 3 (final rapid repolarization); *4* = phase 4 (slow depolarization).

(2) Where fast channels dominate (as in cardiac muscle cells), depolarization occurs quickly. Slow-channel domination (as in the electrical cells of the SA node and AV junction) results in relatively slow depolarization.

3. **Electrocardiography**. The electrical activity occurring during depolarization/repolarization can be transmitted through electrodes attached to the body and transformed by an **electrocardiograph (ECG) machine** into a series of waveforms (ECG waveform). Figure 32-3 shows a normal ECG waveform.
   a. The **P wave** reflects atrial depolarization.
   b. The **PR interval** represents the spread of the impulse from the atria through the Purkinje fibers.
   c. The **QRS complex** reflects ventricular depolarization.
   d. The **ST segment** represents phase 2 of the action potential—the absolute refractory period (part of ventricular repolarization).
   e. The **T wave** shows phase 3 of the action potential—ventricular repolarization.

C. **Classification**. Arrhythmias generally are classified by origin—supraventricular or ventricular.

1. **Supraventricular** arrhythmias stem from enhanced automaticity of the SA node (or another pacemaker region) or from reentry conduction.

2. **Ventricular** arrhythmias occur when an ectopic (abnormal) pacemaker triggers a ventricular contraction before the SA node fires (as from a conduction disturbance or ventricular irritability).

D. **Etiology**

1. **Precipitating causes**. Arrhythmias result from various conditions, including:
   a. Heart disease (e.g., infection, coronary artery disease, valvular heart disease, rheumatic heart disease, or ischemic heart disease)
   b. Myocardial infarction (MI)
   c. Toxic doses of cardioactive drugs (especially digitalis preparations)
   d. Increased sympathetic tone
   e. Decreased parasympathetic tone
   f. Vagal stimulation (e.g., straining at stool)
   g. Increased oxygen demand (e.g., from stress, exercise, or fever)
   h. Metabolic disturbances
   i. Cor pulmonale
   j. Systemic hypertension
   k. Hyperkalemia
   l. Chronic obstructive pulmonary disease (e.g., chronic bronchitis or emphysema)
   m. Thyroid disorders

2. **Mechanisms of arrhythmias**. Abnormal impulse formation, abnormal impulse conduction, or a combination of these may give rise to an arrhythmia.
   a. **Abnormal impulse formation** may stem from:
      (1) Depressed automaticity, as in escape beats and bradycardia
      (2) Increased automaticity, as in premature beats, tachycardia, and extrasystole
      (3) Depolarization and triggered activity, leading to sustained ectopic firing
   b. **Abnormal impulse conduction** results from:
      (1) A conduction block or delay
      (2) **Reentry**. This occurs when an impulse is rerouted through certain regions in which it has already traveled. The impulse thus depolarizes the same tissue more than once, producing an additional impulse (Fig. 32-4 and Fig. 32-5).
         (a) For reentry to occur, the following conditions must exist:
            (i) Markedly shortened refractoriness or a slow conduction area that allows an adequate delay so that depolarization recurs
            (ii) Unidirectional conduction

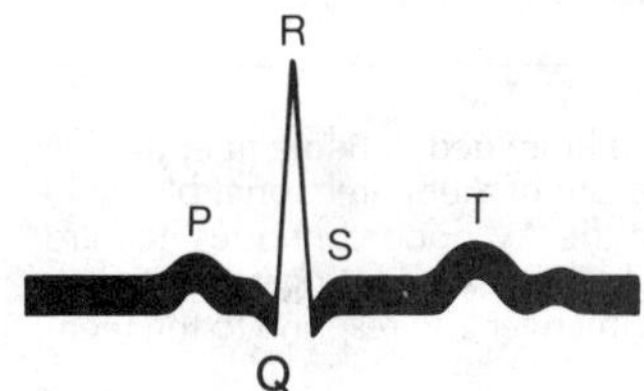

Figure 32-3. Normal ECG waveform.

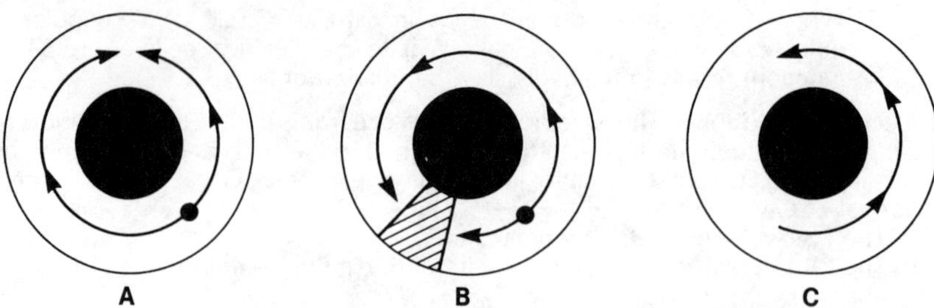

Figure 32-4. Reentry arrhythmias. *A* shows two waves of excitation going in opposite directions; *B* represents a unidirectional wave of excitation; *C* shows reexcitation of tissue in a slow conduction area.

(b) Reentry sites include the SA and AV nodes as well as various accessory pathways in the atria and ventricles (Fig. 32-6).

E. Pathophysiology. Arrhythmias may decrease cardiac output, reduce blood pressure, and disrupt perfusion of vital organs. Specific pathophysiologic consequences depend on the arrhythmia present (see section IV).

F. Clinical evaluation

1. Physical findings. Although some arrhythmias are silent, most produce signs and symptoms. Only an ECG can definitively identify an arrhythmia; however, physical findings may suggest which arrhythmia is present. They also yield information about the patient's clinical status and may help identify associated complications. Signs and symptoms that typically accompany arrhythmias include:

a. Chest pain
b. Anxiety and confusion (from reduced brain perfusion)
c. Dyspnea
d. Skin pallor or cyanosis

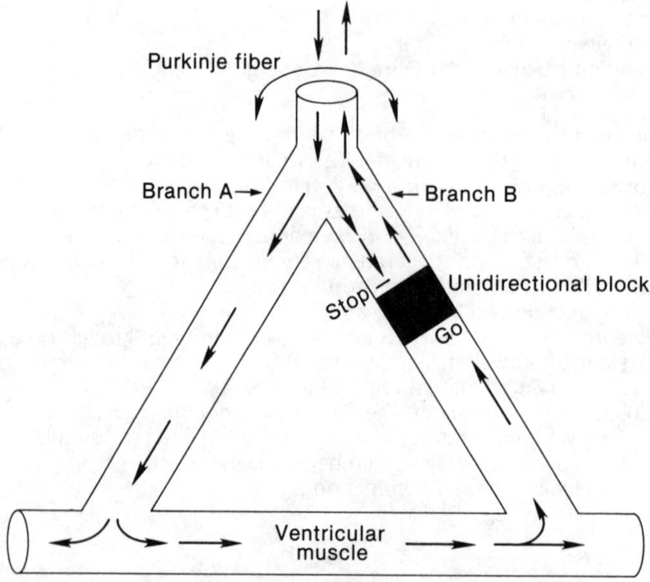

Figure 32-5. Ventricular reentry. This diagram shows a branched Purkinje fiber joining ventricular muscle. The darkened area represents the site of a unidirectional block; in this depolarized region, the impulse heading toward the AV node continues upward while the impulse traveling toward the muscle is blocked. Because retrograde conduction in branch **B** is slow, cells in branch **A** have time to recover and respond to the reentrant impulse.

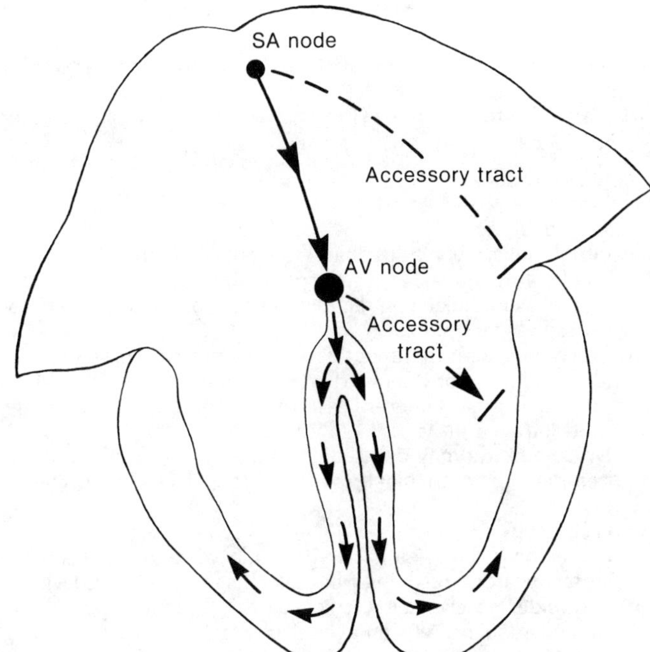

Figure 32-6. Reentry sites.

e. Abnormal pulse rate, rhythm, or amplitude
f. Reduced blood pressure
g. Palpitations
h. Syncope
i. Weakness
j. Convulsions
k. Hypotension
l. Decreased urinary output

2. **Diagnostic test results**
   a. An **ECG** can identify a specific arrhythmia; usually, a 12-lead ECG is used. (For ECG findings in specific arrhythmias, see section IV.)
   b. **Electrophysiologic (EP) testing.** This intracardiac procedure determines the location of ectopic foci and bypass tracts and may help assess therapeutic response to antiarrhythmic drug therapy. It also can determine the need for a pacemaker or surgical intervention.
      (1) Intracardiac catheters and pacing wires are placed transvenously or transarterially.
      (2) The heart is divided into imaginary sections and each section is stimulated until an arrhythmia is induced. The section in which the arrhythmia occurs is identified as the origin of the ectopic foci.
   c. **His bundle study**, a type of EP testing, can locate the origin of a heart block or reentry pattern.
   d. **Laboratory findings**. Some arrhythmias result from electrolyte abnormalities—most commonly, hyperkalemia and hypocalcemia.
      (1) A serum potassium level above 5 mEq/L reflects hyperkalemia; a serum calcium level below 4.5 mEq/L signifies hypocalcemia.
      (2) An ECG tracing may suggest an electrolyte abnormality. For example, prolonged QRS complexes, tented T waves, and lenghthened PR intervals may signal hyperkalemia; prolonged QT intervals and flattened or inverted T waves suggest hypocalcemia.

II. TREATMENT OBJECTIVES

A. Terminate or suppress the arrhythmia, if it causes hemodynamic compromise or disturbing symptoms

B. Maintain adequate cardiac output and tissue perfusion

C. Correct or maintain fluid balance (some arrhythmias cause hypervolemia)

III. THERAPY

A. Antiarrhythmic agents. These drugs directly or indirectly alter the duration of the myocardial action potential. Most antiarrhythmics fall into one of four classes, depending on their specific effects on the heart's electrical activity (Table 32-1). Class I drugs are further subdivided into three groups.

1. Class I antiarrhythmics

a. Indications

(1) Class IA drugs

(a) Quinidine is given to treat and prevent acute and chronic ventricular and supraventricular arrhythmias, especially premature supraventricular tachycardias (PSVTs), premature ventricular contractions (PVCs), premature atrial contractions (PACs), and ventricular tachycardia.

(b) Procainamide is therapeutic for the same arrhythmias for which quinidine is given. It is used more frequently than quinidine because it can be administered intravenously and in sustained-release oral preparations. Quinidine poses concern when used intravenously.

(c) Disopyramide may be used as an alternative to quinidine or procainamide in the treatment of ventricular arrhythmias (e.g., PVCs and moderate ventricular tachycardia).

(2) Class IB drugs

(a) Lidocaine is therapeutic for ventricular arrhythmias (especially PVCs and ventricular tachycardia) resulting from digitalis therapy, acute MI, and open-heart surgery.

(b) Tocainide, closely related to lidocaine, is given to suppress ventricular arrhythmias, including frequent PVCs and ventricular tachycardia. It may be given after an acute MI.

(c) Phenytoin most commonly is used to treat digitalis-induced ventricular and supraventricular arrhythmias. It also is given to suppress ventricular arrhythmias associated with an acute MI or open-heart surgery or ventricular arrhythmias that are refractory to lidocaine or procainamide, but its efficacy is less significant than in digitalis-induced arrhythmias.

(d) Mexiletine, another drug with a close resemblance to lidocaine, is used to suppress ventricular arrhythmias, including those following an acute MI. It has proven to be effective against ventricular tachycardia that has not responded to other antiarrhythmics.

(3) Class IC drugs

(a) Encainide is given to treat life-threatening ventricular arrhythmias and to prevent or suppress frequent PVCs and nonsustained ventricular tachycardia when these are refractory to first-line agents.

(b) Flecainide also suppresses PVCs and ventricular tachycardia; it may be used to treat some arrhythmias that are refractory to other agents.

b. Mechanism of action. Class I antiarrhythmics slow impulse conduction through the AV node by depressing the flow of sodium ions into cells during phase 0 of the action potential. Class I subgroups (IA, IB, and IC) differ in the degree and onset of their myocardial depressant action and in their effects on the duration of the action potential and/or repolarization phase.

(1) Class IA drugs moderately reduce the depolarization rate and prolong repolarization or the refractory period.

Table 32-1. Currently Available Antiarrhythmic Agents

Class	Agents
IA	Quinidine, procainamide, disopyramide
IB	Lidocaine, phenytoin, tocainide, mexiletine
IC	Flecainide, encainide
II*	Propranolol, esmolol, metoprolol, nadolol, atenolol, timolol, pindolol, labetalol, acebutolol
III	Amiodarone, bretylium
IV†	Verapamil, diltiazem, nifedipine

*Only propranolol and esmolol are currently approved for use as antiarrhythmics.
†Diltiazem and nifedipine are used primarily as antianginal agents.

(2) **Class IB** drugs shorten repolarization or the refractory period; they weakly affect the repolarization rate.
(3) **Class IC** drugs strongly depress depolarization but have a negligible effect on the duration of repolarization or the refractory period.

c. Administration and dosage

(1) **Quinidine** is administered orally, usually in three or four daily doses of 200 to 300 mg. (In special circumstances, it cautiously can be given intravenously or intramuscularly.) To rapidly achieve an effective plasma concentration, a loading dose of 600 to 1000 mg may be administered, in doses of 200 mg every 2 hours, to a maximum of 1000 mg.
(2) **Procainamide** is available for oral, intravenous (IV), or intramuscular use.
  (a) For **acute therapy**, IV administration is preferred.
    (i) **Intermittent** IV administration calls for infusion of 100 mg over 2 to 4 minutes, repeated every 5 minutes until the arrhythmia is abolished, side effects occur, or 1 g has been given. The usual effective dose is 500 to 1000 mg.
    (ii) **Rapid** IV administration calls for infusion of 1 to 2.5 g at a rate of 20 mg/min.
    (iii) Once the arrhythmia is terminated, 2 to 6 mg is given as a **continuous** infusion.
  (b) For **long-term therapy**, the oral route is used. The usual daily dosage is 3 to 6 g, given at intervals of 3 to 6 hours, or less frequently with the sustained-release form of the drug.
(3) **Disopyramide** is available only in oral form. Usually, 400 to 800 mg/day is administered in divided doses. (A loading dose of 200 to 300 mg may be given to rapidly attain an effective plasma level.)
(4) **Lidocaine** may be administered intravenously or intramuscularly.
  (a) An IV loading dose rapidly achieves a therapeutic plasma level.
    (i) Initially, 1 to 1.5 mg/kg is administered.
    (ii) A second injection of half the initial dose may be required 5 minutes later.
  (b) **Continuous** IV infusion of 1 to 4 mg/min produces an effective plasma level in 7 to 10 hours.
  (c) In an emergency, an **intramuscular injection** rapidly achieves an effective plasma level. The usual dosage is 4 to 5 mg/kg.
(5) **Tocainide** is administered orally. Initially, 400 mg is given every 8 hours; then, 1200 to 1800 mg/day is given in two to three divided doses.
(6) **Phenytoin** is given orally or in intermittent IV doses.
  (a) For **oral** administration, a loading dose of 1 g is divided over the first 24 hours; for the next 2 days, 500 mg/day is administered. The maintenance dosage is 300 to 400 mg/day.
  (b) For **intermittent** IV administration, 100 mg is given every 5 minutes, at a rate not exceeding 50 mg/min, until the arrhythmia disappears, adverse effects develop, or 1 g has been given. The usual effective dosage is 700 mg.
(7) **Mexiletine** is given orally in an initial dosage of 200 to 400 mg, followed by 200 mg every 8 hours. If this fails to control the arrhythmia, the dosage may be increased to 400 mg every 8 hours. (Alternatively, doses may be given every 12 hours.)
(8) **Flecainide** is administered orally in a dosage of 50 to 100 mg every 12 hours. To obtain satisfactory arrhythmia control, the dosage may be increased in twice-daily increments of 50 mg every 4 days, to a maximum of 400 mg/day.
(9) **Encainide** is given orally in an initial dosage of 25 mg every 8 hours. If necessary, the dosage may be increased to 35 mg every 8 hours after 3 to 5 days, then increased to 50 mg every 8 hours after another 3 to 5 days.

d. Precautions and monitoring effects

(1) **Quinidine**
  (a) This drug is contraindicated in patients with complete AV block with an AV nodal pacemaker site.
  (b) An increase of 50% or more in the duration of the QRS complex necessitates dosage reduction.
  (c) Quinidine has a narrow therapeutic index. Toxicity may cause acute cardiac effects, such as pronounced slowing of conduction in all heart regions; this, in turn, may lead to SA block or arrest, ventricular tachycardia, or asystole.
  (d) Quinidine should be avoided in patients with marked prolongation of the QT interval or "long QT syndrome" because ventricular tachyarrhythmias (torsades de pointes) may arise, resulting in "quinidine syncope" (syncope or sudden death).
  (e) The ECG should be monitored during quinidine therapy to detect signs of cardiotoxicity. To counteract quinidine-induced ventricular tachyarrhythmias, catecholamines, glucagon, or sodium lactate may be given.
  (f) In patients receiving quinidine for atrial tachyarrhythmias, vagolytic effects may increase impulse conduction at the AV node, resulting in an accelerated ventricular

response. To prevent this, agents that slow AV nodal conduction (e.g., verapamil, digoxin) may be administered.

(g) The dosage should be reduced in patients with hepatic dysfunction or congestive heart failure (CHF).

(h) Embolism may occur upon restoration of normal sinus rhythm after prolonged atrial fibrillation. To prevent or minimize this complication, anticoagulants may be administered before quinidine therapy begins.

(i) Quinidine may cause cinchonism, manifested by tinnitus, hearing loss, blurred vision, and gastrointestinal disturbances. In severe cases, nausea, vomiting, diarrhea, headache, confusion, delirium, photophobia, diplopia, and psychosis may occur.

(j) Gastrointestinal reactions are the most common adverse reactions to quinidine. About 30% of patients experience diarrhea; nausea and vomiting may also occur. Arising almost immediately after the first dose, these symptoms sometimes warrant drug discontinuation.

(k) Hypersensitivity reactions include anaphylaxis, thrombocytopenia, respiratory distress, and vascular collapse.

(l) Plasma quinidine levels of 2 to 6 μg/ml are therapeutic.

(m) Significant interactions

(i) Quinidine may increase the toxic effects of **digitalis**.

(ii) Severe orthostatic hypotension may occur with concomitant administration of **vasodilators** (e.g., nitroglycerin).

(iii) Phenytoin, **rifampin**, and **barbiturates** may antagonize quinidine activity and reduce its therapeutic efficacy.

(iv) Nifedipine may reduce plasma quinidine levels.

(v) Antacids, **sodium bicarbonate**, and **sodium acetazolamide** may increase plasma quinidine levels, possibly resulting in toxicity.

(vi) Quinidine may produce additive hypoprothrombinemic effects with coumarin anticoagulants.

(2) Procainamide

(a) This drug is contraindicated in patients with hypersensitivity to procaine and related drugs, myasthenia gravis, or second- or third-degree AV block with no pacemaker.

(b) An increase of 50% or more in the duration of the QRS complex necessitates dosage reduction.

(c) Procainamide has a narrow therapeutic index. Toxicity may cause acute cardiac effects, such as pronounced slowing of conduction in all heart regions; this, in turn, may lead to SA block or arrest, ventricular tachycardia, or asystole.

(d) High serum procainamide levels may induce ventricular arrhythmias (e.g., PVCs, ventricular tachycardia or fibrillation). The ECG should be monitored continuously to detect these problems. Catecholamines, glucagon, or sodium lactate may be administered to counteract these arrhythmias.

(e) Hypotension may occur with rapid IV administration.

(f) Gastrointestinal effects are less common than with quinidine therapy.

(g) Hypersensitivity reactions are the most frequent adverse effects of procainamide. These reactions include fever, agranulocytosis, and **systemic lupus erythematosus (SLE)-like syndrome**.

(i) SLE-like syndrome is manifested by fatigue, arthralgia, myalgia, and low-grade fever.

(ii) Antinuclear antibody titer is positive in 50% to 80% of patients receiving procainamide. However, only 20% to 30% of these patients develop symptoms of SLE-like syndrome.

(iii) Drug discontinuation usually is necessary when symptomatic SLE-like syndrome occurs.

(h) *N*-Acetylprocainamide (NAPA), an active procainamide metabolite, may accumulate in patients with renal dysfunction, increasing the risk of drug toxicity.

(i) The dosage should be reduced and given over 6 hours to patients with renal or hepatic impairment (drug half-life is increased in these patients).

(j) Lower doses may be needed in patients with CHF to adjust for the lower volume of distribution.

(k) Embolism may occur upon restoration of normal sinus rhythm after prolonged atrial fibrillation. An anticoagulant may be administered before procainamide therapy begins, to prevent this complication.

(l) Plasma levels of both procainamide and NAPA should be monitored. Generally, a procainamide level of 4 to 8 μg/ml and a NAPA level of 15 to 25 μg/ml are considered therapeutic.

(m) **Significant interactions**. **Amiodarone** and **cimetidine** may increase plasma procainamide levels, possibly leading to drug toxicity.

(3) Disopyramide

(a) This drug may cause marked hemodynamic compromise and ventricular dysfunction. It is contraindicated in patients with cardiogenic shock or second- or third-degree AV block with no pacemaker.

(b) Disopyramide should be avoided or used with extreme caution in patients with CHF. It should be used cautiously in patients with urinary tract disorders, myasthenia gravis, and renal or hepatic dysfunction.

(c) In patients receiving this drug for atrial tachyarrhythmias, vagolytic effects may increase impulse conduction at the AV node, resulting in an accelerated ventricular response. To prevent this, agents that slow AV nodal conduction (e.g., verapamil, digoxin) may be given.

(d) Anticholinergic effects of this drug include dry mouth, constipation, urinary hesitancy or retention, and blurred vision.

(e) Therapeutic plasma levels range from 2 to 4 μg/ml.

(f) **Significant interactions**. **Phenytoin** accelerates disopyramide metabolism, possibly reducing its therapeutic efficacy.

(4) Lidocaine

(a) This drug may cause hemodynamic compromise in patients with severe cardiac dysfunction. Generally, however, it has few untoward cardiovascular effects.

(b) Lidocaine should be used cautiously and in reduced dosage in patients with CHF or renal or hepatic impairment.

(c) CNS reactions are the most pronounced adverse effects of lidocaine. These reactions may range from light-headedness and restlessness to confusion, tremors, stupor, and convulsions.

(d) Tinnitus, blurred vision, and anaphylaxis have been reported.

(e) Plasma lidocaine levels of 1.5 to 6.5 μg/ml are therapeutic.

(f) Lidocaine's metabolites—glycinexylidide and monoethylglycinexylidide—may have neurotoxic and antiarrhythmic effects.

(g) **Significant interactions**

(i) **Phenytoin** may increase the cardiodepressant effects of lidocaine.

(ii) **Beta-blockers** (class II antiarrhythmics) may reduce lidocaine metabolism, possibly leading to drug toxicity.

(5) Tocainide

(a) This drug is contraindicated in patients with hypersensitivity to lidocaine and related agents.

(b) Tocainide must be used cautiously in patients with CHF or reduced cardiac reserve.

(c) CNS effects include light-headedness, paresthesias, restlessness, confusion, and tremors.

(d) Nausea, vomiting, epigastric pain, and diarrhea have been reported.

(e) Other adverse effects of tocainide include hypotension, blurred vision, aplastic anemia, hepatitis, and skin rash.

(f) Dosage reduction may be necessary in patients with renal or hepatic impairment.

(g) Plasma tocainide levels of 6 to 12 μg/ml are therapeutic.

(h) Allopurinol, as an enzyme inhibitor, may prolong the half-life of tocainide.

(6) Phenytoin

(a) This drug is contraindicated in patients with sinus bradycardia or heart block.

(b) Phenytoin must be used cautiously in patients with CHF, renal or hepatic impairment, myocardial insufficiency, respiratory depression, or hypotension.

(c) During acute therapy, this drug may cause CNS reactions (e.g., drowsiness, vertigo, nystagmus, ataxia, nausea). Cardiotoxicity also may occur, especially with fast IV infusion rates.

(d) Chronic phenytoin administration may lead to vestibular and cerebellar effects, behavioral changes, gastrointestinal distress, gingival hyperplasia, megaloblastic anemia, and osteomalacia.

(e) Hypersensitivity reactions may be manifested by liver, skin, and hematologic problems.

(i) Toxic hepatitis may occur.

(ii) Skin reactions include exfoliative dermatitis, Stevens-Johnson syndrome, scarlatiniform or morbilliform rash, lupus erythematosus, and toxic epidermal necrolysis.

(iii) Hematologic reactions include agranulocytosis, megaloblastic anemia, leukopenia, thrombocytopenia, and pancytopenia.

(f) Therapeutic plasma phenytoin levels range from 10 to 20 μg/ml.

(g) **Significant interactions**

(i) The risk of phenytoin toxicity increases with concomitant administration of **diazepam, antihistamines, isoniazid, chloramphenicol, dicumarol, cimetidine, salicylates, sulfisoxazole, phenylbutazone, amiodarone**, and **valproate**.

(ii) **Carbamazepine** may enhance phenytoin metabolism and thus reduce plasma phenytoin levels and therapeutic efficacy. (Phenytoin has the same effect on carbamazepine.)

(7) Mexiletine

(a) This drug is contraindicated in patients with cardiogenic shock or second- or third-degree AV block with no pacemaker.

(b) Tremor is an early sign of mexiletine toxicity. Dizziness, ataxia, and nystagmus indicate an increasing plasma drug concentration.

(c) Hypotension, bradycardia, and widened QRS complexes may develop during mexiletine therapy.

(d) Adverse gastrointestinal effects include nausea and vomiting.

(e) Therapeutic serum levels range from 0.75 to 2.0 μg/ml.

(f) Significant interactions. Phenobarbital, rifampin, and **phenytoin** reduce plasma mexiletine levels and may decrease therapeutic efficacy.

(8) Flecainide

(a) This drug is contraindicated in patients with cardiogenic shock or second- or third-degree AV block with no pacemaker.

(b) The ECG should be monitored during flecainide therapy because this drug may exacerbate existing arrhythmias or precipitate new ones.

(c) This drug has a significant negative inotropic effect and may bring on or worsen CHF and cardiomyopathy.

(d) Adverse CNS effects (e.g., dizziness, headache, tremor) and gastrointestinal effects (e.g., nausea, abdominal pain) may occur.

(e) Blurred vision and dyspnea have been reported.

(9) Encainide

(a) This drug may exacerbate existing arrhythmias or precipitate new ones. It also may increase the frequency of PVCs and severe ventricular tachycardia (especially when the daily dose exceeds 200 mg). To reduce these risks, the dosage should not be increased until the fourth day of therapy.

(b) Chest pain and palpitations may occur.

(c) Dizziness, insomnia, headache, dyspnea, and blurred vision have been reported.

(d) Adverse gastrointestinal effects of encainide include nausea, vomiting, constipation, and dry mouth.

(e) Significant interactions. Cimetidine may increase plasma encainide levels, possibly causing drug toxicity.

2. Class II antiarrhythmics

a. Indications. These drugs—β-adrenergic blockers—are used mainly to treat systemic hypertension. Among the drugs in this class, propranolol and esmolol are approved for antiarrhythmic use. (The use of class II drugs in the treatment of hypertension is discussed in Chapter 33.)

(1) Propranolol may be given to:

(a) Control supraventricular arrhythmias (e.g., atrial fibrillation or flutter, PSVTs)

(b) Treat tachyarrhythmias caused by catecholamine stimulation (e.g., as in hypothyroidism or during anesthesia)

(c) Suppress severe ventricular arrhythmias in prolonged QT syndrome

(d) Treat digitalis-induced ventricular arrhythmias

(e) Terminate certain ventricular arrhythmias (e.g., PVCs in patients without structural heart disease)

(2) Esmolol is used to treat supraventricular tachycardias; it possesses a very short (9-minute) half-life.

b. Mechanism of action. Class II antiarrhythmics reduce sympathetic stimulation of the heart, decreasing impulse conduction through the AV node and lengthening the refractory period. As a result, the heart rate slows, resulting in a decrease in myocardial oxygen demand.

c. Administration and dosage

(1) Propranolol may be given intravenously or orally when used as an antiarrhythmic.

(a) Emergency therapy calls for **IV** administration of 1 to 3 mg diluted in 50 ml dextrose 5% in water or normal saline solution. This dose is infused slowly (no faster than 1 mg/min). A second dose of 1 to 3 mg may be given 2 minutes later.

(b) For **oral** therapy, 40 to 800 mg/day is given in three or four doses. (However, 1000 mg or more may be required for resistant arrhythmias.)

(2) Esmolol is given intravenously. A loading dose of 500 μg/kg/min is infused over 1 minute, followed by a 4-minute maintenance infusion of 50 μg/kg/min. If a satisfactory response is not achieved within 5 minutes, the loading dose is repeated and followed by a maintenance infusion of 100 μg/kg/min.

d. Precautions and monitoring effects

(1) Propranolol

(a) This drug is contraindicated in patients with sinus bradycardia, second- or third-degree AV block, cardiogenic shock, diabetes mellitus, or asthma.

(b) The β-blocking effects of this drug may lead to marked hypotension, exacerbation of CHF and left ventricular failure, or cardiac arrest.

(c) Blood pressure, heart rate, and the ECG should be monitored during IV infusion.

(d) Embolism may occur upon restoration of normal sinus rhythm after sustained atrial fibrillation. An anticoagulant may be given before propranolol therapy begins, to prevent this complication.

(e) Propranolol may depress AV node conduction and ventricular pacemaker activity, resulting in AV block or asystole.

(f) This drug may mask the signs and symptoms of hypoglycemia. It also may mask signs of shock.

(g) Fatigue, lethargy, increased airway resistance, and skin rash have been reported.

(h) Nausea, vomiting, and diarrhea may occur.

(i) Sudden withdrawal of propranolol may lead to acute MI, arrhythmias, or angina in cardiac patients.

(j) Significant interactions

(i) Severe vasoconstriction may occur with concomitant **epinephrine** administration.

(ii) Digitalis preparations can cause excessive bradycardia and additive myocardial depression.

(iii) Calcium-channel blockers (e.g., diltiazem and verapamil) and other **negative inotropic and/or chronotropic drugs** will add to the depressant effects of propranolol.

(2) Esmolol

(a) This drug is contraindicated in patients with CHF or sinus bradycardia.

(b) Hypotension occurs in approximately 50% of patients receiving esmolol. This effect can be reversed by reducing the dosage or stopping the infusion.

(c) This drug is for short-term use only and should be replaced by a longer-acting antiarrhythmic once the patient's heart stabilizes.

(d) Dizziness, headache, fatigue, and agitation may occur.

(e) Other adverse effects include nausea, vomiting, and bronchospasm.

(f) Significant interactions. Morphine may raise plasma esmolol levels.

3. Class III antiarrhythmics

a. Indications

(1) Amiodarone is given to control refractory ventricular arrhythmias and may be used prophylactically against ventricular tachycardia and fibrillation. It usually is reserved for arrhythymias that are nonresponsive to first- and second-line agents as a last-line agent.

(2) Bretylium is used solely to treat life-threatening ventricular arrhythmias (including ventricular fibrillation) that have not responded to other agents. It should be given only in intensive care facilities.

b. Mechanism of action. Class III antiarrhythmics prolong the refractory period and action potential; they have no effect on myocardial contractility or conduction time.

c. Administration and dosage

(1) Amiodarone is available for oral use; IV administration is investigational.

(a) For **oral** therapy, 800 to 1600 mg is given daily for 1 to 3 weeks until a satisfactory response occurs. Then, a maintenance dose of 200 to 400 mg/day is given.

(b) IV therapy calls for administration of a loading dose of 5 to 10 mg/kg infused via a central line, followed by 10 mg/kg/day for 3 to 5 days.

(2) Bretylium is used for short-term IV or intramuscular therapy.

(a) For ventricular fibrillation, 5 mg/kg is given by **rapid IV** injection. As needed, the dosage may be increased to 10 mg/kg and repeated every 15 to 30 minutes, up to a total of 30 mg/kg.

(b) For other ventricular arrhythmias, 500 mg is diluted to 50 ml with dextrose or normal saline solution and infused intravenously at 5 to 10 mg/kg over more than 8 minutes. The dose may be repeated in 1 to 2 hours, then given every 6 to 8 hours.

(c) Bretylium has also been used successfully as a continuous infusion at a rate of 1 to 2 mg/min, after diluting 500 mg in 50 ml dextrose 5% in water or normal saline solution.

(d) **Intramuscular therapy** calls for administration of 5 to 10 mg/kg undiluted. As needed, the dose may be repeated in 1 to 2 hours, then given every 6 to 8 hours.

d. Precautions and monitoring effects

(1) Amiodarone

(a) Life-threatening pulmonary toxicity may occur during amiodarone therapy, especially in patients receiving more than 400 mg/day.

(b) Most patients develop corneal microdeposits 1 to 4 months after amiodarone therapy begins. However, this reaction rarely causes visual disturbance.

(c) Blood pressure and heart rate and rhythm should be monitored.

(d) Hepatic dysfunction, thyroid disorders, and photosensitivity may develop.

(e) CNS reactions include fatigue, malaise, peripheral neuropathy, and extrapyramidal effects.

(f) Nausea and vomiting have been reported.

(g) This drug has an extremely long half-life (up to 50 days). Therapeutic response may be delayed for weeks after oral therapy begins; adverse reactions may persist up to 4 months after therapy ends.

(h) **Significant interactions**. Amiodarone may increase the plasma levels of **quinidine**, **procainamide**, **diltiazem**, and **digitalis**.

(i) It may increase the pharmacologic effect of β-blockers as well as calcium-channel blockers.

(2) Bretylium

(a) This drug is contraindicated in digitalis-induced arrhythmias.

(b) Severe hypotension (especially orthostatic hypotension) may develop when bretylium is administered intravenously for the treatment of acute arrhythmias.

(c) Rapid IV injection may cause severe nausea and vomiting.

(d) Patients with renal impairment may require dosage reduction.

(e) **Significant interactions**. **Antihypertensives** may potentiate bretylium-induced hypotension.

4. Class IV antiarrhythmics

a. Indications

(1) **Verapamil** is used mainly to treat and prevent supraventricular arrhythmias.

(a) It is a first-line agent for the suppression of PSVTs stemming from AV nodal reentry or Wolff-Parkinson-White syndrome.

(b) Verapamil can immediately control the ventricular response to atrial flutter and fibrillation.

(2) **Diltiazem** and **nifedipine**, the other drugs in this class, are used mainly to control angina. For information on these agents, see Chapter 31.

b. Mechanism of action. Class IV antiarrhythmics are calcium-channel blockers. They inhibit AV node conduction by depressing the SA and AV nodes, where calcium channels predominate.

c. Administration and dosage

(1) To control atrial arrhythmias, verapamil usually is administered intravenously. A dose of 5 to 10 mg is given over at least 2 minutes and may be repeated in 30 minutes if necessary.

(2) To prevent PSVTs, verapamil may be given orally in four daily doses of 80 to 120 mg each.

d. Precautions and monitoring effects

(1) Verapamil is contraindicated in patients with AV block, left ventricular dysfunction, or severe hypotension.

(2) This drug must be used cautiously in patients with CHF, sick sinus syndrome, MI, or hepatic or renal impairment.

(3) Because of its negative chronotropic effect, verapamil must be used cautiously in patients who have slow heart rates or who are receiving β-blockers or digitalis.

(4) The ECG (especially the RR interval) should be monitored during verapamil therapy.

(5) Patients over age 60 should receive reduced dosages and slower injection rates.

(6) Constipation and nausea have been reported.

(7) **Significant interactions**

(a) Concomitant administration of **β-blockers** or **disopyramide** may precipitate heart failure.

(b) **Quinidine** may increase the risk of verapamil-induced hypotension.

5. Other antiarrhythmics. **Atropine** is an unclassified antiarrhythmic.

a. Indications. Atropine is therapeutic for symptomatic sinus bradycardia and junctional rhythm.

b. Mechanism of action. An anticholinergic, atropine blocks vagal effects on the SA node, promoting conduction through the AV node and increasing the heart rate.

c. **Administration and dosage**. For antiarrhythmic use, atropine is administered in a dose of 0.5 to 1 mg by IV push; the dose is given every 5 minutes to a maximum of 2 mg.

d. **Precautions and monitoring effects**

(1) Thirst and dry mouth are the most common adverse effects of atropine.

(2) CNS reactions (e.g., restlessness, headache, disorientation, dizziness) may occur with doses greater than 5 mg.

(3) Tachycardia and ophthalmic disturbances (e.g., mydriasis, blurred vision, photophobia) may occur with doses of 1 mg or more.

(4) Initial doses may induce a reflex bradycardia due to incomplete suppression of vagal impulses.

IV. MAJOR ARRHYTHMIAS

A. Supraventricular arrhythmias

1. Sinus bradycardia

a. **Description**. The heart rate is less than 60 beats/min; impulses originate in the SA node. This arrhythmia may cause such signs and symptoms as light-headedness, palpitations, and fatigue.

b. **Causes** include hyperkalemia, drugs, vagal stimulation, severe pain, and MI. (In well-conditioned athletes, sinus bradycardia is considered normal.)

c. **Therapy**

(1) Asymptomatic sinus bradycardia usually requires no treatment.

(2) When this arrhythmia leads to hemodynamic compromise, atropine may be administered intravenously in a dose of 0.5 to 1.0 mg every 5 to 10 minutes until the desired heart rate is attained.

(3) Artificial pacing may be indicated in some cases.

2. Sinus tachycardia

a. **Description**. The heart rate ranges from 100 to 160 beats/min; impulses originate from the SA node. Sinus tachycardia commonly causes palpitations.

b. **Causes** include decreased vagal tone, increased sympathetic tone, digitalis toxicity, and increased myocardial oxygen demand as well as fever, stress, and inflammation. Nonpathologic causes include caffeine and alcohol consumption.

c. **Therapy**. A class II antiarrhythmic (e.g., propranolol) may be given if treatment is required.

3. Sinus arrest

a. **Description**. This arrhythmia occurs when the SA node fails to initiate an electrical impulse. On ECG, the P wave is dropped or absent and the PP interval is not a multiple of the sinus rhythm.

b. **Causes** include MI, digitalis toxicity, increased vagal tone, and degenerative heart disease.

c. **Therapy**. The underlying cause should be treated if symptomatic bradycardia develops.

4. Sick sinus syndrome

a. **Description**. In this conduction disturbance (also known as Stokes-Adams syndrome), tachycardia and bradycardia alternate; these arrhythmias are interrupted by a long sinus pause. Signs and symptoms include dizziness and syncope.

b. **Causes** include cardiomyopathy, atherosclerosis, MI, neuromuscular disorders, and drug therapy.

c. **Therapy**. Chronic sick sinus syndrome may warrant drugs (digitalis or propranolol), permanent pacing, or both.

5. Premature atrial contraction (PAC)

a. **Description**. PAC occurs when an ectopic pacemaker generates premature beats before the SA node fires again. On the ECG, the P wave is premature and abnormal (possibly buried in the preceding T wave); PR intervals are abnormally short or long. A **nonconducted PAC**, which occurs when the impulse reaches the ventricles during the absolute refractory period, causes absent QRS complexes. PACs typically produce an irregular pulse and palpitations.

b. **Causes** include coronary heart disease, valvular heart disease, drug therapy (e.g., procainamide, digitalis), infection, and inflammation. Nonpathologic causes include fatigue, stress, and caffeine or alcohol consumption.

c. **Therapy**. Usually, PAC is clinically insignificant and does not require treatment. However, when it occurs frequently or leads to prolonged tachycardia, therapy with digitalis, propranolol, or another drug that prolongs the atrial refractory period may be given.

6. Paroxysmal supraventricular tachycardia (PSVT)

a. **Description**. This category includes two tachyarrythmias originating above the bundle of

His bifurcation: paroxysmal atrial tachycardia (PAT) and paroxysmal junctional tachycardia (PJT). These arrhythmias result from an AV nodal reentry mechanism.

(1) The heart rate is from 140 to 240 beats/min; the rhythm is regular.

(2) On the ECG, PSVTs are manifested by aberrant QRS complexes and a P wave contour that deviates from that of sinus beats.

(3) PSVTs may cause no symptoms or may produce mild chest pain, palpitations, nausea, and dyspnea.

b. Causes include digitalis toxicity, primary cardiac disease (e.g., MI or congenital heart disease), hyperthyroidism, and cor pulmonale.

c. Therapy. Most PSVTs subside spontaneously.

(1) In patients with underlying cardiac disease or if PSVTs cause hemodynamic compromise, an emergency mechanical measure (e.g., the Valsalva maneuver, carotid sinus massage, synchronized cardioversion) or drug therapy (verapamil) may be needed.

(2) Chronic PSVTs may warrant maintenance therapy with digitalis, a class II or class IV antiarrhythmic, or permanent pacing.

7. Atrial flutter

a. Description

(1) Ectopic impulses occur at a rate of 220 to 350/min. However, a protective mechanism at the AV node allows only some of these impulses to reach the ventricles. The ventricular rate determines how much danger this arrhythmia poses.

(2) On the ECG, sawtoothed "F" (flutter) waves appear; the ratio of atrial to ventricular contractions may be constant or variable.

b. Causes include MI, valvular heart disease, cor pulmonale, coronary artery disease, cardiac infection, CHF, COPD, thyrotoxicosis, and quinidine therapy.

c. Therapy

(1) Atrial flutter causing a rapid ventricular rate and decreased cardiac output calls for emergency measures, such as:

(a) Synchronized cardioversion

(b) A class IV antiarrhythmic (e.g., verapamil)

(2) Chronic atrial flutter may warrant digoxin, possibly given in combination with verapamil or a β-blocker.

8. Atrial fibrillation

a. Description. In this arrhythmia, many ectopic foci fire at different times. However, the AV node blocks many impulses from reaching the ventricles.

(1) The atrial rate is 400 to 600 beats/min.

(2) The atrial rhythm is chaotic.

b. Causes include valvular, ischemic, or rheumatic heart disease; coronary artery disease; systemic hypertension; cardiomyopathy; thyrotoxicosis; COPD; CHF; and MI.

c. Therapy. The treatment goal is to control the ventricular response.

(1) Immediate synchronized cardioversion is necessary in hemodynamically unstable patients.

(2) Verapamil (administered intravenously) is the drug of choice in acute atrial fibrillation.

(3) Digoxin frequently is used in chronic atrial fibrillation. It may be administered in combination with verapamil or a β-blocker.

(4) Type I antiarrhythmics may be useful in converting atrial fibrillation to sinus rhythm or preventing recurrence.

B. Preexcitation syndromes. This arrhythmia category includes Wolff-Parkinson-White (WPW) syndrome and Lown-Ganong-Levine (LGL) syndrome.

1. Description. In these arrhythmias, early ventricular depolarization occurs.

a. In **WPW syndrome**, the ECG shows a PR interval of less than 0.12 second and a QRS complex greater than 0.12 second.

(1) The ventricular rate may be as high as 300 beats/min. At rates of 180 or more, atrial fibrillation may develop.

(2) Delta waves, the hallmark of WPW, appear as a slurring of the initial portion of the QRS complex.

b. In **LGL syndrome**, the ECG shows short but constant PR intervals and normal P waves and QRS complexes.

2. Cause. Preexcitation syndromes result from abnormal conduction of impulses from the atria to the ventricles. Impulses travel along accessory pathways, which connect the atria and ventricles at abnormal locations and provide a reentry route for impulses.

3. Therapy

a. In an emergency, vagotonic maneuvers or drugs (e.g., propranolol, procainamide, verapamil, lidocaine) may be necessary. If no response occurs, cardioversion may be used.

b. Long-term management may involve administration of a class IA antiarrhythmic (to increase refractoriness in the bypass tract), a class II or IV antiarrhythmic, or digoxin.
c. In resistant cases, electrophysiologic testing and surgical ablation of the bypass tract are necessary.

C. Ventricular arrhythmias

1. Premature ventricular contractions (PVCs)

a. Description. These common arrhythmias cause a slow heart rate and a regular rhythm.
(1) A premature beat occurs, followed by a compensatory pause (as evidenced on heart auscultation or radial pulse palpation).
(2) On the ECG, PVCs appear as wide, bizarre QRS complexes; absent P waves; and large, wide T waves pointing in the direction opposite the QRS complexes.
(3) PVCs occur in the following patterns:
(a) Couplet, consisting of two consecutive PVCs
(b) Salvo (run of ventricular tachycardia), consisting of three or more consecutive PVCs
(c) Ventricular bigeminy, consisting of a PVC following each normal beat
(d) Ventricular trigeminy, consisting of two normal beats followed by a PVC
(4) PVCs may be **unifocal** or **multifocal**.
(a) In **unifocal PVCs**, QRS complexes are identical in configuration, reflecting a single ectopic ventricular pacemaker.
(b) In **multifocal PVCs**, QRS complexes have varying configurations, reflecting two ectopic ventricular pacemakers.
(5) The **R-on-T phenomenon** occurs when the PVC falls on the T wave of the preceding beat.

b. Causes include cardiomyopathy, coronary artery disease, and mitral valve prolapse. In persons with normal hearts, PVCs may arise from caffeine or alcohol consumption or tobacco use. The mechanism underlying this arrhythmia is unknown.

c. Therapy
(1) Treatment is **always** required for the following types of PVCs:
(a) Multifocal PVCs
(b) Bigeminy
(c) Couplets or salvos
(d) R-on-T phenomenon
(2) Treatment may involve a class IA, IB, or IC antiarrhythmic (lidocaine is commonly given).
(3) Asymptomatic patients with benign PVC types and no underlying heart disease do not require treatment.

2. Ventricular tachycardia

a. Description. This dangerous arrhythmia, which may be brief or sustained, is defined as three or more consecutive PVCs.
(1) Uncoordinated atrial and ventricular activity may lead to a drastic reduction in cardiac output; ventricular fibrillation may occur.
(2) The ventricular rate is 150 to 240 beats/min; the rhythm is fairly regular.
(3) On the ECG, QRS complexes are wide and bizarre, P waves are absent, T waves appear in the direction opposite the QRS complexes, and RR intervals are regular or slightly irregular.

b. Causes. Ventricular tachycardia results from myocardial irritability or ischemia (e.g., from MI, valvular heart defects, cardiomyopathy, or heart failure).

c. Therapy
(1) Immediate intervention is necessary to prevent acute ventricular tachycardia from evolving into ventricular fibrillation.
(a) In unconscious patients, cardiopulmonary resuscitation (CPR) and defibrillation are warranted.
(b) In less acute cases, lidocaine is given.
(2) Long-term drug therapy may include quinidine, procainamide, disopyramide, tocainide, mexiletine, flecainide, encainide, and finally amiodarone.

3. Ventricular fibrillation

a. Description. This deadly arrhythmia is the most common cause of cardiac arrest after an acute MI. The ventricles quiver rather than contract; as a result, cardiac output is interrupted and death may ensue.
(1) Typically, the patient is pulseless and apneic and may have seizures. Acidosis and hypoxemia develop.
(2) The ECG shows a rapid, chaotic ventricular rhythm and an undulating baseline; P waves, T waves, and QRS complexes cannot be discerned.

b. **Causes**. PVCs and ventricular tachycardia most commonly cause this arrhythmia. Rarely, it arises spontaneously.

c. **Therapy**. Ventricular fibrillation calls for immediate emergency measures, such as CPR and defibrillation. Emergency IV drug therapy may include epinephrine, lidocaine, bretylium, procainamide, or propranolol.

D. **AV blocks**. These arrhythmias reflect disturbances in impulse conduction from the atria to the ventricles. AV block occurs in three major variations—first degree, second degree, and third degree.

1. **Description**

a. In **first-degree** AV block, all supraventricular impulses are delayed. On the ECG, the PR interval is prolonged (greater than 0.20 second) but constant, QRS complexes are normal, and the rhythm is regular.

b. In **second-degree** AV block, some impulses are blocked at the AV node. Second-degree AV block occurs in two types.

(1) In **Type I** (also called **Mobitz I** or **Wenckebach**), each successive impulse is conducted at an earlier stage of the refractory period, until one impulse arrives during the absolute refractory period and cannot be conducted. The next impulse, arriving during the relative refractory period, is conducted normally. The dropped ventricular beats have a predictable pattern. ECG evidence of this arrhythmia includes grouped beating, an irregular rhythm, progressively lengthening PR intervals, progressively shortening RR intervals, and constant PP intervals.

(2) In **Type II** (also called **Mobitz II**), abnormal conduction in the bundle of His and the bundle branches causes dropped ventricular beats at unpredictable times. ECG manifestations include a sudden dropped beat with normal PR intervals and QRS complexes.

c. In **third-degree AV block** (also known as **complete heart block**), all supraventricular impulses are blocked at the AV junction. As a result, the atria and ventricles beat independently of one another.

(1) An ectopic pacemaker in the AV junction or the ventricles stimulates ventricular contractions.

(2) On the ECG, QRS complexes may be wide or narrow, depending on the location of the secondary pacemaker, PP intervals are constant, and P waves have no relationship to QRS complexes.

(3) Usually, the ventricular rate exceeds 45 beats/min.

2. **Causes**. AV heart block typically results from drug toxicity (e.g., digitalis, quinidine), degenerative disease of myocardial conductive tissue, acute MI, rheumatic fever, or severe coronary artery disease. In some cases, this arrhythmia is congenital.

3. **Therapy**

a. First- and second-degree AV blocks usually do not require treatment. If the underlying cause is drug toxicity, the offending drug will be withdrawn. If the arrhythmia reduces cardiac output, atropine may be given.

b. Type II second-degree AV block may warrant drug therapy to maintain cardiac output if the patient is hypotensive. Long-term management may involve artificial pacing to prevent ventricular standstill.

c. Third-degree AV block may warrant drug therapy (atropine or isoproterenol) if the arrhythmia has compromised cardiac output. Artificial pacing frequently is necessary.

STUDY QUESTIONS

Directions: Each question below contains five suggested answers. Choose the **one best** response to each question.

1. Strong anticholinergic effects limit the antiarrhythmic use of

A. quinidine
B. procainamide
C. tocainide
D. flecainide
E. disopyramide

2. A pronounced slowing in phase 0 of the myocardial action potential would be reflected on the electrocardiogram as a

A. shortened QRS complex
B. shortened P wave
C. prolonged QRS complex
D. flipped T wave
E. ST segment depression

3. Which of the following class I antiarrhythmics would be most capable of inducing the torsades de pointes type of ventricular tachycardia?

A. Lidocaine
B. Amiodarone
C. Quinidine
D. Flecainide
E. Diltiazem

4. A patient receiving a class I antiarrhythmic agent on a chronic basis complains of fatigue, low-grade fever, and joint pain suggestive of systemic lupus erythematosus. The patient is most likely receiving

A. lidocaine
B. procainamide
C. quinidine
D. flecainide
E. propranolol

5. Class IA antiarrhythmics do all of the following to the cardiac cell's action potential EXCEPT

A. slow the rate of rise for phase 0 depolarization
B. delay the fast-channel conductance of sodium ions
C. prolong phases 2 and 3 repolarization
D. inhibit the slow-channel conductance of calcium ions
E. prolong the refractory period of the action potential

6. Which of the following drugs is a class IV antiarrhythmic that is primarily indicated for the treatment of supraventricular tachyarrhythmias?

A. Nifedipine
B. Mexiletine
C. Verapamil
D. Quinidine
E. Propranolol

7. Sinus tachycardia is characterized by a heart rate

A. in excess of 100 with impulses initiated by the AV node
B. in excess of 60 with impulses initiated by the SA node
C. less than 60 with impulses initiated by the AV node
D. less than 60 with impulses initiated by the SA node
E. in excess of 100 with impulses initiated by the SA node

8. Which of the following agents has a direct effect on the AV node, delaying calcium-channel depolarization?

A. Lidocaine
B. Verapamil
C. Bretylium
D. Quinidine
E. Nifedipine

9. Which of the following is a class III antiarrhythmic agent that is effective in the acute management of ventricular tachycardia, including ventricular fibrillation?

A. Bretylium
B. Lidocaine
C. Metoprolol
D. Disopyramide
E. Diltiazem

10. All of the following problems represent concerns when patients are started on amiodarone EXCEPT

A. extremely long elimination half-life
B. need for multiple daily doses
C. development of hyper- or hypothyroidism
D. development of pulmonary fibrosis
E. interactions with other antiarrhythmic drugs

Directions: The group of questions below consists of lettered choices followed by several numbered items. For each numbered item select the **one** lettered choice with which it is **most** closely associated. Each lettered choice may be used once, more than once, or not at all.

Questions 11–15

For each description of a phase of an action potential in Purkinje fibers, choose the corresponding letter in the accompanying diagram.

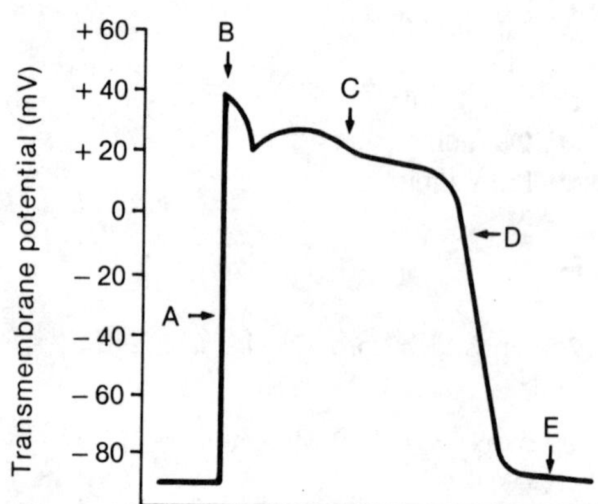

11. Slow-channel depolarization—calcium influx
12. Resting phase—diastole
13. Rapid repolarization
14. Fast-channel depolarization—sodium influx
15. Early repolarization

ANSWERS AND EXPLANATIONS

1. The answer is E. [*III A 1 d (3) (d)*] Disopyramide has anticholinergic actions about one-tenth the potency of atropine. Effects include dry mouth, constipation, urinary retention, and blurred vision. Therefore, it cannot be used in patients with glaucoma or with conditions causing urinary retention. Moreover, disopyramide has a negative inotropic effect and must therefore be used with great caution, if at all, in patients with preexisting ventricular failure.

2. The answer is C. (*I B 2 b, 3*) A slowing in phase 0 of the myocardial action potential corresponds to a slowing down of depolarization within the myocardium. This results in a prolongation of either atrial depolarization (causing a prolonged P wave on the electrocardiogram) or ventricular depolarization (causing a prolonged QRS complex).

3. The answer is C. [*III A 1 d (1) (d)*] Torsades de pointes is a form of ventricular tachyarrhythmia characterized by electrocardiographic changes known as the R-on-T phenomenon and a markedly prolonged QT interval. This potentially fatal reaction to quinidine causes syncopal episodes (quinidine syncope) or sudden death. Therefore, quinidine should not be used in patients whose QT interval is long or shows a marked prolongation in response to quinidine administration.

4. The answer is B. [*III A 1 d (2) (e)*] The patient's complaints are typical of a systemic lupus erythematosus (SLE)–like hypersensitivity reaction to procainamide. Symptoms of an SLE-like syndrome include fatigue, arthralgia, myalgia, a low-grade fever, and a positive antinuclear antibody titer. The patient's symptoms should subside if procainamide therapy is stopped and an alternative antiarrhythmic agent is given instead.

5. The answer is D. (*III A 1 b*) Class IA antiarrhythmic agents delay phase 0 depolarization. Fast-channel conduction of sodium and phases 2 and 3 repolarization are also slowed. The net effect is to extend the refractory period of myocardial tissue. Class IA antiarrhythmic agents do not inhibit the slow-channel conductance of calcium ions; that is an action of class IV agents such as verapamil.

6. The answer is C. [*III A 4 a (1)*] Of the agents listed, verapamil and nifedipine are calcium-channel blockers and along with diltiazem, represent the class IV antiarrhythmics. Verapamil, but not nifedipine, has been used for its direct-acting effects on impulse conduction throughout the heart. Thus, verapamil is used to treat and prevent supraventricular arrhythmias, while diltiazem and nifedipine are used mainly to control angina pectoris. Mexiletine is a class IB drug that closely resembles lidocaine. Quinidine is a class IA drug, and propranolol, a β-adrenergic blocker, is class II. Mexiletine, quinidine, and propranolol are all also effective for supraventricular arrhythmias.

7. The answer is E. (*IV A 2*) The term sinus tachycardia denotes a rapid heart rate with impulses originating in the sinoatrial (SA) node. In sinus tachycardia, the heart rate ranges from 100 to 160 beats per minute

8. The answer is B. [*I B 2 d (2); III A 4 b*] Verapamil, a calcium-channel blocker, inhibits calcium influx through slow channels into myocardial cells. Verapamil's direct actions on the slow-channel–dependent SA node and AV node, along with its availability in injection form, make it an ideal agent for the acute IV treatment of such reentry arrhythmias as paroxysmal supraventricular tachyarrhythmias.

9. The answer is A. [*III A 3 a (2)*] Bretylium and amiodarone are class III antiarrhythmic agents. Class III agents prolong the refractory period and myocardial action potential; they are used to treat ventricular arrhythmias. Bretylium is considered a second-line drug for controlling ventricular fibrillation. When used intravenously, bretylium requires close monitoring for hypotension, especially orthostatic hypotension, and may cause severe nausea and vomiting.

10. The answer is B. [*III A 3 c (1), d (1)*] Amiodarone, like bretylium, is a class III antiarrhythmic agent and acts by prolonging repolarization of cardiac cells. Amiodarone is given orally, often in once-a-day or twice-a-day maintenance dosage. Because of its very long elimination half-life, therapeutic response may be delayed for weeks. Therefore, an initial loading phase is often advisable. This requires hospitalization with close monitoring for desired effects, untoward reactions, and adjustments in dosage. Amiodarone may increase the plasma levels of quinidine, procainamide, diltiazem, and digitalis. During therapy with amiodarone, patients may develop hypo- or hyperthyroidism, pulmonary disorders, hepatic dysfunction, and various other unwanted effects. Because of amiodarone's extremely long half-life, adverse reactions may persist for months after therapy ends.

11–15. The answers are: 11-C, 12-E, 13-D, 14-A, 15-B. (*I B 2 b*) The action potential of cardiac Purkinje fibers reflects the depolarization and repolarization of the cardiac cells. This electrical activity involves the transport of sodium, calcium, and potassium ions across the cell membrane. The action potential has five phases. Phase 0 (rapid depolarization) is primarily dependent on the conduction of sodium ions into the cell through fast channels. Phase 0 is followed by phase 1 (early repolarization), which precedes phase 2, a slight notch that represents the inward flow of calcium ions into the cardiac cell via slow channels. Phase 3 (rapid repolarization) represents the inward flow of potassium ions. Phase 4 (slow depolarization), ending the action potential, represents electrical diastole.

33
Systemic Hypertension

Alan H. Mutnick

I. GENERAL CONSIDERATIONS

A. Definition. Hypertension is an elevation of the blood pressure necessary to perfuse tissues and organs. Elevated systemic blood pressure is usually defined as a systolic reading greater than 140 mm Hg and a diastolic reading greater than 90 mm Hg.

B. Classification of hypertension, regardless of type, is shown in Table 33-1.

C. Incidence

1. **Hypertension is the most common cardiovascular disorder.** Approximately 60 million Americans have blood pressure measurements exceeding 140/90 mm Hg.
2. **Primary** (or essential) **hypertension**—in which no specific cause can be identified—constitutes approximately 90% of all cases of systemic hypertension. The average age of onset is about 35 years.
3. **Secondary hypertension**—resulting from an identifiable cause, such as renal disease—accounts for the remaining 10% of patients with systemic hypertension. This type usually develops before age 35 or after age 55.

D. Physiology

1. Blood pressure = (stroke volume × heart rate) × total peripheral resistance. Altering any of the factors on the right side of the blood pressure equation will result in a change in blood pressure, as shown in Figure 33-1.
2. **Sympathetic nervous system. Baroreceptors** (pressure receptors) in the carotids and aortic arch respond to changes in blood pressure and influence vasodilation or vasoconstriction. When stimulated to vasoconstriction, the contractile force strengthens, increasing the heart rate and augmenting peripheral resistance, thus increasing cardiac output. If pressure remains elevated, then baroreceptors reset at the higher levels, sustaining the hypertension.
3. **Renin-angiotensin-aldosterone system.** Decreased renal perfusion pressure in afferent arterioles stimulates the release of renin from the juxtaglomerular cells. The renin reacts with circulating angiotensinogen to produce angiotensin I (a weak vasoconstrictor). This in turn is hydrolyzed to form angiotensin II (the most powerful natural vasoconstrictor). This vasopressor stimulates aldosterone release, with a resulting increase in sodium reabsorption and fluid volume.
4. **Fluid volume regulation. Increased fluid volume** increases venous system distention and venous return, affecting cardiac output and tissue perfusion. These changes lead to **alterations in vascular resistance**, increasing the blood pressure.

Table 33-1. Classification of Hypertension

Type	Diastolic Blood Pressure (mm Hg)
Mild	90–104
Moderate	105–129
Severe	130–140
Hypertensive emergency	Above 140

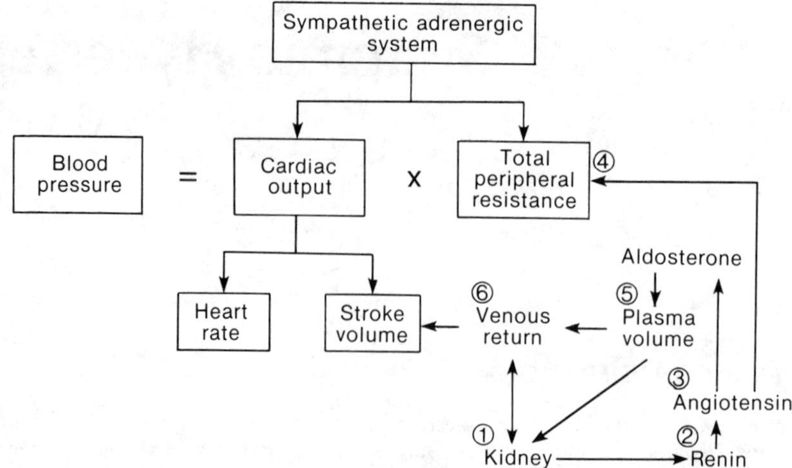

Figure 33-1. Blood pressure regulation. This figure depicts the various determinants of blood pressure as they relate to cardiac output and total peripheral resistance. Angiotensin, a potent vasopressor, not only increases total peripheral resistance but, by stimulating aldosterone release, leads to an increase in plasma volume, venous return, stroke volume, and ultimately an increase in cardiac output.

E. Complications. Untreated systemic hypertension, regardless of cause, results in inflammation and necrosis of the arterioles, narrowing blood vessels and restricting blood flow to major body organs (Table 33-2). When blood flow is severely compromised, organ damage ensues.

1. Cardiac effects

a. Increased cardiac work load is compensated for by development of left ventricular hypertrophy. Signs and symptoms of heart failure occur, and the increased oxygen requirements of the enlarged heart may produce angina pectoris.

b. Hypertension can be caused by accelerated atherosclerosis. Atheromatous lesions in coronary arteries lead to decreased blood flow, resulting in angina pectoris. Myocardial infarction and sudden death may ensue.

2. Renal effects

a. Decreased blood flow leads to an increase in renin–aldosterone secretion, which heightens the reabsorption of sodium and water and increases blood volume.

b. Accelerated atherosclerosis causes a decreased oxygen supply, leading to renal parenchymal damage with decreased filtration capability and to azotemia. The atherosclerosis also causes decreased blood flow to the renal arterioles, leading to nephrosclerosis and, ultimately, renal failure.

Table 33-2. Findings in Hypertension

Findings	Basis of Findings
Cardiovascular	
Blood pressure persistently above 140/90	Arterioles are constricted, causing abnormal resistance to blood flow
Angina pain	Insufficient blood flow to coronary vasculature
Dyspnea on exertion	Left-sided heart failure
Edema of extremities	Right-sided heart failure
Intermittent claudication	Decrease in blood supply from the peripheral vessels to the legs
Neurologic	
Severe occipital headaches with nausea and vomiting; drowsiness; giddiness; anxiety; mental impairment	Vessel damage within the brain, characteristic of severe hypertension
Renal	
Polyuria; nocturia; diminished ability to concentrate urine; protein and red blood cells in urine	Arteriolar nephrosclerosis (hardening of arterioles within the kidney)
Ocular	
Retinal hemorrhage and exudates	Damage to arterioles that supply the retina

3. **Cerebral effects.** Decreased blood flow, decreased oxygen supply, and weakened blood vessel walls lead to transient ischemic attacks, cerebral thromboses, and the development of aneurysms with hemorrhage. There are alterations in mobility, weakness, paralysis, and memory deficits.

4. **Retinal effects.** Decreased blood flow with retinal vascular sclerosis and increased arteriolar pressure with the appearance of exudates and hemorrhage result in visual defects, such as blurred vision, spots, and blindness.

II. SECONDARY HYPERTENSION

A. Clinical evaluation. Since most patients presenting with high blood pressure will prove to have primary rather than secondary hypertension, extensive screening is unwarranted. A thorough history and physical examination, along with evaluation of common laboratory tests, should rule out most causes of secondary hypertension. If a secondary cause is not found, then the patient should be considered to have essential hypertension.

1. **History or physical findings requiring further evaluation** because they suggest an underlying cause of hypertension include:
   - **a.** Weight gain, round face, and truncal obesity (may signal Cushing's syndrome)
   - **b.** Weight loss, episodic flushing, and diaphoresis (suggest pheochromocytoma)
   - **c.** Steroid or estrogen intake, including oral contraceptives (suggests drug-induced hypertension)
   - **d.** Repeated urinary tract infections (may signal renal involvement)
   - **e.** Abdominal bruits (indicate renal artery stenosis)

2. **Laboratory findings**
   - **a.** Blood urea nitrogen (BUN) and creatinine elevations suggest renal disease.
   - **b.** Increased urinary excretion of catecholamine or its metabolites (vanillylmandelic acid and metanephrine) confirms pheochromocytoma.
   - **c.** Serum potassium evaluation revealing hypokalemia suggests primary aldosteronism.

3. **Diagnostic test results**
   - **a.** Renal arteriography or renal venography may show evidence of renal artery stenosis.
   - **b.** Electrocardiography may reveal left ventricular hypertrophy or ischemia.

B. Examples of diagnosable causes

1. **Primary aldosteronism.** Hypersecretion of aldosterone by the adrenal cortex yields increased distal tubular sodium retention, expanding blood volume, which increases total peripheral resistance.

2. **Pheochromocytoma.** A tumor of the adrenal medulla stimulates hypersecretion of epinephrine and norepinephrine, which results in increased total peripheral resistance.

3. **Renal artery stenosis.** Decreased renal tissue perfusion results in the activation of the renin-angiotensin-aldosterone system (see section I D 3).

C. Treatment. Secondary hypertension requires treatment of the underlying cause, as through surgical intervention, possibly accompanied by supplementary control of hypertensive effects (see section III B).

III. ESSENTIAL (PRIMARY) HYPERTENSION

A. Clinical evaluation requires a thorough history and physical examination followed by a careful analysis of common laboratory test results.

1. **Objectives**
   - **a.** To rule out uncommon secondary causes of hypertension
   - **b.** To determine the presence and extent of hypertensive vascular disease
   - **c.** To determine the presence of other cardiovascular risk factors

2. **Predisposing factors**
   - **a.** Family history of essential hypertension
   - **b.** Patient history of intermittent blood pressure elevations
   - **c.** Racial predisposition (common among blacks)
   - **d.** Obesity
   - **e.** Smoking
   - **f.** Stress

g. High dietary intake of saturated fats or sodium
h. Sedentary life-style
i. Diabetes mellitus
j. Hyperlipidemia

3. Physical findings

a. Serial blood pressure readings above 140/90 mm Hg should be obtained (on at least two occasions) before specific therapy is warranted—unless the diastolic level exceeds 120 mm Hg. A single elevated reading is an insufficient basis for a diagnosis.

b. Essential hypertension usually does not become clinically evident—other than through serial blood pressure elevations—until vascular changes affect the heart, brain, kidneys, or ocular fundi.

c. Examination of the ocular fundi is valuable; their condition can indicate the duration and severity of the hypertension.

(1) Early stages. Hard shiny deposits, tiny hemorrhages, and elevated arterial blood pressure occur.

(2) Late stages. Cotton-wool patches, exudates, retinal edema, papilledema due to ischemia and capillary insufficiency, hemorrhages, and microaneurysms become evident.

B. Treatment

1. General principles

a. Candidates for treatment

(1) Virtually all patients with a diastolic pressure of 105 mm Hg or above should receive antihypertensive drug therapy.

(2) For those with diastolic pressures of 90 to 104 mm Hg, treatment should be individualized, with risk factors considered.

(3) Borderline hypertensives. This term describes patients who are relatively young and have normal blood pressure (140/90 or less) most of the time but at other times register elevated values. These patients are considered to be in the "gray" area between individuals with normotension and those with mild essential hypertension.

b. Treatment goals

(1) To prevent or reverse organ damage

(2) To lower blood pressure toward "normal" with a minimum of side effects

c. Nonspecific measures. Prior to initiating antihypertensive drug therapy, the patient should be encouraged to eliminate or minimize—through life-style and dietary changes—the controllable risk factors among those listed in section III A 2.

d. Stepped-care drug therapy. Minimalism is the root philosophy of stepped care, which is a layered, add-on approach based on therapeutic response (as illustrated in Figure 33-2). If the step-one agent fails to achieve the desired effect, a step-two agent is added to the regimen, and so on. The treatment of chronic hypertension relies heavily on this program of pharmacologic adjustment. The drugs most commonly used are listed in Table 33-3.

e. General monitoring guidelines. (Specific monitoring parameters for the various drug categories are covered in sections III B 2 to 5.)

(1) Blood pressure should be monitored on a routine basis to determine therapeutic response and to encourage patient compliance.

(2) The clinician must be alert to, and try to elicit, information indicating the occurrence of adverse drug effects. Many patients do not mention side effects because they lack the knowledge to link occurrences to drug therapy or are embarrassed to discuss them (as with instances relating to sexual function). This is especially true of effects that appear later in therapy, rather than as an early response.

f. Patient compliance

(1) Because hypertension is usually a symptomless disease, how the patient "feels" probably does not reflect the blood pressure level. In fact, the patient may actually report "feeling more normal" with an elevated blood pressure than during a hypotensive episode, which is more likely to be noticed because of the lightheadedness associated with a sudden drop in blood pressure. Essential hypertension usually requires a lifelong drug regimen. For these reasons, it can be difficult to impress on the patient the need for consistent compliance.

(2) Recognition of the seriousness of possible consequences of noncompliance is key. The patient should know that although "symptomless" for a while, prolonged, untreated hypertension can affect the heart, brain, kidneys, and ocular fundi. That is why it has come to be known as "the silent killer." Reinforcing this reputation can provide an excellent motivator in promoting patient compliance.

2. Diuretics

a. Thiazide diuretics—hydrochlorothiazide and chlorothiazide—are generally used as step-

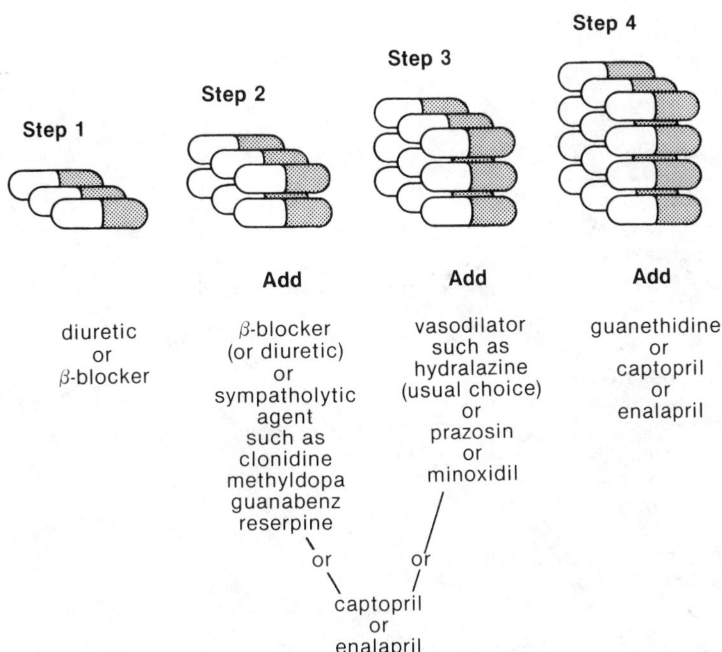

Figure 33-2. The stepped-care approach uses a layering of drugs and dosages in stages until the desired effect is achieved with a minimum of adverse effects. An unsatisfactory therapeutic response must be evaluated for factors other than pharmacologic inadequacy **at each stage** before proceeding to the next. These factors include poor patient compliance, increased sodium intake or retention, self-dosing with vasoconstricting drugs (such as common cold remedies), and undiagnosed secondary hypertension. At press time, the National High Blood Pressure Education Program was finalizing the 1988 report of the Joint National Committee on Detection, Evaluation, and Treatment of High Blood Pressure. Current recommendations are based on the 1984 report of the Joint National Committee.

one antihypertensives. Once initiated, the thiazide should almost always be continued when additional agents are added.

(1) **Actions**. Antihypertensive effects are produced by direct dilation of the arterioles and reduction of the total fluid volume. Thiazides increase urinary excretion of sodium and water by inhibiting sodium and chloride reabsorption in the distal renal tubules. Thiazides also increase urinary excretion of potassium and, to a lesser extent, bicarbonate. Thiazides enhance the effectiveness of other antihypertensive agents by preventing re-expansion of extracellular and plasma volumes.

(2) **Significant interactions**. Nonsteroidal anti-inflammatory drugs (NSAIDs) such as the now common over-the-counter forms of ibuprofen, interact to diminish the antihypertensive effects of thiazide diuretics.

(3) **Precautions and monitoring effects**

(a) **Potassium** ion depletion may require supplementation, increased dietary intake, or the use of a potassium-sparing diuretic.

(b) **Uric acid** retention may occur; this is of potential significance in the patient who is predisposed to gout and related disorders.

(c) **Blood glucose** levels may increase, which may be significant in the diabetic patient.

(d) **Calcium** levels may increase due to the potential for calcium ion retention.

(e) Patients with known **allergies to sulfa-type drugs** should be questioned to determine the significance of the allergy.

(f) **Other common effects** include fatigue, headache, palpitations, rash, vertigo, and transitory impotence.

b. Loop (high-ceiling) diuretics

(1) **Indications**. These agents are primarily indicated when the patient is unable to tolerate thiazides, experiences a loss of thiazide effectiveness, or has impaired renal function (clearance < 30 ml/min).

(2) **Actions. Furosemide**, **ethacrynic acid**, and **bumetanide** act primarily in the loop of Henle (thus "loop" diuretics). Their action is more intense but of shorter duration than that of the thiazides; they are also more expensive.

Table 33-3. Common Antihypertensive Drugs

Diuretics	Sympatholytics
Thiazide diuretics	β-Adrenergic blocking agents
Hydrochlorothiazide	Propranolol
Chlorothiazide	Metoprolol
Loop diuretics	Nadolol
Furosemide	Atenolol
Ethacrynic acid	Timolol
Bumetanide	Pindolol
Potassium-sparing diuretics	Labetalol
Amiloride	Acebutolol
Triamterene	Esmolol
Spironolactone	Centrally acting agents
	Methyldopa
Vasodilators	Clonidine
Hydralazine	Guanabenz
Nitroprusside	Postganglionic adrenergic neuron blockers
Diazoxide	Reserpine
Minoxidil	Guanethidine
Prazosin	Guanadrel
Angiotensin-converting enzyme (ACE) inhibitors	α-Adrenergic blocking agent
Captopril	Prazosin
Enalapril	
Lisinopril	

(3) **Significant interactions**. As with the thiazides, the antihypertensive effect of loop diuretics may be diminished by NSAIDs.

(4) **Precautions and monitoring effects**. Loop diuretics have the same effects as the thiazides [see section III B 2 a (3)] in addition to the following:

(a) Loop diuretics have a complex influence on renal hemodynamics; thus, therapy with these agents requires that the patient be monitored closely for signs of **hypovolemia**.

(b) Because these agents should be used cautiously in patients with **episodic or chronic renal impairment**, BUN and serum creatinine levels should be routinely checked.

(c) **Transient deafness** has occurred. If the patient is taking a potentially ototoxic drug (e.g., an aminoglycoside antibiotic), another class of diuretic (such as a thiazide) should be administered.

c. Potassium-sparing diuretics

(1) **Indications**. The diuretics in this group—**spironolactone**, **amiloride**, and **triamterene**—are indicated primarily for patients in whom potassium loss is significant and supplementation is not feasible. These agents are often used with a thiazide diuretic because they potentiate the effects of the thiazide while minimizing potassium loss. **Spironolactone** is particularly useful in patients with hyperaldosteronism as it has direct antagonistic effects on aldosterone.

(2) **Actions**. The drugs in this group have slightly different mechanisms through which they achieve their diuretic effects (which tend to be less potent than the thiazide and loop diuretics). Their most pertinent shared feature is promotion of potassium retention.

(3) **Significant interactions**. Coadministration with angiotensin-converting enzyme (ACE) inhibitors or potassium supplements significantly increases the risk of hyperkalemia.

(4) **Precautions and monitoring effects**

(a) As a group, these agents should be avoided in patients with acute renal failure and used with caution in the presence of impaired renal function or diabetes.

(b) **Triamterene** should not be used in patients with a history of kidney stones or gout.

(c) **Hyperkalemia** is a major risk, requiring routine monitoring of serum electrolytes. BUN and serum creatinine levels should be routinely checked to monitor kidney function and signal incipient excess potassium retention.

d. Combination products. Four products are now available that combine a thiazide and a potassium-sparing diuretic.

(1) Aldactazide (spironolactone/hydrochlorothiazide)
(2) Moduretic (amiloride/hydrochlorothiazide)
(3) Dyazide (triamterene/hydrochlorothiazide)
(4) Maxzide (triamterene/hydrochlorothiazide)

3. Sympatholytics

a. β-Adrenergic blockers

(1) Indications. These agents are used as step-one or step-two antihypertensives.

(2) Actions. Proposed mechanisms of action include the following:

(a) Stimulation of renin secretion is blocked.

(b) Cardiac contractility is decreased, thus diminishing cardiac output.

(c) Sympathetic output is decreased.

(d) β-blockers action may combine all of the above mechanisms.

(3) Significant interactions. β-Adrenergic blockers interact with numerous agents, requiring cautious selection, administration, and monitoring.

(4) Precautions and monitoring effects

(a) Patients must be monitored for signs and symptoms of **cardiac decompensation** (increasingly reduced cardiac output) because decreased contractility can trigger compensatory mechanisms leading to congestive heart failure.

(b) Electrocardiograms should be monitored routinely because all β-blockers have the ability to **decrease electrical conduction** within the heart.

(c) Relative cardioselectivity is dose-dependent and is lost as dosages are increased. Therefore, no β-blocker is totally safe in patients with **bronchospastic disease**.

(d) Sudden cessation of β-blocker therapy puts the patient at risk for a **withdrawal syndrome** that may produce:

(i) Exacerbated anginal attacks, particularly in patients with coronary artery disease

(ii) Myocardial infarction

(iii) A life-threatening rebound of blood pressure to levels exceeding pretreatment readings

(e) β-Blocker therapy should be **used with caution** in patients with the following conditions:

(i) Diabetes. β-Blockers can mask hypoglycemic symptoms, such as tachycardia.

(ii) Raynaud's phenomenon or peripheral vascular disease. Vasoconstriction can occur.

(iii) Neurologic disorders. Several β-blockers enter the central nervous system, potentiating related side effects.

(5) β-Blocker terms

(a) Relative cardioselective activity. Relative to propranolol, these agents have a greater tendency to occupy the β_1-receptor in the heart, rather than the β_2-receptors within the lungs.

(b) Intrinsic sympathomimetic activity. These agents have the ability to release catecholamine and the ability to maintain a satisfactory heart rate. It has also been speculated that intrinsic sympathomimetic activity prevents bronchoconstriction and other direct β-blocking actions.

(6) Individual agents

(a) Propranolol was the first β-blocking agent shown to block both β_1- and β_2-receptors.

(b) Metoprolol was the first β-blocking agent with relative cardioselective blocking activity.

(c) Nadolol was the first β-blocking agent with once-daily dosing. It blocks both β_1- and β_2-receptors.

(d) Atenolol was the first β-blocking agent to combine once-daily dosing with relative cardioselective blocking activity.

(e) Timolol was the first β-blocking agent shown to be effective after myocardial infarction for the prevention of sudden death. It blocks both β_1- and β_2-receptors.

(f) Pindolol was the first β-blocking agent shown to have intrinsic sympathomimetic activity.

(g) Labetalol was the first β-blocking agent shown to possess both α- and β-blocking activity.

(h) Acebutolol was the first β-blocking agent combining efficacy with once-daily dosing, possessing intrinsic sympathomimetic activity, and having relative cardioselective blocking activity.

(i) Esmolol was the first β-blocking agent to have an ultrashort duration of activity.

b. Centrally acting α_2-adrenergic blocking agents are used mainly as step-two antihypertensives. They act primarily within the central nervous system on α_2-receptors to decrease sympathetic outflow to the cardiovascular system.

(1) Methyldopa

(a) Actions. Methyldopa decreases total peripheral resistance while having little effect on cardiac output or heart rate (except in older patients).

(b) Precautions and monitoring effects

(i) **Common untoward effects** include orthostatic hypotension, fluid accumulation (in the absence of a diuretic), and rebound hypertension upon abrupt withdrawal. Sedation is a common finding upon initiating therapy and when increasing doses; however, the degree of sedation usually lessens with continued therapy.

(ii) **Fever** and other **flu-like symptoms** occasionally occur and may represent hepatic dysfunction. Liver function tests should be followed routinely to monitor for this dysfunction.

(iii) A **positive Coombs' test** develops in as many as 20% of patients with chronic use (longer than 6 months). Fewer than 1% of these patients develop a hemolytic anemia (red blood cells, hemoglobin, and blood count indices should be checked). The anemia is reversible with discontinuation of the drug.

(iv) **Other effects** include dry mouth, subtly decreased mental activity, sleep disturbances, depression, impotence, and lactation in either sex.

(2) Clonidine

(a) Indications. Clonidine is effective in patients with renal impairment, although they may require a dose reduction or a prolongation of the dosing interval.

(b) Precautions and monitoring effects

(i) Intravenous administration causes an initial paradoxical increase in pressure (diastolic and systolic); however, this transient increase is followed by a more prolonged drop. As with methyldopa, abrupt withdrawal can cause rebound hypertension.

(ii) Sedation and dry mouth are common but usually disappear with continued therapy.

(iii) More than methyldopa, clonidine has a tendency to cause or worsen depression. It also heightens the depressant effects of alcohol and other sedating substances.

(3) Guanabenz. The actions and effects of guanabenz are similar to those of clonidine, although rebound hypertension occurs less often than with clonidine.

c. Postganglionic adrenergic neuron blockers

(1) Reserpine

(a) General considerations

(i) Due to the high incidence of adverse effects, other step-two agents are usually chosen first. If used, reserpine is given in low doses and in conjunction with other antihypertensive agents. Reserpine in very low doses (0.05 mg) combined with a diuretic such as chlorothiazide (50 to 100 mg) may prove a likely alternative to traditional 0.1 to 0.25 mg/day doses.

(ii) Reserpine acts centrally as well as peripherally by depleting catecholamine stores in the brain and in the peripheral adrenergic system.

(b) Precautions and monitoring effects

(i) **A history of depression is a contraindication** for reserpine. Even low doses, such as 0.25 mg/day, can trigger a range of psychic responses, from nightmares to suicide attempts. Drug-induced depression may linger for months after the last dose.

(ii) **Peptic ulcer also contraindicates** reserpine use. Even a single dose of reserpine tends to increase gastric acid secretion.

(iii) **Common adverse effects** include drowsiness, dizziness, weakness, lethargy, memory impairment, sleep disturbances, and weight gain. Nasal congestion is also common but may decrease with continued therapy.

(2) Guanethidine

(a) Actions. Guanethidine acts in peripheral neurons, where it first produces a sympathetic blockade. With chronic administration, its cumulative effect reduces tissue concentrations of norepinephrine. This lasts several days after discontinuation of the drug.

(b) Significant interactions

(i) Patients should be cautioned to avoid over-the-counter preparations that contain **sympathomimetic substances** (found in cold medicines, for example) because the combination potentiates an acute hypertensive crisis.

(ii) **Tricyclic antidepressants** and **chlorpromazine** antagonize the therapeutic effect of guanethidine.

(c) Precautions and monitoring effects

(i) **Pheochromocytoma contraindicates** guanethidine use due to the risk of a severe hypertensive reaction.

(ii) **Postural and exercise hypotension** are common and may be heightened by heat (e.g., hot weather and hot showers) and alcohol ingestion. The patient should be warned of these effects with changes in body position, particularly upon standing.

(iii) Fluid retention can occur, diminishing the antihypertensive effect and usually requiring a diuretic to be added to the drug regimen.

(iv) Sexual dysfunction (primarily inhibition of ejaculation) can occur and should be considered before initiating therapy.

d. Peripheral α-adrenergic blocker—prazosin

(1) Actions. Prazosin is a quinazoline derivative that acts postsynaptically as a selective α_1-adrenergic antagonist, causing vasodilation of both arteries and veins. An additional benefit is that the incidence of reflex tachycardia is lower with prazosin than with the vasodilator hydralazine. Prazosin is most effective when combined with a diuretic, a β-blocker, or both.

(2) Precautions and monitoring effects

(a) Prazosin should be avoided or used with caution in patients with severe congestive heart failure, pheochromocytoma, or hypertensive crisis.

(b) First-dose phenomenon. A syncopal episode may occur within 30 to 90 minutes of the first dose; similarly associated are postural hypotension, nausea, dizziness, headache, palpitations, and sweating. To minimize this effect, the first dose should be limited to 1.0 mg and administered just before bedtime.

(c) Additional reported adverse effects include diarrhea, weight gain, peripheral edema, dry mouth, urinary urgency, constipation, and priapism.

4. Vasodilators. Primarily, these drugs are used as step-three or step-four agents in patients refractory to previous therapy. Vasodilators work by directly relaxing peripheral vascular smooth muscle—arterial, venous, or both.

a. Hydralazine

(1) Actions. Hydralazine directly relaxes arterioles, decreasing peripheral vascular resistance. It is also used intravenously or intramuscularly in hypertensive crisis management.

(2) Precautions and monitoring effects

(a) Because this vasodilator triggers compensatory reactions that counteract its antihypertensive effects, it is most useful when combined with a diuretic and a sympatholytic drug, as a latter-step agent.

(b) Reflex tachycardia is common and should be considered prior to initiating therapy.

(c) Hydralazine may induce **angina**, especially in patients with coronary artery disease and those not receiving a β-blocker.

(d) Drug-induced systemic lupus erythematosus (SLE) may occur.

(i) Baseline and serial complete blood counts with antinuclear antibody titers should be followed routinely to aid detection of this effect.

(ii) Slow acetylators of this drug have an increased incidence of SLE; their risk may be reduced by administering doses of less than 200 mg/day.

(iii) Patients should report symptoms such as fatigue, malaise, low-grade fever, and joint aches because these may signal SLE.

(e) Other adverse effects may include headache, peripheral neuropathy, nausea, and vomiting.

b. Minoxidil

(1) Actions. A more potent vasodilator than hydralazine, minoxidil relaxes arteriolar smooth muscle directly, decreasing peripheral resistance. It also decreases renal vascular resistance while preserving renal blood flow. Effective in most patients, minoxidil is commonly used to treat patients with severe hypertension that has been refractory to conventional drug regimens.

(2) Precautions and monitoring effects

(a) Peripheral dilation results in a reflex activation of the sympathetic nervous system and an increase in heart rate, cardiac output, and renin secretion.

(b) Because this agent promotes sodium and water retention, particularly in the presence of renal impairment, patients should be monitored for fluid accumulations and signs of cardiac decompensation. Administering minoxidil along with a sympatholytic agent and a potent diuretic (such as furosemide) minimizes increased sympathetic stimulation and fluid retention.

(c) Hypertrichosis (excessive hair growth) is a common side effect, particularly if the drug is continued for more than 4 weeks.

c. Nitroprusside

(1) A direct-acting peripheral dilator, this agent has potent effects on both the arterial and venous systems. It is usually used only in short-term emergency treatment of acute hypertensive crisis, when a rapid effect is required. Onset of action is almost instantaneous and is maximal in 1 to 2 minutes. Nitroprusside is administered intravenously with continuous blood pressure monitoring.

(2) **Precautions and monitoring effects.** To prevent acute hypotensive episodes, initial doses should be very low, followed by slow titration upward until the desired effect is achieved.

(a) Once the solution is prepared, it should be protected from light. Color changes are a signal that replacement is needed.

(b) **Thiocyanate toxicity** may develop with long-term treatment—particularly in patients with reduced renal activity—but can be treated with hemodialysis. Symptoms may include fatigue, anorexia, disorientation, nausea, psychotic behavior, or muscle spasms.

(c) **Cyanide toxicity** can occur (rarely) with long-term, high-dose administration. It may present as altered consciousness, convulsions, tachypnea, or even coma.

d. Diazoxide

(1) **Indications.** Diazoxide exerts a direct action on the arterioles but has little effect on venous capacity. It is used intravenously in the emergency treatment of acute hypertensive crisis.

(2) **Administration**

(a) Because the antihypertensive effect of diazoxide increases with the speed of infusion, recent recommendations suggest that slow infusion (spread over 15 to 30 minutes) may achieve more predictable, controllable hypotensive effects than rapid, large-dose administration.

(b) Alternatively, maximal reductions in mean arterial pressure may be obtained after 2 minutes through bolus injections of 0.05 to 1.0 mg/kg for 5 to 10 seconds, with repetition of this dose every 5 to 10 minutes.

(3) **Precautions and monitoring effects**

(a) Diazoxide is closely related to the thiazides chemically; therefore, patients with thiazide sensitivity will cross-react to diazoxide. In patients with impaired cerebral or cardiac function, the risks may outweigh the benefits of diazoxide administration.

(b) Diazoxide also produces transient hyperglycemia, requiring caution if administered to diabetic patients.

(c) Hypotensive reactions may be severe.

(d) Unlike the thiazides, this agent promotes sodium and water retention, potentiating edema.

5. Angiotensin-converting enzyme (ACE) inhibitors

a. General considerations. Captopril and enalapril are quite similar; however, enalapril is more potent and, although slower in onset of action, its duration of action is longer. Enalapril is an inactive substance that requires metabolism (de-esterification) in the liver before conversion to the active substance enalaprilate. Unlike captopril, enalapril is not a sulfhydryl compound; therefore, associated side effects should be minimized with enalapril.

b. Indications. Although the use of ACE inhibitors was initially restricted to patients with refractory hypertension or for use as a step-four agent, it is gaining favor as a step-two agent or as a "floating" alternative to agents used in step two, three, or four (see Figure 33-2).

c. Actions

(1) Basically, these agents inhibit conversion of angiotensin I (a weak vasoconstrictor) to angiotensin II (a highly effective vasoconstrictor) or interfere with utilization of angiotensin II.

(2) ACE inhibitors indirectly inhibit fluid volume increases when interfering with angiotensin II because angiotensin II stimulates the release of aldosterone, which promotes sodium and water retention.

d. Significant interactions. The antihypertensive effect of ACE inhibitors may be diminished by NSAIDs (such as over-the-counter forms of ibuprofen).

e. Precautions and monitoring effects

(1) **Neutropenia** is rare (especially with enalapril) but serious; there is an increased incidence in patients with renal insufficiency or autoimmune disease.

(2) **Proteinuria; nephrotic syndrome**. This occurs particularly in patients with a history of renal disease. Urinary proteins should be monitored regularly.

(3) **Hyperkalemia.** Serum potassium levels should be monitored regularly. The mechanism of action tends to increase potassium levels somewhat. Patients with renal dysfunction are at increased risk.

(4) **Renal insufficiency** can occur in patients with predisposing factors, such as renal stenosis, and when enalapril is administered with hydrochlorothiazide. Renal function should be monitored (e.g., serum creatinine and BUN).

Table 33-4. Rapid-Acting Parenteral Antihypertensive Agents

Drug	Mode of Administration	Dose	Onset of Action	Duration of Action	Precautions	Side Effects
Sodium nitroprusside	IV drip	Titration 0.1 mg/ml	Instantaneous	2–3 minutes after cessation of drip	Use fresh solution every 4–8 hours; shield solution from light; constant monitoring is needed	Nausea; vomiting; hypotension; thiocyanate intoxication; sodium retention
Diazoxide	IV bolus (usually 10–30 seconds)	300 mg	2–5 minutes	1–18 hours	Use with care in cerebral vascular disease, coronary artery disease, aortic dissections. Blood glucose monitoring is necessary	Hyperglycemia; hyperuricemia; hypotension; tachycardia; chest pain; nausea; vomiting; sodium retention
Trimethaphan camsylate	IV drip	Titration 1 mg/ml	2–5 minutes	5 minutes after cessation of drip	Requires constant monitoring; resistance develops in 24–48 hours; not advised for postoperative patients or those with a history of allergies	Paresis of the bowel, bladder; hypotension; visual blurring; dry mouth; sodium retention
Hydralazine	IM or IV	10–20 mg	30–45 minutes	4-6 hours	Relatively contraindicated in patients with angina pectoris, aortic dissections	Flushing; headache; tachycardia; nausea; vomiting; possible aggravation of angina

IV = intravenous; IM = intramuscular.

(5) A **dry cough** may occur. If it is drug-related, the cough will disappear within a few days after the ACE inhibitor is discontinued.

(6) **Other untoward effects** include rashes, alteration in sense of taste (dysgeusia), vertigo, headache, fatigue, first-dose hypotension, and minor gastrointestinal disturbances.

IV. HYPERTENSIVE EMERGENCIES

A. Definition. A hypertensive emergency is a severe elevation of blood pressure (more than 200 mm Hg systolic or greater than 140 mm Hg diastolic) that demands either immediate (within minutes) or prompt (within hours) reduction.

1. Conditions requiring **immediate** reduction include hypertensive encephalopathy and acute left ventricular failure.

2. Conditions requiring **prompt** reduction include malignant or accelerated hypertension.

B. Treatment

1. Although the goal is to decrease blood pressure, the **reduction must be gradual** (e.g., a 15% decrease in mean arterial pressure over the first hour) rather than precipitous in order to avoid compromising perfusion of critical organs, particularly cerebral perfusion.

2. **Diuretics should be avoided initially** (they may exacerbate hypovolemia and induce severe vasoconstriction) unless intravascular fluid overload has been demonstrated. They may be introduced later to treat sodium and fluid retention resulting from drug therapy with agents such as diazoxide or sodium nitroprusside.

3. **Individual agents** used in hypertensive crises are shown in Table 33-4; for further information on vasodilators, see section III B 4.

STUDY QUESTIONS

Directions: Each question below contains five suggested answers. Choose the **one best** response to each question.

1. Which of the following β-adrenergic blockers would be the best treatment for a hypertensive patient suffering from sinus bradycardia?

A. Propranolol
B. Atenolol
C. Nadolol
D. Pindolol
E. Metoprolol

2. Reflex tachycardia, headache, and postural hypotension are adverse effects that limit the use of which of the following antihypertensive agents?

A. Prazosin
B. Captopril
C. Methyldopa
D. Guanethidine
E. Hydralazine

3. Mr. Benson is a 60-year-old white man with moderate hypertension that is refractory to diuretics, β-blockers, and methyldopa. He is found to have renovascular hypertension, with elevated renin levels confirmed on laboratory evaluation. This patient's antihypertensive regimen would be enhanced best by the addition of which of the following agents?

A. Prazosin
B. Hydralazine
C. Enalapril
D. Nitroprusside
E. Clonidine

4. A hypertensive patient being managed with stepped-care therapy is being considered for treatment with a step-three agent. No evidence of toxicity has been noted during the course of treatment with step-one and step-two agents. What is the proper step to be taken at this point in the patient's treatment?

A. Increase the dosages of the step-one and step-two agents while adding the new agent
B. Decrease the dosages of the step-one and step-two agents while adding the new agent
C. Remove the step-two agent to prevent the development of excess hypotension
D. Maintain the step-one and step-two agents at their current dosages while adding the new agent
E. Remove the step-one and step-two agents prior to adding the step-three agent

5. Long-standing hypertension leads to tissue damage in all of the following organs EXCEPT

A. the heart
B. the lungs
C. the kidneys
D. the brain
E. the eyes

6. A hypertensive patient who is asthmatic and very noncompliant would be best treated with which of the following β-blocking agents?

A. Timolol
B. Nadolol
C. Esmolol
D. Acebutolol
E. Propranolol

Directions: Each question below contains three suggested answers of which **one or more** is correct. Choose the answer

A if **I only** is correct
B if **III only** is correct
C if **I and II** are correct
D if **II and III** are correct
E if **I, II, and III** are correct

7. A patient being treated with a thiazide diuretic should be monitored regularly for altered plasma levels of

I. potassium
II. glucose
III. uric acid

8. Before antihypertensive therapy begins, secondary causes of hypertension should be ruled out. Laboratory findings that suggest an underlying cause of hypertension include

I. a decreased serum potassium level
II. an increased urinary catecholamine level
III. an increased blood cortisol level

9. In an otherwise healthy adult with mild hypertension, appropriate initial antihypertensive therapy would be

I. hydrochlorothiazide
II. furosemide
III. hydralazine

Directions: The groups of questions below consist of lettered choices followed by several numbered items. For each numbered item select the **one** lettered choice with which it is **most** closely associated. Each lettered choice may be used once, more than once, or not at all.

Question 10–14

Match the adverse effects with the antihypertensive agent that is most likely to cause them.

A. Captopril
B. Methyldopa
C. Nitroprusside
D. Prazosin
E. Propranolol

10. Thiocyanate intoxication, hypotension, convulsions

11. Bradycardia, bronchospasm, cardiac decompensation

12. Dysgeusia, skin rash, proteinuria

13. Postural hypotension, fever, positive Coombs' test

14. First-dose syncope, postural hypotension, palpitations

Question 15–19

Match each description of a β-blocker with the most appropriate β-adrenergic blocking agent.

A. Esmolol
B. Labetalol
C. Metoprolol
D. Nadolol
E. Pindolol

15. A β-blocker with intrinsic sympathomimetic activity

16. A β-blocker that also blocks α-adrenergic receptors

17. A β-blocker with an ultrashort duration of action

18. A β-blocker with a long duration of action

19. A β-blocker with relative cardioselective blocking activity

ANSWERS AND EXPLANATIONS

1. The answer is D. [*III B 3 a (5) (b), (6) (f)*] Pindolol is a nonselective β-adrenergic blocking agent with intrinsic sympathomimetic activity, as evidenced by a lesser decrease in cardiac output and heart rate than is seen with other β-blockers (e.g., propranolol, atenolol, nadolol, metoprolol). As a result, pindolol would be a good choice of treatment for a hypertensive patient with sinus bradycardia.

2. The answer is E. (*III B 4 a*) Hydralazine is a vasodilator that works by directly relaxing arterioles, thereby reducing peripheral vascular resistance. Its effectiveness as an antihypertensive agent is compromised, however, by the compensatory reactions it triggers (i.e., reflex tachycardia) and by its other adverse effects (e.g., headache, postural hypotension, nausea, palpitations). Fortunately, the unwanted effects of hydralazine are minimized when it is used in combination with a diuretic agent and a β-blocker. Thus, hydralazine is most effective as a step-three antihypertensive drug.

3. The answer is C. (*III B 5*) Enalapril, an angiotensin-converting enzyme (ACE) inhibitor, acts by inhibiting the conversion of angiotensin I (a weak vasoconstrictor) to angiotensin II (a potent vasoconstrictor). As this patient has renovascular hypertension, a response would be expected from an ACE inhibitor, such as enalapril; enalapril will work directly on the renin-angiotensin system, which is activated by renal artery stenosis.

4. The answer is D. (*III B 1; Figure 33-2*) Although controversial and waning somewhat in popularity, the stepped-care regimen remains an often-used approach to antihypertensive therapy. The primary goal of this therapeutic approach is to control blood pressure using the fewest drugs at the lowest dosages. Typically, treatment begins with a small dose of a step-one drug, and the dosage is increased until blood pressure is controlled or the maximal therapeutic dose is reached. If blood pressure is not controlled at the maximal therapeutic dose, a step-two drug is added at a low dosage while maintaining the step-one drug at its maximal dosage. The dosage of the step-two drug is increased, again, until blood pressure is controlled or the maximal therapeutic dose is reached. If blood pressure is not controlled by the step-one and step-two drugs at their maximal therapeutic doses, a step-three drug is added. The addition of drugs continues in this way until blood pressure is controlled.

5. The answer is B. (*I E; Table 33-2*) Left untreated, hypertension can be lethal due to its progressively destructive effects on major organs, such as the heart, kidneys, and brain. The eyes also suffer damage; the lungs, however, do not. End-organ damage caused by hypertension includes left ventricular hypertrophy, congestive heart failure, angina pectoris, myocardial infarction, renal insufficiency due to atherosclerotic lesions, nephrosclerosis, cerebral aneurysm and hemorrhage, retinal hemorrhage, and papilledema.

6. The answer is D. [*III B 3 a (6)*] The β-adrenergic blocking agents are employed as step-one or step-two agents in the treatment of hypertension. A major feature of some of these agents is their relative selectivity for β_1-receptors (in the heart) rather than for β_2-receptors (in the lung), which provides advantages in the treatment of certain patients (e.g., asthmatic patients). Of the β-blockers listed in the question, acebutolol is less likely than the rest to block β_2-receptors, due to its relative cardioselective blocking activity. Acebutolol also has a long duration of action, which could be helpful in the noncompliant patient by requiring fewer doses per day. Nadolol also has a long duration of action but is nonselective (i.e., it is equally effective in blocking β_1- and β_2-receptors).

7. The answer is E (all). (*III B 2 a*) Thiazide diuretics act directly on the kidneys by increasing the excretion of sodium and water and, to a lesser extent, the excretion of potassium. Patients who are treated with thiazides should be monitored for hypokalemia, which may require potassium supplementation or the addition of a potassium-sparing diuretic to the antihypertensive regimen. Thiazide diuretics have the opposite effect on uric acid and glucose excretion. Thus, patients receiving these drugs also should be monitored for increased plasma levels of uric acid (especially if they are predisposed to gout) and glucose (especially if they are predisposed to diabetes).

8. The answer is E (all). (*II A*) Low serum potassium levels in a hypertensive patient suggest primary aldosteronism. Elevated urinary catecholamines suggest a pheochromocytoma; other signs and symptoms of this tumor include weight loss, episodic flushing, and sweating. Elevated serum cortisol levels suggest Cushing's syndrome; the patient is also likely to show a round face and truncal obesity. Secondary hypertension requires treatment of the underlying cause; supplementary antihypertensive drug therapy may also be needed.

9. The answer is A (I). [*III B 2 a, b (1), 3 a (1), 5 b; Figure 33-2*] Thiazide diuretics, such as hydrochlorothiazide, are indicated as first-line antihypertensive agents for the treatment of mild to moderate hypertension. A β-blocker, such as propranolol, also would be appropriate initial therapy. Furosemide is a diuretic that acts primarily in the loop of Henle, with a shorter but more intense action than that of thiazide diuretics; it is reserved for patients who cannot tolerate thiazides, who have experienced a loss of thiazide function, or who have impaired renal clearance. Hydralazine is a vasodilator that is used at the third step in antihypertensive therapy.

10–14. The answers are: 10-C, 11-E, 12-A, 13-B, 14-D. [*III B 3 a (4), b (1) (b), d (2), 4 c (2), 5 e*] The goal of treatment in hypertension is to lower blood pressure toward ''normal'' with a minimum of side effects. All antihypertensive drugs can cause adverse effects. Therefore, the stepped-care approach has evolved, on the principle that combination therapy allows the use of lower doses of each drug and thus reduces the risk of adverse effects while providing optimal therapeutic benefits.

15–19. The answers are: 15-E, 16-B, 17-A, 18-D, 19-C. [*III B 3 a (6)*] The β-adrenergic blocking agents are valuable in the management of hypertension and are used as step-one or step-two antihypertensives. The β-blockers are sympathetic antagonists: They act by blocking various receptors of the sympathetic nervous system. The β-blockers differ in their selectivity for these sympathetic receptors. For example, β_1-blockers have relative cardioselective activity; that is, they block β_1-receptors (in the heart) rather than β_2-receptors (in bronchial smooth muscle) and, therefore, are highly useful antihypertensive agents. Intrinsic sympathomimetic activity also appears to reduce the problem of bronchoconstriction; moreover, drugs with this property also have the ability to maintain a satisfactory heart rate.

34 Congestive Heart Failure

Alan H. Mutnick

I. INTRODUCTION

A. Definition

1. **Congestive heart failure** (CHF) is a condition in which an abnormality in myocardial function results in the inability of the ventricles to deliver adequate quantities of blood to the metabolizing tissues during normal activity or at rest.
2. The condition is termed **congestive because of the edematous state** commonly produced by the fluid backup resulting from poor pump function.

B. The **mortality** rate is high; according to the Framingham Heart Disease Epidemiology Study, of those who were diagnosed as having CHF, less than 50% of the men and less than 60% of the women survived 5 years after the initial diagnosis.

C. Etiology

1. Although the disease occurs most commonly among the elderly, it may appear at any age as a consequence of underlying cardiovascular disease (Table 34-1).
2. CHF should not be considered an independent diagnosis, as it is superimposed on an underlying cause.
   a. Hypertension and coronary artery disease are the two major underlying causes of CHF development.
   b. Myocardial stress may be caused by trauma, disease, or another abnormal state such as pulmonary embolism, infection, anemia, pregnancy, drug use or abuse, fluid overload, and arrhythmias.

D. Forms of heart failure

1. **Low-output versus high-output failure**
   a. If metabolic demands are within normal limits but the heart is unable to meet them, the failure is designated **low output** (the most common type).
   b. If metabolic demands increase (e.g., as in hyperthyroidism and anemia), and the heart is unable to meet them, the failure is designated **high output**.
2. **Left-sided versus right-sided failure**
   a. **Left-sided failure**
      (1) In this form of failure, blood cannot be adequately pumped from the left ventricle to the peripheral circulation; therefore, it accumulates within the left ventricle.
      (2) Given this accumulation, the left ventricle is unable to accept blood from the left atrium and lung; therefore, the fluid portion of the blood backs up into the pulmonary alveoli, producing pulmonary edema.

Table 34-1. Cardiac Diseases Commonly Underlying Congestive Heart Failure

Age Range (Years)	Common Underlying Causes
20–40	Rheumatic fever, rheumatic heart disease
40–50	Myocardial infarction, hypertension, pulmonary disease
Over 50	Calcific aortic stenosis

b. Right-sided failure

(1) When blood cannot be pumped from the right ventricle into the lungs, it accumulates within the right ventricle.

(2) When blood is not pumped from the right ventricle, the fluid portion of the blood backs up throughout the body (e.g., in the veins, liver, legs, and bowels), producing systemic edema.

(1) The signs and symptoms of heart failure usually result from the effects of blood backing up behind the failing ventricle (except in heart failure due to increased body demands).

(2) Initially, the signs and symptoms tend to be specific to failure of one side of the heart, but eventually bilateral involvement will be evidenced.

(3) This progression occurs because the cardiovascular system is a closed system (Fig. 34-1); thus over time, right-sided failure will cause left-sided failure and vice versa.

II. PATHOPHYSIOLOGY.

Heart failure and decreases in cardiac output trigger a complex scheme of compensatory mechanisms designed to normalize cardiac output (cardiac output = stroke volume × heart rate).

A. Compensatory mechanisms are represented schematically in Figure 34-2.

1. Sympathetic responses. Inadequate cardiac output stimulates reflex activation of the sympathetic nervous system and an increase in circulating catecholamines. The heart rate increases, and blood flow is redistributed to ensure perfusion of the most vital organs (the brain and heart).

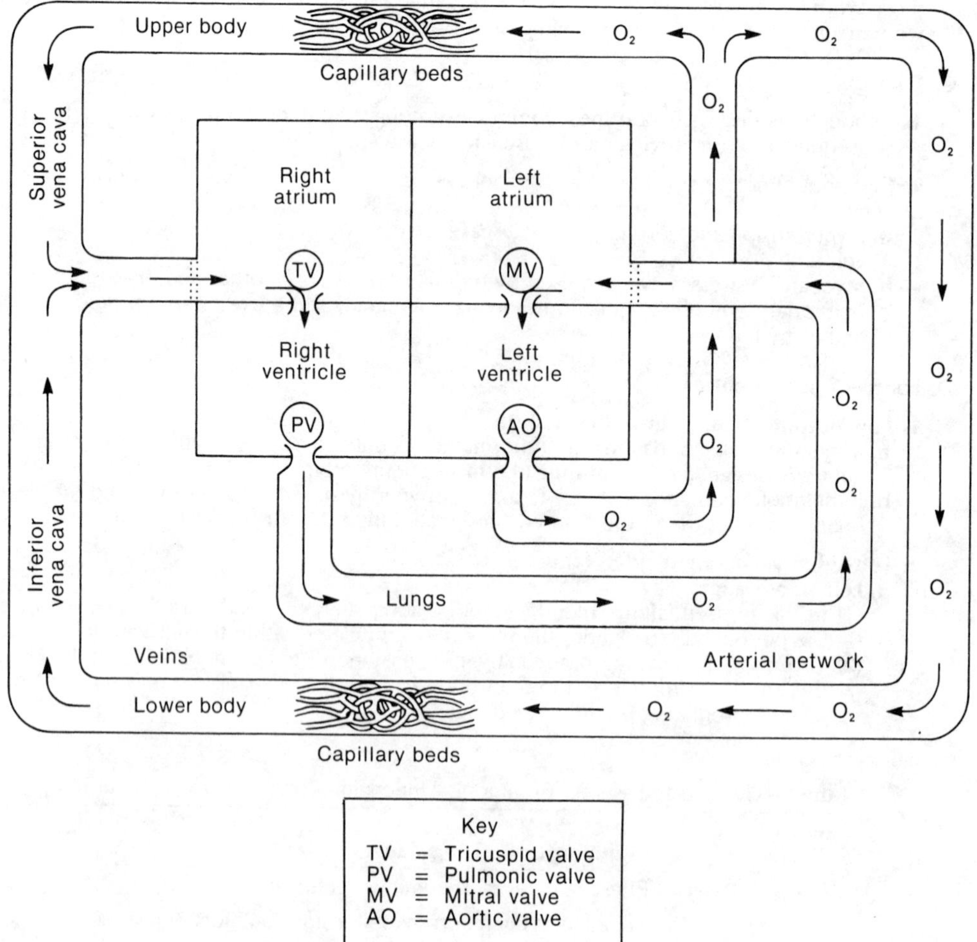

Figure 34-1. This figure presents an overview of blood flow through the cardiovascular system.

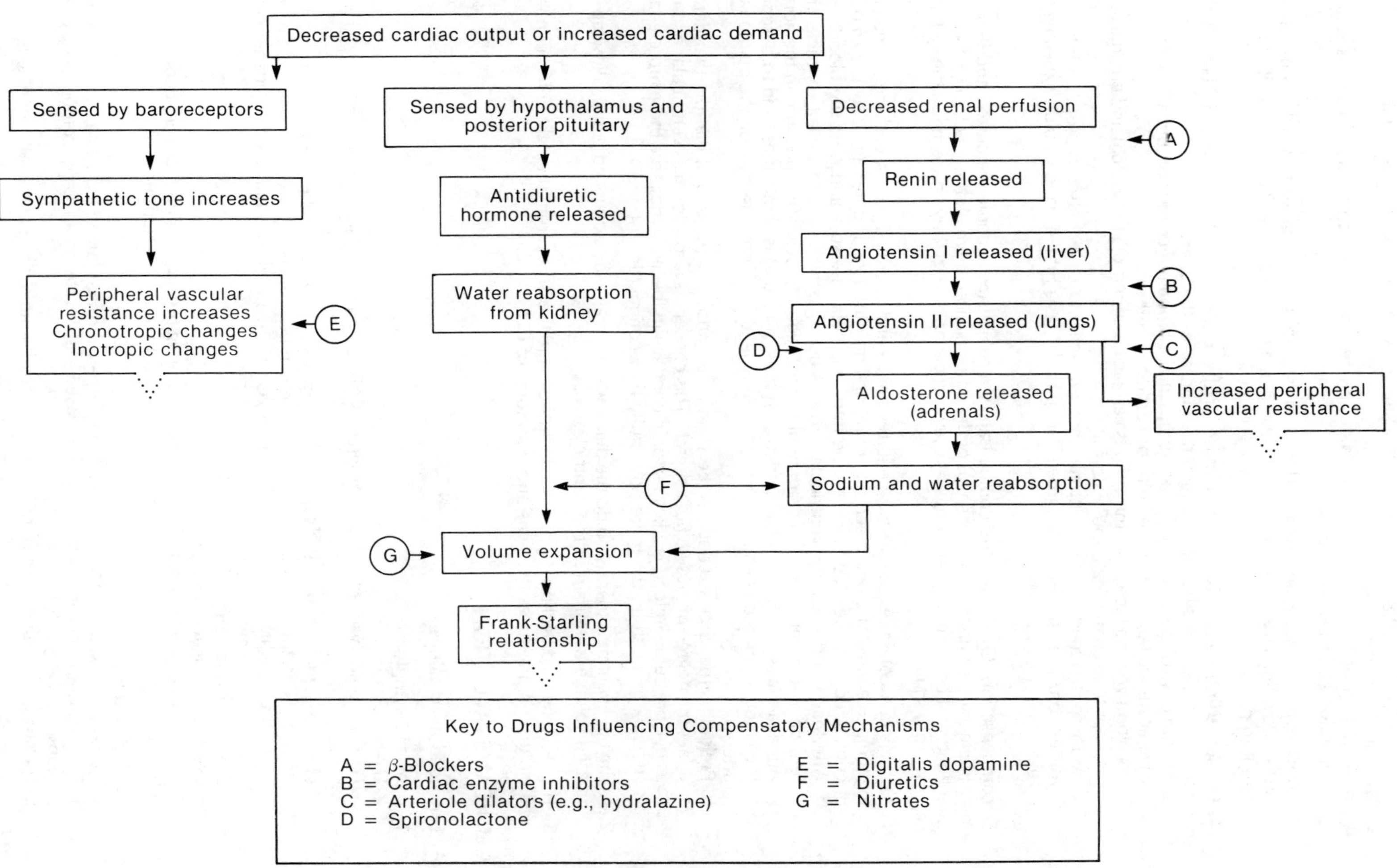

Figure 34-2. Compensatory mechanisms in congestive heart failure (CHF).

2. **Hormonal stimulation**. The redistribution of blood flow results in reduced renal perfusion, which decreases the glomerular filtration rate (GFR). Reduction in GFR results in:
   a. Sodium and water retention
   b. Activation of the renin-angiotensin-aldosterone system, which further enhances sodium retention and thus volume expansion

3. **Concentric cardiac hypertrophy**. This term describes a mechanism that thickens cardiac walls, providing larger contractile cells and diminishing the capacity of the cavity in an attempt to precipitate expulsion at lower volumes.

4. **Frank-Starling mechanism**. The premise of this response is that increased fiber dilation heightens the contractile force, which then increases the energy released.
   a. Within physiologic limits, the heart pumps all the blood it receives without allowing excessive accumulation within the veins or cardiac chambers.
   b. As blood volume increases, the various cardiac chambers dilate (stretch) and enlarge in an attempt to accommodate the excess fluid.
   c. As these stretched muscles contract, the contractile force increases in proportion to their distension. Then the extended fibers "snap back" (as a rubber band would), expelling the extra fluid into the arteries.

B. **Decompensation**. Over time, the compensatory mechanisms become exhausted and increasingly ineffective, entering a vicious spiral of decompensation in which the mechanisms surpass their limits and become self-defeating—as they work ever harder, they only exhaust the system's capacity to respond.

1. As the strain continues, total peripheral resistance and afterload increase, thereby decreasing the percentage of blood ejected per unit of time. Afterload is determined by the amount of contractile force needed to overcome intraventricular pressure and eject the blood.
   a. **Afterload** is the tension in ventricular muscles during contraction. In the left ventricle, this tension is determined by the amount of force needed to overcome pressure in the aorta. Afterload (also known as intraventricular systolic pressure) is sometimes used to describe the amount of force needed in the right ventricle to overcome pressure in the pulmonary artery.
   b. **Preload** is the force exerted on the ventricular muscle at the end of diastole that determines the degree of muscle fiber stretch. This concept is also known as ventricular end-diastolic pressure. Preload is a key factor in contractility because the more these muscles are stretched in diastole, the more powerfully they contract in systole.

2. As the fluid volume expands, so do the demands on an already exhausted pump, allowing increased volume to remain in the ventricle.

3. The resulting fluid backup (from the left ventricle into the lungs; from the right, into peripheral circulation) produces the signs and symptoms of CHF.

III. CLINICAL EVALUATION

A. Left-sided heart failure

1. Signs and symptoms

a. Dyspnea

(1) **Exertional dyspnea**. As CHF progresses, the amount of exertion required to trigger this response lessens.

(2) **Paroxysmal nocturnal dyspnea; orthopnea**. These difficulties result from volume pooling in the recumbent position; both can be relieved by propping with pillows or sitting upright. (Orthopnea is often gauged by the number of pillows the patient needs to sleep comfortably.)

b. Dry, wheezing cough

c. Exertional fatigue and weakness

d. Nocturia. Edematous fluids that accumulate during the day migrate from dependent areas when the patient is in a recumbent position and renal perfusion increases.

2. Physical findings

a. **Rales** (or crackles) indicate the movement of air through fluid-filled passages.

b. **Tachycardia**, detected through an **increased pulse rate**, is an early compensatory response.

c. **S_3 ventricular gallop**. This vibration is produced by rapid filling of the left ventricle early in diastole.

d. **S_4 atrial gallop** is a vibration produced by increased resistance to sudden, forceful ejection of atrial blood in late diastole; it does not vary with inspiration in left-sided failure.

3. Diagnostic test results

a. Cardiomegaly (heart enlargement), left ventricular hypertrophy, and pulmonary congestion may be evidenced by chest x-ray, electrocardiogram (ECG), and echocardiography.

b. Arm-to-tongue circulation time will be prolonged.

c. Transudative pleural effusion may be suggested by x-ray and confirmed by analysis of aspirated pleural fluid.

B. Right-sided heart failure

1. Signs and symptoms

a. Patient complaints of tightness and swelling (e.g., "My ring is too tight"; "My skin feels too tight") suggest edema.

b. Nausea, vomiting, anorexia, bloating, or abdominal pain on exertion may reflect hepatic and visceral engorgement, resulting from venous pressure elevation.

2. Physical findings

a. Jugular vein distension reflects increased venous pressure and is a cardinal sign of CHF.

b. S_3 ventricular gallop is described in section III A 2 c.

c. S_4 atrial gallop intensifies on inspiration in right-sided failure.

d. Hepatomegaly (a tender, enlarged liver) is revealed when pushing on the edge of the liver results in a fluid reflux into the jugular veins, causing bulging (positive hepatojugular reflux).

e. Edema. Bilateral leg edema is an early sign of right-sided heart failure; pitting ankle edema signals more advanced heart failure. However, edema is common to many disorders, and a pattern of associated findings, such as concurrent neck vein distension, is required for differential diagnosis.

3. Laboratory findings. Elevated levels of hepatic enzymes [e.g., serum glutamic-pyruvic transaminase (SGPT)] reflect hepatic congestion.

IV. TREATMENT GOALS. CHF requires a two-pronged therapeutic approach, the overall goals of which are:

A. To remove or mitigate the underlying cause; for example, by eliminating ingestion of certain drugs or other substances (Table 34-2) that can produce or exacerbate CHF or by correcting an anemic syndrome, which can increase cardiac demands.

B. To relieve the symptoms and improve pump function by:

1. Reducing metabolic demands through rest and relaxation

2. Reducing fluid volume excess through dietary and pharmaceutic controls

3. Administering digitalis and other inotropic substances

4. Promoting patient compliance and self-regulation through education

V. THERAPY

A. Bed rest

1. Advantages

a. Rest reduces cardiac workload by reducing metabolic needs.

b. Reduced workload, in turn, reduces pulse rate and dyspnea.

Table 34-2. Substances that May Exacerbate Congestive Heart Failure

Promote Sodium Retention	Produce Osmotic Effect	Decrease Contractility
Androgens	Albumin	Antiarrhythmic agents (e.g., quinidine, disopyramide, procainamide, flecainide)
Corticosteroids	Glucose	β-Adrenergic blocking agents
Diazoxide	Mannitol	Daunomycin
Estrogens	Saline	
Guanethidine	Urea	
Licorice		
Lithium carbonate		
Methyldopa		
Phenylbutazone		
Salicylates		

c. Bed rest also helps decrease excess fluid volume by promoting diuresis.

2. **Disadvantages.** The risk of venous stasis increases with bed rest and can result in thromboembolism. Antiembolism stockings help minimize this risk, as do passive or active leg exercises, when the patient's condition permits.

3. Adequate bed rest should be followed by progressive ambulation.

B. Dietary controls

1. The patient should receive frequent (4 to 6 daily) **small meals** that are low in calories and residue so that they provide nourishment without unduly increasing metabolic demands.

2. **Sodium restriction** is a primary tool in reducing central volume in CHF.
   a. Renal function should be evaluated to assess sodium conservation if severe sodium restriction is contemplated.
   b. Moderate sodium restriction (2 to 4 g of dietary sodium/day) can be achieved with relative ease by limiting the addition of salt during cooking and at the table.
   c. The patient should be advised about medications and common products that contain sodium and cautioned about their use (e.g., antacids, such as Alka-Seltzer; sodium bicarbonate or baking soda; commercial diet food products; and water softeners). Table 34-2 lists other substances that promote sodium retention.

C. Digitalis glycosides. Digitalis usually is considered a mainstay of CHF treatment, but its use, particularly in chronic CHF, has become somewhat controversial. Some authorities feel that digitalis use should be reserved for cases refractory to therapy combining rest, dietary controls, diuretics, and vasodilators.

1. **Therapeutic effects**
   a. **Positive inotropic effects** provide most of the benefits:
      (1) Increased cardiac output
      (2) Decreased cardiac filling pressure
      (3) Decreased venous and capillary pressure
      (4) Decreased heart size
      (5) Increased renal blood flow
      (6) Deactivation of renin-angiotensin-aldosterone compensation, promoting diuresis
      (7) Decreased fluid volume
      (8) Diminished edema
   b. **Negative chronotropic effects** accrue from the effect of digitalis on the sinoatrial (S-A) node when given in doses that produce high total body stores (e.g., 15 to 18 μg/kg).

2. **Choice of agent.** All of the digitalis glycosides have similar properties; thus, selection is based on absorption, elimination kinetics, speed of onset, and duration of effect. Overall, digoxin is the most versatile and widely used and will, therefore, be used as the therapeutic prototype.
   a. Digoxin is available in tablet, injection, elixir, and capsule forms.
   b. Calculation of doses must factor in the differences in systemic availability among these forms. For example, Lanoxicaps are more bioavailable than Lanoxin tablets; therefore, 0.125-mg tablets are equivalent to 0.1-mg capsules.

3. **Dosage and administration**
   a. The range between therapeutic and toxic doses is extremely narrow.
   b. There is no "magic threshold" level for digitalis therapy, but serum concentration levels of 0.8 to 2.0 ng/ml for digoxin (10 to 35 ng/ml for digitoxin) have been associated with therapeutic response and minimal toxicity.
   c. **Rapid digitalization**
      (1) In this method, the effects (and steady-state levels) are achieved within 24 hours—but the actual administration rate is usually slow and delivered in divided doses.
      (2) In the presence of an acute need for an immediate effect, intravenous (IV) digitalization with digoxin may be required—if the patient has not received any digitalis in the previous 2 weeks. (IV digitoxin is not usually used in an acute situation because it has a long latency period.)
   d. **Slow digitalization.** When urgency is not the driving force, oral administration of maintenance doses should achieve steady-state levels in 7 to 8 days for the average patient (3 to 4 weeks in a patient with renal dysfunction).

4. **Precautions and monitoring effects**
   a. **Potassium** seems to antagonize digitalis preparations.
      (1) Decreased potassium levels favor digoxin binding to cardiac cells and increase its effect, thus increasing the likelihood of digitalis toxicity. This antagonism is particularly

significant for the CHF patient who is receiving a diuretic (many of which decrease potassium levels).

(2) Conversely, increased potassium levels seem to decrease digoxin binding and decrease its effect. This is likely in a patient taking potassium or a captopril-like agent (which increases potassium reabsorption).

b. **Calcium** ions act synergistically with digoxin, and increased levels will increase the force of myocardial contraction. At excessive levels, arrhythmias and systolic standstill can develop.

c. **Magnesium** levels are inversely related to digoxin activity. As magnesium levels decrease, the predisposition to toxicity increases and, within reason, vice versa.

d. **Serum digoxin levels**

(1) In cardiac glycoside therapy, the patient's clinical state is the most practical barometer of a successful regimen. However, should questions arise as to compliance, absorption, or a drug–drug interaction, serum digoxin levels may be helpful.

(2) After oral ingestion of digoxin, the serum levels rise rapidly, then drop sharply as the drug enters the myocardium and other tissues. Therefore, a meaningful evaluation requires a determination of the relationship between serum digoxin levels and myocardial tissue levels.

(3) The most meaningful results are obtained if serum samples are taken after steady-state has been reached and 6 to 8 hours after an oral dose (3 to 4 hours after an IV dose).

e. **Renal function studies**. Because the kidney is the primary metabolic route **for digoxin**, renal function studies such as serum creatinine levels aid evaluation of elimination kinetics for digoxin. (**For digitoxin**, which is eliminated primarily through the liver, evaluation of metabolizing capabilities is more difficult.)

5. **Digitalis toxicity** is a fairly common occurrence because of the narrow therapeutic range and can be fatal in a significant percentage of patients experiencing a toxic reaction.

a. The risk of toxicity increases with coadministration of quinidine, verapamil, and amiodarone and is influenced by the electrolyte effects described in section V C 4 a–c.

b. **Signs of toxicity** include:

(1) Anorexia, a common and early sign
(2) Fatigue, headache, malaise
(3) Nausea and vomiting
(4) Mental confusion and disorientation
(5) Alterations in visual perception, such as blurring, yellowing, or a halo effect
(6) Cardiac effects include:
(a) Premature ventricular contractions; ventricular tachycardia and fibrillation
(b) S-A and A-V block
(c) Atrial tachycardia with A-V block

c. **Treatment of digitalis toxicity**

(1) Digitalis is discontinued immediately, as is any potassium-depleting diuretic.

(2) If the patient is hypokalemic, potassium supplements are administered and serum levels are monitored to avoid hyperkalemia through overcompensation. However, potassium supplements are contraindicated in a patient with severe A-V block.

(3) Arrhythmias are treated with lidocaine (usually a 100-mg bolus, followed by infusion at 2 to 4 mg/min) or phenytoin (as a slow IV infusion of 25 to 50 mg/min, to a maximum of 1.0 g).

(4) Cholestyramine, which binds to digitalis glycosides, may help prevent absorption and reabsorption of digitalis in the bile.

(5) Those patients with very high serum digoxin levels (such as those resulting from a suicidal overdose) may benefit from the use of purified digoxin-specific Fab fragment antibodies (Digibind).

D. **Diuretics** (see Chapter 33, section III B 6)

1. All diuretics reduce excess sodium and water. Thus, they reduce preload by decreasing venous return, which is essential in managing CHF.

2. The **thiazide diuretics** are highly effective and commonly used, but they deplete potassium stores in the process.

3. The loop diuretic **furosemide** has the same effect plus the added advantage of reducing venous return independent of diuresis. Also, because its action is more intense, it is useful as a rapid-acting IV agent in reversing acute pulmonary edema, due to its direct dilating effects on pulmonary vasculature.

4. **Potassium-sparing diuretics** may help avoid the exacerbating effects of hypokalemia, but they have a weaker diuretic effect.

E. Vasodilators (see Chapter 33, section III B 8)

1. These agents reduce pulmonary congestion and increase cardiac output by reducing preload and afterload.

2. Because of the complexity of vasodilator actions in patients with CHF, their use requires close hemodynamic monitoring and individualized adjustments to avoid excessive vasodilation and its adverse effects.

3. Generally, vasodilators seem more effective in treating acute heart failure than chronic failure requiring long-term therapy.

4. Some vasodilators exert their action primarily on the veins (preload reduction) or on the arteries (afterload reduction); others act on venous and arterial beds almost equally, providing a balanced effect (preload–afterload reduction).

5. **Individual agents**
   a. **Nitroprusside** (see Chapter 33, section III B 8 e) is administered intravenously to provide potent dilation of both arteries and veins.
   b. **Hydralazine** (see Chapter 33, section III B 8 c)
      (1) This arteriole dilator decreases afterload and increases cardiac output in patients with CHF.
      (2) Effective long-term therapy has been achieved with doses of 75 to 100 mg taken orally up to four times daily.
   c. **Prazosin** (see Chapter 33, section III B 8 d)
      (1) This α-adrenergic blocker acts as a balanced arteriovenous dilator.
      (2) It has been shown to be effective in long-term therapy in doses of 2 to 10 mg taken up to four times daily.
   d. **Nitrates** (see Chapter 33, section II H)
      (1) Venous dilation by nitrates increases venous pooling, which decreases preload.
      (2) Their arterial effects seem to result in decreased afterload with continued therapy.
      (3) Nitrates are available in many forms and doses. Because individual reactions vary widely, dosages have to be adjusted, but, in general, will be higher for CHF than for angina. Table 34-3 provides examples of nitrate doses used in CHF patients.
   e. **Combination therapy**. Hydralazine has been used with isosorbide dinitrate to reduce afterload (or with nitroglycerin to reduce preload) in treatment of chronic CHF.
   f. **Converting enzyme inhibitors** (see Chapter 33, section III B 9)
      (1) **Captopril and enalapril** inhibit conversion of angiotensin I to angiotensin II (a potent vasoconstrictor). This inhibitory action significantly decreases total peripheral resistance, which aids in reducing afterload.
      (2) Inhibiting production of angiotensin II interferes with stimulation of aldosterone release, thus indirectly reducing retention of sodium and water, which decreases venous return and preload.

F. Inotropic agents have been used in the emergency treatment of patients with CHF and in patients refractory to, or unable to take, digitalis.

1. **Dopamine**
   a. **Low doses** of 2 to 5 μg/kg/min seem to stimulate specific dopamine receptors within the kidney to increase renal blood flow.
   b. **Moderate doses** of 5 to 10 μg/kg/min increase cardiac output in CHF patients.
   c. **High doses**
      (1) As doses are raised above 10 μg/kg/min, alpha peripheral activity increases, resulting in increased total peripheral resistance and pulmonary pressures.
      (2) When the infusion exceeds 8 to 9 μg/kg/min, the patient should be monitored for tachycardia. If the infusion is slowed or interrupted, the adverse effect should disappear, as dopamine has a very short half-life in plasma.

Table 34-3. Examples of Nitrate Use in Congestive Heart Failure

Form	Typical Dose	Interval
Nitroglycerin ointment	1–3 inches	4–6 hours
Sublingual nitroglycerin	0.4 mg	1–2 hours
Oral isosorbide dinitrate	20–40 mg	4–6 hours
Sublingual isosorbide dinitrate	5–10 mg	4 hours

2. Dobutamine

a. Patients who are unresponsive to or adversely affected by dopamine may benefit from dobutamine in doses of 5 to 20 μg/kg/min.

b. Although dobutamine resembles dopamine chemically, its actions differ somewhat. For example, dobutamine does not have a direct effect on renal receptors and, therefore, does not act as a renal vasodilator. It only increases urinary output through increased cardiac output.

c. Serious arrhythmias are a potential occurrence, although less likely to occur than with dopamine. Slowing or interrupting the infusion usually reverses this effect, as it does for dopamine.

3. Combination therapy. Dobutamine and dopamine have been used together to treat cardiogenic shock, but similar use in CHF has yet to be accepted.

4. Amrinone

a. A derivative of bipyridine, amrinone has both a positive inotropic effect and a vasodilating effect.

b. It is the newest of a new class of drugs referred to as nonglycoside, nonsympathomimetic inotropic agents.

c. By inhibiting phosphodiesterase located specifically in the cardiac cells, it increases the amount of cyclic adenosine monophosphate (cAMP).

d. Amrinone has been used in patients with heart failure that has been refractory to treatment with other inotropic agents.

e. Effective regimens have used loading infusions of 0.75 mg/kg over 3 to 4 minutes followed by maintenance infusions of 5 to 10 μg/kg/min.

f. Precautions and monitoring effects

(1) Amrinone is unstable in dextrose solutions and should be added to saline solutions instead. Because of fluid balance concerns, this may be a potential problem in patients with CHF.

(2) Because of the peripheral dilating properties, patients should be monitored for hypotension.

(3) Thrombocytopenia and proteinuria have occurred with chronic therapy.

(4) Ventricular rates may increase in patients with atrial flutter or fibrillation.

G. Patient education

1. The patient should be made aware of the importance of taking the digitalis glycoside (and any other medications) exactly as prescribed and should be advised to watch for signs of toxicity (see section V C 5 b).

2. Dietary sodium restrictions should be emphasized.

3. The patient should understand the need for regular checkups and be able to recognize symptoms that require immediate physician notification; for example, an unusually irregular pulse rate, palpitations, shortness of breath, swollen ankles, visual disturbances, or weight gain exceeding 3 to 5 lb in 1 week.

STUDY QUESTIONS

Directions: Each question below contains five suggested answers. Choose the **one best** response to each question.

1. A patient who presents with aortic valve stenosis (stiffness of a valve causing backup of blood) would most likely have a diagnosis of

A. right-sided heart failure
B. left-sided heart failure
C. high-output heart failure
D. high-output, right-sided heart failure
E. low-output, right-sided heart failure

2. Which of the following groups of symptoms is most often associated with a patient who has right-sided heart failure?

A. Nocturia, rales, paroxysmal nocturnal dyspnea
B. Paroxysmal nocturnal dyspnea, pedal edema, jugular venous distension, hepatojugular reflux
C. Jugular venous distension, hepatojugular reflux, pedal edema, shortness of breath
D. Hepatojugular reflux, jugular venous distension, pedal edema, abdominal distension
E. Paroxysmal nocturnal dyspnea, jugular venous distension, abdominal distension, shortness of breath

3. Which of the following combinations of drugs when used together reduce both preload and afterload?

A. Nitroglycerin and isosorbide dinitrate
B. Nitroglycerin and hydralazine
C. Captopril and methyldopa
D. Prazosin and angiotensin II
E. Hydralazine and methyldopa

4. When digitalis glycosides are used in the patient with congestive heart failure, they work by exerting a positive effect on

A. stroke volume
B. total peripheral resistance
C. heart rate
D. blood pressure
E. venous return

Questions 5 and 6

A 60-year-old white hypertensive woman is currently being treated with propranolol, nitroglycerin, nifedipine, aspirin, and dipyridamole. She is admitted with a diagnosis of congestive heart failure (CHF).

5. Which agent is most likely to be discontinued in this patient?

A. Nifedipine
B. Propranolol
C. Aspirin
D. Nitroglycerin
E. Dipyridamole

6. It is later found that the patient has developed CHF as a result of a serious anemia due to aspirin-induced bleeding. What type of heart failure does the patient have?

A. High-output
B. Low-output
C. Left-sided
D. Right-sided
E. Low-output, left-sided

7. Because of direct dilating effects on the lung, certain agents aid in the treatment of congestive heart failure (CHF) patients suffering from pulmonary congestion. Which of the following agents is in this category?

A. Hydrochlorothiazide
B. Triamterene
C. Furosemide
D. Metolazone
E. Spironolactone

8. All of the following have been shown to be effective in the acute management of digitalis toxicity EXCEPT

A. cholestyramine resin
B. lidocaine or phenytoin
C. potassium administration
D. digoxin-specific Fab fragment antibodies
E. sodium administration

9. Which of the following vasodilators is an orally effective preload–afterload reducer in the patient with congestive heart failure (CHF)?

A. Hydralazine
B. Diltiazem
C. Isosorbide dinitrate
D. Prazosin
E. Nitroprusside

10. For treating the patient with congestive heart failure (CHF), which of the following dosages of dopamine is selected for its positive inotropic effects?

A. 2.0 μg/kg/min
B. 5 to 10 μg/kg/min
C. 10 to 20 μg/kg/min
D. 40 μg/kg/min
E. greater than 40 μg/kg/min

11. The use of converting enzyme inhibitors in congestive heart failure (CHF) centers around their ability to cause

A. direct reduction in renin levels with a resultant decrease in angiotensin II and aldosterone levels
B. indirect reduction in angiotensin II and aldosterone levels due to inhibition of the converting enzyme
C. direct reduction in aldosterone secretion and angiotensin I production by inhibiting the converting enzyme
D. increase in afterload due to an indirect decrease in angiotensin II as well as a decrease in preload due to an indirect reduction in aldosterone secretion
E. indirect increase in renin levels, secondary to a secondary hyperaldosteronism

Directions: Each question below contains three suggested answers of which **one or more** is correct. Choose the answer

A if **I only** is correct
B if **III only** is correct
C if **I and II** are correct
D if **II and III** are correct
E if **I, II, and III** are correct

12. Situations that predispose a digitalis-treated patient to toxicity include

I. hypercalcemia
II. hyperkalemia
III. hypermagnesemia

13. Guidelines necessary for monitoring the patient with congestive heart failure (CHF) include which of the following questions?

I. Does the patient have therapeutic blood levels of digoxin in the range of 0.8 to 2.0 ng/ml?
II. Is the patient taking a product that may decrease the effectiveness of therapy (e.g., Alka-Seltzer or baking soda)?
III. Does the patient have signs of digitalis toxicity or a digoxin–drug interaction?

14. Correct statements about dobutamine include which of the following?

I. Doses of 5 to 20 μg/kg/min have been associated with a positive inotropic effect in treating the patient with congestive heart failure (CHF)
II. Patients receiving dobutamine should be monitored for increases in peripheral vascular resistance
III. Dobutamine is considered a nonglycoside, nonsympathomimetic positive inotropic agent

ANSWERS AND EXPLANATIONS

1. The answer is B. (*I D 2 a; Figure 34-1*) The aortic valve is located on the left side of the heart; therefore, stenosis will result in the backup of blood behind the failing valve and, thus, left-sided, low-output failure will result.

2. The answer is D. (*III B 2*) A patient with right-sided heart failure would present with symptoms and signs of peripheral edema, due to the backup of fluid behind the failing right ventricle. The patient's symptoms and signs result from the peripheral accumulation of fluid within the liver, the legs, the abdomen, and the venous system in general. Pulmonary signs (e.g., rales, shortness of breath, paroxysmal nocturnal dyspnea) are more the consequence of the backup of fluid behind the failing left ventricle, characteristically seen in left-sided heart failure.

3. The answer is B. (*V E 5 d–e*) The venous dilating properties of nitroglycerin (preload) in conjunction with the arteriolar dilating effects of hydralazine (afterload) make this combination of agents effective in reducing both preload and afterload.

4. The answer is A. (*V C 1 a*) Digitalis glycosides are used in congestive heart failure as positive inotropic agents to increase stroke volume. By increasing stroke volume, digitalis glycosides increase the cardiac output by increasing the right side of the following equation:

$$\text{Cardiac output} = \text{stroke volume} \times \text{heart rate}$$

5. The answer is B. (*IV A, B; Table 34-2*) Because they produce negative inotropic effects, β-adrenergic receptor blockers, such as propranolol, must be used very cautiously in patients who develop congestive heart failure (CHF). All β-blockers have the potential to reduce cardiac output. The physician must determine whether the benefit of such therapy for a patient with angina, hypertension, arrhythmia, and so forth is worth the risk of inducing heart failure. In many situations, the risk is worth taking; in other situations, it may not be if alternative therapy is available.

6. The answer is A. (*I D 1 b*) In anemia, the lack of oxygen-carrying capacity by the red blood cells puts an added stress on the heart, which must work harder to provide better oxygenation to the metabolizing tissues. Initially, the heart may be able to compensate, either by increasing the heart rate or by increasing stroke volume through cardiac dilation and hypertrophy. However, if the anemia is allowed to continue, the heart is unable to meet the metabolic demands placed on it, resulting in the signs and symptoms of heart failure.

7. The answer is C. (*V D 3*) Furosemide has been shown to possess direct pulmonary dilating effects, which are independent of a diuretic effect and which occur prior to the diuretic effect.

8. The answer is E. (*V C 5 c*) Cholestyramine resin has been used in the acute situation to decrease the absorption of digoxin within the gastrointestinal tract. This results in lower digoxin levels if the resin is administered before all the digoxin has been absorbed. Digoxin-specific antibodies have been shown to be effective in binding free digoxin in the blood and thereby reducing the potential for digoxin toxicity. Potassium administration has been shown to be effective in protecting the myocardium from the toxic effects of digoxin while toxic levels return to normal. Both lidocaine and phenytoin have been shown to be useful in preventing and treating toxic arrhythmias associated with digitalis toxicity.

9. The answer is D. (*V E 5 c*) Prazosin acts as an α-adrenergic blocking agent. The physiologic response seen includes both arteriolar and venous dilation. Prazosin has been shown to produce a balanced dilating effect, making it a useful agent in the ambulatory setting. Unlike hydralazine (which produces afterload reduction), isosorbide dinitrate (producing preload reduction), and nitroprusside (a parenteral agent), prazosin is effective orally in reducing both preload and afterload when used alone.

10. The answer is B. (*V F 1*) Dopamine has shown great versatility in its effects. At doses of 2–5 μg/kg/min, it increases renal blood flow through its dopaminergic effects. At doses of 5–10 μg/kg/min, it increases cardiac output through its β-adrenergic stimulating effect. At doses of 10–20 μg/kg/min, it increases peripheral vascular resistance through its α-adrenergic stimulating effects. There is no specific cutoff for any of these effects, so close titration is required to provide for individual response.

11. The answer is B. [*V E 5 f (2); Figure 34-2*] By directly inhibiting the converting enzyme, production of angiotensin II is reduced, as is angiotensin II-mediated secretion of aldosterone from the adrenal gland.

12. The answer is A (I). (*IV C 4 a–c*) Calcium ions act synergistically with digitalis. Therefore, when hypercalcemia occurs, digitalis exerts an added pharmacologic effect on the heart. This may present itself as toxic arrhythmias, cardiac standstill, and even death. Elevated potassium levels or elevated magnesium levels seem to aid in the prevention of digitalis-induced toxicity. There is building evidence that digitalis preparations need calcium ions in order to work, and consequently low calcium levels may negate the pharmacologic potential of digitalis.

13. The answer is E (all). (*V B 2 c; C 3 b, 5 a–b; G 1–3*) Digitalis has a narrow therapeutic range; serum levels of 0.8 to 2.0 ng/ml provide a therapeutic response with minimal toxicity. Monitoring serum digoxin levels is especially helpful during initial dosage titrations and when questions arise as to compliance, absorption, or a drug–drug interaction. Patients with congestive heart failure (CHF) must be informed of the need to take their medication appropriately and accurately so that blood levels for all drugs will be within the therapeutic range. Patients must also be told to inform their pharmacist of any additional drugs they are taking since these could aggravate the disease or interact with digoxin or with other drugs. Patients should also be monitored for those symptoms related to CHF that effective therapy should prevent. Reporting symptoms such as swollen legs or shortness of breath will enable the physician to add different drugs or increase the dosage of current medications.

14. The answer is A (I). (*V F 2 a*) Dobutamine in doses of 5 to 20 μg/kg/min is an inotropic agent that is useful in the treatment of congestive heart failure (CHF). Dobutamine does not have the versatility that dopamine offers, lacking comparable effects on renal blood flow or peripheral vascular resistance. Rather, dobutamine has a peripheral dilating effect that offers a benefit to patients who have reduced cardiac output due to elevated peripheral resistance.

35 Infectious Diseases

Paul F. Souney
Cheryl A. Stoukides

I. GENERAL PRINCIPLES OF ANTI-INFECTIVE THERAPY

A. Definition. Anti-infective agents treat infection by suppressing or destroying the causative microorganisms—bacteria, mycobacteria, fungi, protozoa, or viruses. Anti-infective agents derived from natural substances are called **antibiotics**; those produced from synthetic substances are called **antimicrobials**. (However, these two terms are now used interchangeably.)

B. Indications for anti-infective therapy. Anti-infective agents should be used only when:

1. A significant infection has been diagnosed or is strongly suspected
2. An established indication for prophylactic therapy exists

C. Gram stain, microbiologic culturing, and susceptibility tests. These tests should be performed before anti-infective therapy is initiated. Test materials must be obtained by a method that avoids contamination of the specimen by the patient's own flora.

1. **Gram stain**. Performed on all specimens except blood cultures, the Gram stain helps to immediately identify the cause of infection. By determining if the causative agent is gram-positive or gram-negative, the test allows a better choice of drug therapy, especially when an anti-infective regimen must begin without delay.
   a. **Gram-positive** microorganisms stain **blue** or **purple**.
   b. **Gram-negative** microorganisms stain **red** or **rose–pink**.
   c. The Gram stain also identifies many **fungi**.

2. **Microbiologic cultures**. To identify the specific causative agent, specimens of body fluids or infected tissue are collected for analysis.

3. **Susceptibility tests**. Different strains of the same pathogenic species may have widely varying susceptibility to a particular anti-infective agent. Susceptibility tests help determine microbial susceptibility to a given drug and thus can be used to predict whether the drug will effectively combat the infection.
   a. In the **microdilution method** of susceptibility testing, the drug is diluted serially in various media containing the test microorganism.
      (1) The lowest drug concentration that prevents microbial growth after 18 to 24 hours of incubation is called the **minimum inhibitory concentration (MIC)**.
      (2) The lowest drug concentration that reduces bacterial density by 99.9% is called the **minimum bactericidal concentration (MBC)**.
   b. The **Kirby-Bauer disk diffusion technique** (cheaper but less reliable than the microdilution method) provides qualitative susceptibility information.
      (1) Filter paper disks impregnated with specific drug quantities are placed on the surface of agar plates streaked with a microorganism culture. After 18 hours, the size of a clear inhibition zone is determined; drug activity against the test strain is then correlated to zone size.
      (2) The Kirby-Bauer technique does not reliably predict therapeutic effectiveness against certain microorganisms (e.g., *Staphylococcus aureus* and *Shigella*).

D. Choice of agent. An anti-infective agent should be chosen on the basis of its pharmacologic properties and spectrum of activity as well as on various host (patient) factors.

1. **Pharmacologic properties**. These include the drug's ability to reach the infection site and to attain a desired level in the target tissue.

2. **Spectrum of activity**. To treat an infectious disease effectively, an anti-infective drug must be active against the causative pathogen. Susceptibility testing or clinical experience in treating a given syndrome may suggest that a particular drug will be effective.

3. **Patient factors**. Selection of an anti-infective drug regimen must take various patient factors into account. Such factors help determine which type of drug should be administered, the correct drug dosage and administration route, and the potential for adverse drug effects.
   a. **Immunologic status**. A patient with **impaired immune mechanisms** may require a drug that rapidly destroys pathogens (i.e., a **bactericidal** agent) rather than one that merely suppresses a pathogen's growth or reproduction (i.e., a **bacteriostatic** agent).
   b. **Presence of a foreign body**. The effectiveness of anti-infective therapy is reduced in patients who have prosthetic joints or valves, cardiac pacemakers, and various internal shunts.
   c. **Age**. A drug's pharmacokinetic properties may vary widely in patients of different ages. In very young and very old patients, drug metabolism and excretion commonly decrease. Elderly patients also have an increased risk of suffering ototoxicity when receiving certain antibiotics.
   d. **Underlying disease**
      (1) Preexisting **kidney or liver disease** increases the risk of nephrotoxicity or hepatotoxicity during the administration of some antibacterial drugs.
      (2) Patients with **central nervous system (CNS) disorders** may suffer neurotoxicity (motor seizures) during penicillin therapy.
      (3) Patients with **neuromuscular disorders** (e.g., myasthenia gravis) are at increased risk for developing neuromuscular blockade during aminoglycoside or polymyxin B therapy.
   e. **History of drug allergy or adverse drug reactions**. Patients who have had previous allergic or other untoward reactions to a particular antibiotic have a higher risk of experiencing the same reaction during subsequent administration of that drug. Except in life-threatening situations, patients who have had serious allergic reactions to penicillin, for example, should not receive the drug again.
   f. **Pregnancy and lactation**. Because drug therapy during pregnancy and lactation can cause unwanted effects, the mother's need for the antibiotic must be weighed against the drug's potential harm.
      (1) Pregnancy can increase the risk of adverse drug effects—for both mother and fetus. Also, plasma drug concentrations tend to decrease in pregnant women, reducing a drug's therapeutic effectiveness.
      (2) Most drugs, including antibiotics, appear in the breast milk of nursing mothers and may cause adverse effects in infants. For example, sulfonamides may lead to toxic bilirubin accumulation in a newborn's brain.
   g. **Genetic traits.** Sulfonamides may cause hemolytic anemia in patients with glucose-6-phosphate deficiency (G6PD); patients who rapidly metabolize drugs (rapid acetylators) may develop hepatitis when receiving the antitubercular drug isoniazid.

E. **Empiric therapy**. In serious or life-threatening disease, anti-infective therapy must begin before the infecting organism has been identified. In this case, the choice of drug (or drugs) is based on clinical experience suggesting that a particular agent will be effective in a given setting.

1. A **broad-spectrum** antibiotic usually is the most appropriate choice until the specific organism has been determined.

2. In all cases, culture specimens must be obtained **before therapy begins.**

F. **Multiple antibiotic therapy**. A combination of drugs should be given only when clinical experience has shown such therapy to be more effective than single-agent therapy in a particular setting. A multiple-agent regimen can increase the risk of toxic drug effects and, in a few cases, may result in drug antagonism and subsequent therapeutic ineffectiveness. Indications for multiple-agent therapy include:

1. **Need for increased antibiotic effectiveness**. The **synergistic** (intensified) effect of two or more agents may allow a dosage reduction or a faster or enhanced drug effect.

2. **Treatment of an infection caused by multiple pathogens** (e.g., intra-abdominal infection)

3. **Prevention of proliferation of drug-resistant organisms** (e.g., during treatment of tuberculosis)

G. **Duration of anti-infective therapy**. To achieve the therapeutic goal, anti-infective therapy must continue for a sufficient duration.

1. Treatment for an **acute uncomplicated infection** generally should continue until the patient has been afebrile and asymptomatic for at least 72 hours.

2. Treatment of a **chronic infection** (e.g., endocarditis, osteomyelitis) may require a longer duration (4 to 6 weeks), with follow-up culture analyses to assess therapeutic effectiveness.

H. **Monitoring therapeutic effectiveness**. To assess the patient's response to anti-infective therapy, appropriate specimens should be cultured and the following parameters monitored.

1. **Fever curve**. An important assessment tool, the fever curve may be a reliable indication of response to therapy. Defervescence usually indicates favorable response.

2. **White blood cell (WBC) count**. In the initial stage of infection, the neutrophil count from a peripheral blood smear may rise above normal (neutrophilia) and immature neutrophil forms (''bands'') may appear (''left shift''). In patients who are elderly, debilitated, or suffering overwhelming infection, the WBC count may be normal or subnormal.

3. **Radiographic findings**. Small effusions, abscesses, or cavities may appear on x-ray and indicate focus of infection.

4. **Pain and inflammation** (as evidenced by swelling, erythema, and tenderness) may occur when the infection is superficial or within a joint or bone, also indicating possible focus of infection.

I. **Lack of therapeutic effectiveness**. When an antibiotic drug regimen fails, other drugs should not be added indiscriminately or the regimen otherwise changed. Instead, the situation should be reassessed and diagnostic efforts intensified. Causes of therapeutic ineffectiveness include:

1. **Misdiagnosis**. The isolated organism may have been misidentified by the laboratory or may not be the causative agent for infection (e.g., the patient may have an unsuspected infection).

2. **Improper drug regimen**. The drug dosage, administration route, dosing frequency, or duration of therapy may be inadequate or inappropriate.

3. **Inappropriate choice of antibiotic agent**. As discussed in section I D, patient factors and the pharmacologic properties and spectrum of activity of a given drug must be considered when planning anti-infective drug therapy.

4. **Microbial resistance**. By acquiring resistance to a specific antibiotic, microorganisms can survive in the drug's presence. Many gonococcal strains, for instance, now resist penicillin. Drug resistance is especially common in geographic areas where a particular drug has been used excessively (and perhaps improperly).

5. **Unrealistic expectations**. Antibiotics are ineffective in certain circumstances.
   a. Patients with conditions that require **surgical drainage** frequently cannot be cured by anti-infective drugs until the drainage has been removed. For example, the presence of necrotic tissue or pus in patients with pneumonia, empyema, or renal calculi is a common cause of antibiotic failure.
   b. **Fever** should not be treated with anti-infective drugs unless infection has been identified as the cause. Although fever frequently signifies infection, it sometimes stems from noninfectious conditions (e.g., drug reactions, phlebitis, neoplasms, metabolic disorders, arthritis). These conditions will not respond to antibiotics.

6. **Infection by two or more types of microorganisms**. If not detected initially, an additional cause of infection may lead to therapeutic failure.

II. ANTIBACTERIAL AGENTS

A. **Definition and classification**. Used to treat infections caused by **bacteria**, antibacterial agents fall into several major categories: **aminoglycosides, cephalosporins, erythromycins, penicillins** (including various subgroups), **tetracyclines, sulfonamides, urinary tract antiseptics,** and **miscellaneous antibacterials** (Table 35-1).

B. **Aminoglycosides**. These drugs, containing amino sugars, are used primarily in infections caused by gram-negative enterobacteria and in suspected sepsis. They have little activity against anaerobic and facultative organisms. The toxic potential of these drugs limits their use. Major aminoglycosides include **amikacin, kanamycin, gentamicin, neomycin, netilmicin, streptomycin**, and **tobramycin**.

Table 35-1. Some Important Parameters of Anti-Infective Drugs

Agent	Elimination Route	Half-Life	Administration Route	Common Dosage Range (Adults)
Aminoglycosides				
Amikacin	Renal	2–3 hours	IV, IM	15 mg/kg/day
Gentamicin	Renal	2 hours	IV, IM	3 mg/kg/day
Neomycin	Renal	2–3 hours	Oral, topical	50–100 mg/kg/day (oral); 10–15 mg/day (topical)
Netilmicin	Renal	2.7 hours	IV, IM	3–6 mg/kg/day
Streptomycin	Renal	2–3 hours	IM	15 mg/kg/day*
Tobramycin	Renal	2–5 hours	IV, IM	3–5 mg/kg/day
Cephalosporins				
First-generation				
Cefadroxil	Renal	1.5 hours	Oral	1–2 g/day
Cefazolin	Renal	1.4–2.2 hours	IV	250 mg–1 g q 8 hours
Cephalexin	Renal	0.9–1.3 hours	Oral	250–500 mg q 6 hours
Cephalothin	Renal (H)	0.5–0.9 hours	IV, IM	500 mg–2 g q 4–6 hours
Cephapirin	Renal (H)	0.6–0.8 hours	IV, IM	500 mg–2 g q 4–6 hours
Cephradine	Renal	1.3 hours	Oral, IV	250–500 mg q 6 hours
Second-generation				
Cefaclor	Renal (H)	0.8 hours	Oral	250–500 mg q 8 hours
Cefamandole	Renal	1 hour	IV	500 mg–1 g q 4–8 hours
Cefonicid	Renal	4 hours	IV	1–2 g/day
Ceforanide	Renal	2.2–3 hours	IV	0.5 mg–1 g q 12 hours
Cefoxitin	Renal	0.8 hours	IV	1–2 g q 6–8 hours
Cefuroxime	Renal	1.5–2.2 hours	IV, IM	750 mg–1.5 g q 8 hours
Third-generation				
Cefoperazone	Hepatic	1.6–2.4 hours	IV	2–4 g q 12 hours
Cefotaxime	Renal (H)	1.5 hours	IV	1–2 g q 6–8 hours
Cefotetan	Renal	4.2 hours	IV, IM	1–2 g q 12 hours
Ceftazidime	Renal	1.8 hours	IV, IM	1–2 g q 8–12 hours
Ceftizoxime	Renal	1.7 hours	IV	1–2 g q 8–12 hours
Ceftriaxone	Renal	8 hours	IV, IM	1–2 g/day
Moxalactam	Renal	2.2 hours	IV, IM	2–4 g q 8–12 hours
Erythromycins				
Erythromycin base, estolate, ethylsuccinate, and stearate	Hepatic	1.2–2.6 hours	Oral	250–500 mg q 6 hours
Erythromycin gluceptate and lactobionate	Hepatic	1.2–2.6 hours	IV	0.5–2 g q 6 hours
Natural penicillins				
Penicillin G	Renal (H)	0.5 hours	Oral, IV, IM	200,000–500,000 units q 6–8 hours
Penicillin V	Renal	1 hour	Oral	500 mg–2 g/day
Penicillin G procaine	Renal	24–60 hours	IM	300,000–600,000 units/day
Penicillin G benzathine	Renal	24–60 hours	IM	300,000–600,000 units/day
Penicillinase-resistant penicillins				
Cloxacillin	Renal (H)	0.5 hours	Oral	250–500 mg q 6 hours
Dicloxacillin	Renal (H)	0.5–0.9 hours	Oral	500 mg–1 g/day
Methicillin	Renal (H)	0.5–1 hour	IV, IM	1–2 g q 4–6 hours
Nafcillin	Hepatic (R)	0.5 hours	Oral, IV, IM	0.25–2 g q 6 hours
Oxacillin	Renal (H)	0.5 hours	Oral, IV, IM	500 mg–2 g q 4–6 hours
Aminopenicillins				
Amoxicillin	Renal (H)	0.9–2.3 hours	Oral	250–500 mg q 8 hours
Ampicillin	Renal (H)	0.8–1.5 hours	Oral, IV, IM	250 mg–2 g q 4–6 hours

Continued on next page

Table 35-1. Continued

Agent	Elimination Route	Half-Life	Administration Route	Common Dosage Range (Adults)
Bacampicillin	Renal	1 hour	Oral	400–800 mg q 12 hours
Cyclacillin	Renal (H)	0.5 hours	Oral	250–500 mg q 6 hours
Extended-spectrum penicillins				
Azlocillin	Renal (H)	0.8–1.5 hours	IV	100–300 mg/kg/day
Carbenicillin	Renal (H)	1.5 hours	IM, IV	1–5 g q 4–6 hours
Carbenicillin indanyl	Renal (H)	1.5 hours	Oral	382–764 mg q.i.d.
Mezlocillin	Renal (H)	0.6–1.2 hours	IV, IM	1–3 g q 4–6 hours
Piperacillin	Renal (H)	0.8–1.4 hours	IV, IM	1–1.5 mg/kg q 6–12 hours
Ticarcillin	Renal	0.9–1.5 hours	IV, IM	1–3 g q 4–6 hours
Sulfonamides				
Sulfadiazine	Renal (H)	6 hours	Oral, IV	2–4 g/day
Sulfamethoxazole	Hepatic (R)	9–11 hours	Oral	1–3 g/day
Sulfisoxazole	Renal (H)	3–7 hours	Oral, IV	2–8 g/day
Tetracyclines				
Demeclocycline	Renal	10–17 hours	Oral	300 mg–1 g/day
Doxycycline	Hepatic	14–25 hours	Oral, IV	100–200 mg q 12 hours
Methacycline	Renal	16 hours	Oral	150 mg q 6 hours to 300 mg q 12 hours
Minocycline	Hepatic	12–15 hours	Oral, IV	100–200 mg q 12 hours
Tetracycline	Renal	6–12 hours	Oral, IV, IM	1–2 g/day
Urinary tract antiseptics				
Methenamine hippurate and mandelate	Renal		Oral	0.5–2 g q.i.d.
Nalidixic acid	Renal	8 hours	Oral	4 g/day
Nitrofurantoin	Renal	0.3–1 hour	Oral	5–7 mg/kg/day
Norfloxacin	Hepatic	3–4 hours	Oral	400 b.i.d.
Miscellaneous anti-infectives				
Aztreonam	Renal	1.7 hours	IV, IM	500 mg–2 g q 8–12 hours
Chloramphenicol	Hepatic	1.5–4.1 hours	Oral, IV	50–100 mg/kg/day
Ciprofloxacin	Hepatic (R)	3–5 hours	Oral	250–750 mg q 12 hours
Clindamycin	Hepatic	2–4 hours	Oral, IM, IV	300–900 mg q 6–8 hours
Dapsone	Hepatic (R)	28 hours	Oral	50–100 mg/day
Imipenem	Renal	1 hour	IV	250 mg–1 g q 6 hours
Spectinomycin	Renal	1.2–2.8 hours	IM	2–4 g (single dose)
Trimethoprim	Renal (H)	8–15 hours	Oral	100–200 mg/day
Vancomycin	Renal	6–8 hours	Oral, IV	500 mg q 6 hours
Antifungal agents				
Amphotericin B	Unknown	24 hours	IV	1–1.5 mg/kg/day
Flucytosine	Renal	3–6 hours	Oral	50–150 mg/kg/day
Griseofulvin	Hepatic (R)	9–24 hours	Oral	300–375 mg/day
Ketoconazole	Hepatic	1.5–3.3 hours	Oral	200–400 mg/day
Miconazole	Hepatic	20–24 hours	IV	600 mg–3 g/day
Nystatin	Fecal	Unknown	Oral	500,000–1,000,000 units t.i.d.
Antiprotozoal agents				
Chloroquine				
hydrochloride	Renal	3 days	IM	160–200 mg/day†
phosphate			Oral	500 mg–1 g/day
Diloxanide furoate	Renal		Oral	500 mg t.i.d.
Emetine	Renal	4–7 days	SC, IM	1 mg/kg/day to 60 mg/day maximum

Continued on next page

Table 35-1. Continued

Agent	Elimination Route	Half-Life	Administration Route	Common Dosage Range (Adults)
Metronidazole	Hepatic (R)	6–14 hours	Oral	250–500 q 6–8 hours
Primaquine phosphate	Renal	3–6 hours	Oral	15 mg (base)/day
Pyrimethamine	Renal	4 days	Oral	25 mg/week
Quinacrine	Unknown	5 days	Oral	100 mg/day
Quinine sulfate	Renal	12 hours	Oral	650 q 8 hours‡
Antitubercular agents				
Aminosalicylic acid	Renal	1 hour	Oral	10–12 g/day
Capreomycin	Renal	4–6 hours	IM	15 mg/kg/day to 1 g/day maximum
Cycloserine	Renal	10 hours	Oral	500 mg/day to 1 g/day maximum
Ethambutol	Hepatic	3.3 hours	Oral	15 mg/kg/day
Ethionamide	Hepatic	3 hours	Oral	500 mg/day to 1 g/day
Isoniazid	Hepatic	1–4 hours	Oral, IM	5 mg/kg/day to 300 mg/ day maximum
Pyrazinamide	Hepatic	9–10 hours	Oral	20–35 mg/kg/day to 3 g/day maximum
Rifampin	Hepatic	3 hours	Oral	600 mg/day
Antiviral agents				
Acyclovir	Renal	2.1–3.8 hours	Oral, IV, topical	200 mg q 4 hours (oral); 5 mg/kg q 8 hours (IV)
Amantadine	Renal	12 hours	Oral	100–200 mg/day
Ribavirin	Renal	9.5 hours	Aerosol	6 g q 24 hours
Vidarabine	Renal (H)	1.5 hours	IV, topical	15 mg/kg/day
Zidovudine	Renal (H)	1 hour	Oral	200 mg q 4 hours

(H) = secondary hepatic elimination.
IM = intramuscular.
IV = intravenous.
(R) = secondary renal elimination.
SC = subcutaneous.
*Dosage applies to infections other than tuberculosis; for tuberculosis, dosage is 1 g/day.
†For short-term therapy.
‡For initial therapy.

1. **Mechanism of action**. Aminoglycosides are **bactericidal**; they inhibit bacterial protein synthesis by binding to and impeding the function the 30S ribosomal subunit. (Some aminoglycosides also bind to the 50S ribosomal subunit.) Their mechanism of action is not fully known.

2. **Spectrum of activity**
   a. **Streptomycin** is active against both gram-positive and gram-negative bacteria. However, widespread resistance to this drug has restricted its use to the organisms that cause plague and tularemia; gram-positive streptococci (given in combination with penicillin); and *Mycobacterium tuberculosis* (given in combination with other antitubercular agents, as described in section V C).
   b. **Amikacin, kanamycin, gentamicin, tobramycin, neomycin,** and **netilmicin** are active against many gram-negative bacteria (e.g., *Proteus*, *Serratia*, and *Pseudomonas* organisms).
      (1) **Gentamicin** is active against some *Staphylococcus* strains; it is more active than tobramycin against *Serratia* organisms.
      (2) **Amikacin** is the broadest-spectrum aminoglycoside, with activity against most aerobic gram-negative bacilli as well as many anaerobic gram-negative bacterial strains that resist gentamicin and tobramycin. It is also active against *M. tuberculosis*.
      (3) Compared to gentamicin, **tobramycin** may be more active against *Pseudomonas aeruginosa*.
      (4) **Netilmicin** may be active against gentamicin-resistant organisms; it appears to be less ototoxic than other aminoglycosides.
      (5) In addition to its activity against such gram-negative organisms as *Escherichia coli* and

Klebsiella pneumoniae, **neomycin** is active against several gram-positive organisms (e.g., *S. aureus, M. tuberculosis*). *P. aeruginosa* and most streptococci are now neomycin-resistant.

3. Therapeutic uses

a. Streptomycin is used to treat plague, tularemia, acute brucellosis (given in combination with tetracycline), bacterial endocarditis caused by *Streptococcus viridans* (given in combination with penicillin), and tuberculosis (given in combination with other antitubercular agents, as described in section V C 2).

b. Gentamicin, tobramycin, amikacin, and **netilmicin** are therapeutic for serious gram-negative bacillary infections (e.g., those caused by *Enterobacter, Serratia, Klebsiella,* and *P. aeruginosa*); pneumonia (given in combination with a cephalosporin or penicillin); meningitis; complicated urinary tract infections; osteomyelitis; bacteremia; and peritonitis.

c. Neomycin is used for preoperative bowel sterilization; hepatic coma (as adjunctive therapy); and, in topical form, for skin and mucous membrane infections (e.g., burns).

4. Precautions and monitoring parameters. Aminoglycosides can cause serious adverse effects. To prevent or minimize such problems, blood drug concentrations and blood urea nitrogen (BUN) and serum creatinine levels should be monitored during therapy.

a. Ototoxicity. Aminoglycosides can cause vestibular or auditory damage.

(1) Gentamicin and streptomycin cause primarily **vestibular** damage (manifested by tinnitus, vertigo, and ataxia). Such damage may be bilateral and irreversible.

(2) Amikacin, kanamycin, and neomycin cause mainly **auditory** damage (hearing loss).

(3) Tobramycin can result in both vestibular and auditory damage.

b. Nephrotoxicity. Because aminoglycosides accumulate in the proximal tubule, mild renal dysfunction develops in up to 25% of patients receiving these drugs for several days or more. Usually, this adverse effect is reversible.

(1) Neomycin is the most nephrotoxic aminoglycoside; streptomycin, the least nephrotoxic. Gentamicin and tobramycin are nephrotoxic to about the same degree.

(2) Risk factors for increased nephrotoxic effects include:

(a) Preexisting renal disease

(b) Previous or prolonged aminoglycoside therapy

(c) Concurrent administration of another nephrotoxic drug

(3) Trough levels above 2 μg/ml for gentamicin and tobramycin and above 10 μg/ml for amikacin are associated with nephrotoxicity.

c. Neuromuscular blockade. This problem may arise in patients receiving high-dose aminoglycoside therapy.

(1) Risk factors for neuromuscular blockade include:

(a) Concurrent administration of a neuromuscular blocking agent or an anesthetic

(b) Preexisting hypocalcemia or myasthenia gravis

(c) Intraperitoneal or rapid intravenous (IV) drug administration

(2) Apnea and respiratory depression may be reversed with administration of calcium or an anticholinesterase.

d. Hypersensitivity and local reactions are rare adverse effects of aminoglycosides.

e. Therapeutic levels

(1) Gentamicin and tobramycin peak at 6 to 10 μg/ml. Their trough level is 0.5 to 1.5 μg/ml.

(2) Amikacin peaks at 25 to 30 μg/ml. The trough level is 5 to 8 μg/ml.

5. Drug interactions

a. IV loop diuretics can result in increased ototoxicity.

b. Other aminoglycosides, cephalothin, cisplatin, amphotericin B, and **methoxyflurane** can cause increased nephrotoxicity when given concurrently with streptomycin.

C. Cephalosporins. These agents are known as **β-lactam antibiotics** because their chemical structure consists of a β-lactam ring adjoined to a thiazolidine ring. Cephalosporins generally are classified in three major groups based mainly on their spectrum of activity (Table 35-2).

1. Mechanism of action. Cephalosporins are **bactericidal**; they inhibit bacterial cell wall synthesis, reducing cell wall stability and thus causing membrane lysis.

2. Spectrum of activity

a. First-generation cephalosporins are active against most gram-positive cocci (except enterococci) as well as enteric aerobic gram-negative bacilli (*E. coli, K. pneumoniae*, and *Proteus mirabilis*).

b. Second-generation cephalosporins are active against the organisms covered by first-generation cephalosporins and have extended gram-negative coverage (including β-lactamase-producing strains of *Hemophilus influenzae*).

Table 35-2. Classification of Cephalosporins

First-Generation Cephalosporins	Second-Generation Cephalosporins	Third-Generation Cephalosporins
Cefadroxil* (Duricef, Ultracef)	Cefaclor* (Ceclor)	Cefoperazone (Cefobid)
Cefazolin (Ancef, Kefzol)	Cefamandole (Mandol)	Cefotaxime (Claforan)
Cephalexin* (Keflex)	Cefonicid (Monocid)	Cefotetan (Cefotan)
Cephalothin (Keflin)	Ceforanide (Precef)	Ceftazidime (Fortaz, Tazicef, Tazidime)
Cephapirin (Cefadyl)	Cefoxitin (Mefoxin)	Ceftizoxime (Cefizox)
Cephradine* (Anspor, Velosef)	Cefuroxime (Zinacef)	Ceftriaxone (Rocephin)
	Cefuroxime axetil* (Ceftin)	Moxalactam (Moxam)

*Oral agents.

c. **Third-generation cephalosporins** have wider activity against most gram-negative bacteria; for example, *Enterobacter, Citrobacter, Serratia, Providencia, Neisseria,* and *Hemophilus* organisms (including β-lactamase-producing strains).

d. Each generation of cephalosporin has shifted toward increased gram-negative activity but has lost activity toward gram-positive organisms.

3. Therapeutic uses

a. **First-generation cephalosporins** commonly are administered to treat serious *Klebsiella* infections and gram-positive and some gram-negative infections in patients with mild penicillin allergy. They also are used widely in perioperative prophylaxis. For most other indications, they are not the preferred drugs.

b. **Second-generation cephalosporins** are valuable in the treatment of urinary tract infections resulting from *E. coli* organisms and gonococcal disease caused by organisms that resist other agents.

(1) **Cefaclor** is useful in otitis media and sinusitis in patients who are allergic to ampicillin and amoxicillin.

(2) **Cefoxitin** is therapeutic for mixed aerobic–anaerobic infections, such as intra-abdominal infection.

(3) **Cefamandole** and **cefuroxime** are commonly administered for community-acquired pneumonia.

c. **Third-generation cephalosporins** penetrate the cerebrospinal fluid (CSF) and thus are valuable in the treatment of meningitis caused by such organisms as meningococci, pneumococci, *H. influenzae*, and enteric gram-negative bacilli.

(1) These agents also are used to treat sepsis of unknown origin in immunosuppressed patients and to treat fever in neutropenic immunosuppressed patients (given in combination with an aminoglycoside).

(2) Third-generation cephalosporins are useful in infections caused by many organisms resistant to older cephalosporins.

(3) These agents frequently are administered as empiric therapy for life-threatening infection in which resistant organisms are the most likely cause.

(4) Initial therapy of mixed bacterial infections (e.g., sepsis) commonly involves third-generation cephalosporins.

4. Precautions and monitoring parameters

a. Because all cephalosporins (except cefoperazone) are eliminated renally, doses must be adjusted for patients with renal impairment.

b. Cross-sensitivity with penicillin has been reported in up to 10% of patients receiving cephalosporins. More recent information indicates that true cross-reactivity is rare.

c. Cephalosporins can cause hypersensitivity reactions similar to those resulting from penicillin (see section II E 7 a). Manifestations include fever, maculopapular rash, anaphylaxis, and hemolytic anemia.
d. Other adverse effects include nausea; vomiting; diarrhea; superinfection; nephrotoxicity; with cefoperazone, moxalactam, and cefamandole, bleeding diastheses may occur. Bleeding can be reversed by vitamin K administration.
e. Cephalosporins may cause false-positive glycosuria results on tests using the copper-reduction method.

5. **Drug interactions**
a. **Probenicid** may impair the excretion of cephalosporins (except ceftazidime and moxalactam), causing increased cephalosporin levels and possible toxicity.
b. **Alcohol consumption** may result in a disulfiram-type reaction in patients receiving moxalactam, cefoperazone, and cefamandole.
c. **Aminoglycosides** may cause additive toxicity when administered with cephalothin.

D. **Erythromycins**. The chemical structure of these macrolide antibiotics is characterized by a lactone ring to which sugars are attached. **Erythromycin base** and the **estolate, ethylsuccinate**, and **stearate salts** are given orally; **erythromycin lactobionate** and **gluceptate** are given parenterally.

1. **Mechanism of action**. Erythromycins may be **bactericidal** or **bacteriostatic**; they bind to the 50S ribosomal subunit, inhibiting bacterial protein synthesis.

2. **Spectrum of activity**. Erythromycins are active against many gram-positive organisms, including streptococci (e.g., *Streptococcus pneumoniae*), and *Corynebacterium* and *Neisseria* species as well as some strains of *Mycoplasma*, *Legionella*, *Treponema*, and *Bordetella*. Some *S. aureus* strains that resist penicillin G are susceptible to erythromycins.

3. **Therapeutic uses**
a. Erythromycins are the preferred drugs for the treatment of *Mycoplasma pneumoniae* and *Campylobacter* infections, legionnaires' disease, chlamydial infections, diphtheria, and pertussis.
b. In patients with penicillin allergy, erythromycins are important alternatives in the treatment of pneumococcal pneumonia, *S. aureus* infections, syphilis, and gonorrhea.
c. Erythromycins may be given prophylactically before dental procedures to prevent bacterial endocarditis.

4. **Precautions and monitoring parameters**
a. Serious adverse effects from erythromycins are rare.
b. Gastrointestinal distress (nausea, vomiting, diarrhea, epigastric discomfort) may occur with oral erythromycin forms.
c. Allergic reactions (rare) may present as skin eruptions, fever, and eosinophilia.
d. Cholestatic hepatitis may arise in patients treated for 1 week or longer with erythromycin estolate; symptoms usually disappear within a few days after drug therapy ends. There have been infrequent reports of hepatotoxicity with other salts of erythromycin.
e. Intramuscular injections of over 100 mg produce severe pain persisting for hours.
f. Transient hearing impairment may develop with high-dose erythromycin therapy.

5. **Drug interactions**
a. Erythromycin inhibits the hepatic metabolism of **theophylline**, resulting in toxic accumulation.
b. Erythromycin interferes with the metabolism of **digoxin**, **corticosteroids**, **carbamazepine**, **cyclosporin**, and **lovastatin**, possibly potentiating the effect and toxicity of these drugs.

E. **Natural penicillins**. Like cephalosporins and all other penicillins, natural penicillins are β-lactam antibiotics. Among the most important antibiotics, natural penicillins are the preferred drugs in the treatment of many infectious diseases.

1. **Penicillin G** sodium and potassium salts can be administered orally, intravenously, or intramuscularly.

2. **Penicillin V**, a soluble drug form, is administered orally.

3. **Penicillin G procaine** and **penicillin G benzathine** are repository drug forms. Administered intramuscularly, these insoluble salts allow slow drug absorption from the injection site and thus have a longer duration of action (12 to 24 hours).

4. **Mechanism of action**. Penicillins are **bactericidal**; they inhibit bacterial cell wall synthesis in a manner similar to that of the cephalosporins.

5. Spectrum of activity

a. Natural penicillins are highly active against gram-positive cocci and against some gram-negative cocci.

b. Penicillin G is five to ten times more active than penicillin V against gram-negative organisms and some anaerobic organisms.

c. Because natural penicillins are readily hydrolyzed by penicillinases (β-lactamases), they are ineffective against *S. aureus* and other organisms that resist penicillin.

6. Therapeutic uses

a. Penicillin G is the preferred agent for all infections caused by *Streptococcus pneumoniae* organisms, including:

(1) Pneumonia
(2) Arthritis
(3) Meningitis
(4) Peritonitis
(5) Pericarditis
(6) Osteomyelitis
(7) Mastoiditis

b. Penicillins G and V are highly effective against other streptococcal infections, such as pharyngitis, otitis media, sinusitus, and bacteremia.

c. Penicillin G is the preferred agent in gonococcal infections, syphilis, anthrax, actinomycosis, gas gangrene, and *Listeria* infections.

d. Administered when an oral penicillin is needed, penicillin V is most useful in skin and soft-tissue infections and mild respiratory infections.

e. Penicillin G procaine is effective against syphilis and uncomplicated gonorrhea.

f. Used to treat syphilis infections outside the CNS, penicillin G benzathine also is effective against group A β-hemolytic streptococcal infections.

g. Penicillins G and V may be used prophylactically to prevent streptococcal infection, rheumatic fever, and neonatal gonorrhea ophthalmia. Patients with valvular heart disease may receive these drugs preoperatively.

7. Precautions and monitoring parameters

a. Hypersensitivity reactions. These occur in up to 10% of patients receiving penicillin. Manifestations range from mild rash to anaphylaxis.

(1) The rash may be urticarial, vesicular, bullous, scarlatiniform, or maculopapular. Rarely, thrombopenic purpura develops.

(2) Anaphylaxis is a life-threatening reaction that most commonly occurs with parenteral administration. Signs and symptoms include severe hypotension, bronchoconstriction, nausea, vomiting, abdominal pain, and extreme weakness.

(3) Other manifestations of hypersensitivity reactions include fever, eosinophilia, angioedema, and serum sickness.

(4) Before penicillin therapy begins, the patient's history should be evaluated for reactions to penicillin. A positive history places the patient at heightened risk for a subsequent reaction. In most cases, such patients should receive a substitute antibiotic. (However, hypersensitivity reactions may occur even in patients with a negative history.)

b. Other adverse effects of natural penicillins include gastrointestinal distress (nausea, diarrhea); bone marrow suppression (impaired platelet aggregation, agranulocytosis); and superinfection. With high-dose therapy, seizures may occur, especially in patients with renal impairment.

8. Drug interactions

a. Probenicid increases blood levels of natural penicillins and may be given concurrently for this purpose.

b. Antibiotic antagonism occurs when **erythromycins, tetracyclines**, or **chloramphenicol** is given within 1 hour of the administration of penicillin. The clinical significance of such antagonism is not clear.

c. With penicillin G procaine and benzathine, precaution must be used in patients with a history of hypersensitivity reactions to penicillins since prolonged reactions may occur. Intravascular injection should be avoided. Procaine hypersensitivity is a contraindication to use of procaine penicillin G.

d. Parenteral products contain either potassium (1.7 mEq/million units) or sodium (2 mEq/million units).

F. Penicillinase-resistant penicillins. These penicillins are not hydrolyzed by staphylococcal penicillinases (β-lactamases). These agents include **methicillin, nafcillin**, and the **isoxazolyl penicillins—cloxacillin, dicloxacillin**, and **oxacillin**.

1. **Mechanism of action** (see section II E 4)

2. **Spectrum of activity**. Because these penicillins resist penicillinases, they are active against staphylococci that produce these enzymes.

3. **Therapeutic uses**
   a. Penicillinase-resistant penicillins are used solely in staphylococcal infections resulting from organisms that resist natural penicillins.
   b. They are less potent than natural penicillins against organisms susceptible to natural penicillins and thus make poor substitutes in treatment of infections caused by these organisms.
   c. **Nafcillin** is excreted by the liver and thus may be useful in treating staphylococcal infections in patients with renal impairment.
   d. **Oxacillin, cloxacillin**, and **dicloxacillin** are most valuable in long-term therapy of serious staphylococcal infections (e.g., endocarditis, osteomyelitis) and in the treatment of minor staphylococcal infections of the skin and soft tissues.

4. **Precautions and monitoring parameters**
   a. Like all penicillins, the penicillinase-resistant group can cause hypersensitivity reactions (see section II E 7 a).
   b. Methicillin may cause nephrotoxicity and interstitial nephritis.
   c. Oxacillin may be hepatotoxic.
   d. Complete cross-resistance exists among the penicillinase-resistant penicillins.

5. **Drug interaction. Probenicid** increases blood levels of these penicillins and may be given concurrently for that purpose.

G. **Aminopenicillins**. This penicillin group includes the semisynthetic agents **ampicillin** and **amoxicillin** and their derivatives, **bacampicillin** and **cyclacillin**. Because of their wider antibacterial spectrum, these drugs are also known as **broad-spectrum penicillins**.

1. **Mechanism of action** (see section II E 4)

2. **Spectrum of activity**. Aminopenicillins have a spectrum that is similar to but broader than that of the natural and penicillinase-resistant penicillins. Easily destroyed by staphylococcal penicillinases, aminopenicillins are ineffective against most staphylococcal organisms. Against most bacteria sensitive to penicillin G, aminopenicillins are slightly less effective than this agent.

3. **Therapeutic uses**. Aminopenicillins are used to treat gonococcal infections, upper respiratory infections, uncomplicated urinary tract infections, and otitis media caused by susceptible organisms.
   a. For infections resulting from penicillin-resistant organisms, **ampicillin** may be given in combination with sulbactam.
   b. **Amoxicillin** is less effective than ampicillin in shigellosis.
   c. **Amoxicillin** is more effective against *S. aureus, Klebsiella*, and *Bacteroides fragilis* infections when administered in combination with clavulanic acid (amoxicillin/potassium clavulanate) because clavulanic acid inactivates penicillinases.

4. **Precautions and monitoring parameters**
   a. Hypersensitivity reactions may occur (see section II E 7 a).
   b. Diarrhea is most common with ampicillin.
   c. In addition to urticarial hypersensitivity rash seen with all penicillins, ampicillin and amoxicillin frequently cause a generalized erythematous, maculopapular rash. (This occurs in 5 to 10% of patients receiving ampicillin.)

5. **Drug interaction** (see section II F 5)

H. **Extended-spectrum penicillins**. These agents have the widest antibacterial spectrum of all penicillins. Also called **antipseudomonal penicillins**, this group includes the **carboxypenicillins (carbenicillin, carbenicillin indanyl**, and **ticarcillin)** and the **ureidopenicillins (azlocillin, mezlocillin,** and **piperacillin)**.

1. **Mechanism of action** (see section II E 4)

2. **Spectrum of activity**. These drugs have a spectrum similar to that of the aminopenicillins but also are effective against *Klebsiella* and *Enterobacter* species, some *B. fragilis* organisms, and indole-positive *Proteus* and *Pseudomonas* organisms.
   a. **Carbenicillin** frequently is active against ampicillin-resistant *Proteus* strains and some other gram-negative organisms.

b. **Ticarcillin** is two to four times as active as carbenicillin against *P. aeruginosa*. Combined with clavulanic acid, this drug has enhanced activity against organisms that resist ticarcillin alone.
c. **Azlocillin** and **piperacillin** are 10 times as active as carbenicillin against *Pseudomonas* organisms and are more active than carbenicillin against streptococcal organisms.
d. **Mezlocillin** and **piperacillin** are more active than carbenicillin against *Klebsiella* organisms.

3. **Therapeutic uses**. Extended-spectrum penicillins are used mainly to treat serious infections caused by gram-negative organisms (e.g., sepsis, pneumonia, and infections of the abdomen, bone, and soft tissues).

4. **Precautions and monitoring parameters**
   a. Hypersensitivity reactions may occur (see section II E 7 a).
   b. Carbenicillin and ticarcillin may cause hypokalemia.
   c. The high sodium content of carbenicillin and ticarcillin may pose a danger to patients with congestive heart failure.
   d. All inhibit platelet aggregation, which may result in bleeding.

5. **Drug interaction** (see section II F 5)

I. **Sulfonamides**. Derivatives of sulfanilamide, these agents were the first drugs to prevent and cure human bacterial infection successfully. Although their current usefulness is limited by the introduction of more effective antibiotics and the emergence of resistant bacterial strains, sulfonamides remain the drugs of choice for certain infections. The major sulfonamides are **sulfadiazine, sulfamethoxazole**, and **sulfisoxazole**.

1. **Mechanism of action**. Sulfonamides are **bacteriostatic**; they suppress bacterial growth by triggering a mechanism that blocks folic acid synthesis, thereby forcing bacteria to synthesize their own folic acid.

2. **Spectrum of activity**. Sulfonamides are broad-spectrum agents with activity against many gram-positive organisms (e.g., *Streptococcus pyogenes* and *S. pneumoniae*) and certain gram-negative organisms (*H. influenzae, E. coli*, and *P. mirabilis*). They also are effective against certain strains of *Chlamydia trachomatis, Nocardia, Actinomyces*, and *Bacillus anthracis*.

3. **Therapeutic uses**
   a. Sulfonamides most often are used to treat urinary tract infections caused by *E. coli*, including acute and chronic cystitis, and chronic upper urinary tract infections.
   b. These agents have value in the treatment of nocardiosis, trachoma and inclusion conjunctivitis, and dermatitis herpetiformis.
   c. **Sulfadiazine** may be administered in combination with pyrimethamine to treat toxoplasmosis.
   d. **Sulfamethoxazole** may be given in combination with trimethoprim to treat such infections as *Pneumocystis carinii* pneumonia, *Shigella* enteritis, *Serratia* sepsis, urinary tract infections, respiratory infections, and gonococcal urethritis (see section II L 8 c).
   e. **Sulfisoxazole** is sometimes used in combination with erythromycin ethylsuccinate to treat acute otitis media caused by *H. influenzae* organisms. For the initial treatment of uncomplicated urinary tract infections, sulfisoxazole may be given in combination with phenazopyridine for relief of symptoms of pain, burning, or urgency.
   f. Prophylactic sulfonamide therapy has been used successfully to prevent streptococcal infections and rheumatic fever recurrences.

4. **Precautions and monitoring parameters**
   a. Sulfonamides may cause blood dyscrasias (hemolytic anemia—especially in patients with G6PD, aplastic anemia, thrombocytopenia, agranulocytosis, eosinophilia).
   b. Hypersensitivity reactions to sulfonamides probably result from sensitization and most commonly involve the skin and mucous membranes. Manifestations include various types of skin rash, exfoliative dermatitis, and photosensitivity. Drug fever and serum sickness also may develop.
   c. Crystalluria and hematuria may occur, possibly leading to urinary tract obstruction. (Adequate fluid intake and urine alkalinization can prevent or minimize this risk.) Sulfonamides should be used cautiously in patients with renal impairment.
   d. Life-threatening hepatitis caused by drug toxicity or sensitization is a rare adverse effect. Signs and symptoms include headache, nausea, vomiting, and jaundice.

5. **Drug interactions**. Sulfonamides may potentiate the effects of **phenytoin, oral anticoagulants**, and **sulfonylureas**.

J. **Tetracyclines**. These broad-spectrum agents are effective against certain bacterial strains that resist other antibiotics. Nonetheless, they are the preferred drugs in only a few situations. The major tetracyclines include **demeclocycline, doxycycline, methacycline, minocycline** and **tetracycline**.

1. **Mechanism of action**. Tetracyclines are **bacteriostatic**; they inhibit bacterial protein synthesis by binding to the 30S ribosomal subunit.

2. **Spectrum of activity**. Tetracyclines are active against gram-negative and gram-positive organisms, spirochetes, *Mycoplasma* and *Chlamydia* organisms, rickettsial species, and certain protozoa.
   a. *Pseudomonas* and *Proteus* organisms are now resistant to tetracyclines. Many coliform bacteria, pneumococci, staphylococci, streptococci, and *Shigella* strains are increasingly resistant.
   b. Cross-resistance within the tetracycline group is extensive.

3. **Therapeutic uses**
   a. Tetracyclines are the agents of choice in rickettsial, chlamydial, and mycoplasmal infections; amebiasis; and bacillary infections (e.g., cholera, brucellosis, tularemia, and some *Salmonella* and *Shigella* infections).
   b. Tetracyclines are useful alternatives to penicillin in the treatment of anthrax, syphilis, gonorrhea, Lyme disease, nocardiosis, and *H. influenzae* respiratory infections.
   c. Oral or topical tetracycline may be administered as a treatment for acne.
   d. **Doxycycline** is highly effective in the prophylaxis of "traveler's diarrhea" (commonly caused by *E. coli*). Because the drug is excreted mainly in the feces, it is the safest tetracycline for the treatment of extrarenal infections in patients with renal impairment.
   e. **Demeclocycline** is commonly used as an adjunctive agent to treat the syndrome of inappropriate antidiuretic hormone (SIADH) secretion.

4. **Precautions and monitoring parameters**
   a. Gastrointestinal distress (diarrhea, abdominal discomfort, nausea, anorexia) is a common adverse effect of tetracyclines. This problem can be minimized by administering the drug with food or temporarily decreasing the dosage.
   b. Skin rash, urticaria, and generalized exfoliative dermatitis signify a hypersensitivity reaction. Rarely, angioedema and anaphylaxis occur.
   c. Cross-sensitivity within the tetracycline group is common.
   d. Phototoxic reactions (severe skin lesions) can develop with exposure to sunlight. This reaction is most common with demeclocycline and doxycycline.
   e. Tetracyclines may cause hepatotoxicity, especially in pregnant women. Manifestations include jaundice, acidosis, and fatty liver infiltration.
   f. Patients with renal impairment may suffer nephrotoxicity.
   g. Tetracyclines may induce permanent tooth discoloration, tooth enamel defects, and retarded bone growth in infants and children.
   h. Use of outdated and degraded tetracyclines can lead to renal tubular dysfunction, possibly resulting in renal failure.
   i. Minocycline can cause vestibular toxicity (ataxia, dizziness, nausea, and vomiting).
   j. IV tetracyclines are irritating and may cause phlebitis.

5. **Drug interactions**
   a. Dairy products and other foods, iron preparations, and antacids and laxatives containing aluminum, calcium, or magnesium can cause reduced tetracycline absorption. Absorption of doxycycline is not inhibited by these factors.
   b. **Methoxyflurane** may exacerbate the tetracyclines' nephrotoxic effects.
   c. **Barbiturates** and **phenytoin** decrease the antibiotic effectiveness of tetracyclines.
   d. Demeclocycline antagonizes the action of **antidiuretic hormone** and may be given as a diuretic in patients with SIADH.

K. **Urinary tract antiseptics**. Concentrating in the renal tubules and bladder, these agents exert local antibacterial effects; most do not achieve blood levels high enough to treat systemic infections. [However, some new quinolone derivatives, such as ciprofloxacin and pefloxacin, are valuable in the treatment of certain infections outside the urinary tract (see section II K 3 b).]

1. **Mechanism of action**
   a. **Methenamine** is hydrolyzed to ammonia and formaldehyde in acidic urine; formaldehyde is antibacterial against gram-positive and gram-negative organisms. Mandelic and hippuric acids, with which methenamine is combined, provide supplementary antibacterial action.
   b. **Nitrofurantoin** is **bacteriostatic**; in high concentrations, it may be **bactericidal**. Presumably, it disrupts bacterial enzyme systems.

c. **Quinolones. Nalidixic acid** and its analogues and derivatives—**oxolinic acid, norfloxacin, cinoxacin, ciprofloxacin, pefloxacin**, and others—interfere with deoxyribonucleic acid (DNA) gyrase and inhibit DNA synthesis during bacterial replication.

2. **Spectrum of activity**
   a. **Methenamine** is active against both gram-positive and gram-negative organisms (e.g., *Enterobacter, Klebsiella, Proteus, P. aeruginosa*, and *S. aureus*).
   b. **Nitrofurantoin** is active against many gram-positive and gram-negative organisms, including some strains of *E. coli, S. aureus, Proteus, Enterobacter*, and *Klebsiella*.
   c. **Quinolones**
      (1) **Nalidixic acid** and **oxolinic acid** are active against most gram-negative organisms that cause urinary tract infections, including *P. mirabilis, E. coli, Klebsiella*, and *Enterobacter* organisms. These drugs are not effective against *Pseudomonas* organisms.
      (2) **Norfloxacin** is active against *E. coli, Enterobacter, Klebsiella, Proteus, P. aeruginosa, S. aureus, Citrobacter*, and some *Streptococcus* organisms.
      (3) **Cinoxacin** is active against *E. coli, Klebsiella, P. mirabilis, Proteus vulgaris, Proteus morgani, Serratia*, and *Citrobacter* organisms.

3. **Therapeutic uses**
   a. **Methenamine** and **nitrofurantoin** are used to prevent and treat urinary tract infections.
   b. **Quinolones** are administered to treat urinary tract infections; some also are used in such diseases as osteomyelitis and respiratory tract infections (see section II L).

4. **Precautions and monitoring parameters**
   a. **Methenamine** may cause nausea, vomiting, and diarrhea; in high doses, it may lead to urinary tract irritation (dysuria, frequency, hematuria, albuminuria). Skin rash also may develop.
   b. **Nitrofurantoin** may cause various adverse effects.
      (1) Gastrointestinal distress (nausea, vomiting, diarrhea) is relatively common.
      (2) Hypersensitivity reactions to nitrofurantoin may involve the skin, lungs, blood, or liver; manifestations include fever, chills, hepatitis, jaundice, leukopenia, granulocytopenia, and pneumonitis.
      (3) Adverse CNS effects include headache, vertigo, and dizziness. Polyneuropathy may develop with high doses or in patients with renal impairment.
   c. **Quinolones**
      (1) **Nalidixic acid** and **oxolinic acid** may cause nausea, vomiting, abdominal pain, urticaria, pruritus, skin rash, fever, eosinophilia, and CNS effects (headache, dizziness, confusion, vertigo, drowsiness, weakness).
      (2) **Cinoxacin** may induce nausea, vomiting, diarrhea, headache, insomnia, skin rash, pruritus, and urticaria.

5. **Drug interactions**
   a. The effects of methenamine are inhibited by **alkalinizing agents** and are antagonized by **acetazolamide**.
   b. Nitrofurantoin absorption is decreased by **magnesium-containing antacids**. Nitrofurantoin blood levels are increased and urine levels decreased by **sulfinpyrazone** and **probenicid**, leading to increased toxicity and reduced therapeutic effectiveness.
   c. **Quinolones**
      (1) Cinoxacin urine levels are decreased by **probenicid**, reducing therapeutic effectiveness.
      (2) Norfloxacin is rendered less effective by **antacids**.

L. Miscellaneous antibacterial agents

1. **Aztreonam**. This agent was the first commercially available monobactam (monocyclic β-lactam compound). It resembles the aminoglycosides in its efficacy against many gram-negative organisms but does not cause nephrotoxicity or ototoxicity. Other advantages of this drug include its ability to preserve the body's normal gram-positive and anaerobic flora, activity against many gentamicin-resistant organisms, and lack of cross-allergenicity with penicillin.
   a. **Mechanism of action**. Aztreonam is **bactericidal**; it inhibits bacterial cell wall synthesis.
   b. **Spectrum of activity**. This drug is active against many gram-negative organisms, including *Enterobacter* and *P. aeruginosa*.
   c. **Therapeutic uses**. Aztreonam is therapeutic for urinary tract infections, septicemia, skin infections, lower respiratory tract infections, and intra-abdominal infections resulting from gram-negative organisms.
   d. **Precautions and monitoring parameters**
      (1) Aztreonam sometimes causes nausea, vomiting, and diarrhea.
      (2) Liver enzymes may increase transiently during aztreonam therapy.
      (3) This drug may induce skin rash.

2. **Chloramphenicol**. A nitrobenzene derivative, this drug has broad activity against rickettsia as well as many gram-positive and gram-negative organisms. It also is effective against many ampicillin-resistant strains of *H. influenzae*.
   a. **Mechanism of action**. Chloramphenicol is primarily **bacteriostatic**, although it may be bactericidal against a few bacterial strains.
   b. **Spectrum of activity**. This agent is active against rickettsia and a wide range of bacteria, including *H. influenzae*, *Salmonella typhi*, *Neisseria meningitides*, *Bordetella pertussis*, *Clostridium*, *B. fragilis*, *S. pyogenes*, and *S. pneumoniae*.
   c. **Therapeutic uses**. Because of its toxic side effects, chloramphenicol is used only to suppress infections that cannot be treated effectively with other antibiotics. Such infections typically include:
      (1) Typhoid fever
      (2) Meningococcal infections in cephalosporin-allergic patients
      (3) Serious *H. influenzae* infections, especially in cephalosporin-allergic patients
      (4) Anaerobic infections (e.g., those originating in the pelvis or intestines)
      (5) Anaerobic or mixed infections of the CNS
      (6) Rickettsial infections in pregnant patients, tetracycline-allergic patients, and renally impaired patients
   d. **Precautions and monitoring parameters**
      (1) Chloramphenicol can cause bone marrow suppression (dose-related), with resulting pancytopenia; rarely, the drug leads to aplastic anemia (non–dose-related).
      (2) Hypersensitivity reactions may include skin rash and, in extremely rare cases, angioedema or anaphylaxis.
      (3) Chloramphenicol therapy may lead to gray-baby syndrome in neonates (especially premature infants). This dangerous reaction, which stems partly from inadequate liver detoxification of the drug, is manifested by vomiting, gray cyanosis, rapid and irregular respirations, vasomotor collapse, and, in some cases, death.
   e. **Drug interactions**
      (1) Chloramphenicol inhibits the metabolism of **phenytoin, tolbutamide, chlorpropamide**, and **dicumarol**, leading to prolonged action and intensified effect of these drugs.
      (2) **Phenobarbital** shortens chloramphenicol's half-life, thereby reducing its therapeutic effectiveness.
      (3) **Penicillins** can cause antibiotic antagonism.
      (4) **Acetaminophen** elevates chloramphenicol levels and may cause toxicity.

3. **Clindamycin**. This agent has essentially replaced lincomycin, the drug from which it is derived. It is used to treat skin, respiratory tract, and soft-tissue infections caused by staphylococci, pneumococci, and streptococci.
   a. **Mechanism of action**. Clindamycin is **bacteriostatic**; it binds to the 50S ribosomal subunit, thereby suppressing bacterial protein synthesis.
   b. **Spectrum of activity**. This agent is active against most gram-positive and many anaerobic organisms, including *B. fragilis*.
   c. **Therapeutic uses**. Because of its marked toxicity, clindamycin is used only against infections for which it has proven to be the most effective drug. Typically, such infections include abdominal and female genitourinary tract infections caused by *B. fragilis*.
   d. **Precautions and monitoring parameters**
      (1) Clindamycin may cause rash, nausea, vomiting, diarrhea, and pseudomembranous colitis (as evidenced by fever, abdominal pain, and bloody stools).
      (2) Blood dyscrasias (eosinophilia, thrombocytopenia, leukopenia) may occur.
   e. **Drug interactions.** Clindamycin may potentiate the effects of **neuromuscular blocking agents**.

4. **Dapsone**. A member of the sulfone class, this drug is the primary agent in the treatment of all forms of leprosy.
   a. **Mechanism of action**. Dapsone is **bacteriostatic** for *Mycobacterium leprae*; its mechanism of action probably resembles that of the sulfonamides.
   b. **Spectrum of activity**. This drug is active against *M. leprae* (however, drug resistance develops in up to 40% of patients). Dapsone also has some activity against *P. carinii* organisms and the malarial parasite *Plasmodium*.
   c. **Therapeutic uses**
      (1) Dapsone is the drug of choice in leprosy.
      (2) This agent may be used to treat dermatitis herpetiformis, a skin disorder.
      (3) Maloprim, a dapsone–pyrimethamine product, is valuable in the prophylaxis and treatment of malaria.
   d. **Precautions and monitoring parameters**
      (1) Hemolytic anemia can occur with daily doses above 200 mg. Other adverse hematologic effects include methemoglobinemia and leukopenia.

(2) Nausea, vomiting, and anorexia may develop.
(3) Adverse CNS effects include headache, dizziness, nervousness, lethargy, paresthesias, and psychosis.
(4) Dapsone occasionally results in a potentially lethal mononucleosis-like syndrome.
(5) Paradoxically, this drug sometimes exacerbates leprosy.
(6) Other adverse effects include skin rash, peripheral neuropathy, blurred vision, tinnitus, hepatitis, and cholestatic jaundice.

e. Drug interaction. Probenicid elevates blood levels of dapsone, possibly resulting in toxicity.

5. Fluoroquinolones

a. These are synthetic agents related to nalidixic acid [see section II K 4 c (1)]. They are bactericidal for growing bacteria and inhibit DNAgyrase. They are active against enteric gram-negative bacilli.

(1) **Norfloxacin** is indicated for oral treatment of urinary tract infections. Unapproved indications include therapy of gonorrhea and prostatitis; treatment and prophylaxis of traveler's diarrhea and bacterial gastroenteritis; and prophylaxis of infections in neutropenic patients.
(2) **Ciprofloxacin** is active against many anaerobes, chlamydia, and *M. tuberculosis*. In addition to indications described for norfloxacin, ciprofloxacin is useful for treatment of gram-negative osteomyelitis and respiratory tract infection.
(3) Other agents under investigation include pefloxacin, enoxacin, ofloxacin, amifloxacin.

b. Precautions and monitoring parameters

(1) Adverse reactions include nausea, dyspepsia, headache, dizziness, insomnia, rash, urticaria, leukopenia, and elevated liver enzymes.
(2) Crystalluria occurs with high doses enhanced at alkaline pH.

c. Drug interactions. Ciprofloxacin has been shown to increase serum theophylline levels.

6. Imipenem. Formerly known as thienamycin, imipenem is the first carbapenem compound introduced in the United States. A β-lactam antibiotic, it resists destruction by most β-lactamases. Because it is inhibited by renal dipeptidases, imipenem must be combined with cilastatin sodium, a dipeptidase inhibitor.

a. Mechanism of action. Imipenem is **bactericidal**; it inhibits bacterial cell wall synthesis.

b. Spectrum of activity. This drug has the broadest spectrum of all β-lactam antibiotics. It is active against most gram-positive cocci (including many enterococci), gram-negative rods (including many *P. aeruginosa* strains), and anaerobes. It has good activity against many bacterial strains that resist other antibiotics.

c. Therapeutic uses. Imipenem has most value in the treatment of severe infections caused by drug-resistant organisms susceptible only to imipenem.

d. Precautions and monitoring effects

(1) Imipenem may cause nausea, vomiting, diarrhea, and pseudomembranous colitis.
(2) Seizures, dizziness, and hypotension may develop.
(3) Patients who are allergic to penicillin or cephalosporins may suffer cross-allergy during imipenem therapy.

7. Spectinomycin. An aminocyclitol agent related to the aminoglycosides, this antibiotic is useful against penicillin-resistant strains of gonorrhea.

a. Mechanism of action. Spectinomycin is **bacteriostatic**; it selectively inhibits protein synthesis by binding to the 30S ribosomal subunit.

b. Spectrum of activity. This agent is active against various gram-negative organisms.

c. Therapeutic uses. Spectinomycin is used only to treat gonococcal infections in patients with penicillin allergy or when such infection stems from penicillinase-producing gonococci (PPNG).

d. Precautions and monitoring effects. Because spectinomycin is given only as a single-dose intramuscular injection, it causes few adverse effects. Nausea, vomiting, urticaria, chills, dizziness, and insomnia occur rarely.

8. Trimethoprim. A substituted pyrimidine, trimethoprim is most commonly combined with sulfamethoxazole (a sulfonamide discussed in section II I) in a preparation called co-trimoxazole. However, it may be used alone for certain urinary tract infections.

a. Mechanism of action. Spectinomycin is **bacteriostatic**; it selectively inhibits protein synthesis by binding to the 30S ribosomal subunit.

b. Spectrum of activity. This agent is active against various gram-negative organisms.

(1) Trimethoprim is active against most gram-negative and gram-positive organisms. However, drug resistance may develop when this drug is used alone.
(2) Trimethoprim–sulfamethoxazole is active against a wide variety of organisms, including *S. pneumoniae*, *N. meningitides*, and *Corynebacterium diphtheriae* and some strains

of *S. aureus*, *Staphylococcus epidermis*, *P. mirabilis*, *Enterobacter*, *Salmonella*, *Shigella*, *Serratia*, *Klebsiella* species, and *E. coli*.

(3) The trimethoprim–sulfamethoxazole combination is synergistic; many organisms resistant to one component are susceptible to the combination.

c. Therapeutic uses

(1) Trimethoprim may be used alone or in combination with sulfamethoxazole to treat uncomplicated urinary tract infections caused by *E. coli*, *P. mirabilis*, *Klebsiella*, and *Enterobacter* organisms.

(2) Trimethoprim–sulfamethoxazole is therapeutic for acute gonococcal urethritis, acute exacerbation of chronic bronchitis, shigellosis, and *Salmonella* infections.

(3) Trimethoprim–sulfamethoxazole may be given as prophylactic or suppressive therapy in *P. carinii* pneumonia.

d. Precautions and monitoring parameters

(1) Most adverse effects involve the skin (possibly from sensitization). These include rash, pruritus, and exfoliative dermatitis.

(2) Rarely, trimethoprim–sulfamethoxazole causes blood dyscrasias (acute hemolytic anemia, leukopenia, thrombocytopenia, methemoglobinemia, agranulocytosis, aplastic anemia).

(3) Adverse gastrointestinal effects including nausea, vomiting, and epigastric distress glossitis may occur.

(4) Neonates may develop kernicterus.

(5) Patients with acquired immune deficiency syndrome (AIDS) sometimes suffer fever, rash, malaise, and pancytopenia during trimethoprim therapy.

9. Vancomycin. This glycopeptide destroys most gram-positive organisms.

a. Mechanism of action. Vancomycin is **bactericidal**: It inhibits bacterial cell wall synthesis.

b. Spectrum of activity. This drug is active against most gram-positive organisms, including methicillin-resistant strains of *S. aureus*.

c. Therapeutic uses. Vancomycin usually is reserved for serious infections, especially those caused by methicillin-resistant staphylococci. It is particularly useful in patients who are allergic to penicillin or cephalosporins. Typical uses include endocarditis, osteomyelitis, and staphylococcal pneumonia.

(1) Oral vancomycin is valuable in the treatment of antibiotic-induced pseudomembranous colitis caused by *Clostridium difficile* or *S. aureus* enterocolitis. Since vancomycin is not absorbed after oral administration, it is not useful for systemic infections.

(2) Because 1 g provides adequate blood levels for 7 to 10 days, IV vancomycin is especially useful in the treatment of anephric patients with gram-positive bacterial infections.

d. Precautions and monitoring parameters

(1) Ototoxicity may arise; nephrotoxicity is rare but can occur with high doses.

(2) Vancomycin may cause hypersensitivity reactions, manifested by such symptoms as anaphylaxis or skin rash.

(3) Therapeutic levels peak at 20 to 40 μg/ml. The trough is <10 μg/ml.

(4) "Red neck syndrome" may occur. This is facial flushing and hypotension due to too rapid infusion of the drug. Infusion should be over a minimum of 60 minutes for a 1-g dose.

(5) IV solutions are very irritating to the vein.

III. ANTIFUNGAL AGENTS

A. Definition. These agents treat systemic and local fungal (mycotic) infections—diseases that resist treatment with antibacterial drugs.

B. Amphotericin B. This polyene antibiotic is therapeutic for various fungal infections that frequently proved fatal before the drug became available. It is used increasingly in the empiric treatment of severely immunocompromised patients in certain clinical situations.

1. Mechanism of action. Amphotericin B is both **fungicidal** and **fungistatic**; it binds to sterols in the fungal cell membrane, thereby increasing membrane permeability and permitting leakage of intracellular contents. Other mechanisms may be involved as well.

2. Spectrum of activity. Amphotericin B is a broad-spectrum antifungal agent, with activity against *Histoplasma capsulatum*, *Cryptococcus neoformans*, *Coccidioides immitis*, and *Candida* species. Many strains of *Aspergillus* and *Sporothrix schenckii* also are susceptible.

3. Therapeutic uses. Amphotericin B is the most effective antifungal agent in the treatment of systemic fungal infections, especially in immunocompromised patients.

a. It is therapeutic for meningitis, histoplasmosis, coccidioidomycosis, blastomycosis, cryptococcosis, disseminated moniliasis, aspergillosis, and phycomycosis.

b. This agent may be used to treat coccidioidal arthritis.
c. Topical preparations are given to eradicate cutaneous and mucocutaneous candidiasis.

4. **Precautions and monitoring parameters**. Because amphotericin B can cause many serious adverse effects, it should be administered in a hospital setting—at least during the initial therapeutic stage.
   a. Nephrotoxicity occurs in most patients; those with serious preexisting renal impairment may require dosage reduction or temporary drug discontinuation.
   b. Adverse CNS effects include headache, peripheral neuropathy, and convulsions.
   c. Adverse gastrointestinal effects include nausea, vomiting, diarrhea, anorexia, and cramps.
   d. Fever, malaise, and chills may be minimized by pretreatment with aspirin, acetaminophen, or diphenhydramine or by the addition of hydrocortisone to the IV infusion.
   e. Parenteral administration may cause local pain, thrombophlebitis, burning, stinging, irritation, and tissue damage with extravasation. Addition of heparin (100 units/infusion) helps minimize these effects.

5. **Drug interactions**. Other nephrotoxic drugs may cause additive nephrotoxicity.

C. **Flucytosine**. This fluorinated pyrimidine usually is given in combination with amphotericin B.

1. **Mechanism of action**. Flucytosine penetrates fungal cells and is converted to fluorouracil, a metabolic antagonist. Incorporated into the ribonucleic acid (RNA) of the fungal cell, flucytosine causes defective protein synthesis.

2. **Spectrum of activity**. This drug is active against some strains of *Cryptococcus*, *Candida*, *Aspergillus*, *Torulopsis*, and certain other fungal species. In combination with amphotericin B, flucytosine results in synergistic activity against *Cryptococcus neoformans* and some strains of *Candida tropicalis* and *Candida albicans*.

3. **Therapeutic uses**. Flucytosine is therapeutic for systemic infections (e.g., septicemia, endocarditis, pulmonary and urinary tract infections, meningitis). In most cases, it is given with amphotericin B.

4. **Precautions and monitoring parameters**
   a. Although flucytosine is less toxic than amphotericin B, it may cause serious adverse effects, including bone marrow suppression, severe enterocolitis, and hepatomegaly.
   b. Nausea, vomiting, diarrhea, dizziness, drowsiness, and skin rash also may occur.
   c. Flucytosine may increase serum creatinine values on tests using the EKTACHEM method.

D. **Griseofulvin**. Produced from *Penicillium griseofulvum*, this drug is deposited in the skin, bound to keratin.

1. **Mechanism of action**. This agent is **fungistatic**; it inhibits fungal cell activity by interfering with mitotic spindle structure.

2. **Spectrum of activity**. Griseofulvin is active against various strains of *Microsporum*, *Epidermophyton*, and *Trichophyton*.

3. **Therapeutic uses**. Griseofulvin is effective in tinea infections of the skin, hair, and nails (including athelete's foot) caused by *Microsporum*, *Epidermophyton*, and *Trichophyton*.
   a. Generally, it is given only for infections that do not respond to topical antifungal agents.
   b. Griseofulvin is available only in oral form.

4. **Precautions and monitoring parameters**
   a. Griseofulvin rarely results in serious adverse effects. However, the following problems have been reported:
      (1) Headache, fatigue, confusion, impaired performance, syncope, and lethargy
      (2) Leukopenia, neutropenia, and granulocytopenia
      (3) Serum sickness, angioedema, urticaria, erythema, and hepatotoxicity
   b. The dosage is dependent on the particle size of the product: 250 mg of ultramicrosize is equivalent in therapeutic effects to 500 mg of microsize.

5. **Drug interactions**
   a. Griseofulvin may increase the metabolism of **warfarin**, leading to decreased prothrombin time.
   b. **Barbiturates** may reduce griseofulvin absorption.
   c. **Alcohol consumption** may cause tachycardia and flushing.

E. **Imidazoles**. The substituted imidazole derivatives **ketoconazole** and **miconazole** are valuable in the treatment of a wide range of systemic fungal infections.

1. **Mechanism of action**. Ketoconazole and miconazole inhibit sterol synthesis in fungal cell membranes and increase cell wall permeability; this, in turn, makes the cell more vulnerable to osmotic pressure.

2. **Spectrum of activity**. These agents are active against many fungi, including yeasts, dermatophytes, actinomycetes, and some phycomycetes.

3. **Therapeutic uses**
   a. **Ketoconazole**, an oral agent, successfully treats many fungal infections that previously yielded only to parenteral agents.
      (1) It is therapeutic for systemic and vaginal candidiasis, mucocandidiasis, candiduria, oral thrush, histoplasmosis, coccidioidomycosis, chromomycosis, and paracoccidioidomycosis.
      (2) Because ketoconazole is slow-acting and requires a long duration of therapy (up to 6 months for some chronic infections), it is less effective than other antifungal agents for the treatment of severe and acute systemic infections.
   b. **Miconazole**, primarily administered as a topical agent, also is available in parenteral form.
      (1) Topical miconazole is highly effective in vulvovaginal candidiasis, ringworm, and other skin infections.
      (2) Parenteral miconazole serves as a second-line agent in severe systemic fungal infections only when other antifungal drugs have proven to be ineffective or cannot be tolerated.

4. **Precautions and monitoring parameters**
   a. Ketoconazole may cause nausea, vomiting, diarrhea, abdominal pain, and constipation. Rarely, it leads to headache, dizziness, gynecomastia, and fatal hepatotoxicity.
   b. Parenteral miconazole therapy frequently induces nausea, vomiting, diarrhea, phlebitis, pruritic rash, anaphylactoid reaction, CNS toxicity, and hyponatremia. Dose-related anemia and thrombocytosis may also occur.

5. **Drug interactions**
   a. Both ketoconazole and miconazole may enhance the anticoagulant effect of **warfarin**.
   b. Ketoconazole may antagonize the antibiotic effects of **amphotericin B**.

F. **Nystatin**. A polyene antibiotic, nystatin has a chemical structure similar to that of amphotericin B.

1. **Mechanism of action**. Nystatin is **fungicidal** and **fungistatic**; binding to sterols in the fungal cell membrane, it increases membrane permeability and permits leakage of intracellular contents.

2. **Spectrum of activity**. Nystatin is active against *Candida, Cryptococcus, Histoplasma,* and *Blastomyces* organisms.

3. **Therapeutic uses**
   a. This drug is used primarily as a topical agent in vaginal and oral *Candida* infections.
   b. Oral nystatin is therapeutic for *Candida* infections of the gastrointestinal tract, especially oral and esophageal infections.

4. **Precautions and monitoring parameters**. Oral nystatin occasionally causes gastrointestinal distress (nausea, vomiting, diarrhea). Rarely, hypersensitivity reactions occur.

IV. ANTIPROTOZOAL AGENTS

A. **Classification**. These drugs fall into two main categories: **antimalarial agents**, used to treat malaria infection; and **amebicides and trichomonacides**, used to treat amebic and trichomonal infections.

B. **Antimalarial agents**. Still a leading cause of illness and death in tropical and subtropical countries, malaria results from infection by any of four species of the protozoal genus *Plasmodium*. Antimalarial agents are selectively active during different phases of the protozoan life cycle. Major antimalarial drugs include **chloroquine, primaquine, pyrimethamine**, and **quinine**.

1. **Mechanism of action**
   a. **Chloroquine** binds to and alters the properties of microbial and mammalian DNA.
   b. The mechanism of action of **primaquine** and **quinine** is unknown.
   c. **Pyrimethamine** impedes folic acid reduction by inhibiting the enzyme dihydrofolate reductase.

2. Spectrum of activity

a. Chloroquine, a suppressive agent, is active against the asexual erythrocyte forms of *Plasmodium vivax* and *Plasmodium falciparum* and gametocytes of *P. vivax, Plasmodium malariae*, and *Plasmodium ovale*.

b. Primaquine, a curative agent, is active against liver forms of *P. vivax* and *P. ovale* and the primary exoerythrocyte forms of *P. falciparum*.

c. Pyrimethamine is active against chloroquine-resistant strains of *P. falciparum* and some strains of *P. vivax*.

d. Quinine, a generalized protoplasmic poison, is toxic to a wide range of organisms. In malaria, this drug has both suppressive and curative action against chloroquine-resistant strains.

3. Therapeutic uses

a. Chloroquine is used to suppress malaria symptoms and to terminate acute malaria attacks resulting from *P. falciparum* and *P. malariae* infection.

(1) It is more potent and less toxic than quinine.

(2) Except where drug-resistant *P. falciparum* strains are prevalent, chloroquine is the most useful antimalarial agent.

b. Primaquine is used to cure relapses of *P. vivax* and *P. ovale* malaria and to prevent malaria in exposed persons returning from regions where malaria is endemic.

c. Pyrimethamine is effective in the prevention and treatment of chloroquine-resistant strains of *P. falciparum*. It is now used almost exclusively in combination with a sulfonamide or sulfone.

d. Quinine

(1) Quinine sulfate, an oral form, is therapeutic for acute malaria caused by chloroquine-resistant strains.

(2) Quinine dihydrochloride, a parenteral form, is used in severe cases of chloroquine-resistant malaria. (It is available only from the Centers for Disease Control in Atlanta.)

(3) Quinine is almost always given in combination with another antimalarial agent.

4. Precautions and monitoring parameters

a. Chloroquine

(1) Because this drug concentrates in the liver, it should be used cautiously in patients with hepatic disease.

(2) Chloroquine must be administered with extreme caution in patients with neurologic, hematologic, or severe gastrointestinal disorders.

(3) Visual disturbances, headache, skin rash, and gastrointestinal distress have been reported.

b. Primaquine

(1) This agent is contraindicated in patients with rheumatoid arthritis and lupus erythematosus and in those receiving other potentially hemolytic drugs or bone marrow suppressants.

(2) Primaquine may cause agranulocytosis, granulocytopenia, and mild anemia; in patients with G6PD deficiency, it may cause hemolytic anemia.

(3) Abdominal cramps, nausea, vomiting, and epigastric distress sometimes occur.

c. Pyrimethamine

(1) In high doses, this drug may cause agranulocytosis, megaloblastic anemia, aplastic anemia, and thrombocytopenia.

(2) Erythema multiforme (Stevens-Johnson syndrome), nausea, vomiting, and anorexia may develop during primaquine therapy.

d. Quinine

(1) Quinine is contraindicated in patients with G6PD deficiency, tinnitus, and optic neuritis.

(2) Quinine overdose or hypersensitivity reactions may be fatal. Manifestations of quinine poisoning include visual and hearing disturbances; gastrointestinal symptoms (e.g., nausea, vomiting); hot, flushed skin; headache; fever; syncope; confusion; shallow, then depressed, respirations; and cardiovascular collapse.

(3) Quinine must be used cautiously in patients with atrial fibrillation.

(4) Renal damage and anuria have been reported.

C. Amebicides and trichomonacides. These agents are crucial in the treatment of amebiasis, giardiasis, and trichomoniases—the most common protozoal infections in the United States. The major amebicides include **diloxanide, emetine, metronidazole**, and **quinacrine**.

1. Mechanism of action

a. Diloxanide, a dichloroacetamide derivative, is **amebicidal**; its mechanism of action is unknown. (It is available only from the Centers for Disease Control in Atlanta.)

b. **Emetine**, an alkaloid obtained from ipecac, is **amebicidal**; it kills amebae by inhibiting amebic protein synthesis.

c. **Metronidazole** is a synthetic compound with direct **amebicidal** and **trichomonacidal** action; it works at both intestinal and extraintestinal sites. Its mechanism of action involves disruption of the helical structure of DNA.

d. **Quinacrine** is an acridine derivative that inhibits DNA metabolism.

2. **Spectrum of activity and therapeutic uses**

a. **Diloxanide**

(1) This drug is used to treat asymptomatic carriers of amebic and giardiac cysts.

(2) Diloxanide is therapeutic for invasive and extraintestinal amebiasis (given in combination with a systemic or mixed amebicide).

(3) Diloxanide is not effective as single-agent therapy for extraintestinal amebiasis.

b. **Emetine**

(1) This drug is widely used to treat severe invasive intestinal amebiasis, amebic abscess, and amebic hepatitis.

(2) Because of its toxicity, emetine generally is used only when other drugs are contraindicated or have proven to be ineffective.

(3) Usually, emetine is administered in combination with another amebicidal agent.

c. **Metronidazole**

(1) This agent is the preferred drug in amebic dysentery, giardiasis, and trichomoniasis.

(2) Metronidazole also is active against all anaerobic cocci and gram-negative anaerobic bacilli.

d. **Quinacrine** is useful in the treatment of giardiasis and tapeworms.

3. **Precautions and monitoring parameters**

a. **Diloxanide** rarely causes serious adverse effects. Vomiting, flatulence, and pruritus have been reported.

b. **Emetine**

(1) This drug may induce potentially lethal systemic toxicity. Manifestations may be cardiovascular (e.g., electrocardiogram abnormalities, tachycardia, hypotension, congestive heart failure); gastrointestinal (e.g., nausea, vomiting, diarrhea); or neurologic (e.g., dizziness, headache, changes in central or peripheral nerve function).

(2) Emetine usually is contraindicated in patients with cardiac disease, renal impairment, muscle disease, and polyneuropathy; in children; and in patients who have taken the drug in the past 6 to 8 weeks.

(3) IV injection is contraindicated.

(4) Deep subcutaneous administration (preferred over the intramuscular route) may cause muscle weakness at the injection site.

c. **Metronidazole**

(1) The most common adverse effects of this drug are nausea, epigastric distress, and diarrhea.

(2) Metronidazole is carcinogenic in mice and should not be used unnecessarily.

(3) Headache, vomiting, metallic taste, and stomatitis have been reported.

(4) Occasionally, neurologic reactions (e.g., ataxia, peripheral neuropathy, seizures) develop.

(5) A disulfiram-type reaction may occur with concurrent ethanol use.

d. **Quinacrine**

(1) This drug frequently causes dizziness, headache, nausea, and vomiting. Nervousness and seizures also have been reported.

(2) Quinacrine should not be taken in combination with primaquine because this may increase primaquine toxicity.

(3) Quinacrine should be administered with extreme caution in patients with psoriasis because it may cause marked exacerbation of this disease.

V. ANTITUBERCULAR AGENTS

A. **Definition and classification**. Drugs used to treat tuberculosis suppress or kill the slow-growing mycobacteria that cause this disease. Antitubercular agents fall into two main categories: **first-line** (primary) and **second-line** (secondary). Because the causative organisms tend to develop resistance to any single drug, combination drug therapy has become standard in the treatment of tuberculosis.

B. **First-line antitubercular agents**. These drugs—**isoniazid, rifampin**, and **ethambutol**—usually offer the greatest effectiveness with the least toxicity; they are successful in most tuberculosis patients. Frequently, two or three are administered together; in most cases, the combination of isoniazid and rifampin proves the most effective. In life-threatening or renal tuberculosis, initial therapy may include three antitubercular drugs (typically, a combination of first- and second-line agents) to ensure that the causative organism is susceptible to at least two.

1. **Ethambutol** is a synthetic water-based compound.
   a. **Mechanism of action**. This drug is **bacteriostatic**; its precise mechanism of action is unknown.
   b. **Spectrum of activity and therapeutic uses**. Ethambutol is active against many *M. tuberculosis* strains. However, drug resistance develops fairly rapidly when it is used alone. In most cases, ethambutol is given adjunctively in combination with isoniazid or rifampin.
   c. **Precautions and monitoring parameters**. Rarely, ethambutol causes such adverse effects as reversible dose-related ($\geq$15 mg/kg/day) optic neuritis, drug fever, abdominal pain, headache, dizziness, and confusion.

2. **Isoniazid** is a hydrazide of isonicotinic acid. The mainstay of antitubercular therapy, this drug should be included (if tolerated) in all therapeutic regimens.
   a. **Mechanism of action**. Isoniazid is **bacteriostatic** for resting bacilli, **bactericidal** for rapidly dividing organisms. Its mechanism of action is not fully known; the drug probably disrupts bacterial cell wall synthesis by inhibiting mycolic acid synthesis.
   b. **Spectrum of activity**. Isoniazid is active against most tubercle bacilli; some atypical mycobacteria are resistant.
   c. **Therapeutic uses**
      (1) The most widely used antitubercular agent, isoniazid should be given in combination with another antitubercular drug (such as rifampin or ethambutol) to prevent drug resistance.
      (2) For uncomplicated pulmonary tuberculosis, isoniazid therapy may last 9 months to 2 years.
      (3) Prophylactic isoniazid may be administered alone for 1 year in children who have a positive tuberculin test result but lack active lesions.
   d. **Precautions and monitoring parameters**
      (1) The most common adverse effects of isoniazid are skin rash, fever, jaundice, and peripheral neuritis.
      (2) Hepatitis, an occasional reaction, can be severe and, in some cases, fatal. The risk of hepatitis increases with the patient's age and rises with alcohol abuse.
      (3) Blood dyscrasias (e.g., agranulocytosis, aplastic or hemolytic anemia, thrombocytopenia) may occur.
      (4) Adverse gastrointestinal effects include nausea, vomiting, and epigastric distress.
      (5) CNS toxicity may result from pyridoxine deficiency. Signs and symptoms include insomnia, restlessness, hyperreflexia, and convulsions.
   e. **Drug interactions**
      (1) With concurrent **phenytoin** therapy, blood levels of both phenytoin and isoniazid may increase, possibly causing toxicity.
      (2) **Aluminum-containing antacids** may reduce isoniazid absorption.
      (3) Concurrent **carbamazepine** therapy may increase the risk of hepatitis.

3. **Rifampin** is a complex macrocyclic agent.
   a. **Mechanism of action**. This drug is **bactericidal**; it impairs bacterial RNA synthesis by binding to DNA-dependent RNA polymerase.
   b. **Spectrum of activity**. Rifampin is active against most gram-negative and many gram-positive organisms.
   c. **Therapeutic uses**
      (1) The combination of rifampin and isoniazid is the most effective therapy for tuberculosis. Rifampin should not be administered alone because this can lead to the emergence of highly drug-resistant organisms.
      (2) Prophylactic rifampin is effective when administered to carriers of meningococcal disease caused by *H. influenzae* organisms.
   d. **Precautions and monitoring effects**
      (1) Serious hepatotoxicity may result from rifampin therapy.
      (2) In rare cases, this drug induces an influenza-like syndrome.
      (3) Other adverse effects include skin rash, drowsiness, headache, fatigue, confusion, nausea, vomiting, and abdominal pain.
      (4) Rifampin colors urine, sweat, tears, saliva, and feces orange–red.
   e. **Drug interactions**
      (1) Rifampin induces hepatic microsomal enzymes and thus may decrease the therapeutic effectiveness of **corticosteroids, warfarin, oral contraceptives, quinidine, digitoxin**, and **barbiturates**.
      (2) **Probenicid** may increase blood levels of rifampin.

C. **Second-line antitubercular agents**. This category includes **aminosalicylic acid, capreomycin, cycloserine, pyrazinamide**, and **streptomycin.**

1. **Mechanism of action**
   a. **Aminosalicylic acid** is **bacteriostatic**; it probably inhibits the enzymes responsible for folic acid synthesis.
   b. **Cycloserine** can be bacteriostatic or bactericidal, depending on its concentration at the infection site; it impairs amino acid utilization, thereby inhibiting bacterial cell wall synthesis.
   c. The mechanism of action of **capreomycin** (bacteriostatic), **ethionamide** (bactericidal), and **pyrazinamide** (bactericidal) is unknown.
   d. **Streptomycin** (see section II B 2 a)

2. **Spectrum of activity and therapeutic uses**. Second-line antitubercular agents are active against various microorganisms, including *M. tuberculosis*. They generally are reserved for patients with extensive extrapulmonary or drug-resistant disease or for patients who need retreatment. These drugs are almost always administered in combination.

3. **Precautions and monitoring parameters**
   a. Adverse effects of aminosalicylic acid include leukopenia, agranulocytopenia, thrombocytopenia, hemolytic anemia, mononucleosis-like syndrome, malaise, joint pain, fever, and skin rash.
   b. Capreomycin and streptomycin are ototoxic and nephrotoxic; they should not be administered together.
   c. Cycloserine may cause adverse CNS effects, including headache, suicidal and psychotic tendencies, hyperirritability, confusion, paranoia, and nervousness.
   d. Ethionamide may induce nausea, vomiting, orthostatic hypotension, metallic taste, epigastric distress, and peripheral neuropathy.
   e. Pyrazinamide may result in hepatotoxicity and, rarely, hepatic necrosis resulting in death. Anorexia, nausea, vomiting, malaise, and fever have been reported.
   f. Streptomycin (see section II B 4)

VI. ANTIVIRAL AGENTS

A. **Definition**. These drugs alleviate viral disease by influencing viral replication. Because viruses lack independent metabolic activity and can replicate only within living host cells, antiviral agents tend to injure host as well as viral cells. Consequently, few antiviral drugs have been introduced; most are active against only one virus.

B. **Acyclovir** is a synthetic purine nucleoside analogue that is therapeutic for various herpes infections. It is the least toxic antiviral agent.

1. **Mechanism of action**. Acyclovir becomes incorporated into viral DNA and inhibits viral replication.

2. **Spectrum of activity**. This agent is active against herpes viruses, especially herpes simplex type I.
   a. Acyclovir is used to treat mucocutaneous herpes simplex infections in immunocompromised patients and to reduce pain and speed healing of herpes zoster, genital herpes, and neonatal herpes.
   b. This agent is available in topical as well as oral and IV forms. Topical acyclovir is applied directly on herpes lesions in primary herpes infection and in non–life-threatening mucocutaneous herpes simplex infection in immunocompromised patients.
   c. Acyclovir may be administered intravenously in the treatment of initial and recurrent mucocutaneous herpes simplex infection in immunocompromised patients as well as severe initial herpes infection in patients with normal immunity.

3. **Precautions and monitoring parameters**
   a. Oral acyclovir may induce nausea, vomiting, diarrhea, and headache.
   b. IV administration may cause nephrotoxicity, neurologic effects (e.g., lethargy, confusion, tremors, agitation, seizures, coma, obtundation), hypotension, rash, itching, and inflammation and phlebitis at the injection site.
   c. Local discomfort and pruritus may result from topical administration.

4. **Drug interaction. Probenecid** may increase blood concentrations of acyclovir, possibly causing toxicity.

C. Amantadine, a synthetic tricyclic amine with a unique chemical structure, serves as a valuable agent against influenza A viral infection.

1. **Mechanism of action**. Amantadine inhibits replication of the influenza A virus by interfering with viral attachment and uncoating.

2. **Spectrum of activity and therapeutic uses**
   a. Amantadine is effective in the prophylaxis and treatment of influenza A virus.
   b. Clinicians recommend that all nonimmunized high-risk patients receive this drug at the first sign of community influenza A activity.
   c. Suppressive therapy should continue for 24 to 48 hours after influenza symptoms disappear or, if necessary, up to 90 days for repeated exposure to the virus.
   d. This drug may be used to treat some patients with parkinsonism.

3. **Precautions and monitoring parameters**
   a. The most pronounced adverse effects of amantadine are ataxia, nightmares, and insomnia. Other CNS effects include depression, confusion, dizziness, fatigue, anxiety, and headache. Patients with a history of epilepsy and psychiatric disorders should be monitored closely during therapy.
   b. Anticholinergic reactions (dry mouth, blurred vision, tachycardia) have been reported.

D. Ribavirin is a synthetic nucleoside analogue that plays a key role in the treatment of respiratory syncytial virus.

1. **Mechanism of action**. Ribavirin may inhibit RNA and DNA synthesis by depleting intracellular nucleotide reserves.

2. **Spectrum of activity**. This agent is active in vitro against RNA and DNA viruses, such as influenza A and B, respiratory syncytial virus, and herpes simplex.

3. **Therapeutic uses**. Administered in aerosol form, ribavirin is used to relieve symptoms and speed recovery in young adults with influenza A and B and in children with respiratory syncytial virus.

4. **Precautions and monitoring parameters**
   a. Ribavirin must be administered only with a specific small-particle aerosol generator (Viratek SPAG-2).
   b. This agent is contraindicated in patients using respirators because it may precipitate on respirator valves and tubing, causing lethal malfunction. (However, use of a prefilter may permit ribavirin therapy in such patients.)
   c. Serious adverse effects include cardiac arrest, deterioration of pulmonary function, bacterial pneumonia, and apnea.
   d. Rash, conjunctivitis, and reticulocytosis have been reported.

E. Vidarabine, an adenosine analogue, is useful in the treatment of serious herpes infections.

1. **Mechanism of action**. Vidarabine inhibits viral multiplication by becoming incorporated into viral DNA.

2. **Spectrum of activity and therapeutic uses**. Vidarabine is effective against herpes simplex encephalitis (administered intravenously) and herpes simplex keratoconjunctivitis (administered as a topical ophthalmic agent). In immunocompromised patients, it is given intravenously to treat herpes zoster infection.

3. **Precautions and monitoring parameters**
   a. The most common adverse effects of vidarabine are nausea, diarrhea, and rash.
   b. Dose-related CNS toxicity (manifested by tremors, dizziness, confusion, and ataxia) may develop.
   c. IV administration requires dilution in a large volume of fluid, posing a danger to patients with cardiac or renal disease.
   d. Vidarabine may be carcinogenic and mutagenic.

4. **Drug interaction. Allopurinol** increases the risk of CNS toxicity.

F. Zidovudine is a synthetic thymidine analogue. Formerly called azidothymidine (AZT), this agent is the first available drug for the treatment of human immunodeficiency virus (HIV) infection in patients with AIDS and AIDS-related complex (ARC).

1. **Mechanism of action**. Zidovudine inhibits the enzyme reverse transcriptase, terminating synthesis of viral DNA and preventing HIV replication.

2. **Spectrum of activity and therapeutic uses**. Zidovudine has been shown to slow virus production, alleviate symptoms, and prolong life in some patients with AIDS and ARC. The drug may decrease HIV excretion and infectivity.

3. **Precautions and monitoring parameters**
   a. Zidovudine can cause severe bone marrow suppression leading to anemia, granulocytopenia, and thrombocytopenia. Patients may require blood transfusions to reverse anemia.
   b. Other adverse effects include headache, agitation, confusion, anxiety, insomnia, rash, and itching.

4. **Drug interactions**
   a. **Co-trimoxazole** (trimethoprim–sulfamethoxazole) may impair zidovudine metabolism, causing increased zidovudine toxicity.
   b. Other **cytotoxic drugs** can cause additive bone marrow suppression.
   c. Fatigue and lethargy may develop with concurrent **acyclovir** therapy.

STUDY QUESTIONS

Directions: Each question below contains five suggested answers. Choose the **one best** response to each question.

1. Isoniazid is a primary antitubercular agent that

A. requires pyridoxine supplementation
B. may discolor the tears, saliva, urine, or feces orange–red
C. causes ocular complications that are reversible if the drug is discontinued
D. may be ototoxic and nephrotoxic
E. should never be used due to hepatotoxic potential

2. All of the following factors may increase the risk of nephrotoxicity from gentamicin therapy EXCEPT

A. age over 70 years
B. prolonged courses of gentamicin therapy
C. concurrent amphotericin B therapy
D. trough gentamicin levels below 2 μg/ml
E. concurrent cisplatin therapy

3. Which of the following groups contains four drugs that warrant careful monitoring for drug-related seizures in high-risk patients?

A. Penicillin G, imipenem, amphotericin B, metronidazole
B. Penicillin G, chloramphenicol, tetracycline, vancomycin
C. Imipenem, tetracycline, vancomycin, sulfadiazine
D. Cycloserine, metronidazole, vancomycin, sulfadiazine
E. Metronidazole, imipenem, doxycycline, erythromycin

4. Spectinomycin is an aminoglycoside-like antibiotic indicated for the treatment of

A. gram-negative bacillary septicemia
B. tuberculosis
C. penicillin-resistant gonococcal infections
D. syphilis
E. gram-negative meningitis due to susceptible organisms

5. Robert O. has an *Escherichia coli* bacteremia with a low-grade fever (101.6° F). Appropriate management of his fever would be to

A. give acetaminophen 650 mg orally every 4 hours
B. give aspirin 650 mg orally every 4 hours
C. give alternating doses of aspirin and acetaminophen every 4 hours
D. withhold antipyretics and use the fever curve to monitor his response to antibiotic therapy
E. use tepid water baths to reduce the fever

6. Elsie F. has an upper respiratory infection. Six years ago she experienced an episode of bronchospasm following penicillin V therapy. The cultures now reveal a strain of *Streptococcus pneumoniae* that is sensitive to all of the following drugs. Which of these drugs would be the best choice for this patient?

A. Augmentin (amoxicillin/clavulanate)
B. Erythromycin
C. Ampicillin
D. Cefaclor
E. Cyclacillin

7. All of the following drugs are suitable oral therapy for a lower urinary tract infection due to *Pseudomonas aeruginosa* EXCEPT

A. norfloxacin
B. trimethoprim–sulfamethoxazole
C. ciprofloxacin
D. carbenicillin
E. methenamine mandelate

8. Julia C.'s neglected hangnail has developed into a mild staphylococcal cellulitis. Which of the following regimens would be appropriate oral therapy?

A. Dicloxacillin 125 mg q6h
B. Vancomycin 250 mg q6h
C. Methicillin 500 mg q6h
D. Cefazolin 1g q8h
E. Penicillin V 500 mg q6h

Directions: Each question below contains three suggested answers of which **one or more** is correct. Choose the answer

- **A** if **I only** is correct
- **B** if **III only** is correct
- **C** if **I and II** are correct
- **D** if **II and III** are correct
- **E** if **I, II, and III** are correct

9. Drugs usually active against penicillinase-producing *Staphylococcus aureus* include which of the following?

I. Timentin (ticarcillin–clavulanate)
II. Augmentin (amoxicillin–clavulanate)
III. Oxacillin

Directions: The groups of questions below consist of lettered choices followed by several numbered items. For each numbered item select the **one** lettered choice with which it is **most** closely associated. Each lettered choice may be used once, more than once, or not at all.

Questions 10–14

For each description of activity or therapeutic use given below, select the anti-infective agent that it best describes.

A. Demeclocycline
B. Cefaclor
C. Clavulanic acid
D. Methenamine mandelate
E. Amantadine

10. Oral cephalosporin active against *Hemophilus influenzae*

11. A β-lactamase inhibitor

12. Exerts an antibacterial effect by formaldehyde formation

13. Used to treat the syndrome of inappropriate antidiuretic hormone (SIADH) secretion

14. Improves symptoms in patients with Parkinson's disease

Questions 15–19

For each adverse reaction described below, select the anti-infective agent with which it is most likely to be associated.

A. Minocycline
B. Amikacin
C. Chloramphenicol
D. Erythromycin
E. Metronidazole

15. May increase serum theophylline levels

16. Vestibular reactions commonly reported

17. May cause disulfiram-type reaction with alcohol ingestion

18. Nephrotoxicity and ototoxicity are major limiting adverse reactions

19. May cause dose-related bone marrow suppression

ANSWERS AND EXPLANATIONS

1. The answer is A. (*V B 2*) Isoniazid increases the excretion of pyridoxine, which can lead to peripheral neuritis, especially in poorly nourished patients. Pyridoxine (a form of vitamin B_6) deficiency may cause convulsions as well as the neuritis, involving synovial tenderness and swelling. Treatment with the vitamin can reverse the neuritis and prevent or cure the seizures.

2. The answer is D. (*II B 4 b*) Trough serum levels below 2 μg/ml are considered appropriate for gentamicin and are recommended to minimize the risk of toxicity from this aminoglycoside. Because the aminoglycosides accumulate in the proximal tubule of the kidney, nephrotoxicity can occur.

3. The answer is A. [*II E 7 b; L 6 d (2); III B 4 b; IV C 3 c*] Seizures have been attributed to the use of penicillin G, imipenem, amphotericin B, and metronidazole. Seizures are especially likely with high doses in patients with a history of seizures and in patients with impaired drug elimination.

4. The answer is C. (*II L 7*) Although active against various gram-negative organisms, spectinomycin is approved only for the treatment of gonorrhea and is particularly recommended for treatment of uncomplicated forms of the disease.

5. The answer is D. (*I H 1*) The fever curve is very useful for monitoring a patient's response to antimicrobial therapy. Antipyretics can be used to reduce high fever in patients at risk for complications (e.g., seizures) or, in some cases, to make the patient more comfortable.

6. The answer is B. (*II D 3*) Amoxicillin, ampicillin, and cyclacillin are all penicillins and should be avoided in patients with histories of hypersensitivity to other penicillin compounds. While the risk of cross-reactivity with cephalosporins (e.g., cefaclor) is now considered very low, most clinicians avoid the use of these agents in patients with histories of type I hypersensitivity reactions (anaphylaxis, bronchospasm, giant hives).

7. The answer is B. (*II H 3, I 3 d, K, L 8 b*) Norfloxacin, ciprofloxacin, carbenicillin, and methenamine mandelate achieve urine concentrations high enough to treat urinary tract infection due to *Pseudomonas aeruginosa*. Trimethoprim–sulfamethoxazole is not useful for infection due to this organism, although the combination is useful for certain other urinary tract infections.

8. The answer is A. (*II C 3 a; E 5 c; F 2, 3; L 9 c; Table 35-1*) Although vancomycin, methicillin, and cefazolin have excellent activity against staphylococci, they are not effective orally for systemic infections. Vancomycin is prescribed orally for infections limited to the gastrointestinal tract, but because it is poorly absorbed orally, it is not effective for systemic infections. Most hospital- and community-acquired staphylococci are currently resistant to penicillin V. Thus, of the drugs listed in the question, the most appropriate for oral therapy of staphylococcal cellulitis is dicloxacillin.

9. The answer is E (all). (*II F 2; G 2, 3*) Timentin and augmentin each include a β-lactamase inhibitor, combined with ticarcillin and amoxicillin, respectively. These combinations offer activity against *Staphylococcus aureus* similar to that of the penicillinase-resistant penicillins, such as oxacillin.

10–14. The answers are: 10-B, 11-C, 12-D, 13-A, 14-E. (*II C 2, D 3 a, E 6 a, G 3 c, J 3 e, K 1 a; VI C 2 d; Table 35-1*) Anti-infective agents treat infection by suppressing or destroying the causative microorganisms. These agents differ widely in their mechanisms of anti-microbial action. For example, cephalosporins and penicillins inhibit bacterial cell wall synthesis; aminoglycosides and erythromycins inhibit protein synthesis within the bacterial cell. Methenamine is hydrolyzed to ammonia and formaldehyde in acidic urine, and formaldehyde has an antibacterial action. Penicillins, cephalosporins, and certain other antibacterials have a β-lactam ring in their chemical structure. Some bacteria, most notably staphylococci, produce β-lactamases. These enyzmes destroy the β-lactam ring and thereby inactivate the antimicrobial drug. Some β-lactam antimicrobials (e.g., amoxicillin) can be combined with a β-lactamase inhibitor, such as clavulanic acid; this maintains their antimicrobial effectiveness against β-lactamase–producing organisms. Sometimes the pharmacologic actions of a drug will suggest its potential value for a disease unrelated to the drug's primary uses. Thus, for example, the effects of demeclocycline on the kidney make it useful for treating patients with an excess of antidiuretic hormone. Sometimes the ancillary pharmacologic benefits of a drug are unexpected, as when the antiviral agent amantadine was found to improve the symptoms of patients with Parkinson's disease.

15–19. The answers are: 15-D, 16-A, 17-E, 18-B, 19-C. [*II B 4, D 5 b, J 4 i, L 2 d (1); IV C 3 c (5); V B 2 d, 3 d*] The unwanted effects of drugs are all too many and highly varied in both nature and severity.

Sometimes a likely side effect can be predicted from a drug's known pharmacologic effects or from clinical experience with a related drug. Sometimes the relationship between a drug and an untoward event can only be established by cumulated clinical statistics. The pharmacist can play an important role in anticipating and forestalling known adverse drug reactions by acquiring a broad knowledge of drug effects, interactions between drugs, and the way that patient factors alter the expected effects of drugs.

36
Seizure Disorders

Glenda P. Meneilly

I. GENERAL CONSIDERATIONS

A. Definitions

1. **Seizure** is a sudden brief episode of abnormal sensory or somatosensory phenomena, unusual motor or autonomic nervous system activity, or alteration in consciousness.

2. **Epilepsy** is a chronic disorder characterized by recurrent seizures.

B. Classification.
The International Classification of Epileptic Seizures* is a universally accepted system that divides seizures into four main categories and their subgroups (Table 36-1). Seizures also may be classified according to their etiology, as discussed in section I D.

1. **Partial seizures** are the most common seizure type, occurring in approximately 80% of epileptics.
   a. They begin locally but may extend to other or all brain areas.
   b. Partial seizures sometimes involve loss of consciousness.
   c. Manifestations depend on the site of the epileptogenic focus in the brain.

2. **Generalized seizures** are diffuse, affecting both cerebral hemispheres.
   a. These seizures begin in a deeper brain region than do partial seizures.
   b. Consciousness is usually impaired.
   c. Manifestations include bilateral motor disturbances.

C. Incidence

1. Epilepsy affects roughly 1% to 2% of the United States population. According to some estimates, 1 in every 15 children experiences a seizure by age 7.

2. Approximately 70% of epileptics have only one seizure type; the remainder have two or more seizure types.

D. Etiology.
Some seizures arise secondary to other conditions. However, in most cases, the cause of the seizure is unknown.

1. **Primary (idiopathic) seizures** have no identifiable cause.
   a. This type of seizure affects about 75% of epileptics.
   b. Onset of primary seizures typically occurs before age 20.
   c. Birth trauma, hereditary factors, and unexplained metabolic disturbances have been proposed as possible causes of primary seizures.

2. **Secondary seizures** (also called **symptomatic** or **acquired seizures**) occur secondary to an identifiable cause.
   a. Disorders that may lead to seizures include:
      (1) Intracranial neoplasms
      (2) Infectious diseases, such as meningitis, influenza, toxoplasmosis, mumps, measles, and syphilis
      (3) High fever (in children)
      (4) Head trauma
      (5) Congenital diseases
      (6) Metabolic disorders, such as hypoglycemia and hypocalcemia
      (7) Alcohol or drug withdrawal

---

*Commission on the Classification and Terminology of the International League Against Epilepsy, 1981. Reprinted with permission from Adams RD, Victor M: *Principles of Neurology*, 3rd ed. New York, McGraw-Hill, 1985.

Table 36-1. International Classification of Epileptic Seizures

I. Partial seizures (seizures beginning locally)
  A. Simple partial seizures (consciousness not impaired)
    1. With motor symptoms
    2. With somatosensory or special sensory symptoms
    3. With autonomic symptoms
    4. With psychic symptoms
  B. Complex partial seizures (with impairment of consciousness)
    1. Simple partial onset followed by impairment of consciousness
    2. With impairment of consciousness at onset
      a. Impairment of consciousness only
      b. Automatisms accompanying impairment of consciousness
  C. Partial seizures evolving to secondary generalized seizures
    1. Simple partial seizures with generalized evolution
    2. Complex partial seizures with generalized evolution

II. Generalized seizures (bilaterally symmetric and without local onset)
  A. Absence seizures (petit mal)
  B. Myoclonic seizures
  C. Clonic seizures
  D. Tonic seizures
  E. Tonic–clonic seizures (grand mal)
  F. Atonic seizures

III. Unclassified seizures (due to incomplete data)

(8) Lipid storage disorders
(9) Developmental abnormalities

b. Age at seizure onset suggests the precipitating cause (Table 36-2).

E. Pathophysiology. Seizures reflect a sudden, abnormal, excessive neuronal discharge in the cerebral cortex.

1. The mechanisms underlying the discharge are poorly understood. The following theories have been offered.

a. Epileptics may have a deficiency of γ-aminobutyric acid (GABA), the major inhibitory neurotransmitter.

b. A diencephalic nerve group that normally suppresses excessive brain discharge may be deafferentated, hypersensitive, and vulnerable to activation by various stimuli in epileptics.

c. Epileptics may be genetically predisposed to a lower seizure threshold.

2. The abnormal electrical brain activity occurring during a seizure usually produces characteristic changes on the electroencephalogram (EEG), as discussed in section I F 2 b.

Table 36-2. Probable Causes of Recurrent Seizures by Age Group

Age at Seizure Onset	Probable Cause of Seizure
Birth–1 month	Birth injury or anoxia, congential or hereditary disease, metabolic disorder
1–6 months	As above, plus infantile spasms
6 months–3 years	Infantile spasms, febrile convulsions, birth injury or anoxia, meningitis, head trauma
3–10 years	Birth injury or anoxia, meningitis, cerebral vessel thrombosis, idiopathic epilepsy
10–18 years	Idiopathic epilepsy, head trauma
18–25 years	Idiopathic epilepsy, trauma, neoplasm, withdrawal from alcohol or drugs
35–60 years	Trauma, neoplasm, vascular disease, withdrawal from alcohol or drugs
Over 60 years	Vascular disease, neoplasm, degenerative disease, trauma

3. At the **neuronal level**, the following events take place during a seizure.

a. The glial cell fails to maintain extracellular potassium concentrations at a normal level.

b. Potassium leakage at the dendrite leads to abnormal neuronal excitability.

c. Increased cell membrane permeability causes impaired potassium pumping, leading to rapid, repetitive depolarization.

d. Reverse activation occurs across the synapse.

4. Seizure phases. Seizure activity may include three major phases.

a. A **prodrome** may precede the seizure by hours or days.

(1) Prodromal changes in behavior or mood typically occur.

(2) This phase may include an **aura**—a subjective sensation, such as an unusual smell or flashing light.

b. The **ictal phase** is the seizure itself. In some cases, its onset is heralded by a scream or cry.

c. The **postictal phase** takes place immediately after the seizure.

(1) Extensor plantar reflexes may appear.

(2) The victim typically exhibits lethargy, confusion, and behavioral changes.

F. Clinical evaluation

1. Physical findings during a seizure vary with the seizure type and phase. An **eyewitness account** of the seizure is crucial to differential diagnosis.

a. Partial seizures. Manifestations reflect the local origin of the abnormal brain activity.

(1) Simple partial seizures generally do not cause loss of consciousness.

(a) Signs and symptoms of simple partial seizures may be primarily motor, sensory, somatosensory, autonomic, or psychic.

(i) Motor signs include convulsive jerking, chewing motions, and lip smacking.

(ii) Sensory and **somatosensory manifestations** include paresthesias and auras.

(iii) Sweating, flushing, and pupil dilatation are common **autonomic signs**.

(iv) Psychic manifestations, which are sometimes accompanied by impaired consciousness, include déjà vu experiences, structured hallucinations, and dysphasia.

(b) Signs and symptoms may help pinpoint the site of the abnormal brain discharge. For example, localized numbness or tingling reflects a dysfunction in the sensory cortex, located in the parietal lobe.

(2) Complex partial seizures are accompanied by impaired consciousness (however, in some cases, the impairment precedes or follows the seizure). These seizures have variable manifestations.

(a) Purposeless behavior is common.

(b) The affected person may have a glassy stare and may wander aimlessly and speak unintelligibly.

(c) Psychomotor (temporal lobe) epilepsy may lead to aggressive behavior (e.g., outbursts of rage or violence).

(d) Postictal confusion usually persists for 1 to 2 minutes after the seizure ends.

(e) Automatisms (e.g., picking at clothes) are common and may follow visual, auditory, or olfactory hallucinations.

b. Generalized seizures may cause either minor or major signs and symptoms.

(1) Absence (petit mal) seizures present as alterations of consciousness (absences) lasting 10 to 30 seconds.

(a) Staring (with occasional eye blinking) and loss or reduction in postural tone are typical. If the seizure takes place during conversation, the victim may break off in midsentence.

(b) Enuresis and other autonomic components may occur during absence seizures.

(c) Some patients experience 100 or more absences daily.

(d) Onset of this seizure type occurs from ages 3 to 16; in most patients, the seizures disappear by age 40.

(2) Myoclonic (bilateral massive epileptic myoclonus) seizure presents as involuntary jerking of the facial, limb, or trunk muscles, possibly in a rhythmic manner.

(3) Clonic seizures are characterized by sustained muscle contractions alternating with relaxation.

(4) Tonic seizures involve sustained tonic muscle extension (stiffening).

(5) Generalized (grand mal) tonic–clonic seizures cause sudden loss of consciousness.

(a) The victim becomes rigid and falls to the ground. Respiration is interrupted. The legs extend and the back arches; contraction of the diaphragm may induce grunting. This **tonic phase** lasts for about 1 minute.

(b) A **clonic phase** follows, marked by rapid bilateral muscle jerking, muscle flaccidity, and hyperventilation. Incontinence, tongue biting, tachycardia, and heavy salivation sometimes occur.

(c) During the postictal phase, the victim may experience headache, confusion, disorientation, nausea, drowsiness, and muscle soreness. This phase may last for hours.

(d) Some epileptics have **serial grand-mal seizures**, regaining consciousness briefly between attacks. In some cases, grand-mal seizures occur repeatedly, with no recovery of consciousness between attacks. Called **status epilepticus**, this disorder is discussed in section IV A.

(6) Atonic seizures (drop attacks) are characterized by sudden loss of postural tone so that the victim falls to the ground. They occur primarily in children.

2. Diagnostic test results

a. Laboratory findings

(1) Blood analysis

(a) Complete blood count (CBC), blood chemistry assays, and serum glucose and electrolyte measurement are useful in detecting the underlying cause of seizures.

(b) Measurement of **serum drug levels** may reveal ingestion of drugs (e.g., antidepressants, amphetamines) as the cause of seizures.

(2) **Liver** and **kidney function tests** may suggest that seizures stem from hepatic or renal impairment.

b. An **EEG** can confirm epilepsy by identifying paroxysmal brain dysrhythmias. However, a normal EEG does not rule out epilepsy because the abnormalities usually are intermittent. Epileptic EEG patterns contain **focal waves**, **slow waves**, or **spikes**.

c. **Computed tomography (CT)** and **magnetic resonance imaging (MRI) scans** may indicate brain abnormalities, including tumors and temporal horn atrophy (typical of psychomotor epilepsy).

d. **Skull x-rays** may suggest trauma-induced asymmetries or pineal body calcification as the cause of seizures.

e. **Radionuclide brain scans** may detect such seizure causes as subdural hematoma or arteriovenous malformation.

f. **Pneumoencephalogram** may indicate a cerebrospinal fluid (CSF) obstruction—also a possible seizure cause.

g. **Lumbar puncture** may be done to examine CSF for evidence of an infectious disease as the precipitating cause.

II. TREATMENT OBJECTIVES

A. To prevent or suppress seizures or reduce their frequency through drug therapy

B. To control or eliminate the factors that cause or precipitate seizures

C. To prevent serious consequences of seizures (such as anoxia, airway occlusion, or injury) by protecting the tongue and placing a pillow under the victim's head

D. To encourage a normal lifestyle and prevent an invalid attitude

III. THERAPY

A. Drug therapy

1. Approximately 50% of epileptics achieve complete seizure control through drug therapy. In another 25%, drugs reduce the frequency of seizures.

2. Epileptics generally require drug therapy on a continuing basis for at least 4 seizure-free years.

3. New antiseizure drugs have helped to refine epilepsy therapy and provide treatment for previously unresponsive seizure types.

4. Widespread access to accurate methods for monitoring serum drug concentrations has reduced the incidence of adverse effects and toxicity from antiseizure drugs.

5. The specific antiseizure drug used varies with the seizure type. Some patients with mixed seizure types require a combination of drugs.

6. The drug regimen must be further individualized through a system of **pyramidal drug administration**.

a. Initially, a single first-line agent with proven efficacy against the patient's specific seizure type is given at a low dosage.

b. The dosage is increased gradually until one of the following occurs:

(1) Seizures are suppressed.

(2) The serum drug level reaches the upper limit of the therapeutic range.
(3) Serious adverse effects occur.

c. If seizures recur after the maximum tolerated dosage is reached, a second antiseizure drug is added at a low dosage.
(1) The dosage of the second drug is increased until a therapeutic level is reached.
(2) The first drug is maintained until the optimal dosage of the second drug is determined. Then, the first drug is discontinued. **Withdrawal must be gradual** because rapid withdrawal may trigger seizure activity.

7. **Serum drug level monitoring**. Steady-state levels of antiseizure drugs must be measured regularly to ensure safe and effective therapy.
a. Levels should be measured when therapy begins in order to establish an appropriate drug regimen.
b. During ongoing therapy, serum monitoring is necessary if seizure control is poor, adverse effects develop, the dosage must be adjusted, or a new drug is added.
c. Regular monitoring also helps evaluate patient compliance. For therapeutic serum levels of major antiseizure drugs, see Table 36-3 and section III A 8.

8. **Specific antiseizure agents**. Drugs used to control seizures fall into four main groups—hydantoins, barbiturates, benzodiazepines, and succinimides—and a miscellaneous category.
a. **Hydantoins** include **phenytoin**, **mephenytoin**, and **ethotoin**.
(1) **Mechanism of action**. These agents stabilize neuronal membranes and restrict the spread of the seizure discharge by reducing influx or enhancing efflux of sodium ions across motor cortex cell membranes.
(2) **Indications**
(a) **Phenytoin** is a first-line agent for most seizure types, including generalized tonic–clonic seizures and partial seizures (both simple and complex). It is not effective for absence seizures. Phenytoin also is used as an antiarrhythmic (see Chapter 32).

Table 36-3. Drugs of Choice and Alternatives for Major Seizure Disorders

Seizure Disorder	Drug Therapy	Usual Daily Adult Dosage (mg)	Therapeutic Serum Range (μg/ml)
Generalized tonic–clonic seizure (grand mal)	**Preferred drug**		
	Carbamazepine	600–1200	6–12
	or		
	Phenytoin	300–400	10–20
	or		
	Valproate	1000–3000	50–100
	Alternatives		
	Phenobarbital	120–250	15–35
	or		
	Primidone	750–1500	6–12
Partial seizure	**Preferred drug**		
	Carbamazepine	600–1200	6–12
	or		
	Phenytoin	300–400	10–20
	Alternatives		
	Phenobarbital	120–250	15–35
	or		
	Primidone	750–1500	6–12
Absence seizure (petit mal)	**Preferred drug**		
	Ethosuximide	750–2000	40–100
	or		
	Valproate	1000–3000	50–100
	Alternative		
	Clonazepam	1.5–20	0.013–0.072
Atypical absence, myoclonic, or atonic seizure	**Preferred drug**		
	Valproate	1000–3000	50–100
	Alternative		
	Clonazepam	1.50–20	0.013–0.072

(b) **Mephenytoin**, a hydantoin derivative, has a spectrum similar to that of phenytoin.
(c) **Ethotoin**, also a hydantoin derivative, has some value in generalized seizures and complex partial seizures. However, it is much less effective than phenytoin and thus is used mainly as an adjunctive agent in combination with other antiseizure drugs.

(3) Administration and dosage

(a) Phenytoin

(i) The usual adult daily dosage is 300 to 400 mg, with adjustments made as needed.
(ii) The usual daily dosage for children is 4 to 7 mg/kg, divided every 12 hours.
(iii) Phenytoin sodium is available as capsules and parenteral solution. Phenytoin is available as tablets and oral suspension.
(iv) Regular daily dosages above 500 mg are poorly tolerated.
(v) For adults, a loading dose of 900 mg to 1.5 g may be given intravenously. (For children, the loading dose is 15 mg/kg.) The infusion rate should not exceed 50 mg/min. (Alternatively, an oral loading dose may be given.)

(b) **Mephenytoin** is given orally in a usual adult dosage of 200 to 600 mg/day. Children typically receive 100 to 400 mg/day.
(c) **Ethotoin**, also an oral agent, is administered in a usual adult daily dosage of 2 to 3 g, divided four times. For children, the maximum dosage is 250 mg given two to four times per day.

(4) Precautions and monitoring effects

(a) Hydantoins are contraindicated in patients with hydantoin hypersensitivity; they should be used cautiously in patients receiving more than one hydantoin compound.
(b) CBC should be monitored regularly for evidence of megaloblastic anemia.
(c) Dose-related adverse effects involving the central nervous system (CNS) include nystagmus, ataxia, confusion, slurred speech, and drowsiness. These reactions are most common with phenytoin
(d) Nausea, vomiting, and gingival hyperplasia may occur.
(e) Agranulocytosis, skin rash, exfoliative dermatitis, toxic epidermal necrolysis, and Stevens-Johnson syndrome have been reported.
(f) Liver function tests should be monitored because hepatic granuloma or hepatitis may develop.
(g) **Therapeutic serum levels** for phenytoin are 10 to 20 μg/ml; for mephenytoin, 25 to 40 μg/ml. A phenytoin level above 25 μg/ml may exacerbate seizures.
(h) **Significant interactions**

(i) Hydantoin activity may increase, resulting in toxicity, when hydantoins are given concurrently with **antihistamines**, **chloramphenicol**, **isoniazid**, **salicylates**, **valproate**, **oral anticoagulants**, **cimetidine**, **diazoxide**, **sulfamethizole**, or **diazepam**.
(ii) **Alcohol** and **folic acid** may lead to reduced hydantoin activity and consequent reduction in therapeutic efficacy.

b. Barbiturate compounds currently used for seizure disorders include **phenobarbital**, **mephobarbital**, and **primidone** (a deoxybarbiturate).

(1) Mechanism of action

(a) **Phenobarbital** and **mephobarbital** inhibit monosynaptic and polysynaptic transmission and raise the seizure threshold in the motor cortex.
(b) **Primidone** has an unknown mechanism; its antiseizure activity may be partly attributable to phenobarbital, its active metabolite.

(2) Indications

(a) **Phenobarbital** is therapeutic for generalized tonic–clonic seizures and is the preferred agent for children under age 5 with this seizure type. It also is used for complex partial seizures and febrile seizures in children.
(b) **Mephobarbital** is a second-line agent with a spectrum similar to that of phenobarbital.
(c) **Primidone** is used to treat all seizure types except absence seizures.

(3) Administration and dosage

(a) When used in the treatment of seizures, **phenobarbital** usually is administered orally to adults at 120 to 250 mg/day (in three divided doses or as a single bedtime dose). Children typically receive 3 to 6 mg/kg/day in two divided doses. Adjustment is made as needed.
(b) **Mephobarbital** is available in oral form. The usual adult dosage is 400 to 600 mg/day (it can be taken in divided doses). The usual children's dosage is 6 to 12 mg/kg/day, divided every 6 to 8 hours.

(c) **Primidone** is given orally at 750 to 1500 mg/day in four divided doses (adults) or 10 to 25 mg/kg/day in four divided doses (children).

(4) **Precautions and monitoring effects**

(a) These drugs are contraindicated in patients with barbiturate sensitivity or porphyria. Phenobarbital and mephobarbital are additionally contraindicated in patients with respiratory disease accompanied by dyspnea or obstruction. Phenobarbital also is contraindicated in patients with hepatic dysfunction or nephritis and in lactating women.

(b) Phenobarbital and mephobarbital may cause drowsiness, lethargy, hangover, and confusion. Primidone may cause drowsiness, ataxia, nystagmus, and diplopia.

(c) Barbiturates may induce nausea and vomiting.

(d) Skin reactions (e.g., rash, urticaria, Stevens-Johnson syndrome) have been reported.

(e) CBC should be monitored for evidence of blood dyscrasias.

(f) Liver function tests should be monitored for nonspecific hepatic changes.

(g) **Therapeutic serum levels** are 15 to 35 μg/ml for phenobarbital and mephobarbital and 6 to 12 μg/ml for primidone. (In patients receiving primidone, phenobarbital levels also should be measured; 15 to 35 μg/ml is the therapeutic range.)

(h) **Significant interactions**

(i) Primidone may elevate phenobarbital levels when given concomitantly.

(ii) Excessive CNS depression may result when barbiturates are given with **other CNS depressants** or **alcohol**.

(iii) **Monoamine oxidase (MAO) inhibitors** potentiate the barbiturate effect when given concurrently with phenobarbital or mephobarbital.

(iv) Concurrent administration of **carbamazepine** with primidone may cause primidone toxicity.

(v) **Rifampin** may decrease the effects of phenobarbital and mephobarbital.

(vi) **Valproate** increases phenobarbital levels.

(vii) **Diazepam** causes increased effects of both phenobarbital and diazepam when given concurrently.

c. **Benzodiazepines** approved for use in the long-term treatment of seizure disorders are **clonazepam** and **clorazepate**. (Diazepam, another benzodiazepine, is sometimes used in absence seizures and other minor motor seizures as well as in status epilepticus, as discussed in section IV A 2.)

(1) **Mechanism of action**. The antiseizure effects of these agents apparently stem from their action on the limbic system, thalamus, and hypothalamus.

(2) **Indications**

(a) **Clonazepam** is used to treat absence, atonic, and myoclonic seizures.

(b) **Clorazepate** is an adjunctive agent given in combination with other drugs in the treatment of partial seizures.

(3) **Administration and dosage**

(a) **Clonazepam**, an oral agent, may be given in an initial dosage of 1.5 mg/day for adults or 0.01 to 0.03 mg/day for children; preferably, the dose is divided two or three times. The dosage may be increased to a maximum of 20 mg/day for adults or 0.2 mg/kg/day for children.

(b) **Clorazepate** is administered orally in a maximum initial dosage of 22.5 mg/day in three divided doses for adults; 15 mg/day in two divided doses for children. The dosage may be increased to a maximum of 90 mg/day for adults or 60 mg/day for children.

(4) **Precautions and monitoring effects**

(a) Both drugs are contraindicated in patients with narrow-angle glaucoma. Clorazepate is further contraindicated in patients with psychosis or depression.

(b) Adverse CNS effects include drowsiness, lethargy, ataxia, hangover, and muscle incoordination.

(c) Behavioral disturbances and salivation may develop in children receiving clonazepam.

(d) **Therapeutic serum levels** of clonazepam are 0.013 to 0.072 μg/ml. The range for clorazepate has not been clearly defined.

(e) **Significant interaction**. **Cimetidine** may increase the sedative effect of clorazepate.

d. **Succinimide compounds** used in the treatment of seizure disorders include **ethosuximide**, **methsuximide**, and **phensuximide**.

(1) **Mechanism of action**. These agents increase the seizure threshold; by depressing nerve transmission in the motor cortex, they also reduce the spike and wave EEG patterns that characterize absence seizures.

(2) **Indications**. Succinimides are therapeutic for absence seizures; methsuximide is used primarily for refractory cases.

(3) **Administration and dosage**

(a) **Ethosuximide** is given orally in an initial dosage of 500 mg/day in adults and older children; 250 mg/day in children ages 3 to 6. The dosage may be raised by 250 mg every week, to a maximum of 1.5 g/day (adults) or 750 to 1000 mg/day (children).

(b) **Methsuximide**, also an oral drug, is administered in an initial dosage of 300 mg/day (adults and children). This may be increased by 300 mg weekly, to a maximum of 1.2 g/day, given in divided doses. The usual adult daily dosage is 600 to 1200 mg.

(c) **Phensuximide** is given orally in a usual dosage of 500 mg to 1 g two or three times per day (adults and children).

(4) **Precautions and monitoring effects**

(a) These agents are contraindicated in patients with succinimide hypersensitivity.

(b) Dose-related adverse effects include drowsiness, lethargy, dizziness, headache, nausea, and vomiting.

(c) Patients with preexisting psychiatric disorders may exhibit behavioral disturbances (e.g., agitation, anxiety, aggression).

(d) Skin rash and urticaria have been reported.

(e) Blood dyscrasias (e.g., agranulocytosis, aplastic anemia) may develop, especially with ethosuximide.

(f) **Therapeutic serum levels** of ethosuximide are 40 to 100 μg/ml; for methsuximide, 0.04 to 0.08 μg/ml for the parent drug or 20 to 40 μg/ml for the active *N*-demethyl metabolite.

e. **Miscellaneous antiseizure agents** include **carbamazepine**, **acetazolamide**, and **valproate**.

(1) Mechanism of action

(a) **Carbamazepine** stabilizes neuronal membranes and inhibits the spread of seizure activity by reducing influx or enhancing efflux of sodium ions across motor cortex cell membranes.

(b) **Acetazolamide** presumably limits carbonic anhydrase in the CNS and reduces abnormal electrical discharge.

(c) **Valproate** may enhance brain concentrations of GABA, thereby inhibiting CNS nerve impulses.

(2) **Indications**

(a) **Carbamazepine** is therapeutic for generalized tonic–clonic seizures and partial seizures (both simple and complex).

(b) **Acetazolamide** is given for refractory generalized tonic–clonic seizures, absence seizures, myoclonic seizures, and mixed seizures. (It is also used as a diuretic.)

(c) **Valproate** is especially therapeutic for absence seizures. It also is used to treat mixed seizures, myoclonic seizures, and, on an investigational basis, major motor seizures.

(3) **Administration and dosage**

(a) **Carbamazepine** is given initially in an oral dosage of 200 mg twice daily (adults and children over age 12). This may be increased gradually to 600 to 1200 mg/day (usually given in three divided doses). Children under age 12 usually receive 10 to 20 mg/kg/day in two, three, or four divided doses.

(b) **Acetazolamide** is available in oral and parenteral form. Adults receive 375 mg to 1 g/day (or, when used in combination with other drugs, 250 mg/day). Children receive 8 to 30 mg/kg/day, in three or four divided doses, increased to a maximum of 1.5 g/day.

(c) **Valproate** is administered orally in a usual dosage of 1000 to 3000 mg/day (adults) or 15 to 60 mg/kg/day (children), divided into two or three doses.

(4) **Precautions and monitoring effects**

(a) **Carbamazepine** is contraindicated in patients with hypersensitivity to this drug or tricyclic antidepressants and in patients with bone marrow depression.

(b) **Acetazolamide** is contraindicated in patients with sulfonamide sensitivity, Addison's disease, renal or hepatic impairment, chronic respiratory disease, or metabolic imbalance (e.g., hyponatremia, hypokalemia).

(c) **Valproate** is contraindicated in patients with hepatic dysfunction.

(d) CBC should be monitored for evidence of hematologic toxicity.

(i) **Carbamazepine** may cause aplastic anemia, agranulocytosis, leukocytosis, and thrombocytopenia.

(ii) Aplastic anemia and leukopenia have been reported with the use of **acetazolamide**.

(iii) **Valproate** may lead to thrombocytopenia, increased bleeding time, and inhibited platelet aggregation.

(e) Nausea and vomiting may occur with any of these agents.

(f) Skin rash may develop with **carbamazepine** and **acetazolamide**.
(g) **Valproate** therapy may result in hepatic enzyme elevations or toxic hepatitis.
(h) **Therapeutic serum levels** for carbamazepine are 6 to 12 μg/ml; valproate, 50 to 100 μg/ml.
(i) **Significant interactions**
(i) Carbamazepine levels may increase with concomitant use of **propoxyphene**, **erythromycin**, **isoniazid**, or **troleandomycin**. Carbamazepine levels may decrease with concomitant use of **nicotinic acid**.
(ii) Acetazolamide may antagonize the effect of **methenamine**.
(iii) Valproate toxicity may occur if this drug is administered concurrently with **antacids** or **salicylates**.

B. Surgery. If seizures do not respond to drug therapy, surgery may be performed to remove the epileptogenic brain region.

1. **Indications** for surgery are intractable or disabling seizures recurring for 6 to 12 months.

2. **Stereotaxic surgery** may be used. In this technique, the surgeon uses three-dimensional coordinates to guide a needle through a hole drilled in the skull, then destroys abnormal pathways via small intracerebral incisions.

3. **Other surgical approaches** include temporal lobe resection, removal of the temporal lobe tip, and cerebral hemispherectomy.

IV. COMPLICATIONS

A. Convulsive status epilepticus. This disorder is characterized by rapid repetition of generalized tonic–clonic seizures, with no recovery of consciousness between seizures. This life-threatening condition may persist for hours or even days; if it lasts longer than 1 hour, severe permanent brain damage may result.

1. **Causes** of status epilepticus include poor therapeutic compliance, intracranial infection or neoplasm, alcohol withdrawal, drug overdose, and metabolic imbalance.

2. **Management**
a. A patent airway must be maintained.
b. If the cause of the condition is unknown, 50% dextrose in water (25 to 50 ml) is given intravenously in case hypoglycemia is the cause.
c. If seizures persist, **diazepam** (10 mg) is administered intravenously at a rate not exceeding 2 mg/min, until seizures stop or a total of 20 mg has been given.
d. **Phenytoin** is then administered intravenously no faster than 50 mg/min, to a maximum dose of 11 to 18 mg/kg. Blood pressure is monitored to detect hypotension.
e. If these measures do not stop the seizures, **one** of the following drugs is given.
(1) **Diazepam** via intravenous (IV) drip, as 50 to 100 mg diluted in 500 ml dextrose 5% in water, infused at 40 ml/hr until seizures stop
(2) **Phenobarbital** as an IV infusion of 8 to 20 mg/kg, given no faster than 100 mg/min
f. If seizures continue despite these measures, one of the following steps is then taken.
(1) **Paraldehyde** is given intravenously in a dosage of 0.10 to 0.15 ml/kg diluted to a 4% solution in normal saline solution.
(2) **Lidocaine** is given in an IV loading dose of 50 to 100 mg, followed by an infusion of 1 to 2 mg/min.
(3) **General anesthesia** is induced, with ventilatory assistance and neuromuscular junction blockade.

B. Nonconvulsive status epilepticus. This condition presents as repeated absence seizures or complex partial seizures. The patient's mental state fluctuates; confusion, impaired responses, and automatisms are prominent. **Initial management** typically involves IV diazepam. Complex partial status epilepticus may also necessitate administration of such drugs as phenytoin or phenobarbital.

STUDY QUESTIONS

Directions: Each question below contains five suggested answers. Choose the **one best** response to each question.

1. Phenytoin is effective for treatment of all of the following types of seizures EXCEPT

A. generalized tonic–clonic
B. simple partial
C. complex partial
D. absence
E. grand mal

2. Which of the following anticonvulsants is contraindicated in patients with a history of hypersensitivity to tricyclic antidepressants?

A. Phenytoin
B. Ethosuxamide
C. Acetazolamide
D. Carbamazepine
E. Phenobarbital

3. Which anticonvulsant drug requires therapeutic monitoring of phenobarbital serum levels as well as its own serum levels?

A. Phenytoin
B. Primidone
C. Clonazepam
D. Ethotoin
E. Carbamazepine

ANSWERS AND EXPLANATIONS

1. The answer is D. [*III A 8 a (2) (a)*] Phenytoin (diphenylhydantoin) is the most commonly prescribed hydantoin for seizure disorders. It is one of the preferred drugs for generalized tonic–clonic (grand mal) seizures and for partial seizures, both simple and complex. However, phenytoin is not effective for absence (petit mal) seizures.

2. The answer is D. [*III A 8 e (4) (a)*] Carbamazepine is structurally related to the tricyclic antidepressants (amitriptyline, desipramine, imipramine, nortriptyline, protriptyline) and should not be administered to patients with hypersensitivity to any of the tricyclic antidepressants.

3. The answer is B. [*III A 8 b (4) (g)*] Primidone's antiseizure activity may be partly attributable to phenobarbital. In patients receiving primidone, serum levels of both primidone and phenobarbital should be measured.

37
Parkinson's Disease

Glenda P. Meneilly

I. DEFINITION. Parkinson's disease is a slowly progressive degenerative neurologic disease characterized by tremor, rigidity, bradykinesia (sluggish neuromuscular responsiveness), and postural instability.

II. INCIDENCE

A. It is one of the most common neurologic disorders that occur after age 50 (with an incidence of 100–150/100,000 population).

B. Onset generally occurs between ages 50 and 65; usually in the 60s.

III. PATHOGENESIS

A. The **feedback mechanism** that helps control voluntary movement, coordination, and posture is based in the striatal tract of the substantia nigra (part of the basal ganglia) and relies primarily on two neurotransmitters: dopamine and acetylcholine.

B. Any **disturbance in the balance** between dopaminergic agents (inhibitory agents) and cholinergic agents (excitatory agents) seems to result in movement disorders.

C. Parkinson's disease involves either direct influence on neurotransmitters (as by dopamine agonists) or a slow degeneration of the substantia nigra, both of which result in **changes in neurotransmitter levels**, including:

1. **Dopamine deficiency**, the primary neurotransmitter defect, which results in rigidity and bradykinesia
2. **Relative increase in acetylcholine levels** (in relation to dopamine levels), which results in tremors
3. **Norepinephrine deficiency**, which adds to bradykinesia
4. **Serotonin and gamma-aminobutyric acid (GABA) deficiencies**, which may lessen symptoms

IV. ETIOLOGY. Several forms of Parkinson's disease have been recognized.

A. Primary (idiopathic) Parkinson's disease

1. This is also called classic Parkinson's disease or paralysis agitans.
2. The cause is unknown, and while treatment may be palliative, the disease is incurable.
3. Most patients suffer from this type of parkinsonism.

B. Secondary parkinsonism—due to a known cause

1. Only a small percentage of cases are secondary, and many of these are curable.
2. Secondary parkinsonism may be caused by drugs, including dopamine antagonists, such as:
   a. Phenothiazines (e.g., chlorpromazine, perphenazine)
   b. Butyrophenones (haloperidol)
   c. Reserpine
3. Poisoning by chemicals or toxins may be the cause, including:
   a. Carbon monoxide poisoning

b. Heavy metal poisoning, such as that by manganese or mercury
c. MPTP (N-methyl-4-phenyl-1,2,3,6-tetrahydropyridine), a commercial compound used in organic synthesis and found (as a side product) in an illegal meperidine analogue

4. Infectious causes include:
a. Encephalitis (viral)
b. Syphilis

5. Other causes include:
a. Arteriosclerosis
b. Degenerative diseases of the central nervous system (CNS), such as progressive supranuclear palsy
c. Metabolic disorders, such as Wilson's disease

V. SIGNS AND SYMPTOMS

A. Tremor

1. There are regular, rhythmic pill-rolling or bread-crumbling muscular contractions.

2. The tremor occurs at rest and increases with anxiety or stress but disappears with purposeful movement and during sleep.

B. Muscle rigidity

1. There is resistance to passive movement, beginning in the neck and shoulders and progressing to the face and limbs.

2. The rigidity may be uniform (**lead-pipe rigidity**) or jerky, as in a free movement followed by a sudden catch (**cog-wheel rigidity**).

C. Bradykinesia

1. There is a sluggish response potentially progressing in later stages to inability to initiate movement.

2. Fine motor movements are reduced.

3. A masklike (blank) facial expression occurs, with poor blink reflex and eyes wide open.

4. Drooling may result from dysphagia (difficulty in swallowing) or excessive salivation.

5. Slowed, monotonous, slurred speech may become severely dysarthric.

D. Abnormalities of gait and posture

1. Parkinsonism inflicts a characteristic gait: shuffling steps that become more rapid (the patient seems to be trying to keep from falling forward).

2. An inability to maintain the trunk in an upright position and an increasing postural tilt toward the unaffected side heighten ambulation difficulties.

3. The patient may suddenly freeze while walking and be temporarily unable to resume motion.

4. Uneven or absent correlative motion of the arms is also characteristic.

VI. TREATMENT GOAL. Therapy is aimed at overcoming the dopamine deficiency (see section III), either by stimulating dopamine receptors or by decreasing the excess acetylcholine with anticholinergic agents.

VII. INDIVIDUAL AGENTS

A. Anticholinergic agents

1. General

a. Indications

(1) These agents are most useful in treating the parkinsonian tremor (it may improve by up to 20%); they may also ease rigidity and bradykinesia.

(2) Patients who have a levodopa intolerance (because of side effects or contraindications) or who experience no therapeutic effect from levodopa may benefit from an anticholinergic regimen.

(3) These drugs are also used to supplement levodopa.
(4) Anticholinergic agents are useful for parkinsonian symptoms induced by antipsychotic agents.
(5) Patients with minimal symptoms usually benefit from anticholinergic therapy.
(6) Antihistamines may be better tolerated in the elderly because they produce fewer side effects.

b. These agents are equally effective; none has been shown to outperform the others. The choice of agent depends on the effects—therapeutic and adverse—obtained in each patient.

c. Anticholinergics should be administered one drug at a time, starting with a low dose that is gradually increased until maximum therapeutic benefit is reached or side effects become unacceptable.

d. If therapeutic effect is lacking or unsatisfactory, or the patient develops unacceptable side effects, changing to another agent may help. This is also advisable for patients whose response has diminished after prolonged treatment with one agent.

2. Dosage (Table 37-1)

3. Precautions and monitoring effects

a. Anticholinergics should be used with **caution** in patients with obstruction of the gastrointestinal or genitourinary tracts, narrow-angle glaucoma, or severe cardiac disease.

b. Side effects include:
(1) Peripheral: dry mouth, blurred vision, constipation, urinary retention, tachycardia
(2) Central: hallucinations, ataxia, mental slowing, confusion, memory impairment

c. Side effects may be potentiated by other drugs with anticholinergic activity, such as antihistamines, antidepressants, and phenothiazines.

d. Drugs must be withdrawn gradually to avoid a severe exacerbation of parkinsonian symptoms, which may result in total immobility.

e. Patients on high doses of anticholinergics in combination with levodopa should be watched for decreased levodopa activity due to a delayed gastric emptying time.

f. The sedative side effects of antihistamines may be of benefit in some patients.

B. Dopaminergic agents

1. General. Dopaminergic drugs combat the dopamine deficiency by one of several **mechanisms**:

a. Exogenously replenishing striatal dopamine (**levodopa**)
b. Directly stimulating dopamine receptors (**bromocriptine**)
c. Stimulating presynaptic dopamine release (**amantadine**)

Table 37-1. Drugs for the Treatment of Parkinsonism

Type	Generic Name	Trade Name	Average Daily Dosage Range
Anticholinergic	Benztropine	Cogentin	0.5–6 mg/day
	Biperiden	Akineton	2–8 mg/day
	Cycrimine	Pagitane	1.25–15 mg/day
	Procyclidine	Kemadrin	5–20 mg/day
	Trihexyphenidyl	Artane	2–20 mg/day
Antihistamine	Chlorphenoxamine	Phenoxene	50–400 mg/day
	Diphenhydramine	Benadryl	50–150 mg/day
	Orphenadrine	Disipal	50–300 mg/day
Dopaminergic	Amantadine	Symmetrel	100–300 mg/day
	Bromocriptine	Parlodel	2.5–150 mg/day
	Carbidopa-levodopa	Sinemet	30/300–200/2000 mg/day
	Levodopa	Larodopa, Dopar	500 mg–8 g/day

2. Levodopa

a. General

(1) Dopamine does not cross the blood–brain barrier, so its precursor levodopa is introduced for conversion to dopamine.

(2) Levodopa is metabolized to dopamine by dopa-decarboxylase, both centrally and peripherally.

(3) Levodopa is not generally the first-line treatment because long-term use almost inevitably produces side effects, and the efficacy of levodopa declines after 3 to 5 years. For these reasons, it is usually held in reserve until anticholinergics and antihistamines are insufficient and the patient's symptoms impose some degree of functional disability.

b. Dosage (see Table 37-1)

(1) Levodopa should be given orally, with food.

(2) The starting dosage should be between 500 mg and 1 g daily, followed by gradual incremental increases every few days until either a desirable response is achieved or side effects are not tolerated.

(3) The maximum daily dosage should be 8 g, given in divided doses, at least three times a day.

(4) Maximum benefit is seen after 6 months of treatment.

c. Precautions and monitoring effects

(1) Levodopa has **no defined therapeutic level**.

(2) It should be avoided in patients with a history of melanoma or suspicious skin lesions because levodopa may activate a malignant melanoma.

(3) Gastrointestinal

(a) Nausea and vomiting may occur, especially on initiation of treatment. This can be managed by increasing doses gradually or administering with food. Some patients require a dosage reduction to make nausea tolerable. In patients with severe nausea and vomiting, electrolytes should be monitored.

(b) Gastrointestinal ulceration and bleeding are possible; patients with a history of active peptic ulcer disease should be monitored for signs of internal bleeding.

(c) Bowel irregularity

(4) Cardiovascular

(a) Arrhythmias may develop secondary to tachycardia, so electrocardiogram (ECG) monitoring is advisable.

(b) Postural hypotension may occur, to which tolerance develops. Blood pressure should be monitored, and the patient should be advised that standing up slowly and wearing elastic stockings will help.

(5) Psychiatric. Confusion, agitation, hallucinations, sleep disturbances, and depression affect up to half of all patients on long-term therapy. These symptoms usually respond to dose reduction. Patients with a history of depression or psychoses should be monitored.

(6) Neurologic. Long-term levodopa therapy exacerbates or induces movement disorders in most patients. These involuntary choreiform movements respond to dose reduction but produce a corresponding reduction in control of parkinsonian symptoms.

d. Drug interactions

(1) Antipsychotic agents neutralize the effect of levodopa.

(a) Reserpine, by depleting dopamine

(b) Phenothiazines and butyrophenones, by blockading dopamine receptors

(2) Pyridoxine is a coenzyme for dopa-decarboxylase. Most **multiple vitamin preparations** contain pyridoxine and thus increase decarboxylase activity, increasing peripheral side effects and decreasing the central desired effect of levodopa.

(3) Monoamine oxidase (MAO) inhibitors and levodopa should not be given concurrently. A 2-week interval between drugs is advised.

3. Carbidopa–levodopa

a. General

(1) Levodopa, when given by itself, requires large-dose therapy to treat Parkinson's disease as only a small percentage of it enters the brain. Carbidopa inhibits peripheral decarboxylation of levodopa to dopamine. Because carbidopa does not cross the blood–brain barrier, it makes more levodopa available for transport to the brain while reducing the peripheral side effects.

(2) Carbidopa administration reduces the amount of required levodopa by about 75%.

b. Dosage (see Table 37-1)

(1) Between 75 and 160 mg/day is required to inhibit peripheral dopa-decarboxylase in most patients. Daily doses greater than 200 mg have no advantage. At least 75 mg/day of carbidopa is required for therapeutic effect.

(2) The carbidopa–levodopa combination is **available in**:
(a) **Ratios of 1:10** (carbidopa 10 mg: levodopa 100 mg and carbidopa 25 mg: levodopa 250 mg)
(b) **Ratios of 1:4** (carbidopa 25 mg: levodopa 100 mg)
(3) The dosage should be titrated to relieve symptoms while avoiding unacceptable side effects.
(4) **Suggested regimens for initiating therapy** include:
(a) One tablet of 25/100 three times daily, increased by one tablet daily or every other day to a maximum of six tablets daily.
(b) One tablet of 10/100 three to four times daily, increased by one tablet every other day to a maximum of eight tablets daily.
(5) **Maintenance doses** should be adjusted according to response. If more carbidopa is required, 25/100 tablets can be used. If more levodopa is needed, 25/250 tablets are used.
(6) When a patient is transferred from levodopa to carbidopa–levodopa, the levodopa should be discontinued for at least 8 hours before starting the combination product. The levodopa dose in the combination product should be 25% of the previous levodopa dose.

c. Monitoring effects
(1) The incidence of nausea and vomiting is much less with the combination product.
(2) There is no decrease in the central side effects (such as movement disorders or mental disturbances) experienced with levodopa. In fact, these effects may develop earlier in the therapy and at lower dosages because more dopamine reaches the brain with the combination product.
(3) The monitoring parameters are the same as those for levodopa alone.

d. Drug interactions. Pyridoxine does not interfere with the effectiveness of the combination product because peripheral decarboxylation is inhibited.

4. Bromocriptine

a. General
(1) Bromocriptine is a dopamine agonist that stimulates dopamine receptors directly. It also stimulates dopamine release and inhibits dopamine reuptake.
(2) Bromocriptine is most useful in patients whose response to levodopa is limited or those who experience severe on–off phenomenon (see section VIII).
(3) It is often used as an adjunct to levodopa therapy.
(4) As with levodopa, the duration of benefit is limited to about 2 years.

b. Dosage (see Table 37-1)
(1) After a test dose of 1.25 mg, the initial dosage is 2.5 mg four times daily.
(2) This dose may be increased gradually by 2.5-mg increments until maximum therapeutic response is achieved.
(3) Patient response is extremely variable. Many patients show a dopamine **antagonist response** at both low and high doses with the desirable **agonist response** in the midrange.
(4) Patients on levodopa usually show an improvement of symptoms when bromocriptine is added; therefore, the levodopa dose may be decreased. (If levodopa alone is used, the levodopa dose may be slowly decreased by 40%. If a carbidopa–levodopa combination is used, the amount of levodopa may be decreased by 20%.)
(5) All dosage reductions should be very gradual (i.e., 5 mg every few days).

c. Precautions and monitoring effects
(1) Bromocriptine may cause a **first-dose phenomenon** that can trigger sudden cardiovascular collapse. It should be used with caution in patients with a history of myocardial infarction or arrhythmias.
(2) **Early in therapy**, dizziness, drowsiness, and fainting may occur, so patients should be cautious about driving or operating machinery.
(3) **Postural hypotension**, to which tolerance develops, may occur. Blood pressure should be monitored, particularly for patients taking antihypertensive agents.
(4) **Gastrointestinal disturbances** may be decreased by taking this drug with food.
(5) **Confusion, hallucinations, and psychoses** may be manifested. Patients with an underlying dementia or psychiatric illness should be monitored because bromocriptine may exacerbate these conditions.
(6) The incidence of the side effects listed in (3)–(5) is significantly higher than that with levodopa.
(7) Long-term treatment has been associated with reversible pulmonary changes (such as pulmonary infiltrates, pleural effusion, and pleural thickening), so pulmonary function should be monitored in patients treated for longer than 6 months.

d. Drug interactions. Concurrent administration of dopamine antagonists, such as phenothiazines, and reserpine may decrease the effectiveness of bromocriptine.

5. Amantadine

a. General

(1) Amantadine increases dopamine supplies by releasing endogenous dopamine from presynaptic nerve terminals and, possibly, by inhibiting reuptake.

(2) It may also have some anticholinergic activity.

(3) While more beneficial than the anticholinergics, amantadine is less effective than levodopa. Many patients gain a significant effect when amantadine and levodopa are used in combination.

(4) Amantadine therapy is most efficacious in the first few weeks; its effectiveness declines by the sixth to eighth week.

(5) Patients who do not respond initially may do so later on rechallenge.

b. Dosage (see Table 37-1)

(1) Amantadine should be started at 100 mg/day. This may be increased to 200–300 mg/day as a maintenance dose.

(2) Patients experiencing a decline in response may benefit from either:

(a) Discontinuing the drug for a few weeks, then restarting, or

(b) Using the drug episodically, only when the patient's condition most needs a therapeutic boost

c. Precautions and monitoring effects

(1) Withdrawal of amantadine, or dose reductions, should be done gradually to avoid precipitating a parkinsonian crisis.

(2) This agent should be used cautiously, and in lower doses, in patients with a history of renal impairment or congestive heart failure.

(3) Peripheral effects include edema, urinary retention, orthostatic hypotension, congestive heart failure, dry skin, rash, and livedo reticularis (a benign, blotchy, red-to-purple skin discoloration) usually in the lower extremities. Blood pressure and ECG readings should be monitored, especially in patients with a history of myocardial infarction or arrhythmias.

(4) Central effects include confusion, hallucinations, and depressive psychoses, especially in the elderly. Patients with an underlying psychiatric illness should be monitored for precipitation of symptoms.

(5) Anticholinergic use in combination with amantadine increases the incidence of side effects, such as confusion and pupil dilation.

(6) Convulsions have been reported in patients receiving very high doses of amantadine.

(7) Periodic complete blood counts should be done for patients on long-term therapy.

VIII. ON–OFF PHENOMENON

A. Definition

1. The on–off phenomenon refers to wide swings in drug response to levodopa or dopamine agonists.

2. During "on" periods, patients are symptom-free, while during "off" periods, there is a sudden loss of drug effectiveness, resulting in full-blown symptoms including akinesia.

B. Mechanism

1. The mechanism by which the on–off phenomenon occurs is unknown, but possibilities include the following:

a. Dopamine-receptor sensitivity may be altered due to long-term overstimulation.

b. Blood levels of levodopa may fluctuate.

c. Metabolites of drugs may compete for receptor sites.

C. Types. Several different variations of the phenomenon may occur and include:

1. Early morning rigidity, which may respond to long-acting preparations of drugs or to a drug holiday (see section IX)

2. Freezing episodes (hesitation on initiation of a movement), which do not appear to respond to alterations in medication and may be a sign of progression of the disease itself

3. End-of-dose deterioration, in which symptoms return hours before the next dose (decreasing the dose while increasing the frequency of dopaminergic medications or a drug holiday may be helpful)

IX. DRUG HOLIDAY

A. Definition. Temporary drug withdrawal—a drug holiday—may benefit some patients who experience loss of drug effectiveness with long-term therapy.

B. Procedure. Generally, the patient must be hospitalized in anticipation of function loss and potential complications caused by symptom exacerbation when the drugs (usually levodopa) are withdrawn. After a drug-free period of about 1 week, the drug is reintroduced in gradually increasing doses, titrated to response.

C. Outcome. For many patients, the drug holiday results in a reduction in dosage required for symptom control, a lessening of side effects, and fewer on–off episodes.

STUDY QUESTIONS

Directions: Each question below contains five suggested answers. Choose the **one best** response to each question.

1. The maximum recommended daily dose of levodopa is

A. 500 mg
B. 1 g
C. 2 g
D. 4 g
E. 8 g

2. When administered with carbidopa, the dosage of levodopa is usually decreased by

A. 75%
B. 50%
C. 40%
D. 20%
E. 10%

3. Which of the following agents should not be used concurrently with levodopa?

A. Diphenhydramine
B. Benztropine
C. Amantadine
D. Monoamine oxidase inhibitors
E. Carbidopa

Directions: Each question below contains three suggested answers of which **one or more** is correct. Choose the answer

A if **I only** is correct
B if **III only** is correct
C if **I and II** are correct
D if **II and III** are correct
E if **I, II, and III** are correct

4. Levodopa is associated with which of the following problems?

I. Gastrointestinal side effects
II. Involuntary movements
III. A decline in efficacy after 3–5 years

5. Amantadine has which of the following advantages over levodopa?

I. More rapid relief of symptoms
II. Higher success rate
III. Better long-term effects

ANSWERS AND EXPLANATIONS

1. The answer is E. [*VII B 2 b (3)*] The maximum total daily dose of levodopa should be 8 g, administered in divided doses at least three times a day. Levodopa is used in the treatment of Parkinson's disease to replenish the brain's supply of dopamine, the neurotransmitter that is deficient in this disorder. Dopamine itself does not cross the blood–brain barrier, and therefore its precursor, levodopa, is administered. Levodopa is metabolized to dopamine in the body by dopa decarboxylase. Dosage of levodopa must be carefully titrated for each patient in order to produce the maximum improvement with the least side effects.

2. The answer is A. [*VII B 3 a (2)*] Administering carbidopa in combination with levodopa reduces the required dose of levodopa by about 75%. When levodopa is given alone, much of the dose is metabolized before the drug reaches the brain. Therefore, large doses are required, and these are apt to cause unwanted side effects. Carbidopa inhibits the peripheral decarboxylation of levodopa. This action simultaneously reduces the likelihood of peripheral side effects and allows more levodopa to reach the brain. Since carbidopa does not cross the blood–brain barrier, the levodopa in the brain is converted there to dopamine. Thus, coadministration of carbidopa plus levodopa allows a significant reduction of levodopa dosage without reducing the desired effects.

3. The answer is D. [*VII B 2 d (3)*] Levodopa causes a significant rise in blood pressure as well as flushing and palpitations when given to patients receiving monoamine oxidase inhibitors. Levodopa can be used in combination with any of the other agents listed in the question without adverse interactions. Amantadine causes an increase in the body's dopamine supply, and carbidopa prevents decarboxylation of levodopa. Diphenhydramine (an antihistamine) and benztropine have anticholinergic effects; they are used to treat Parkinson's disease because they decrease the body's acetylcholine supply.

4. The answer is E (all). (*VII B 2 a, c*) Levodopa can cause gastrointestinal side effects such as nausea and vomiting, particularly on initiation of treatment. Bowel irregularity and gastrointestinal bleeding can also occur. With long-term levodopa therapy, involuntary choreiform movements can develop, and the efficacy of the drug declines. Other unwanted effects of levodopa include tachycardia and cardiac arrhythmias, postural hypotension, and psychiatric disturbances such as confusion or depression.

5. The answer is A (I). (*VII B 5*) Amantadine is most efficacious within the first few weeks, while benefits from levodopa may not be seen for weeks to months. Amantadine is more beneficial than the anticholinergics, but is less effective than levodopa. Unfortunately, the efficacy of amantadine declines after 6 to 8 weeks of therapy. The efficacy of levodopa declines after 3 to 5 years of therapy.

38
Schizophrenia

Robert J. Cersosimo

I. GENERAL CONSIDERATIONS

A. Definition. Schizophrenia is a group of disorders involving disruption of thought and disintegration of personality. Symptoms involve alterations in behavior, thought, affect, and perception. Schizophrenia is characterized by the following disturbances in the content and form of thought:

1. Hallucinations
2. Detachment from reality
3. Diminished or inappropriate affect
4. Abnormal motor behavior

B. Incidence. Schizophrenia occurs in about 0.5% to 1% of the general population. Onset is usually between the ages of 15 and 45 years, with distribution between men and women considered about equal.

C. Etiology. Although the actual cause of schizophrenia remains unproven, theorized etiologies can be categorized broadly as genetic, biologic, and psychosocial.

1. **Genetic**. Studies have provided significant data supporting a genetic basis for schizophrenia. The risk factor in the general population is 0.5% to 1% but increases to 5% to 10% if one parent has a history of schizophrenia and may be as high as to 46% if both parents have been affected.
2. **Biologic**. Suspicion of a chemical alteration or imbalance drives this research. The predominant theory, the **dopamine hypothesis**, suggests that dopamine overactivity in the brain is responsible. Additional theories in this category focus on other neurotransmitters.
3. **Psychosocial**. Theories of psychosocial origin abound. Among the proposed causes are stress, lack of interpersonal skills, conflicting and contradictory family communication, and socioeconomic influences. Each theory has its supporters, but none is definitive.

D. Clinical presentation

1. **The four A's**. Characterization of the disorder has not been standardized. Swiss psychiatrist Eugen Bleuler (1857–1939) described the following four "A's" of schizophrenia; however, these have been criticized as fundamental symptoms because they are seen occasionally in nonschizophrenics.
   a. **Association defect**. Impaired thinking is evidenced by illogical or idiosyncratic thought processes. One idea is not obviously connected with the next, and verbalization ranges from subtly confusing to grossly disorganized.
   b. **Affect**. The patient experiences an alteration of mood or feelings; the affect may be flat, with no emotional responsiveness, or inappropriate.
   c. **Ambivalence**. Opposing attitudes may exist simultaneously, or there may be rapid fluctuations among contradictory emotions.
   d. **Autism**. The patient may withdraw into a private world, absorbed in inner thoughts.
2. **Additional features** of importance include the following:
   a. **Hallucinations**. Sensory perceptions may be abnormal, occurring without external stimuli. Any sense may be affected, but auditory hallucinations are the most common.
   b. **Delusions.** Firmly held but false beliefs are expressed that have absolutely no basis in fact.

These may be simple or multiple, poorly or well organized, and bizarre or seemingly realistic. Often they feature persecutory content. Patients may complain that their thoughts are being read by others or are being broadcast to others, that people are spying on them or talking about them, or that they are being controlled.

E. Diagnostic criteria. The current approach to diagnostic criteria is based on the *Diagnostic and Statistical Manual of Mental Disorders*, 3rd ed.—revised (*DSM-III-R*)*, as summarized below.

1. During a phase of the illness, at least one of the following must be present:
   a. Delusions of a bizarre nature
   b. Delusions without persecutory or jealous content
   c. Delusions with persecutory or jealous content and hallucinations
   d. Auditory hallucinations
   e. Loose associations, incoherence, illogical thinking, or poverty of content of speech if associated with at least one of the following: delusions or hallucinations; blunted, flat, or inappropriate affect; or catatonic or other disorganized behavior

2. Deterioration of function must be evidenced in such areas as social relations, self-care, and work.

3. Symptoms must be present continuously for at least 6 months at some time during the patient's life.

4. Organic or affective mental disorders and mental retardation must be ruled out.

5. Onset of illness must occur before age 45 years.

F. Classification of schizophrenia is based on the symptoms predominating at the time of evaluation, but these syndromes may change over time.

1. **Disorganized (hebephrenic) schizophrenia** is characterized by marked incoherence with inappropriate responses or unresponsiveness. Delusions or hallucinations are disorganized and fragmented. The patient may giggle, grimace, and act in an incongruous or silly manner. Hypochondriacal behavior may be present.

2. **Catatonic schizophrenia** is distinguished by marked psychomotor disturbances. The patient may demonstrate rigidity, immobility, or posturing and may also be withdrawn and silent. At the other extreme is characteristic excitement, such as pacing and shouting. Fluctuations between these behavioral extremes may occur.

3. **Paranoid schizophrenia** is identified by its most prominent characteristics: delusions of grandeur or persecution, during which the patient may be extremely aggressive and argumentative, even violent. Many of these patients are intensely concerned with homosexual impulses in themselves or others.

4. **Undifferentiated schizophrenia** may incorporate prominent delusions, hallucinations, incoherence, or grossly disorganized behavior, but the overall picture either does not meet the criteria for one of the specific types or meets the criteria for more than one type.

5. **Residual schizophrenia** designates a patient who, while not currently acutely psychotic, has a history of at least one prior episode of prominent psychotic symptoms. Residual symptoms such as loose or vague associations, illogical thinking, withdrawal, or inappropriate affect may be present, and daily living skills may be impaired.

II. TREATMENT OBJECTIVES

Because there is no known cure for schizophrenia, treatment is primarily symptomatic. The two major therapeutic approaches—psychotherapy and pharmacotherapy with antipsychotic (neuroleptic) agents—share these goals: (A) Bring the patient's thoughts and behavior under control, (B) prevent self-inflicted harm, (C) restore contact with reality, (D) return the patient to society, and (E) prevent a relapse.

III. THERAPY: ANTIPSYCHOTIC AGENTS

A. Choice of agent. All antipsychotic agents are therapeutically equivalent when administered in appropriate doses, but response varies from patient to patient and drug to drug. Consideration should be given to prior medical experience, if applicable. A patient who has failed to respond to a particular drug in the past is not likely to respond to that drug at any time. The major difference among these agents is their adverse effects (see section III F).

*American Psychiatric Association: *Diagnostic and Statistical Manual of Mental Disorders*, 3rd ed.—revised. Washington, DC, 1987.

B. Mechanism of action. Antipsychotic agents are thought to exert their effects through blockade of dopamine receptors in the brain.

C. Specific agents (Table 38–1)

D. Administration and dosage

1. General guidelines

a. A drug response history should be obtained, and potential side effects should be considered.

b. Therapy should be initiated using a single drug administered in divided doses.

c. The first symptoms to respond are usually aggressiveness, paranoia, and irritability; later symptoms to be reduced are hallucinations and changes in social skills.

d. Once the patient has been stabilized, attempts should be made to lower the dose. The lowest possible dose should be used for maintenance.

e. When discontinuing therapy, withdrawal should be tapered.

2. Gradual control method. This is the standard therapeutic method.

a. Initial doses should be at the lower end of the usual daily dose schedule (see Table 38–1), such as 300 to 400 mg of chlorpromazine daily. Doses should be divided initially to allow for observation of effect and toxicity.

b. If no improvement is noted after 1 week, doses may be increased by 25% to 33% weekly if necessary. Increases should be smaller in the elderly and in others known to be at particular risk for adverse effects. For patients who are acutely psychotic and agitated, increases may be larger.

c. Maximal improvement may take 6 to 8 weeks; longer if this is not the initial therapy.

d. Once a patient's response and tolerance have been determined, the drug may be administered in one or two daily doses.

3. Rapid control method. This approach usually is reserved for patients who are acutely psychotic with agitation.

a. High-potency agents, such as fluphenazine or haloperidol, usually are injected intramuscularly. For example, haloperidol may be initiated at a dose of 5 to 10 mg every hour until the acute symptoms are controlled, adverse effects occur, or the patient falls asleep.

b. Once control has been established, therapy should be converted to oral administration. The physician may elect to administer the same agent, but in oral form, at a dose appropriate for initial therapy. Dosage may then be adjusted in accordance with the patient's response.

4. Maintenance therapy to prevent relapse has less clear guidelines.

a. Some practitioners suggest that therapy be continued for 6 months after an acute episode before drug withdrawal is considered. Signs favoring discontinuation of therapy include the following:

(1) Continued control of symptoms during maintenance therapy

(2) No history of relapse ensuing from drug withdrawal

(3) Willingness of the patient to discontinue therapy

Table 38-1. Currently Available Antipsychotic Agents

Agent	Nonproprietary Name	Brand Name	Approximate Equivalent Dose	Usual Daily Dose Range (mg/day)	
				Acute	Maintenance
Phenothiazines					
Aliphatics	Chlorpromazine	Thorazine	100	300–800	100–300
Piperidines	Mesoridazine	Serentil	50	25–400	30–150
	Thioridazine	Mellaril	100	300–800	100–300
Piperazines	Acetophenazine	Tindal	25	40–120	20–40
	Fluphenazine	Prolixin	2	6–60	2–8
	Perphenazine	Trilafon	6–10	16–24	8–24
	Trifluoperazine	Stelazine	3–5	15–60	5–15
Thioxanthenes	Chlorprothixene	Taractan	100	300–600	75–400
	Thiothixene	Navane	3–5	10–60	4–30
Butyrophenones	Haloperidol	Haldol	2	1–100	1–15
Dihydroindolones	Molindone	Moban	10	15–225	15–100
Dibenzoxazepines	Loxapine	Loxitane	15	20–100	60–100

b. Another suggested guideline is to maintain therapy for 6 months in a patient who has had one episode, for 1 year after a second episode, and indefinitely after a third episode.

c. Long-acting (depot) preparations are primarily for maintenance therapy and are administered intramuscularly. Depot preparations may improve compliance and help to prevent relapse.

(1) While the three preparations currently available are therapeutically equivalent, they differ in duration of action and in therapeutic dose.

(a) Fluphenazine decanoate has a longer duration of action than fluphenazine enanthate and may produce fewer extrapyramidal effects. A dose may last 3 to 4 weeks.

(b) Fluphenazine enanthate may require administration every 2 weeks.

(c) Haloperidol decanoate may be administered every 4 weeks.

(2) Therapy should be initiated at low doses to minimize adverse effects.

(3) If the patient has been receiving oral therapy, continuing the oral medication for the first few weeks of depot therapy may be beneficial while the blood levels of the depot preparation accumulate to steady-state levels.

(4) Before converting to long-acting preparations, it would be helpful if the patient were first converted to oral fluphenazine or haloperidol. Several formulas are available to guide the conversion, but they are only rough guidelines for initation of therapy.

(5) Once depot therapy has begun, the patient must be monitored carefully to facilitate dosage adjustments.

E. Evaluation of patient response should focus on target symptoms to determine therapeutic effectiveness. So-called positive symptoms, such as hallucinations, delusions, hostility, and hyperactivity, are most likely to respond to antipsychotic agents. Negative symptoms, such as poor judgment, apathy, social incompetence, and withdrawal, are less likely to respond.

F. Precautions and monitoring effects. (Table 38–2 lists the association of the major side effects with specific antipsychotic agents.)

1. Sedative effects are common, particularly with the **phenothiazines.**

2. Extrapyramidal effects

a. Dystonic reactions involve sudden muscle spasms of the neck, face, or trunk. These reactions include torticollis (neck twisting), trismus (clenched jaw), and oculogyric crisis (fixed upward gaze). The risk of dystonias is highest during the first 24 to 48 hours of therapy and when the dose is increased; they are most likely to occur in the young, in males, and in patients receiving high doses. Dystonias can be managed initially through intramuscular or intravenous (IV) administration of anticholinergic agents, such as diphenhydramine or benztropine mesylate. Further reactions may be prevented by a short course of oral anticholinergic therapy.

b. Akathisia is associated with an inner tension or agitation that is relieved by activity. Patients usually manifest this restlessness in an inability to keep their legs and feet still. This side effect most commonly appears within the first few weeks of therapy and may respond to anticholinergic agents or diazepam. If not, a change in neuroleptic agent or discontinuation of therapy may be necessary.

c. Drug-induced parkinsonism includes parkinsonian symptoms such as akinesia, rigidity, resting tremor, shuffling gait, mask-like facial expression, and slowed speech. The onset of

Table 38-2. Likelihood of Adverse Effects with Antipsychotic Agents

Agent	Sedative	Extrapyramidal	Anticholinergic	Cardiovascular (Alpha Blockade)
Acetophenazine	Medium	High	Medium	Low
Chlorpromazine	High	Medium	High	High
Chlorprothixene	High	Medium	Medium	Medium
Fluphenazine	Low	High	Low	Low
Haloperidol	Medium	High	Low	Low
Loxapine	Medium	High	Low	Medium
Mesoridazine	High	Low	Medium	Medium
Molindone	Low	High	Low	Low
Perphenazine	Low	High	Medium	Low
Thioridazine	High	Low	High	High
Thiothixene	Low	High	Low	Low
Trifluoperazine	Low	High	Low	Low

symptoms may occur within weeks or months. A related but less common effect, known as the **rabbit syndrome**, compels the patient to movements resembling the chewing motions typical of rabbits. Anticholinergic agents should manage these effects.

d. Tardive dyskinesia

(1) This disorder is characterized by abnormal facial movements with chewing, tongue protrusion, and puckering of the mouth. The reaction may progress to the extremities and trunk, producing involuntary movements, disturbance of the gag reflex, or respiratory distress.

(2) A late-onset effect, tardive dyskinesia usually does not appear for months or years. It is thought to be due to prolonged dopamine receptor blockade, which leads to increased receptor sensitivity, so that dopamine stimulation tends to produce movement disorders. The syndrome may begin when drugs are discontinued; in fact, a short drug holiday may reveal symptoms, allowing early detection.

(3) Treatment. Anticholinergics do not alleviate the syndrome and may even worsen it. Treatment attempts have been aimed at increasing cholinergic activity (using such compounds as physostigmine, lecithin, and choline) or decreasing dopamine activity. Agents that increase GABA (γ-aminobutyric acid) activity have had some success. No definitive treatment has been identified; the emphasis is on prevention.

(a) Antipsychotics and anticholinergics should be used only when needed and in the lowest possible doses.

(b) Patients should be examined for early signs of dyskinesia (e.g., fine worm-like movements when the tongue is at rest, facial tics, and increased frequency of blinking). If any are discovered, antipsychotics should be discontinued gradually, if feasible. Nevertheless, symptoms may persist for months to years and may be irreversible.

(c) If the patient's condition necessitates continuing the medication, the lowest therapeutic dosage should be used.

3. Anticholinergic effects include dry mouth, blurred vision, constipation, and urinary retention. Administering the dose at night or reducing the dosage may reduce significant or persistent effects.

4. Cardiovascular effects include orthostatic hypotension resulting from alpha blockade. Other potential effects include reflex tachycardia and electrocardiogram abnormalities, specifically S-T depression, flattened T waves, Q-T prolongation, and the appearance of U waves.

5. Ocular effects

a. Degenerative pigmentary retinopathy may occur with high doses of **thioridazine** (the maximum daily dose should be 800 mg).

b. Corneal lens opacities have been associated with antipsychotic therapy, especially with **chlorpromazine**. Slit-lamp examination helps detect deposits in the cornea or lens. These deposits usually do not affect vision and may resolve within months after discontinuation of the drug.

6. Decreased seizure threshold may occur with neuroleptics, and they should be used cautiously in a patient with a seizure disorder. Anticonvulsant dose increases may be necessary.

7. Neuroleptic malignant syndrome is an uncommon but serious—potentially life-threatening—complication of therapy. It is a complex of extrapyramidal effects, hyperthermia, altered consciousness, and autonomic changes (e.g., tachycardia, unstable blood pressure, diaphoresis, and incontinence). The onset is sudden, and recovery may take 5 to 10 days after discontinuation of therapy. Specific management includes discontinuation of the drug; supportive measures, such as temperature control; and drug therapy with dantrolene or bromocriptine.

8. Additional effects

a. Temperature regulation may be impaired, causing the patient to assume the environmental temperature; this can result in hyperthermia or hypothermia.

b. Sexual dysfunction may include impotence, inability to ejaculate, retrograde ejaculation, diminished libido, amenorrhea, galactorrhea, and gynecomastia. These effects are seen most commonly with **thioridazine**.

c. Photosensitivity in the form of gray to purple pigmentation has been reported with **chlorpromazine**, **thioridazine**, and the **thiothixenes**. A correlation has been noted between skin and ocular pigmentation; patients with a photosensitive reaction should have an ocular examination.

STUDY QUESTIONS

Directions: Each question below contains five suggested answers. Choose the **one best** response to each question.

1. All of the following statements concerning antipsychotic agents are true EXCEPT

A. studies have proven chlorpromazine to be the most effective antipsychotic agent
B. patients who have responded to a particular drug in the past are likely to respond to re-treatment with that same drug
C. the major differences among antipsychotic drugs are their side effects
D. any given patient may or may not respond to any given antipsychotic drug
E. newly diagnosed, young patients tend to respond to drugs better than older chronic schizophrenic patients

2. The four "A's" that Bleuler used to characterize schizophrenia include all of the following EXCEPT

A. anxiety
B. ambivalence
C. association defect
D. autism
E. alteration of affect

3. Which of the following is an example of a delusion?

A. Hearing strange voices
B. Seeing someone who is not really there
C. The feeling that ants are crawling all over the body
D. The lack of any emotional response to any situation
E. The belief that an advertisement on television is speaking directly to the individual with a secret message

4. Schizophrenia, according to the biologic theory, is thought to be due to

A. excess of acetylcholine
B. excess of dopamine
C. excess of calcium
D. dopamine deficiency
E. zinc deficiency

5. The earliest movement disorder to appear during neuroleptic therapy is

A. pseudoparkinsonism
B. dystonia
C. tardive dyskinesia
D. akathisia
E. resting tremor

6. Specific therapy for an acute extrapyramidal reaction to chlorpromazine is

A. physostigmine
B. diphenhydramine
C. bethanechol
D. propranolol
E. metoclopramide

Directions: The group of questions below consists of lettered choices followed by several numbered items. For each numbered item select the **one** lettered choice with which it is **most** closely associated. Each lettered choice may be used once, more than once, or not at all.

Questions 7–11

Match the drug with the phrase that most accurately describes it.

A. Used in depot preparations
B. Used in the management of neuroleptic malignant syndrome
C. High doses may cause degenerative pigmentary retinopathy
D. Counteracts dystonias
E. Produces minimal sedative effects

7. Thioridazine
8. Benztropine mesylate
9. Dantrolene
10. Molindone
11. Haloperidol

ANSWERS AND EXPLANATIONS

1. The answer is A. (*III A*) Those individuals most likely to respond to antipsychotic drugs are young patients. There is no clinically proven superior antipsychotic agent. Any given patient may respond to any given antipsychotic drug; however, when selecting a drug to treat a patient with schizophrenia, a past history of success with a particular drug indicates that the patient will probably respond to that drug again. The major differences among antipsychotic drugs are their side effects.

2. The answer is A. (*I D 1*) Bleuler described the four "A's" of schizophrenia by using the symptoms of association defect, abnormal affect, ambivalence, and autism. Anxiety disorders are a different class of psychological disorders.

3. The answer is E. (*I D 2 b*) A hallucination is an abnormal sensory perception, such as hearing or seeing something that is not there. The lack of an emotional response to any situation is due to an abnormal affect. A delusion is a firmly held but false belief, such as having one's thoughts read or the belief that an advertisement is speaking directly to you with a secret message.

4. The answer is B. (*I C 2*) A leading biochemical theory of the cause of schizophrenia is the dopamine hypothesis, which proposes that schizophrenia is due to excess dopamine activity. This is supported by the evidence that the most effective antipsychotic agents employed in the treatment of schizophrenia interfere with dopamine-associated neurotransmission in the brain. A deficiency of dopamine would therefore be incorrect. The activities of acetylcholine, calcium, and zinc are not part of this hypothesis.

5. The answer is B. (*III F 2 a*) In patients given antipsychotic drugs, dystonic reactions have the earliest onset—the risk is highest during the first 24 to 48 hours of therapy and when the dose is increased. Pseudoparkinsonism, which is characterized in part by a resting tremor, may not begin for weeks to months after initiation of antipsychotic therapy; and tardive dyskinesia is usually not seen for months to years. Akathisia begins within the first few weeks of therapy.

6. The answer is B. (*III F 2 a–c*) Acute extrapyramidal reactions are due to excess cholinergic activity resulting from the blockade of dopamine receptors by the neuroleptic agent. Specific treatment is administration of an agent with anticholinergic activity, such as diphenhydramine.

7–11. The answers are: 7-C, 8-D, 9-B, 10-E, 11-A. (*III D 4 c, F 2 a, 5 a, 7; Table 38-2*) Pigmentary retinopathy may be caused by thioridazine when administered in doses over 800 mg/day. Benztropine mesylate has anticholinergic activity and may be used to manage the extrapyramidal side effects associated with antipsychotic therapy. Dantrolene, through its effects on muscles, may be able to control the signs of neuroleptic malignant syndrome. Although sedation is common to all antipsychotic agents, molindone, thiothixene, and most piperazine phenothiazines are associated with a lower incidence of this effect. Two antipsychotic agents are currently available in depot (long-acting) formulations: fluphenazine (as the decanoate or the enanthate) and haloperidol decanoate.

39
Affective Disorders

Robert J. Cersosimo

I. INTRODUCTION

A. Definition. Affective disorders are characterized by disturbances of mood, such as low and depressed states or periods of exhilaration to the point of mania. Affective disorders are considered in two major classifications.

1. In **unipolar disorder**, the patient experiences depressive episodes.

2. In **bipolar disorder**, the patient experiences depressive and manic episodes or, less commonly, manic episodes alone.

B. Incidence. Affective disorders rank as the **most common psychiatric disorders**.

1. **Unipolar disorder.** Estimates indicate that 18% to 23% of adult women and 8% to 11% of adult men experience at least one major depressive episode. Onset of a major depressive illness may occur at any age but is most common in the late twenties.

2. **Bipolar disorder.** This form of affective disorder is much less common than the unipolar type. Its incidence ranges between 0.4% and 1.2% of the adult population, with approximately equal distribution among men and women. Onset generally occurs before age 30.

C. Etiology. Although no consensus has been achieved on precise causes for affective disorders, theorists focus on genetic, biological, and psychological factors.

1. **Genetic factors**
   a. Research indicates an increased frequency of occurrence in families of patients with affective disorders as compared with the general population.
   b. Studies of monozygotic and dizygotic twins support theories of genetic influence on the development of major affective disorders. However, they also indicate that other factors are involved.

2. **Neurochemical factors**
   a. The **biogenic amine hypothesis** proposes that depression is due to a deficiency of either norepinephrine or serotonin and that mania results from an excess of norepinephrine.
   b. The **permissive hypothesis** states the following:
      (1) Serotonin deficiencies may create a predisposition to a major affective disorder.
      (2) Deficiencies of both serotonin and norepinephrine result in depression.
      (3) A serotonin deficiency accompanied by a norepinephrine excess results in mania.
   c. The **receptor sensitivity theory** proposes that there is an alteration of receptor sensitivity to neurotransmitters; consequently, antidepressants exert their effects by altering receptor sensitivity.

3. **Psychological factors.** Theories proposing a psychological basis for the origin of major depressive episodes abound. For example, one hypothesis suggests that stress or loss may result in an episode of clinical depression, especially if coupled with the patient's inability to cope with the event.

II. CLINICAL EVALUATION

A. General. Diagnosis of an affective disorder requires the following determinations.

1. The mood disturbance (unipolar or bipolar) should be evident.

2. The symptoms should not be superimposed on a schizophrenic disorder.

3. The mood disturbance must not be due to an organic mental disorder or simple bereavement.

B. Unipolar disorders

1. Major depressive illness is characterized by mood depression or loss of interest or pleasure in all or almost all usual activities.
2. The mood disturbance must be prominent and relatively persistent.
3. Differential diagnosis requires that, for 2 weeks, four or more of the following associated signs accompany the mood disturbance:
   a. Appetite loss or increase, with correlative weight change
   b. Insomnia or hypersomnia
   c. Psychomotor retardation or agitation or both
   d. Loss of interest in or gratification from family, sexual activity, work, hobbies, clubs, and other social activities
   e. Feelings of worthlessness or guilt
   f. Loss of energy; feeling of chronic fatigue or lack of pep
   g. Decreased ability to think clearly or concentrate; impaired memory
   h. Suicidal thoughts, plans, or attempts; thoughts focusing on death

C. Bipolar disorders

1. A diagnosis of bipolar disorder requires one or more periods in which the predominant mood is elated, expansive, or irritable.
2. The mood must predominate for a distinct period, although it may alternate with depressive periods.
3. The diagnosis of the manic phase also requires that at least three of the following associated symptoms have been significant and persistent during the period (four if the mood is solely irritable):
   a. Increase in activity or restlessness
   b. Unusual verbosity or rapid or pressured speech
   c. Flight of ideas, characterized by rapid changes in subject; racing thoughts, which can compromise coherence
   d. Ease of distractibility, in which almost anything can disrupt concentration
   e. Inflation of self-esteem, which can reach delusional proportions
   f. Decrease in need for sleep
   g. Impairment of judgment, which may lead to involvement in highly consequential activities such as buying sprees, reckless driving, sexual indiscretions, and flamboyant, intrusive socializing (such as making late-night phone calls or visits)
4. The disorder must be severe enough to interfere with work, relationships, or social activities, or require hospitalization to prevent harmful activities.

III. CLINICAL COURSE

A. Depressive episodes

1. These episodes are usually self-limiting, lasting 6 months or less.
2. With proper and timely therapy, up to 85% of patients who experience depressive episodes may achieve a complete response.
3. The clinical course may be:
   a. **Limited**—to a single episode
   b. **Recurrent**—with two or more episodes separated by intervals of varying lengths (episodes may also occur in clusters)
   c. **Chronic**—in which some symptoms may persist for up to 2 years, with asymptomatic periods of less than 2 months
4. The major risk for these patients is suicide.

B. Manic episodes

1. If untreated, manic episodes may last from days to months.
2. Recurrence intervals are unpredictable, but it is not unusual for episodes to occur at 1- to 2-year intervals.

3. The sequence of episodes in bipolar disorder is also unpredictable. Manic eipsodes are not necessarily followed by depressive periods.

IV. GENERAL TREATMENT GOALS

A. To shorten the episode

B. To prevent recurrence

V. TREATMENT OF UNIPOLAR (DEPRESSIVE) DISORDERS.

Depressive episodes may be managed with pharmacotherapy, psychotherapy, electroconvulsive therapy, or a combination of modalities. This discussion will be limited to pharmacotherapy; specifically, cyclic antidepressants and monoamine oxidase (MAO) inhibitors.

A. Cyclic antidepressants

1. **Indications.** Cyclic antidepressants are considered the first-line agents for unipolar disorders.

2. **Mechanism of action**
   a. These agents are thought to prevent the presynaptic reuptake of neurotransmitters such as norepinephrine or serotonin.
   b. Most agents affect one specific transmitter more than another.
   c. The newer theories proposing a neurochemical basis for these disorders (see section I C 2) suggest that these drugs are effective because they affect receptor sensitivity or regulate neurotransmitter systems.
   d. Currently available antidepressants and the neurotransmitters they affect are listed in Table 39-1.

3. **Choice of agent**
   a. All antidepressants are equally effective when used at appropriate doses. Therefore, the choice of an individual agent should be based on the patient's past experience with the same or related drugs. Consideration should be given to negative or positive tolerance and effectiveness.
   b. If no such drug history exists, consideration should be given to the therapeutic response of blood relatives, if applicable and available.
   c. Potential adverse effects inherent to the drug or due to any previous or current medical conditions should also be weighed.

4. **Administration and dosage**
   a. **Initiation of treatment**
      (1) The recommended daily dosage ranges for antidepressants are presented in Table 39–2. The high end of these dosage ranges is usually reserved for the severely ill hospitalized patient.
      (2) Therapy should be initiated with one-third of the target dose. For example, 50 to 75 mg of amitriptyline should be administered in divided doses to minimize adverse effects.

Table 39-1. Currently Available Antidepressant Agents

Agents	Brand Name(s)	Transmitter Affected
Tricyclics		
Amitriptyline	Elavil, Endep	Serotonin
Nortriptyline	Aventyl, Pamelor	Norepinephrine
Imipramine	Tofranil, Janimine	Serotonin
Desipramine	Norpramin	Norepinephrine
Protriptyline	Vivactil	Norepinephrine
Doxepin	Adapin, Sinequan	Serotonin
Trimipramine	Surmontil	Norepinephrine
Tetracyclics		
Maprotiline	Ludiomil	Norepinephrine
Amoxapine	Asendin	Norepinephrine
Others		
Trazodone	Desyrel	Serotonin
Fluoxetine	Prozac	Serotonin

Table 39-2. Average Daily Antidepressant Doses in Adults

Agents	Daily Dose (mg)	Therapeutic Serum Levels (ng/ml)
Tricyclics		
Amitriptyline	75–300	60–250*
Nortriptyline	50–200	50–150
Imipramine	75–300	100–300*
Desipramine	75–300	40–160
Protriptyline	15–60	100–200
Doxepin	75–300	30–150*
Trimipramine	75–300	180*
Tetracyclics		
Maprotiline	150–300	200–300*
Amoxapine	100–600	180*
Others		
Trazodone	50–600	Unidentified
Fluoxetine	20–80	Unidentified

*Active metabolites included.

(3) The dose may be increased once or twice a week until a response is obtained.
(4) Further increases of 50 mg weekly may be necessary until improvement, toxicity, or the upper end of the dosing range is reached.
(5) After a gradual transition, most of these drugs may be administered in a single daily dose, usually at bedtime.
(6) The elderly and patients with cardiovascular disease require lower initial doses and a slower rate of increase.
(7) Response rate
(a) Physiologic symptoms (such as sleep disturbances, anorexia, psychomotor disturbance) usually respond first—within 1 week.
(b) Psychosocial symptoms respond later—usually after 2 to 4 weeks.
(c) Full response may require about 4 weeks. If there is no response after 4 weeks, serum drug levels should be checked, as discussed in section V A 5 b (1).

b. Maintenance therapy
(1) Therapy is usually maintained for 6 months after recovery to prevent a relapse.
(2) The maintenance dose is 1/3 to 1/2 of the dose needed to achieve remission.
(3) After the 6 months, the drug is tapered off over 4 to 8 weeks.

c. Prophylaxis. A patient with a history of frequent or severe episodes may require prophylactic therapy to prevent future episodes.

5. Precautions and monitoring effects
a. Contraindications
(1) Cyclic antidepressants should be avoided in patients with severely impaired liver function or with cardiac conduction defects.
(2) Coadministration of MAO inhibitors and cyclic antidepressants can result in serious reactions, including hyperpyrexia, seizures, excitation, and death. Such combination therapy is rarely warranted and should be initiated with great caution.
(3) Caution is required with administering these agents to patients with cardiovascular disease, glaucoma, benign prostatic hypertrophy, or a history of seizures or urinary retention.

b. Serum level monitoring
(1) Although therapeutic serum levels have been identified for most antidepressants (see Table 39-2), the correlation between levels and activity is unclear. Therapeutic levels do not guarantee either the desired response or a lack of adverse effects. Patients should therefore be evaluated by their response to therapy.
(2) Orders for serum levels should account for active metabolites, as applicable.
(3) Assessment of serum levels provides several major benefits, such as helping in the detection and management of antidepressant overdose [see section V A 5 c (6)].
(4) Serum level monitoring is particularly useful **in the nonresponsive patient**.
(a) A subtherapeutic or low-end serum level indicates the need for incremental dosage increases.
(b) A lower than expected serum level despite a reasonable dose may reveal patient noncompliance.

(c) **An upper-end serum level** suggests the need to change to a different drug.
(d) **Achieving therapeutic serum levels** without obtaining patient response after 4 weeks suggests the need for reevaluation of the diagnosis. If the physician is confident of the diagnosis, a change in medications is recommended.

c. **Adverse effects** (Table 39-3)
(1) **Sedative effects**, which may be desirable in a patient with insomnia, are usually undesirable in a patient with psychomotor retardation.
(2) **Anticholinergic effects** include dry mouth, constipation, blurred vision, and urinary retention.
(3) **Cardiac effects**
(a) **Orthostatic hypotension** is the most common cardiac effect (with an incidence as high as 20%).
(b) **Tachycardia** of the mild sinus type is common.
(c) **Arrhythmias and electrocardiogram (ECG) disturbances**
(i) ECG changes may include T wave flattening or prolongation of the P-R, QRS, or Q-T intervals.
(ii) Tricyclic compounds may interfere with atrioventricular conduction, similar to the effect of quinidine. In the presence of bundle-branch block or atrioventricular block, these effects can be life-threatening. Therefore, these agents should be avoided in patients with conduction defects.
(4) **Neurologic effects**
(a) **Seizure threshold**. Most cyclic antidepressants tend to lower the seizure threshold.
(i) Cautious administration is required in patients with a history of seizures.
(ii) Anticonvulsant doses may need to be increased.
(iii) Maprotiline has been associated with an increased risk of seizures at doses exceeding 225 mg/day, even in patients without a history of seizures. To minimize this risk, dosage increases should be gradual.
(b) **Neuroleptic effects**, most common with amoxapine, may include:
(i) Severe restlessness and agitation (akathisia)
(ii) Tardive dyskinesia
(iii) Dystonias
(iv) Drug-induced parkinsonism
(v) Neuroleptic malignant syndrome (extrapyramidal signs, changes in blood pressure, altered consciousness, and hyperpyrexia), a rare but serious complication
(5) **Dermatologic effects. Exanthemous rash** may erupt in 4% to 5% of the patients taking maprotiline.
(6) **Overdosage**
(a) **Signs and symptoms** may reflect cardiac, central nervous system, and anticholinergic effects, including arrhythmias, seizures, coma, confusion, respiratory depression, hyperpyrexia, and bladder or bowel dysfunction.
(b) **Treatment** may initially include emesis or gastric lavage and administration of activated charcoal. Additional measures may include phenytoin or diazepam for seizure control and lidocaine or phenytoin for arrhythmias. Physostigmine may be of value in certain cases.

Table 39-3. Incidence of Adverse Effects with Cyclic Antidepressant Use

Agents	Sedation	Constipation	Orthostatic Hypotension	Arrhythmias	Lowered Seizure Threshold
Tricyclics					
Amitriptyline	High	High	Moderate	High	Moderate
Nortriptyline	Moderate	Moderate	Very low	Moderate	Low
Imipramine	Moderate	Moderate	High	High	Moderate
Desipramine	Low	Low	Moderate	Moderate	Low
Protriptyline	Low	Moderate	Low	High	Low
Doxepin	High	Moderate	Low	Low	Moderate
Trimipramine	High	High	Moderate	High	Moderate
Tetracyclics					
Maprotiline	Moderate	Moderate	Low	Moderate	High
Amoxapine	Low	Moderate	Very low	Low	Moderate
Others					
Trazodone	Moderate	Very low	Moderate	Very low	Low
Fluoxetine	Low	Low	Low	Very low	Very low

(7) **Withdrawal symptoms**, such as nausea, headache, and malaise, can be avoided by withdrawing the drug gradually.

B. Monoamine oxidase (MAO) inhibitors

1. **Mechanism of action**. MAO inhibitors block the usual destruction of neurotransmitters by monoamine oxidase, thus creating a buildup of biogenic amine levels in the brain. This increase probably underlies the antidepressant effect.

2. **Indications**. MAO inhibitors are reserved for patients who have not responded to cyclic antidepressants (the first-line agents) or who cannot tolerate their side effects.

3. **Administration and dosage** (Table 39-4)
   a. When a patient is being changed from a cyclic antidepressant to an MAO inhibitor, the MAO inhibitor should be initiated at a low dose. Dosage increments should be made slowly and cautiously.
   b. When changing from an MAO inhibitor to a cyclic antidepressant, wait at least 10 days after stopping the MAO inhibitor before beginning therapy with the cyclic agent, in order to avoid a potentially serious interaction.
   c. Therapeutic effects may not occur for 2 to 3 weeks or longer.

4. **Precautions and monitoring effects**
   a. **Contraindications**
      (1) MAO inhibitors should not be administered to patients who are debilitated or who have a history of hepatic or renal impairment or cardiovascular or cerebrovascular disease.
      (2) Administration is also contraindicated within 7 to 10 days of surgery that requires general anesthesia or a local anesthetic containing cocaine or sympathomimetic vasoconstrictors.
   b. **Interactions**
      (1) **Hypertensive crisis**, the most serious and most likely interaction, results from ingestion of sympathomimetic drugs and foods with a high tyramine content.
         (a) The patient should be given a list of **foods to avoid**, particularly:
            (i) Beer and most wines (except white wine)
            (ii) Caviar and herring
            (iii) Chicken livers
            (iv) Chocolate
            (v) Most cheeses (especially blue, cheddar, mozzarella, and parmesan)
            (vi) Sausage and other smoked meats
         (b) Patients should also be warned not to take any medications—including over-the-counter cold, hay fever, or diet preparations—without first consulting a physician or pharmacist.
         (c) **Early signs** of hypertensive crisis may include:
            (i) Stiff neck
            (ii) Occipital headache
            (iii) Nausea and vomiting
            (iv) Sweating and flushing
            (v) Palpitations
      (2) Coadministration of a cyclic antidepressant and a MAO inhibitor must be undertaken with extreme caution, if at all [see section V A 5 a (2)].
   c. **Adverse effects**
      (1) **Orthostatic hypotension** is common but may be minimized by using smaller incremental dosage increases.
      (2) MAO inhibitors derived from hydrazide may cause **hepatocellular damage**. Although of low incidence, this toxic effect can have serious consequences; therefore, liver func-

Table 39-4. Recommended Daily Doses for Monoamine Oxidase (MAO) Inhibitors

Agents	Brand Name	Usual Daily Dose (mg)
Hydrazides		
Phenelzine	Nardil	60–90
Isocarboxazid	Marplan	10–50
Nonhydrazide		
Tranylcypromine	Parnate	10–60

tion should be monitored after a baseline is established. Administration should be avoided if the patient has a history of hepatic impairment.

(3) **Weight gain, sexual dysfunction,** and **edema** may occur.

d. **Overdosage** may be signalled by palpitations, agitation, frequent headaches, hypertension, or severe orthostatic hypotension.

VI. TREATMENT OF BIPOLAR DISORDERS.

Neuroleptic agents, lithium, and psychotherapy may be used to manage bipolar disorders. Antidepressants are administered with lithium to manage the depressive phase of the illness. Use of antidepressants alone is usually avoided because of their tendency to provoke the reemergence of the manic phase.

A. Neuroleptic agents

1. **Indications.** Neuroleptic agents are used in the acute manic phase to decrease agitation and hyperactivity, the first treatment priority.

2. **Therapeutic effects**
   a. Neuroleptics such as chlorpromazine and haloperidol quickly lower the arousal level while not interfering with intellectual processes.
   b. Emotional or affective displays are reduced; aggressive and impulsive behavior is diminished.

3. **Administration and dosage**
   a. Because lithium efficacy has a delayed onset (see section VI B 2 a), neuroleptics are used until the lithium can achieve a therapeutic effect.
   b. Neuroleptic therapy is usually initiated at the same time as the lithium therapy.
   c. Neuroleptics can be tapered off as symptoms improve and serum lithium levels reach therapeutic concentrations [see section VI B 3 b (3)].
   d. The dosage varies with the severity of the patient's symptoms and whether the patient is treated in the hospital or as an outpatient.
      (1) The usual starting dose of **chlorpromazine** for a hospitalized patient in the manic phase is 25 mg intramuscularly (IM). Doses of 25 to 50 mg IM may be administered hourly if necessary. The dose is gradually increased over the next few days to as much as 400 mg every 4 to 6 hrs if needed.
      (2) **Haloperidol** may be initiated at a dose of 2 to 5 mg IM in an acutely ill patient. Doses may be repeated hourly as needed.
      (3) **Oral** administration should be employed as soon as the patient is calm.

4. **Precautions and monitoring effects**
   a. **Chlorpromazine**
      (1) This agent should be used with extreme caution or not at all in patients with cardiovascular disease, glaucoma, benign prostatic hypertrophy, or a history of seizures.
      (2) Chlorpromazine has a strong sedative effect while bearing only moderate extrapyramidal effects.
   b. **Haloperidol**
      (1) Extrapyramidal effects may be seen with haloperidol administration. These effects include parkinsonian symptoms, akathisia, and dystonic reactions.
      (2) Coadministration of haloperidol (or a phenothiazine) with lithium may result in an acute encephalopathy. Patients should be carefully monitored while receiving this combination.
      (3) Haloperidol tends to have a high incidence of extrapyramidal effects (especially akathisia and dystonias) while having a moderate sedative effect.
   c. **General.** These agents should not be withdrawn suddenly unless intolerably severe adverse effects arise.

B. Lithium

Lithium is the drug of choice for control and prophylaxis of manic episodes.

1. **Mechanism of action.** Although the exact mechanism remains unknown, lithium is thought to:
   a. Affect membrane stabilization
   b. Inhibit norepinephrine release
   c. Accelerate norepinephrine metabolism
   d. Increase presynaptic reuptake of norepinephrine and serotonin
   e. Decrease receptor sensitivity

2. **Administration and dosage**
   a. **General.** Lithium has a very narrow therapeutic index and a significant lag time (3 to 5 days, longer in some patients) before the initial therapeutic effect is observable. Therefore, monitoring serum lithium levels and evaluating the patient for signs of toxicity provide the keys to determining and adjusting the dosage regimen.

b. Initial therapy

(1) The initial dose is usually 900 to 1200 mg/day.

(2) The daily dosage should be divided into 3 or 4 doses to minimize gastrointestinal toxicity.

(3) Doses may be increased once or twice a week until therapeutic serum levels are achieved.

(4) Daily doses of 1200 to 2400 mg may be required to establish control of symptoms.

c. Maintenance therapy

(1) Once the symptoms have diminished, the dose should be decreased to achieve maintenance serum levels [see section VI B 3 b (3) (b)].

(2) Manic attacks are usually self-limiting. Unless there is an indication for chronic therapy, lithium may be discontinued after 3 to 6 months. Long term therapy is indicated for patients with severe or frequent attacks.

3. Precautions and monitoring effects

a. Contraindications

(1) Renal, cardiovascular, and thyroid disorders may preclude the use of lithium or necessitate extremely cautious monitoring.

(2) Lithium is contraindicated during the first trimester of pregnancy because it increases the risk of congenital cardiovascular anomalies, particularly valvular malformations.

b. Serum level monitoring. To minimize the likelihood of lithium toxicity while assuring adequate dosage, the patient's blood levels should be monitored closely.

(1) Levels should be checked several times during the first few weeks of therapy, until they stabilize.

(2) The ideal time to check serum levels is 12 hours after the last dose. Drawing the sample in the morning before the first dose of the day is generally most convenient.

(3) Therapeutic serum level ranges are as follows:

(a) **Initial therapy**: 0.8 to 1.5 mEq/L

(b) **Maintenance therapy**: 0.6 to 1.2 mEq/L

c. Laboratory test results can be affected by lithium intake, including:

(1) Elevations in urinary and serum glucose tests

(2) Decreases in serum uric acid levels and serum protein-bound iodine studies

(3) Increased thyroid-stimulating hormone

(4) Decreased thyroxine levels

d. Breast feeding should be avoided by mothers taking lithium because significant concentrations of the drug have been detected in breast milk.

e. Adverse effects are generally related to increasing serum concentration levels.

(1) Below 1.5 mEq/L, the effects are usually tolerable or manageable by dividing or reducing the dose. These effects include:

(a) Gastrointestinal distress, such as anorexia, nausea, vomiting, and diarrhea (these may be minimized by taking the drug with food or dividing the dose)

(b) Polyuria and polydipsia

(c) Fine hand tremor

(d) Slight muscle weakness

(2) Effects associated with lithium serum levels between 1.5 and 2.5 mEq/L should be considered early **warning signs of toxicity**. These include:

(a) Persistent or recurring gastrointestinal distress

(b) Coarse hand tremor

(c) Hyperirritability

(d) Slurred speech

(e) Confusion or somnolence

(3) **Lithium toxicity** usually occurs when levels exceed 2.5 mEq/L. This is a potentially fatal medical emergency requiring immediate attention.

(a) **Signs and symptoms** include:

(i) Increased deep tendon reflexes

(ii) Irregular pulse

(iii) Hypotension

(iv) Seizures

(v) Stupor or coma

(b) **Treatment** of acute toxicity should include attempts to empty the stomach by emesis or gastric lavage. Supportive treatment should be administered, and diuresis may increase urinary lithium elimination. Hemodialysis may be necessary if serum lithium levels exceed 3 mEq/L or if the patient's condition does not improve or begins to decline.

(4) Some effects occur with ongoing therapy but are unrelated to serum levels. These include:

(a) **Leukocytosis.** White blood cell counts may range from 10,000 to 15,000 mm^3 and may remain elevated throughout therapy.

(b) **Diabetes insipidus syndrome.** Patients may develop an inability to concentrate urine, with increased urine output and increased thirst. Dosage reduction or specific therapy may be needed if urine output becomes excessive.

(c) **Weight gain.** Gain of 10 kg (22 lb) or more may occur.

(d) **Nontoxic goiter.** Clinically evident hypothyroidism or goiter may occur in a few cases.

4. **Drug interactions.** Lithium interacts with many drugs, only a few of which are discussed below. These interactions either increase lithium levels or increase lithium excretion. Lithium is eliminated through the kidneys by glomerular filtration and competes with sodium for reabsorption in the renal tubules.
   a. **Thiazide diuretics** interfere with sodium reabsorption and thus may favor lithium reabsorption, which could lead to lithium toxicity. Care should be given to adjust the dosage of the lithium, and serum levels should be monitored closely. Conversely, lithium doses may need to be increased if the diuretic is discontinued. Furosemide therapy does not present this concern because the increased reabsorption of lithium in the proximal tubule is counteracted by decreased absorption in the loop of Henle.
   b. **Osmotic diuretics, sodium bicarbonate, and theophylline** increase lithium excretion, thereby diminishing the therapeutic effect.

STUDY QUESTIONS

Directions: Each question below contains five suggested answers. Choose the **one best** response to each question.

1. All of the following patterns are associated with a bipolar major affective disorder EXCEPT

A. a history of manic episodes only
B. a history of depressed episodes only
C. a history of several depressed episodes and only one manic episode
D. cycling from manic to depressed episodes with periods of normal mood in between
E. a history of several manic episodes and only one depressed episode

2. Which of the following is a sign of a unipolar affective disorder?

A. Flight of ideas
B. Unusual verbosity
C. Poor judgment leading to reckless driving
D. Loss of interest in the job and family
E. Ease of distractability

3. The proposed mechanism of action of the tricyclic antidepressants is that they

A. have intrinsic adrenergic activity
B. block adrenergic receptors
C. can stimulate dopamine receptors
D. bind to centers of stimulation in the brain
E. prevent the reuptake of synaptic neurotransmitters

4. Therapeutic serum lithium levels during initiation of therapy are defined as

A. 0.4–0.8 mEq/L
B. 0.8–1.5 mEq/L
C. 0.6–1.0 μg/L
D. 0.8–1.0 mg/L
E. 1.2–1.6 μg/L

5. Which of the following relatively mild adverse effects is associated with initiation of lithium therapy?

A. Blurred vision
B. Dystonic reactions
C. Fine hand tremor
D. Pseudoparkinsonism
E. Tinnitus

6. Foods high in tyramine such as pickled herring and most cheeses (especially blue, cheddar, and parmesan) should be avoided in patients who are taking

A. doxepin
B. phenelzine
C. maprotiline
D. alprazolam
E. trazadone

7. Which of the following drugs prescribed for control of a major affective disorder is associated with an almost immediate onset of activity?

A. Lithium carbonate
B. Protriptyline
C. Tranylcypromine
D. Chlorpromazine
E. Isocarboxazid

8. Under the biogenic amine hypothesis, mania is thought to be due to

A. an excess of epinephrine activity
B. an excess of norepinephrine activity
C. an excess of dopamine activity
D. a deficiency of epinephrine activity
E. a deficiency of dopamine activity

ANSWERS AND EXPLANATIONS

1. The answer is B. (*I A 2; II C, 1, 2*) Bipolar depression is characterized by periods of depression and mania, or mania alone. Therefore, someone with a history of depressed episodes only would not fit the definition of a bipolar disorder.

2. The answer is D. (*II B 3 d*) Loss of interest in the job or family is a common sign of a unipolar affective disorder. Flight of ideas, unusual verbosity, poor judgment that could lead to reckless driving, and ease of distractability are all signs of the manic phase of a bipolar affective disorder.

3. The answer is E. (*V A 2*) The proposed mechanism of action of the tricyclic antidepressants is that they prevent the reuptake of synaptic neurotransmitters. These drugs do not have direct adrenergic activity, and they do not block adrenergic receptors. Antidepressants also do not stimulate dopamine receptors or bind to stimulatory centers in the brain.

4. The answer is B. [*VI B 3 b (3) (a)*] Therapeutic serum lithium levels during initiation of lithium therapy range from 0.8 to 1.5 mEq/L. During maintenance therapy, the therapeutic serum level range is 0.6 to 1.2 mEq/L. It is important to monitor serum levels because lithium, like digoxin, has a narrow range between therapeutic and toxic doses. During the first weeks of therapy, serum levels are checked several times a week until the levels have stabilized. During maintenance therapy, serum lithium levels are checked at least once every 2 months.

5. The answer is C. (*VI B 3 e*) The relatively mild adverse effects associated with lithium therapy consist of gastrointestinal disturbances, polyuria and polydipsia, muscle weakness, and fine hand tremor. Pseudoparkinsonism and dystonic reactions do not occur with lithium therapy; tinnitus and blurred vision are not signs of lithium toxicity.

6. The answer is B. (*V B 4 b*) Foods high in tyramine should be avoided in patients who are taking monoamine oxidase (MAO) inhibitors such as phenelzine. The enzyme monoamine oxidase takes part in the oxidative deamination of biogenic amines (e.g., dopamine, norepinephrine, serotonin, and tyramine). MAO inhibitors prevent this enzymatic degradation. (This is considered to be the mechanism of their antidepressant effects.) When a person taking a MAO inhibitor eats foods high in tyramine, the tyramine is not degraded in the body. The tyramine can induce the release of stored catecholamines (e.g., norepinephrine), and this may precipitate an episode of severe hypertension. Doxepin, maprotiline, alprazolam, and trazadone are not MAO inhibitors.

7. The answer is D. [*V A 4 a (7), B 3 c; VI A 2 a, 3 a*] Protriptyline is a tricyclic antidepressant. Full response may require about 4 weeks. Tranylcypromine and isocarboxazid are monoamine oxidase (MAO) inhibitors. The onset of antidepressant effects may be delayed for 2 to 3 weeks. Lithium carbonate has a delayed onset and may take up to 2 weeks for maximum effectiveness. Chlorpromazine is the only agent listed in the question that has an immediate onset of activity.

8. The answer is B. (*I C 2 a*) Under the biogenic amine hypothesis, depression is thought to be due to a deficiency of serotonin or norepinephrine activity, and mania is thought to be due to an excess of norepinephrine activity.

40
Asthma and Chronic Obstructive Pulmonary Disease

Louise Glassner Cohen

I. ASTHMA

A. Definition. Asthma is a condition of tracheobronchial hyperreactivity to various stimuli, leading to episodic bronchospasms and reversible airway obstruction.

B. Classification. Previous classifications for asthma (i.e., intrinsic, extrinsic) are no longer used. It is now recognized that patients respond to a variety of stimuli. An allergic component can be demonstrated in 35% to 55% of asthmatics. Also, 70% to 90% of all asthmatics will experience exercise-induced asthma. The degree of airway hyperreactivity is dependent on whether the asthmatic is in remission.

C. Incidence. Asthma affects approximately 9 million Americans.

1. In about half the cases, the disorder arises before age 10; approximately 33% of the remaining cases are diagnosed before age 40.
2. Up to age 30, asthma is more prevalent in males; after age 30, men and women are equally affected.

D. Etiology

1. **Precipitating factors** of an acute asthma attack include:
   - **a.** Allergens (e.g., pollen, dust, animal dander)
   - **b.** Upper respiratory tract infection (rhinovirus, influenza)
   - **c.** Exercise
   - **d.** Emotions (e.g., anxiety, stress, laughter)
   - **e.** Occupational exposure to such agents as gasoline fumes and fresh paint
   - **f.** Environmental exposure to cold air, sulfur dioxide, and cigarette smoke
   - **g. Drugs.** Two different mechanisms can trigger drug-related asthma.
     - **(1) Hypersensitivity reaction** with release of bronchoactive mediators (e.g., aspirin, ibuprofen, penicillin, products containing tartrazine)
     - **(2) Extension of pharmacologic effect** may develop with such drugs as β-adrenergic blockers and bethanechol.
2. The **mechanism of bronchial hyperreactivity** has not been determined; however, several theories are suggested:
   - **a.** β-Adrenergic defect producing β-blockade: based on the principle that β-blockers alter respiratory function. This has not been proven in asthmatic patients.
   - **b.** Increased cholinergic response: Asthmatic patients seem to be more responsive to bronchoconstriction after inhalation of cholinergic agents. This has not been proven.
   - **c.** Increased sensitivity of mast cells in asthmatic patients: Asthmatics may be more sensitive to the triggers that cause mast cell degranulation.

E. Pathophysiology

1. An **acute asthma attack** is characterized by an inflammatory response that triggers airway obstruction.
   - **a.** In response to a precipitating factor, mediators from mast cells cause bronchial smooth muscle to become spasmodic, leading to bronchoconstriction.
   - **b.** Bronchoconstriction triggers blood vessel engorgement and infiltration of inflammatory cells (neutrophils).
   - **c.** Mucous glands and **goblet cells**, the mucus-secreting cells of the respiratory tract epithelium, become edematous.

d. This leads to increased mucus production, which further narrows the airway.

e. Airway obstruction reduces ventilation to some lung regions; this, in turn, causes a **ventilation/perfusion (V/P) imbalance** that leads to hypoxemia. This is reflected by a reduction in the partial pressure of arterial oxygen (PaO_2) more frequently in a moderate to severe attack.

f. In the early stages, hyperventilation results in a decrease in the partial pressure of arterial carbon dioxide ($PaCO_2$).

g. If the asthma attack progresses and the airways remain narrowed, respiratory muscles suffer fatigue.

h. Respiratory acidosis develops if hypoxemia worsens and the patient's respiratory rate is not maintained; then the $PaCO_2$ level begins to increase.

i. Peak expiratory flow rate (PEFR) and forced expiratory volume (1 second) [FEV_1] may drop in the early stages of an acute asthma attack. As the attack worsens, FEV_1 decreases, resulting in **air trapping** and **lung hyperinflation**.

2. Immunopathologic events. The **adrenergic** and **cholinergic** responses in asthma are governed by the cyclic adenosine monophosphate (cAMP) and cyclic guanosine monophosphate (cGMP) systems within mast cells and other tissues.

a. When an airborne antigen enters the airway, it binds to a receptor on a mast cell.

b. This activates the mast cell, causing an increase in cAMP, an influx of calcium, release of preformed mediators, and synthesis of nonpreformed mediators.

(1) Preformed mediators include histamine, heparin, eosinophil chemotactic factor of anaphylaxis (ECF-A), neutrophil chemotactic factor (NCF), and certain other enzymes.

(2) Nonpreformed mediators include prostaglandin D_2, platelet-activating factor, and leukotrienes C_4 and B_4 [now known to be components of slow-reacting substance of anaphylaxis (SRS-A)].

(3) These mediators cause bronchoconstriction, airway edema, and mucus production, as shown in Figure 40-1.

F. Clinical evaluation

1. Physical findings

a. An **acute attack**, which may have a sudden or gradual onset, produces respiratory distress and wheezing of a variable degree, depending on the severity of the attack (Table 40-1).

b. Other common findings include chest tightness, cough, tachypnea, tachycardia, accessory muscle use, and pulsus paradoxus.

c. Between acute asthma attacks, the patient may be asymptomatic. Physical findings are dependent on the severity of the disease.

2. Diagnostic test results

a. Blood analysis typically shows a slightly elevated white blood cell (WBC) count during an acute attack; eosinophilia also may be present.

b. Sputum analysis may reveal Curschmann's spirals (mucous casts of the small airways), eosinophils, Charcot-Leyden crystals (products of eosinophil breakdown), and bacteria (if there is an infection).

c. Arterial blood gas (ABG) measurements help gauge the severity of the asthma attack (see Table 40-1).

d. Pulmonary function tests help determine the degree of airway obstruction and gas exchange impairment. During an acute asthma attack, FEV_1 decreases while residual volume (RV) and functional residual volume (FRV) increase. Total lung capacity (TLC) may be elevated.

e. An **electrocardiogram (ECG)** may show sinus tachycardia.

f. Chest x-ray is useful in detecting an accompanying pneumothorax or pneumonia.

g. Allergy skin tests may identify allergens that trigger asthma. (Skin tests should not be done during an acute attack.)

G. Treatment objectives

1. Identify and eliminate causative agents, thus reducing the incidence of acute asthma attacks

2. Manage acute asthma attacks by reversing airway obstruction

3. Treat any chronic symptoms

4. Prevent or manage disease complications

5. Teach the patient about the disease state, proper use of medication, and possible side effects, thereby improving compliance and promoting preventive measures

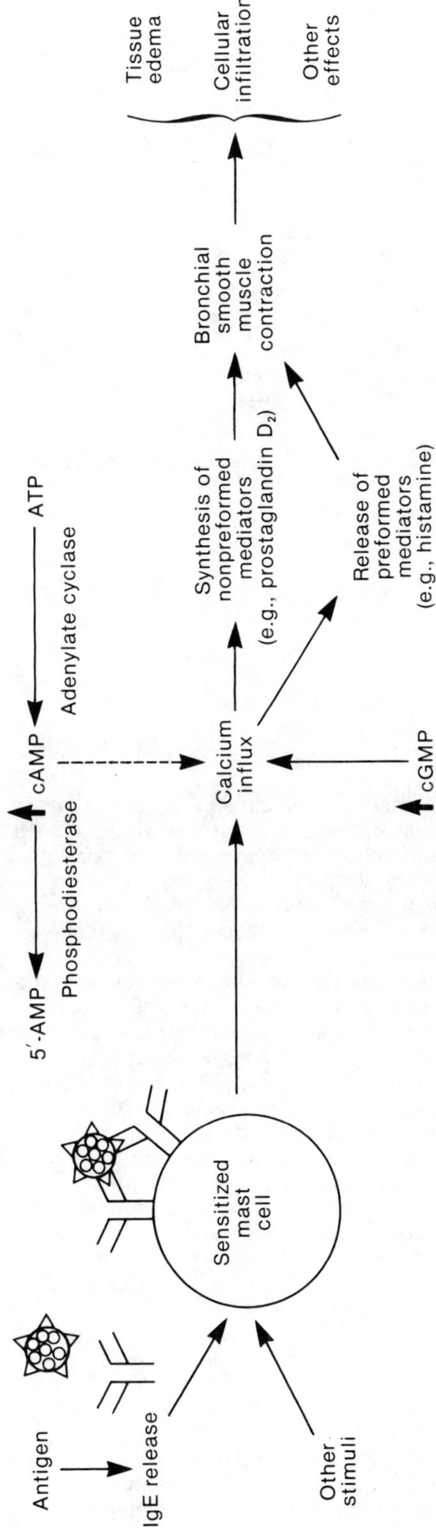

Figure 40-1. Immunopathology of asthma. *IgE* = immunoglobulin E; *5′-AMP* = adenosine-5′-monophosphoric acid; *cAMP* = cyclic adenosine monophosphate; *ATP* = adenosine triphosphate; *cGMP* = cyclic guanosine monophosphate. *Unbroken lines* indicate stimulation; *broken line* indicates inhibition.

Table 40-1. Stages of Severity of an Acute Asthmatic Attack

Stage	Symptoms	FEV_1 or FVC	Arterial pH	PaO_2	$PaCO_2$
I: Mild	Mild dyspnea and wheezing	50%–80% of normal	Normal or ↑	Normal or ↓	Normal or ↓
II: Moderate	Respiratory distress at rest, marked wheezing	50% of normal	↑	↓	↓
III: Severe	Marked respiratory distress, loud wheezing, coughing, difficulty speaking, accessory chest muscle use, chest hyperinflation	25% of normal	Normal or ↓	↓	Normal or ↑
IV: Respiratory failure	Severe respiratory distress, confusion, lethargy, cyanosis, disappearance of breath sounds, pulsus paradoxus > 20–30 mm Hg	10% of normal	↓↓	↓	↑↑

Arrows indicate changes: ↑ = increased; ↓ = decreased; ↑↑ = markedly increased; ↓↓ = markedly decreased.
FEV_1 = Forced expiratory volume in 1 second.
FVC = Forced vital capacity.
PaO_2 = Partial pressure of arterial oxygen.
$PaCO_2$ = Partial pressure of arterial carbon dioxide.

H. Therapy

1. **Management of an acute asthma attack.** A stepped approach is used, with drugs administered in the order discussed below.
   a. **β-Adrenergic agents** (e.g., isoproterenol, epinephrine, metaproterenol, terbutaline) usually are given first (Table 40-2).
      (1) **Therapeutic effects.** Among their various effects, these agents (also called **sympathomimetics**) relieve bronchoconstriction and thus help reverse an acute asthma attack.
      (2) **Mechanism of action.** β-Adrenergics mimic or enhance the effect of sympathetic nervous system stimulation by occupying β-adrenergic receptor sites and increasing norepinephrine release at postganglionic nerve endings. The specific agents used for asthma exert a preferential effect on β_2-receptors and mediate relaxation of bronchial smooth muscle.
      (3) **Administration and dosage.** Whenever possible, these agents are given to asthmatics via nebulizer or metered-dose inhaler (MDI) because of the longer duration of action of this dosage form compared to oral forms. In an emergency situation, a motorized nebulizer should be used. For chronic therapy, they are administered orally only to patients who cannot use aerosols properly. For acute, severe obstruction, parenteral administration is necessary. For dosage information, see Table 40-2.
      (4) **Precautions and monitoring effects**
         (a) These drugs should be used cautiously in patients with a history of arrhythmias, coronary artery disease, hypertension, or diabetes.
         (b) Tremor, nervousness, headache, dizziness, weakness, and insomnia are common central nervous system (CNS) effects of β-adrenergic agents.
         (c) Palpitations and tachycardia occur. Pulse rate should be monitored closely in patients receiving any of the β-adrenergics.
         (d) Excessive use of β_2-adrenergics with some β_1 effects (e.g., metaproterenol) may lead to paradoxical bronchiolar constriction or cardiac arrest.
         (e) Epinephrine and isoproterenol in repeated doses may cause myocardial ischemia and arrhythmias.
         (f) Drug tolerance may occur even with inhaled agents. The mechanism of tolerance is not completely understood, but studies suggest the following:
            (i) There is a decrease in the number of β-receptors.
            (ii) There is a decrease in the sensitivity of β-receptors. This can be reversed by discontinuing the drug or by combining the drug with oral or aerosol corticosteroid therapy.
         (g) **Significant interactions**
            (i) Concomitant use of **monoamine oxidase (MAO) inhibitors** with **ephedrine** or **terbutaline** may lead to severe hypertension.

Table 40-2. *β*-Adrenergics Used in the Treatment of Asthma

Agent	Site of Action	Route/Dosage	Duration of Action	Comments
Isoproterenol	β_1 receptors + + + β_2 receptors + + + +	**Inhalation**: 1–2 puffs during acute attack **IV infusion**: 0.05–2 μg/kg/min	1–2 hours 1–2 hours	Tolerance develops with long-term inhalation therapy; continuous infusion used for severe attacks (mostly in children)
Epinephrine	β_1 receptors + + + β_2 receptors + + +	**Subcutaneous**: Children: 0.01 ml/kg of 1:1000 (maximum 0.3 ml) Adults: 0.2–0.5 ml of 1:1000	15–30 minutes	For use in acute attacks; dose can be repeated every 15–30 minutes until 3 or 4 doses have been given
Isoetharine	β_1 receptors + + β_2 receptors + + +	**Nebulized solution (1%) via mask**: 0.5 ml in 1.5 ml NSS	1–3 hours	Given every 2–3 hours to manage severe attack
Metaproterenol	β_1 receptors + + β_2 receptors + + +	**Inhalation**: 1–3 puffs q 3–4 hours **Nebulizer (5%)**: 0.2–0.3 ml in 2.5 ml NSS **Oral**: Children: 5–10 mg tid or qid Adults: 20 mg tid or qid	3–5 hours	Inhalation route mainly for outpatient use; nebulizer used as alternative for isoetharine; oral route used for long-term therapy
Terbutaline	β_1 receptors + β_2 receptors + + + +	**Subcutaneous (1 mg/ml)**: Children: 0.005–0.01 mg/kg Adults: 0.25 mg **Oral**: Children: 0.05–0.1 mg/kg tid Adults: 2.5–5 mg tid **Inhalation**: 1–2 puffs q 4–6 hours	1.5–5 hours 4–8 hours 6–8 hours	Subcutaneous route used only in emergency; dose can be repeated once q 4 hours
Albuterol	β_1 receptors + β_2 receptors + + + +	**Inhalation**: 1–2 puffs q 4–6 hours **Oral**: 2–4 mg tid	6–8 hours 4–6 hours	For long-term therapy
Bitolterol	β_1 receptors + β_2 receptors + + + +	**Inhalation**: 1–3 sprays q 4–6 hours	6–7 hours	Pro-drug activation by lung esterases
Fenoterol	β_1 receptors + β_2 receptors + + + +	**Inhalation**: 1–2 puffs q 4–6 hours **Oral**: 5–10 mg tid	6–8 hours 4–6 hours	
Pirbuterol	β_1 receptors + β_2 receptors + + + +	**Inhalation**: 1–2 puffs q 4–6 hours	6–8 hours	

NSS = normal saline solution.
IV = intravenous.

(ii) **β-Adrenergic blockers** (e.g., propranolol) block the bronchodilating effect of β-adrenergic agents.

(iii) Vasoconstriction may occur when **epinephrine** is administered concurrently with **propranolol**.

b. Theophylline compounds. These spasmolytic agents are administered if β-adrenergics fail to control an acute asthma attack.

(1) **Therapeutic effects.** Among their various effects, these drugs relax bronchial smooth muscle, reduce mucous secretions, enhance mucociliary transport, and improve diaphragmatic contractility.

(2) **Mechanism of action.** Inhibition of the enzyme phosphodiesterase, resulting in an increase of cAMP, occurs only at toxic concentrations. Other suggested mechanisms include alteration of intracellular calcium and increasd binding of cAMP to its binding protein.

(3) **Administration and dosage**

(a) **Intravenous therapy.** Theophylline and aminophylline both are available.

(i) **Theophylline.** The usual loading dose for adults and children is 6 mg/kg, based on lean body weight, administered over 30 minutes. Loading doses for obese patients (weight greater than 20% over standard weight per insurance tables) should be based on total body weight.

(ii) **Aminophylline.** Aminophylline contains 80% theophylline. Dosage for aminophylline is therefore approximately 1.2 times that of theophylline.

(b) The **maintenance dose** is administered by continuous infusion and is adjusted by monitoring theophylline serum levels (Table 40-3). Maintenance dosage for obese patients should be based on lean body weight.

(c) **Oral therapy**

(i) Oral loading doses of theophylline and aminophylline can be given when the situation is not an emergency one. The initial dose of theophylline for adults and children over age 1 year is the lesser of 400 mg/day or 16 mg/kg/day. The dose can be titrated slowly upward and the serum level monitored until a therapeutic level is obtained. The maximum dose varies with age, from 24 mg/kg/day for children aged 1 to 9 years, to 16 mg/kg/day for adults.

(ii) Other theophylline "salts" are available; dosing is based on theophylline content. These products claim fewer side effects but are comparable when used in equivalent doses (Table 40-4).

(iii) Sustained release forms of theophylline are available to increase the dosing interval and improve compliance. The products can vary in their time to peak concentration (see Table 40-4).

(4) **Precautions and monitoring effects**

(a) These drugs are contraindicated in patients with hypersensitivity to xanthine compounds and in those with a history of arrhythmias.

(b) Cautious use is indicated in patients with peptic ulcer disease, gout, coronary artery disease, and diabetes mellitus.

(c) These agents may cause such adverse CNS effects as dizziness, restlessness, insomnia, and convulsions.

(d) Palpitations and sinus tachycardia have been reported, even in the therapeutic dosage range.

(e) Adverse gastrointestinal effects include nausea, vomiting, and anorexia. These effects should be carefully differentiated from theophylline toxicity, which can occur with serum levels > 20 μg/ml.

(f) Because individuals metabolize theophylline compounds at different rates, serum drug levels should be monitored to ensure a level in the therapeutic range (10 to 20 μg/ml). Levels should be monitored at steady-state (about 4 to 5 half-lives of drug).

Table 40-3. Theophylline Maintenance Doses

Age and Circumstance	Infusion Rate (mg/kg/hr)
Young child (1–9 years old)	0.8
Older child (9–16 years old)	0.7
Adult (older than 16 years)	0.4
Adult smoker	0.7
Adult with cardiac decompensation, cor pulmonale, liver dysfunction, or a combination of these	0.2

Table 40-4. Selection of Theophylline Products

Salt	Theophylline Content (%)	Equivalent Dose (mg)
Theophylline anhydrous	100	100
Theophylline monohydrate	91	110
Aminophylline anhydrous	86	116
Aminophylline dihydrate	79	127
Oxtriphylline	64	156
Theophylline sodium glycinate	46	217
Formulation	**Time to Peak**	**Dosing Interval**
Uncoated tablets	1–2 hours	q 6 hours
Oral liquids	1–2 hours	q 6 hours
Sustained release		
capsule	3–6 hours	q 8 hours
tablet	4–10 hours	q 12 hours
capsule	11–15 hours	q 24 hours

During infusion therapy, levels can be measured at 32 to 40 hours after the start or change in infusion. During oral therapy, a trough level is taken before the dose is given after the first 1½ to 2 days.

(g) Drug clearance may be altered by various factors, including significant drug interactions (Table 40-5).

c. **Corticosteroids** (e.g., beclomethasone, betamethasone, hydrocortisone, prednisone) may be given if bronchoconstriction fails to respond to β-adrenergics or theophylline compounds.

(1) Therapeutic effects. When used to treat asthma, corticosteroids suppress the inflammatory response.

(2) Mechanism of action. The multiple mechanisms of corticosteroids include stimulation of β_2-receptor synthesis in various tissues.

(3) Administration and dosage

(a) Aerosol corticosteroids. Beclomethasone, dexamethasone, flunisolide, triamcinolone, and budesonide are available in aerosol form (preferred because of the lower incidence of adverse effects). Alternatively, corticosteroids may be administered intravenously (for acute attacks) or orally (most appropriate for maintenance therapy).

(b) Oral corticosteroids. Prednisone and prednisolone are the preferred agents—especially for long-term therapy—because of their shorter duration of action.

(4) Precautions and monitoring effects

(a) Corticosteroids should be used cautiously in elderly and pediatric patients and in those with diabetes mellitus, hypothyroidism, peptic ulcers or other gastrointestinal diseases, chronic infections, Cushing's syndrome, myasthenia gravis, and psychotic tendencies.

(b) Patients receiving daily or alternate-day oral corticosteroid therapy should be monitored closely for adverse systemic effects (Table 40-6).

Table 40-5. Factors That Alter Theophylline Clearance

Factors that increase clearance (causing a reduced serum drug level)
Age < 16
Fever
Smoking
Concurrent use of carbamazepine, isoproterenol, phenobarbital, phenytoin, rifampin
Factors that decrease clearance (causing an increased serum drug level)
Advanced age
Cor pulmonale
Congestive heart failure
Pneumonia
Concurrent use of allopurinol, cimetidine, erythromycin, oral contraceptives, propranolol, troleandomycin

Table 40-6. Systemic Effects of Corticosteroid Therapy

Effect	Clinical Manifestations	Intervention/Prevention
Appetite stimulation	Weight gain	Reduction in caloric intake
Fluid and sodium retention	Edema	Reduction in sodium intake
Hyperacidity	Esophagitis, gastritis	Antacids, histamine$_2$-receptor antagonists (e.g., ranitidine)
Hypertension	Headache, cerebrovascular accident	Blood pressure monitoring
Psychosis	Disruptive behavior	Tranquilizers
Increased intraocular pressure	Glaucoma	Ophthalmologic evaluation
Hypokalemia	Muscle weakness	Potassium replacement therapy
Increased gluconeogenesis	Hyperglycemia	Adjustment of dietary, insulin, or oral hypoglycemic therapy

(c) Inhaled steroids may cause such local effects as dry mouth, hoarseness, and fungal infection of the mouth and throat (spacer devices reduce these adverse effects) and rare systemic side effects.

(d) **Significant interaction**. Concurrent use of **hepatic microsomal enzyme inducers** (e.g., rifampin, barbiturates) causes enhanced corticosteroid metabolism, reducing therapeutic efficacy.

2. **Cromolyn sodium** is used adjunctively to treat severe chronic asthma; it sometimes helps reduce the amount of corticosteroid needed. When used prophylactically, it may prevent exercise-induced asthma and seasonal asthma. It has no value in the treatment of an acute asthma attack.

   a. **Therapeutic effect**. Cromolyn suppresses allergen-induced bronchospasm. When used as maintenance therapy for asthma, it suppresses nonspecific bronchial hyperreactivity.

   b. **Mechanism of action**. Cromolyn acts locally on the lung mucosa, inhibiting the degranulation of sensitized mast cells by prevention of calcium influx that takes place after exposure to specific antigens. It also suppresses the release of histamine and other mediators from mast cells, thereby decreasing the stimulus for bronchospasm.

   c. **Administration and dosage**. Cromolyn is available as 20-mg capsules whose contents are inhaled via a special turboinhaler, as a nebulizer solution (20 mg/2 ml) and as an MDI providing 0.8 mg per inhalation.

   (1) As adjunctive therapy for severe chronic asthma, a 20-mg capsule is given for inhalation four times per day; or the solution is sprayed via nebulizer into each nostril three to six times per day; or two sprays of the MDI are used four times a day.

   (2) **To prevent asthma attacks**, cromolyn is used 10 to 15 minutes before exposure to the triggering factor (e.g., pollen).

   d. **Precautions and monitoring effects**

   (1) Cromolyn is not intended for use during an acute asthma attack or status asthmaticus.

   (2) Generally, this drug is well tolerated; occasionally, the inhaled form causes paradoxical bronchospasm, wheezing, and coughing, as well as nasal congestion and dryness of the throat and trachea. There are fewer side effects with the MDI.

   (3) Rarely, laryngeal edema, urticaria, or anaphylaxis occurs.

3. **Other agents** used in the treatment of asthma include the following:

   a. **Anticholinergics**. Also called **cholinergic blockers**, these drugs cause bronchodilation by inhibiting acetylcholine stimulation of lung receptors.

   (1) **Ipratropium bromide** is given as maintenance therapy for asthma that is poorly controlled by β-adrenergics alone. It is administered by MDI (two to four inhalations every 6 hours).

   (2) **Aerosolized atropine** has become nearly obsolete since the introduction of ipratropium because of its high incidence of adverse effects.

   b. **Antihistamines. Terfenadine** and **astemizole** compete with histamine for histamine$_1$-receptor sites on effector cells and thus help prevent the histamine-mediated responses that influence asthma. However, their use in asthma requires further study.

   c. **Calcium channel blockers** (e.g., verapamil, nifedipine). Theoretically, these agents may have therapeutic effects in asthma. In vitro, these agents cause relaxation of smooth muscle by inhibition of calcium influx. This has not been proved in clinical studies, however, and further investigation is needed.

d. **Humidified oxygen** is administered to all patients with severe, acute asthma to reverse hypoxemia. The fraction of inspired oxygen (FIO_2) administered is based on the patient's ABG status; generally 1 to 3 L/min are given via Venturi mask or nasal cannula.
e. **IV fluids and electrolytes** may be required if the patient is dehydrated.
f. **Antibiotics** are administered if the patient has a known or suspected bacterial infection (as suggested by yellow, green, or brown sputum).

I. Complications of asthma

1. **Status asthmaticus.** This life-threatening condition occurs when a prolonged asthma attack fails to respond to normal treatment.
   a. **Physical findings** include altered consciousness, cyanosis (even with O_2 therapy), and pulsus paradoxus ($>$ 20 to 30 mm Hg).
   b. **Standard therapy** for status asthmaticus involves oxygen, IV fluids and electrolytes, epinephrine subcutaneously, inhaled β-adrenergics (by nebulizer only), and corticosteroids. In some cases, IV aminophylline is added.
   c. **Aggressive therapy** is warranted if standard therapy fails.
      (1) If the patient has respiratory acidosis, **tracheal intubation** and **mechanical ventilation** are necessary.
      (2) If the patient does not respond adequately to these measures, any of the following steps may be taken in addition to mechanical ventilation.
         (a) **Sedatives** (e.g., morphine, diazepam) may be administered.
         (b) **Skeletal muscle paralysis** may be induced via **pancuronium** administration.
         (c) **General anesthesia** may be induced via a bronchodilating anesthetic (e.g., halothane).
         (d) Segmental bronchial lavage may be performed to remove the mucous plugs blocking the airway.

2. **Pneumothorax.** This condition is characterized by accumulation of air in the pleural space, as sometimes occurs during an acute asthma attack.
   a. **Physical findings** include sudden sharp chest pain, dyspnea, tachypnea, hypotension, diaphoresis, pallor, and anxiety.
   b. **Therapy** includes placing the patient in Fowler's position, oxygen therapy, aspiration of pleural air via a chest tube, and analgesics.

3. **Atelectasis.** This disorder, which inhibits gas exchange during respiration, may occur if bronchiolar obstruction causes collapse of lung tissue. In asthmatics, atelectasis usually involves the right middle lobe but sometimes affects the entire lung.
   a. **Physical findings** include diminished breath sounds, mediastinal shift toward the affected side, worsening dyspnea, anxiety, and cyanosis.
   b. **Therapy** includes incentive spirometry, postural drainage, chest percussion, coughing and deep breathing exercises, and bronchodilators. Bronchoscopy may be necessary to remove secretions.

II. CHRONIC OBSTRUCTIVE PULMONARY DISEASE

A. **Definitions. Chronic obstructive pulmonary disease (COPD)** is a general term for conditions characterized by chronic, progressive lower airway obstruction causing reduced pulmonary inspiratory and expiratory capacity. The two major forms of COPD—**chronic bronchitis** and **emphysema**—frequently coexist.

   1. **Chronic bronchitis.** In this disorder, excessive mucus production by the tracheobronchial tree results in airway obstruction due to edema and bronchial inflammation. Bronchitis is considered chronic when the patient has a cough producing more than 30 ml of sputum in 24 hours for at least 3 months of the year for 2 consecutive years.

   2. **Emphysema.** This condition is marked by permanent alveolar enlargement distal to the terminal bronchioles and destructive changes of the alveolar walls.

B. **Incidence.** Approximately 10 million Americans have COPD. More common in men than women, COPD affects about 20% of older men. However, due to the increased number of women smokers, the incidence of emphysema in women is rising.

C. **Etiology.** Various factors have been implicated in the development of COPD.

   1. **Cigarette smoking.** The major causative factor, smoking predisposes an individual to COPD by impairing ciliary action and macrophage function and by causing airway inflammation, increased mucous secretion, alveolar wall destruction, and peribronchiolar fibrosis.

2. **Other proposed etiologic factors** include exposure to irritants such as sulfur dioxide (as in polluted air), noxious gases, and organic or inorganic dusts; a history of childhood respiratory infections; familial and hereditary factors (e.g., α_1-antitrypsin deficiency); and allergy. Asthma rarely leads to COPD.

D. Pathophysiology

1. **Chronic bronchitis**
   a. **Respiratory tissue inflammation** (as from smoking) results in vasodilation, congestion, mucosal edema, and goblet cell hypertrophy. These events trigger goblet cells to produce excessive amounts of mucus.
   b. **Changes in tissue** include increased smooth muscle, cartilage atrophy, infiltration of neutrophils and other cells, and impairment of cilia.
   c. Chronic bronchitis, due to lung impairment, predisposes patients to **lung infections**, both viral and bacterial, which further **destroy small bronchioles.**
   d. As the disease progresses, **airways are blocked** by thick, tenacious mucus secretions, which triggers a productive cough.
   e. As the **airways degenerate**, overall gas exchange is impaired, causing **exertional dyspnea. Hypoxemia** results from ventilation/perfusion imbalance and is reflected in an increasing $PaCO_2$ and hypercapnia.
   f. Over time, sustained hypercapnia desensitizes the brain's respiratory control center and central chemoreceptors. As a result, compensatory action to correct hypoxemia and hypercapnia (i.e., a respiratory rate increase) does not occur.

2. **Emphysema**
   a. This disorder leads to anatomical changes that destroy lung elasticity.
      (1) **Inflammation and excessive mucous secretion** (as from long-standing chronic bronchitis) cause **air trapping in the alveoli**. This contributes to breakdown of the bronchioles, alveolar walls, and connective tissue.
      (2) As clusters of alveoli merge, the number of alveoli diminishes, leading to increased space available for air trapping.
      (3) Destruction of alveolar walls causes collapse of small airways on exhalation and disruption of the pulmonary capillary beds.
      (4) These changes result in **ventilation/perfusion (V/Q) abnormalities**; blood is shunted away from destroyed areas to maintain a constant V/Q ratio, unlike the case in chronic bronchitis.
      (5) **Hypercapnia** and **respiratory acidosis** may develop, causing desensitization of brain centers to hypercapnia. When this occurs, hypoxemia serves as the stimulus for breathing.
   b. The **anatomical changes** characteristic of emphysema typically occur in specific lung regions.
      (1) In **centrilobular emphysema**, associated with chronic bronchitis, the upper lung portions are affected. Typically, bronchioles, but not alveoli, become dilated and merge.
      (2) In **panlobular emphysema**, all lung segments are involved. The alveoli enlarge and atrophy, and the pulmonary vascular bed is destroyed. This emphysema form is associated with α_1-antitrypsin deficiency.
      (3) In **paraseptal emphysema**, the lung periphery adjacent to fibrotic regions is the site of alveolar distention and alveolar wall destruction.

E. Clinical evaluation

1. **Physical findings**
   a. **Predominant chronic bronchitis** typically has an insidious onset after age 45.
      (1) **A chronic productive cough** is the **hallmark** of chronic bronchitis. It occurs first in winter, then progresses to year-round. It is usually worse in the morning.
      (2) **Exertional dyspnea**, the most common presenting symptom, is progressive. However, the severity of this symptom does not reflect the severity of the disease.
      (3) Other common findings include obesity, rhonchi and wheezes on auscultation, cyanosis, prolonged expiration, and a normal respiratory rate. As the disease progresses, the following are also common: jugular venous distention, peripheral edema, hepatomegaly, and cardiomegaly.
   b. **Predominant emphysema** has an insidious onset and symptoms occur after age 55.
      (1) The **cough** is chronic but less productive than in chronic bronchitis.
      (2) **Exertional dyspnea** is progressive, constant, and severe.
      (3) Other common findings include weight loss, tachypnea, pursed-lip breathing, prolonged expiration, accessory chest muscle use, hyperresonance on percussion, diaphragmatic excursion, and diminished breath sounds.

c. Patients may have elements and physical findings from each of these diseases simultaneously.

2. Diagnostic test results

a. Chronic bronchitis

(1) Blood analysis usually reveals an increased hematocrit value and sometimes shows an elevated erythrocyte level. With bacterial infection, the WBC count may be elevated.

(2) Sputum inspection reveals thick purulent or mucopurulent sputum tinged yellow, white, green, or gray; the color change is diagnostic of infection. Microscopic analysis may detect neutrophils and microorganisms.

(3) ABG studies may show a markedly decreased PaO_2 level (45 to 60 mmHg) [hypoxemia] and a $PaCO_2$ level that is normal (50 to 60 mmHg) or elevated (hypercapnia).

(4) Pulmonary function tests may be normal in early disease stages. Later, they show an increased RV, a decreased VC and FEV, and normal diffusing capacity and static lung compliance.

(5) Chest x-ray typically identifies lung hyperinflation and increased bronchovascular markings.

(6) An **ECG** may reveal right ventricular hypertrophy and changes consistent with cor pulmonale.

b. Emphysema

(1) Blood analysis may indicate an increased hemoglobin value in late disease stages; it also may show a decreased α_1-antitrypsin level.

(2) Sputum inspection reveals scanty sputum that is clear or mucoid. Infections are less frequent than in chronic bronchitis.

(3) ABG studies typically indicate a reduced or normal PaO_2 level and, in late disease stages, an increased $PaCO_2$ level.

(4) Pulmonary function tests show normal or increased static lung compliance, reduced diffusing capacity, and increased TLC and RV.

(5) Chest x-ray usually reveals bullae, blebs, a flattened diaphragm, lung hyperinflation, vertical heart, enlarged anteroposterior chest diameter, decreased vascular markings in the lung periphery, and a large retrosternal air space.

F. Treatment objectives

1. Relieve symptoms and thus enable the patient to carry on normal daily activities

2. Improve pulmonary function

3. Control life-threatening disease exacerbations

4. Prevent complications

5. Teach the patient about the disease and the use of medications and thus improve therapeutic compliance

G. Therapy

1. Drug therapy. β-Adrenergics and theophylline compounds are the most commonly used drugs in the treatment of COPD. The anticholinergic agent ipratropium bromide also is valuable and may be used in combination with other drugs to enhance and prolong bronchodilation.

a. Theophylline compounds (see section I H 1 b and Table 40-4) typically are added to the drug regimen after a trial of β-adrenergics.

(1) In COPD, these drugs increase mucociliary clearance, stimulate the respiratory drive, enhance diaphragmatic contractility, and improve the ventricular ejection fraction.

(2) A trial of 1 to 2 months, with the serum drug level maintained at 10 to 20 μg/ml, is needed to assess therapeutic efficacy. An increase in FEV_1 by more than 15% to 20% indicates a positive response.

(3) Serum drug levels should be monitored closely in patients with congestive heart failure or cor pulmonale.

b. β-Adrenergics (see section I H 1 a and Table 40-2) are most effective in COPD patients whose airway obstruction is at least partially reversible. After a therapeutic trial of several months, pulmonary function tests are performed to evaluate the efficacy of these agents.

(1) β-Adrenergics are given via aerosol unless the patient cannot use this drug form properly.

(2) Prolonged use of β-adrenergics may lead to drug tolerance.

c. Ipratropium bromide and atropine. These agents produce bronchodilation by competitively inhibiting cholinergic receptors. Some studies have shown an increased response to these agents in COPD when they are combined with β-adrenergics.

(1) **Ipratropium bromide** is three to five times more potent then atropine and has fewer side effects than atropine. It is administered through two inhalations, four times daily.
(2) **Atropine** is administered by diluting 0.025 mg/kg to 0.05 mg/kg in 2 to 4 ml of normal saline and placing it in a nebulizer for spraying every 6 hours. Side effects include dry mouth, tachycardia, and urinary retention.

d. **Corticosteroids** (see section I H 1 c and Table 40-6) play a less prominent role in COPD than in asthma.
(1) These agents may be added to the drug regimen after maximal β-adrenergic and theophylline therapy.
(2) Candidates for corticosteroid therapy should have a history of positive response to bronchodilator therapy (as evidenced by an FEV_1 increase of more than 15% to 20%) and frequent disease exacerbations accompanied by wheezing.
(3) Corticosteroids may be given via aerosol to minimize adverse effects.
(4) Acute exacerbations can be treated intravenously with methylprednisolone, 0.5 mg/kg every 6 hours for 72 hours, then tapered off.
(5) For oral use, these agents are administered in a dosage of 20 to 40 mg/day for the first 2 to 4 weeks, then titrated to the lowest effective dosage.

e. **Antibiotics** are used only to treat a documented infection or to prevent infection in high-risk patients.
(1) The most common infecting organisms are *Mycoplasma pneumoniae*, *Streptococcus pneumoniae*, and *Haemophilus influenzae*.
(2) Antibiotics commonly used in COPD include:
(a) Ampicillin (500 mg given four times per day)
(b) Amoxicillin (500 mg given three times per day)
(c) Erythromycin (500 mg given four times per day)
(d) Tetracycline (250 to 500 mg given four times per day)
(e) Trimethoprim (80 mg) and sulfamethoxazole (400 mg), given as a combination product twice daily

2. **Other measures**. Depending on individual patient needs, COPD therapy also may include the following:
a. **Fluid administration** helps to liquefy secretions; water is a good expectorant.
b. **Mucolytics** (e.g., acetylcysteine); their use is controversial due to side effects.
c. **Expectorants** (e.g., potassium iodide, ammonium chloride) promote mucus removal but with some side effects.
d. **Oxygen therapy** (administered at a low flow rate) reverses hypoxemia. Patients with severe COPD may require oxygen for at least 15 hr/day, administered at a flow rate of 2 L/min.
e. **Chest physiotherapy** loosens secretions, helps re-expand the lungs, and increases the efficacy of respiratory muscle use. Techniques used include postural drainage, chest percussion and vibration, and coughing and deep breathing.
f. **Physical rehabilitation** improves the patient's exercise tolerance. A rehabilitation program usually includes exercises that improve diaphragmatic and abdominal muscle tone.
g. **Vaccines** (e.g., influenza virus, pneumococcal, and *H. influenzae* type b polysaccharide vaccines) may be administered to prevent infection.

H. Complications of COPD. Patients with COPD have an increased risk for developing several life-threatening complications.

1. **Pulmonary hypertension**. With decreased pulmonary vascular bed space (due to lung congestion), pulmonary arterial pressure increases. In some cases, pressure rises high enough to cause **cor pulmonale** (right ventricular hypertrophy), with consequent heart failure.

2. **Acute respiratory failure**. In advanced stages of emphysema, the brain's respiratory center may become seriously compromised, leading to poor cerebral oxygenation and an increased $PaCO_2$ level. Hypoxia and respiratory acidosis may ensue. If the condition progresses, respiratory failure occurs.

3. **Infection**. In chronic bronchitis, trapping of excessive mucus, air, and bacteria in the tracheobronchial tree sets the stage for infection. In addition, impairment of coughing and deep breathing, which normally cleanse the lungs, leads to respiratory cilia destruction. Once an infection sets in, reinfection can easily occur.

STUDY QUESTIONS

Directions: Each question below contains five suggested answers. Choose the **one best** response to each question.

1. The symptoms of asthma result from

A. increased release of preformed mediators from mast cells
B. increased adrenergic responsiveness of the airways
C. increased vascular permeability of bronchial tissue
D. decreased calcium influx into the mast cell
E. decreased prostaglandin production

2. Acute exacerbations of asthma can be triggered by all of the following EXCEPT

A. bacterial or viral pneumonia
B. hypersensitivity reaction to penicillin
C. discontinuation of asthma medication
D. hot, dry weather
E. stressful emotional events

3. The selection of an oral theophylline product depends primarily on

A. the percentage of theophylline content of the product
B. preexisting disease states (e.g., gout, peptic ulcer disease)
C. theophylline half-life
D. concurrent asthma medication
E. age of the patient

4. In the emergency room, the preferred first-line therapy for asthma is

A. theophylline
B. a β-agonist
C. a corticosteroid
D. cromolyn sodium
E. an antihistamine

5. The primary goals of asthma therapy include all of the following EXCEPT

A. treatment of secondary complications
B. management of acute attacks
C. chronic symptom managment
D. prevention of acute exacerbations
E. prevention of lung tissue distruction

6. In the treatment of chronic obstructive pulmonary disease (COPD), corticosteroids

A. are more effective than in the treatment of asthma
B. are more beneficial when used alone
C. produce more side effects when used in the aerosol form
D. should have dosage titrated upward until side effects are seen
E. should be used for at least 2 weeks before efficacy is assessed

Directions: Each question below contains three suggested answers of which **one or more** is correct. Choose the answer

A if **I only** is correct
B if **III only** is correct
C if **I and II** are correct
D if **II and III** are correct
E if **I, II, and III** are correct

7. The disease process of chronic bronchitis is characterized by

I. the destruction of central and peripheral portions of the acinus
II. an increased number of mucous glands and goblet cells
III. edema and inflammation of the bronchioles

Directions: The group of questions below consists of lettered choices followed by several numbered items. For each numbered item select the **one** lettered choice with which it is **most** closely associated. Each lettered choice may be used once, more than once, or not at all.

Questions 8–10

Match the description with the appropriate agent.

A. Cimetidine
B. Albuterol
C. Ipratropium bromide
D. Epinephrine
E. Atropine

8. Decreases theophylline clearance
9. Has anticholinergic activity with few side effects
10. Has high β_2-adrenergic selectivity

ANSWERS AND EXPLANATIONS

1. The answer is A. [*I E 2 b (1)*] In asthma, airborne antigen binds to the mast cell, activating the immunoglobulin E (IgE)-mediated process. Preformed mediators (e.g., histamine) and nonpreformed mediators (e.g., prostaglandin D_2) are then released, causing bronchoconstriction and tissue edema.

2. The answer is D. (*I D 1; Figure 40-1*) Exacerbations of asthma can be triggered by allergens, respiratory infections, occupational stimuli (e.g., fumes from gasoline or paint), emotions, and environmental factors. Studies have shown that cold air can cause release of mast cell mediators by an undetermined mechanism. Hot, dry air does not cause this release.

3. The answer is A. (*I H 1 b; Table 40-4*) Theophylline or aminophylline products vary in their percentage of active drug, or theophylline content, and in the type of preparation. Sustained-release products decrease the absorption rate and do not alter theophylline half-life.

4. The answer is B. [*I H 1 a (3)*] In an emergency situation, the most rapidly acting agent is used first. Selection of the route of administration depends on the severity of the attack. An inhaled β-agonist administered in a nebulizer or administered as a subcutaneous agent is the most appropriate first-line therapy.

5. The answer is E. (*I E, G; II D*) Asthma is a reversible narrowing of airways in response to specific stimuli. Mast cells release mediators, which trigger bronchoconstruction. After an acute attack, in most cases, symptoms will be minimal and pathologic changes will not be permanent. Unlike asthma, chronic obstructive pulmonary disease (COPD) does cause progressive airway destruction, chronic bronchitis by excessive mucus production and other changes, and emphysema by destruction of the acinus.

6. The answer is E. (*II G 1 d*) In COPD, corticosteroids are used in addition to β-adrenergic agents and/or theophylline compounds after maximal therapy with these agents. Corticosteroids may be used in aerosol form to minimize side effects. If given orally, dosage is reduced after 2 to 4 weeks of therapy to the lowest effective dosage. Since the onset of benefit is unknown, an adequate trial of therapy (at least 2–4 weeks) is needed.

7. The answer is D (II, III). (*II D 1 a, c, 2*) Chronic bronchitis is characterized by an increase in the number of mucous and goblet cells due to bronchial irritation. This results in increased mucus production. Other changes include edema and inflammation of the bronchioles and changes in smooth muscle and cartilage. Emphysema is a permanent destruction of the central and peripheral portions of the acinus distal to the bronchioles. In this disease, adequate oxygen reaches the alveolar duct, but there is inadequate blood perfusion.

8–10. The answers are: 8-A, 9-C, 10-B. (*II G 1 c; Table 40-2; Table 40-5*) Cimetidine, a histamine$_2$-receptor antagonist, decreases theophylline clearance by inhibiting hepatic microsomal mixed-function oxidase metabolism. Theophylline clearance can be decreased by 40% during the first 24 hours of concurrent therapy. Anticholinergic agents such as atropine and ipratropium bromide produce bronchodilation by competitively inhibiting cholinergic receptors. The disadvantages of atropine include dry mouth, tachycardia, and urinary retention. Ipratropium bromide is 3 to 5 times more potent than atropine and does not have these side effects. Albuterol is one of the most β_2-selective adrenergic agents available. Other such agents include terbutaline, bitolterol, fenoterol, and pirbuterol. Agents with β_2-selectivity dilate bronchioles without causing side effects related to β_1-stimulation (e.g., increased heart rate).

41
Rheumatoid Arthritis

Larry N. Swanson

I. DEFINITION. Rheumatoid arthritis (RA) is a chronic systemic inflammatory condition that is most patent in its synovial joint involvement. Inflammation may extend to extra-articular sites such as tendons and organ structures.

II. CLASSIFICATION

A. For uniformity of diagnosis, RA classification is based on the presence of criteria developed by the American Rheumatism Association. Of these 11 criteria, 7 are needed for the diagnosis of "classic" RA, 5 for "definite" RA, and 3 for "probable" RA.

B. The 11 American Rheumatism Association criteria are as follows:

1. Morning stiffness
2. Pain on motion or tenderness in at least one joint
3. Swelling in at least one joint
4. Swelling in at least one other joint
5. Symmetric joint swelling with simultaneous swelling in the paired joint
6. Subcutaneous nodules on bony prominences, extensor surfaces, or in juxta-articular regions
7. X-ray changes typical of RA
8. Presence of rheumatoid factor (see section VII C 1)
9. Poor mucin precipitate from synovial fluid
10. Characteristic histologic changes in synovium
11. Characteristic histologic changes in nodules

III. INCIDENCE. RA is **more common in females** than in males, occurring in a female to male ratio of between 2:1 and 3:1. The condition occurs in approximately 1% to 3% of the general adult population, with the peak incidence of onset between the ages of 30 and 50 years.

IV. ETIOLOGY. Although the cause of this disease remains unknown, the two major lines of research into the etiology of RA focus on the following:

A. Immune system abnormalities. Studies of abnormalities in the immune system and its regulation have shown a possible genetic predisposition to RA.

B. Infectious agents. For many years, investigators have noted the occurrence of polyarthritis in association with microbial organisms, including bacteria. However, no specific agent has been identified.

V. PATHOLOGY

A. The initial event inciting synovial inflammation (the earliest synovial response) is unknown. Vasodilation, edema, sensation of heat, and loss of function result. Synovial fluid production increases, with a resultant accumulation of an effusion. If untreated, the synovitis of RA becomes self-perpetuating and chronic. The synovium becomes thickened and boggy.

B. Inward overgrowth of the enlarged synovium across the surface of the articular cartilage results in the formation of **pannus** (an exuberant synovial thickening). The inflammatory reaction at the cartilage–pannus junction may eventually result in articular cartilage degradation, loss of adjacent bone, and characteristic marginal erosions, which are observable on x-ray.

C. The effect of degradation of cartilage is bone rubbing against bone in the joint, producing crepitus and pain.

VI. CLINICAL PRESENTATION

A. Usually, RA presents as symmetric synovitis affecting similar joints bilaterally. Occasionally, the disease may present as arthritis in only one joint or in an asymmetric pattern affecting a few joints. Over time, however, the arthritis is additive and assumes a symmetric pattern.

B. Another commonly observed presentation is frank joint inflammation in a previously healthy individual.

C. A third, but uncommon, presentation is a rapidly progressive arthritis affecting many joints, accompanied by organ system involvement.

D. The least common type of occurrence presents as organ system involvement without clinically evident joint inflammation.

VII. CLINICAL EVALUATION

A. Physical findings

1. Very early symptoms may be vague and lack evidence of synovial inflammation. The presenting complaints may include variable aching, multiple joint pain, and fatigue.
2. Early involvement occurs most often in the hands, with swelling, warmth, and tenderness affecting mainly the proximal interphalangeal and metacarpophalangeal joints.
3. Although hand and foot involvement is the most common initial presentation, synovitis can be prominent in the large joints of the knee, ankle, and elbow, as well as in the intervertebral and temporomandibular joints.
4. The hallmark of RA is maximal pain and stiffness upon awakening; this so-called morning gel typically lasts for more than 30 minutes and may persist for hours.
5. Joint system evaluation reveals swelling, synovial thickening, tenderness, pain, and reduced range of motion in peripheral joints.
6. Rheumatoid nodules (firm, round, rubbery masses that are pathognomonic for RA) are found in about 20% of patients with RA. These nodules are most commonly located in subcutaneous tissues at sites prone to external pressure (e.g., the elbow), but they may affect other organs.

B. X-rays of involved joints may reveal only soft-tissue swelling initially. If inflammation is entrenched, the films may reveal juxta-articular osteoporosis, symmetrical joint space narrowing, and erosions near the joint capsular attachments.

C. Laboratory findings

1. **Rheumatoid factors** (a heterogeneous group of antibodies produced in most patients with RA) are detectable through various serologic techniques, such as the latex fixation test. The most commonly found rheumatoid factors are **immunoglobulin G (IgG)** and **immunoglobulin M (IgM)**. Patients with RA who are seropositive for rheumatoid factors generally follow a more serious disease course than those who are seronegative.
2. **Erythrocyte sedimentation rate increases** reflect the inflammatory response.
3. **Normochromic, normocytic anemia** is indicative of chronic disease.

VIII. CLINICAL COURSE. The course of RA is highly variable but usually follows one of three patterns.

A. Sporadic. This is the most common course; it is distinguished by periods of spontaneous remission and has the most favorable prognosis.

B. Gradual and steady. A gradual but steady and persistent progression of joint inflammation is furthered by periodic debilitating flares. These flares are accompanied by severe polyarticular pain, marked synovial inflammation, joint effusion, stiffness, low-grade fever, and extreme exhaustion.

C. Malignant. This course is less common but more rapid and aggressive. It is characterized by severe, multiple joint synovitis, rheumatoid nodules, weight loss, and very high titers of rheumatoid factor. Complications are common and include involvement of the skin (vasculitis), eyes (scleritis, corneal ulcers), lungs (pleural effusions, nodules, interstitial fibrosis), heart (pericarditis), blood (anemia, thrombocytosis), and nervous system (neuropathies).

IX. TREATMENT OBJECTIVES

A. Provide pain relief

B. Reduce or suppress inflammation

C. Avoid, minimize, or eliminate adverse effects resulting from therapy

D. Preserve or restore function

E. Maintain the patient's life-style

X. THERAPY.

The treatment of RA combines two approaches: mechanical and pharmacologic. Mechanical therapy includes a balanced program of rest and exercise. The pharmacologic component now includes both symptomatic and disease-modifying therapy, which usually requires the combining of agents.

A. Mechanical therapy. The patient is educated in a balanced daily program of exercise and rest.

1. Initially, the joints are rested.
2. Exercises are then introduced to strengthen muscles and increase the range of motion without undue joint strain.
3. Alignment of the joints in a position of function is ensured during sleep through use of specially designed lightweight splints.
4. Complete immobilization is avoided.
5. When preventive measures fail, surgery to improve function of the hands and knees is sometimes beneficial.

B. Drug therapy

1. **Aspirin and aspirin-like agents.** The choice of a drug among these agents is usually empirical because patient response varies widely. Further decisions on drug regimen should be based on the therapeutic effect after 2 to 3 weeks. However, an inadequate response to one drug in this group may not reflect the patient's response to another. Furthermore, adverse effects or toxicity may override an adequate therapeutic response.
   a. **Aspirin** is the first-line agent, administered initially as an analgesic; then, in higher doses, as an anti-inflammatory agent. Aspirin is as effective as any other nonsteroidal anti-inflammatory drug (NSAID) and is much less expensive.
      (1) **Mechanism of action.** In common with other NSAIDs, aspirin appears to work, at least in part, by inhibiting prostaglandin synthesis and release.
      (2) **Dosage.** The usual total dose is 3.6 to 5.4 g daily.
      (3) **Precautions and monitoring effects**
         (a) Aspirin interferes with platelet function and can cause serious bleeding; this effect may persist for 4 to 7 days after the drug has been discontinued.
         (b) Tinnitus and, rarely, hepatitis or renal damage can occur with high-dose aspirin therapy.
         (c) The intolerable gastrointestinal effects experienced by some patients may be avoided by using an agent with an enteric coating.
   b. **Other NSAIDs** (including ibuprofen, naproxen, sulindac, and indomethacin). Many patients tolerate effective doses of the NSAIDs better than high-dose aspirin therapy. However, the newer drugs are much more expensive. No clinical evidence has proven that any one of these drugs is consistently more effective than another, but research shows that a patient who does not respond to one NSAID may respond to another.

(1) **Mechanism of action** [see section X B 1 a (1)]

(2) **Precautions and monitoring effects.** The NSAIDs differ somewhat in adverse effects, with none demonstrably safer in all patients. **Phenylbutazone** is the exception and is usually avoided because of its association with aplastic anemia and agranulocytosis.

(a) NSAIDs should be avoided in asthmatic patients sensitive to aspirin because they may trigger bronchospasm and respiratory failure.

(b) All NSAIDs interfere with **platelet function** and prolong **bleeding time**. However, unlike the effect with aspirin, this effect is quickly reversible with discontinuation of the drug.

(c) All produce **gastrointestinal effects**, including peptic ulceration. The combined effect of gastrointestinal irritation and platelet interference can yield severe gastric hemorrhage.

(d) **Renal blood flow** is decreased somewhat by these agents, and renal failure may ensue in some patients. The potential for renal damage increases when NSAIDs are used in patients at risk for decreased intravascular volume, as occurs in such conditions as congestive heart failure and diuretic use. (This risk may be lower with sulindac.)

(e) Mild **hepatic dysfunction** and, rarely, severe hepatitis may occur.

(f) All NSAIDs can cause adverse **central nervous system (CNS) effects** such as drowsiness, dizziness, anxiety, tinnitus, and confusion initially, but these symptoms usually disappear with continued use. CNS effects, including severe headache, occur more frequently with **indomethacin** (especially in high doses).

(g) Rarely, these agents may cause blood dyscrasias.

c. **Nonacetylated salicylates** (including choline salicylate and salsalate) are safer for aspirin-sensitive patients. They usually will not trigger the respiratory effects produced by aspirin and other NSAIDs, as stated in section X B 1 b (2) (a). Nonacetylated salicylates have less effect on platelet function than aspirin and other NSAIDs, but they may also have less anti-inflammatory effect.

2. **Slow-acting antirheumatic drugs.** Patients with sustained disabling arthritis may require more than an anti-inflammatory agent. Altering the course of the disease is attempted through use of gold compounds, penicillamine, and hydroxychloroquine.

a. **General considerations**

(1) Although their precise mechanisms in RA remain undetermined, these agents attempt to modulate the immune response. Progression of erosion may be delayed or prevented in some patients. Alteration of disease progression evolves slowly and gradually, and therapeutic effect—if it occurs—may not be evident for months.

(2) Generally, the agents in this group are tried one at a time, in combination with a NSAID. If a drug proves ineffective, it is discontinued before another is introduced. No consensus has been formed as to which agent should be tried first; however, most rheumatologists tend to favor gold as the initial agent.

(3) All of these agents potentiate severe adverse reactions and therefore require careful patient monitoring.

b. **Gold compounds** may be administered in oral or intramuscular form.

(1) **Oral agents. Auranofin** may be slightly less toxic but slightly less effective than other forms of gold.

(a) **Administration and dosage.** The initial regimen for auranofin consists of 3 mg twice a day for 6 months. If there is no response, the dosage is increased to 3 mg three times daily (9 mg/day). If there is still no response after 3 more months, the agent should be discontinued.

(b) **Precautions and monitoring effects.** Common, reversible side effects include diarrhea, abdominal pain, rash, stomatitis, and proteinuria.

(2) **Intramuscular agents** (gold sodium thiomalate and aurothioglucose)

(a) **Administration and dosage.** Initially, a test dose of 10 mg is administered, followed by 25 to 50 mg in weekly intervals for up to 20 weeks. Once the cumulative dosage has reached 1500 mg and there is a therapeutic effect, treatment intervals are lengthened to every 2 weeks; then, every 3 weeks, and finally to regular monthly administration.

(b) **Precautions and monitoring effects**

(i) The most common side effects are rash and proteinuria. Pruritus usually precedes stomatitis and a diffuse rash, which can progress to generalized exfoliation; therefore, the drug should be discontinued when pruritus occurs. Lower-dose therapy may be tried later if pruritus does occur. Leukopenia, thrombocytopenia, and aplastic anemia have been reported. Anaphylaxis, angioneurotic edema, glossitis, and interstitial pneumonitis can also occur.

(ii) **Aurothioglucose** (fat-soluble) may be safer than gold thiomalate (water-soluble), which is more likely to cause vasodilation and nitritoid reactions. These reactions are rare and usually mild, but hypotension, syncope, and myocardial infarction have been reported.

c. **Penicillamine.** The effectiveness of this agent as an anti-inflammatory may result from its effect on the altered immune response.

(1) **Administration and dosage.** Penicillamine should be given on an empty stomach because food decreases absorption. Initially, 125 to 250 mg should be administered once daily. Then, the dosage should be increased (by the same amount) at 4- to 12-week intervals until an effective daily dose has been achieved (usually, 750 mg/day; rarely, 1000 to 1500 mg/day).

(2) **Precautions and monitoring effects.** Penicillamine has a high incidence of toxic effects. Adverse effects (usually reversible) include rash, fever, hematuria, proteinuria, dysgeusia, and aphthous ulcers. Of more serious consequence are potential hematologic effects such as leukopenia, thrombocytopenia and aplastic anemia. Autoimmune conditions such as systemic lupus erythematosus, Goodpasture's syndrome, and pemphigus have occurred.

d. **Hydroxychloroquine**

(1) **Administration and dosage.** Hydroxychloroquine should be given in dosages of 400 mg/day or 6.5 mg/kg/day—whichever is less.

(2) **Precautions and monitoring effects**. Hydroxychloroquine can cause severe and sometimes irreversible adverse effects on the eyes, skin, CNS, and bone marrow, but these are rare with recommended doses. An ophthalmologist should check for loss of visual acuity every 6 months. Toxicity can generally be avoided if the drug is discontinued promptly at the first signs of retinal toxicity.

e. **Sulfasalazine** recently has been shown to be useful in the treatment of RA. In a limited number of trials, it has been shown to be as effective as gold and penicillamine and with fewer side effects. In one trial, sulfasalazine was found to be more effective than hydroxychloroquine in preventing progression of joint damage. Common side effects include gastrointestinal disturbances and rash. Serious reactions such as blood dyscracias and hepatitis are rare.

3. **Immunosuppressive drugs**

a. **General considerations.** These agents exert an immunosuppressive effect by inhibiting normal cell metabolism. They are used most often to treat neoplastic diseases or as adjuncts in organ transplants. Because of their toxicity, these agents are usually reserved for severe erosive RA that is unresponsive to other antiarthritic drugs.

b. **Methotrexate** is a folic acid antagonist.

(1) **Administration and dosage**. Initially, the weekly regimen should consist of three doses of 2.5 mg at 12-hour intervals (totaling 7.5 mg/week). This can be increased slowly—at monthly intervals—to 15 mg/week. An alternate regimen is 5 mg once weekly, increased gradually.

(2) **Precautions and monitoring effects**

(a) Aspirin (and possibly other NSAIDs) may increase the toxicity of methotrexate by slowing its rate of excretion.

(b) Adverse effects associated with methotrexate include hepatic toxicity, interstitial pneumonitis, bone marrow suppression, and gastrointestinal ulceration and bleeding. Because 80% to 90% of the drug is excreted unchanged in the urine, methotrexate should be used with extreme caution and at a reduced dosage in patients with renal impairment.

c. **Azathioprine**

(1) **Administration and dosage.** Initially, 50 to 100 mg (about 1 mg/kg) should be given once or twice daily. After 6 to 8 weeks, and then every 4 weeks, the doses can be increased by 0.5 mg/kg/day up to a maximum of 2.5 mg/kg/day. A maintenance regimen should use the lowest effective dose. The dosage should be reduced in patients with renal dysfunction.

(2) **Precautions and monitoring effects.** Adverse effects include nausea, vomiting, abdominal pain, hepatitis, and reversible bone marrow depression. Increased risk of carcinoma and severe infections are potential effects.

d. **Cyclophosphamide** has been used primarily as an antineoplastic agent but may be used in refractory RA. However, cyclophosphamide is significantly more toxic than other immunosuppressive agents.

(1) **Administration and dosage.** The usual initial dose is 1.5 to 3.0 mg/kg/day.

(2) **Precautions and monitoring effects.** Serious toxic effects include bone marrow depression, hemorrhagic cystitis, sterility, alopecia, and malignant diseases (e.g., bladder cancer).

4. Corticosteroids

a. General considerations. In severe progressive RA, prednisone may afford some degree of control, but corticosteroids are usually recognized as agents of last resort. They occasionally may be used for acute flare-ups of the disease or during the interim before the therapeutic effects of slow-acting drugs are observed.

b. Administration and dosage

(1) Oral prednisone in a dose of 5 to 10 mg/day may benefit some patients. Because adverse effects are related to dose and duration, an effort must be made to keep the dose as low as possible.

(2) If painful symptoms are restricted to one or a few acutely inflamed joints, **intra-articular injections** may provide relief.

c. Precautions and monitoring effects. Long-term administration may produce gastrointestinal bleeding, poor wound healing, myopathy, cataracts, hyperglycemia, hypertension, and osteoporosis.

STUDY QUESTIONS

Directions: Each question below contains five suggested answers. Choose the **one best** response to each question.

1. A 50-year-old woman is admitted to the hospital with a chief complaint of bilateral swelling of her knees for 3 days, early morning stiffness, and lethargy. She is not responding to 650 mg of aspirin three times daily. The patient is an obese white woman who states that her ability to move about has slowly regressed due to the stiffness and swelling. She has also noticed a progressive swelling of the hands and wrists. A diagnosis of rheumatoid arthritis is made. Initial suggestion for drug therapy of this patient is

A. hydroxychloroquine 200 mg daily
B. steroid injections into all swollen joints
C. aspirin 975 mg four times a day
D. D-penicillamine 250 mg four times a day
E. gold injections 50 mg intravenously once weekly

2. Which of the following agents and dosage regimens is the best choice of treatment for a patient with rheumatoid arthritis who is considered sensitive to aspirin?

A. Ibuprofen 800 mg three times per day
B. Acetaminophen 650 mg every 4 hours
C. Gold injections 10 to 50 mg intramuscularly once a week
D. Azathioprine 75 mg per day
E. Methotrexate 2.5 mg every 12 hours for 3 doses (total 7.5 mg/week)

3. Which of the following statements best describes the usual course of rheumatoid arthritis? It is

A. an acute exacerbation of joint pain treated with short-term anti-inflammatory therapy
B. a chronic disease characterized by acute changes within nonsynovial joints
C. an acute disease that is characterized by rapid synovial changes due to inflammation
D. a chronic disease characterized by acute exacerbations followed by remissions, with consequences associated with chronic inflammatory changes
E. a joint disease characterized by a marked loss of calcium from the bones and a resultant thinning of the bones

Directions: The groups of questions below consists of lettered choices followed by several numbered items. For each numbered item select the **one** lettered choice with which it is **most** closely associated. Each lettered choice may be used once, more than once, or not at all.

Questions 4–8

Match the drug characteristic with the appropriate agent.

A. Corticosteroids
B. Ibuprofen
C. Aspirin
D. Auranofin
E. Penicillamine

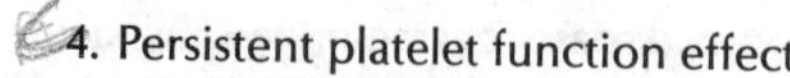

4. Persistent platelet function effect
5. Oral form of gold
6. Given on an empty stomach
7. May be used intra-articularly
8. May cause drowsiness

Questions 9–13

Match the phrase below with the appropriate rheumatoid arthritic agent.

A. Phenylbutazone
B. Aspirin
C. Hydroxychloroquine
D. Methotrexate
E. Cyclophosphamide

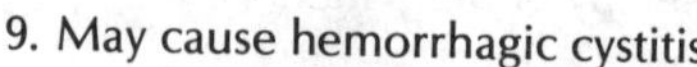

9. May cause hemorrhagic cystitis

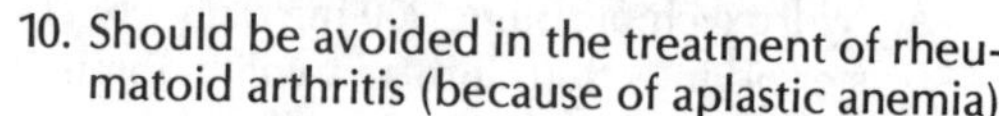

10. Should be avoided in the treatment of rheumatoid arthritis (because of aplastic anemia)
11. Enteric-coated form may be useful in treating some patients
12. Aspirin may slow this drug's rate of excretion
13. Vision should be monitored every 6 months

ANSWERS AND EXPLANATIONS

1. The answer is C. (*X B 1 a*) Unless there are contraindications to the use of salicylates, aspirin administered in anti-inflammatory doses is the agent of choice for initial treatment of the patient with rheumatoid arthritis. The patient in the question has only been taking analgesic doses of aspirin; that is, 650 mg three times a day (1950 mg/day). Parenteral gold preparations are given by intramuscular injection, not intravenously.

2. The answer is C. [*X B 1 b, 2 a (2) (a)*] Patients with nasal polyps, hay fever, or asthma have an increased incidence of aspirin hypersensitivity. In these patients, aspirin administration may result in rhinorrhea, bronchospasm, or anaphylaxis. Patients who are intolerant of aspirin may also show a cross-sensitivity to ibuprofen and other nonsteroidal anti-inflammatory drugs (NSAIDs). Acetaminophen has essentially no anti-inflammatory properties and therefore would not be a good alternative choice for a patient with rheumatoid arthritis. Most rheumatologists would use gold injections (10 mg as a test dose and 25 to 50 mg at weekly intervals) as the next most appropriate agent. Azathioprine and methotrexate would usually be reserved for later therapy.

3. The answer is D. (*I; VIII A*) Rheumatoid arthritis is a chronic disease that most often follows a sporadic course of acute exacerbations of synovial inflammation followed by remissions, with eventual joint manifestations of chronic inflammation.

4–8. The answers are: 4-C, 5-D, 6-E, 7-A, 8-B. [*X B 1 a (3) (a), b (f), 2 b (1), c (1), 4 b (2)*] Both aspirin and other NSAIDs interfere with platelet function; with aspirin, the effect may persist for 4 to 7 days after the drug has been discontinued, whereas platelet function usually returns quickly to normal after stopping other NSAID therapy. Most gold preparations are given by intramuscular injection, but auranofin is given orally. Penicillamine is given on an empty stomach because food decreases its absorption. Intra-articular injection of a corticosteroid is helpful when painful symptoms are restricted to one or a few joints. Ibuprofen, like other NSAIDs, may cause drowsiness and other central nervous system effects, but these usually subside with continuing use.

9–13. The answers are: 9-E, 10-A, 11-B, 12-D, 13-C. [*X B 1 a (3) (c), b (2), 2 d (2), 3 b (2) (a), d*] Phenylbutazone should not be selected for long-term treatment of rheumatoid arthritis because of its association with aplastic anemia. There are many other less toxic NSAIDs that can be used. Many patients taking high doses of aspirin cannot tolerate regular aspirin but can take the enteric-coated form. Because hydroxychloroquine can cause ophthalmic adverse effects, patients receiving this drug should have their vision checked at least every 6 months. Aspirin administration may slow the excretion of methotrexate; this can increase the latter drug's toxicity. Cyclophosphamide is significantly more toxic than other immunosuppressive agents; one of its serious side effects is hemorrhagic cystitis.

42
Hyperuricemia and Gout

Larry N. Swanson

I. INTRODUCTION

A. Definitions

1. **Hyperuricemia** refers to a serum uric acid level that is elevated more than 2 standard deviations above the population mean. In most laboratories, the upper limit of normal is 7 mg/dl (uricase methods). However, the level varies with the laboratory method used. With either method, the upper limit of normal is about 1 mg/dl lower for women than for men.
   a. **Uricase methods** are specific for uric acid and are not subject to interference by drugs.
   b. **Phosphotungstic acid (colorimetric) methods** are nonspecific for uric acid; they are subject to interference (false elevation) by drugs.
2. **Gout** is a disease that is characterized by recurrent acute attacks of urate crystal-induced arthritis. It may include **tophi**—deposits of monosodium urate—in and around the joints and cartilage and in the kidneys, as well as uric acid nephrolithiasis.

B. Incidence

1. Gout affects approximately 0.2% to 1.5% of the United States population.
2. Most gout victims are men (approximately 95% of cases); most women with the disease are postmenopausal.
3. The mean age at disease onset is 47 years.
4. The risk of developing gout increases as the serum uric acid level rises. Virtually all gout patients have a serum uric acid level above 7 mg/dl.
5. Recent research shows that among patients with a serum uric acid level above 9 mg/dl, the cumulative incidence of gout reached 22% after 5 years.
6. Gout has a familial tendency; 10% to 60% of cases occur in family members of patients with the disease.
7. Obesity, heavy alcohol consumption, and certain other life-style factors can increase the chance for developing gout.

C. Uric acid production and excretion

1. An end product of **purine metabolism**, uric acid is produced from both dietary and endogenous sources. Its formation results from the conversion of adenine and guanine moieties of nucleoproteins and nucleotides (Fig. 42-1).
2. **Xanthine oxidase** catalyzes the reaction that occurs as the final step in the degradation of purines to uric acid.
3. The body ultimately excretes uric acid via the kidneys (300 to 600 mg/day; two-thirds of total uric acid) and via the gastrointestinal tract (100 to 300 mg/day; one-third of total uric acid).
4. Uric acid has no known biologic function.
5. The body has a total uric acid content of 1.0 to 1.2 g; the daily turnover rate is approximately 600 to 800 mg.
6. At a pH of 4.0 to 5.0 (i.e., in urine), uric acid exists as a poorly soluble free acid; at physiologic pH, it exists primarily as **monosodium urate salt**.
7. Uric acid filtration, reabsorption, and secretion sites are shown in Figure 42-2.

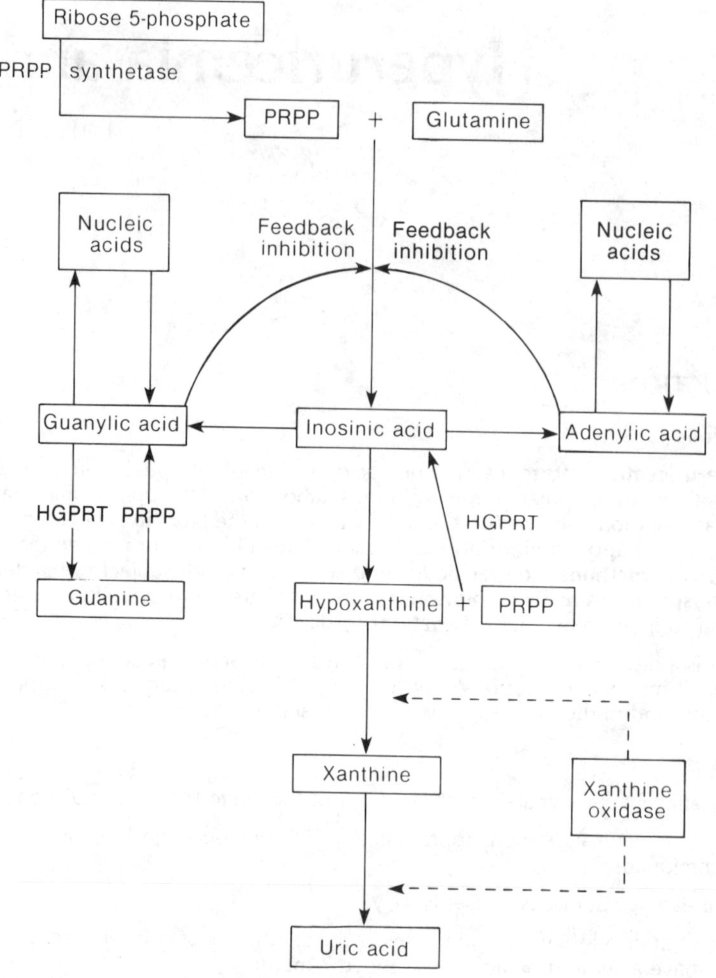

Figure 42-1. Uric acid formation. *PRPP* = phosphoribosyl-1-pyrophosphate; *HGPRT* = hypoxanthine–guanine phosphoribosyltransferase. (Redrawn with permission from DiPiro J, Talbert R, Hayes P, et al: *Pharmacotherapy—A Pathophysiologic Approach*. New York, Elsevier, 1988, p 913.)

D. Etiology. Hyperuricemia and gout may be primary or secondary.

1. **Primary hyperuricemia and gout** apparently result from an innate **defect in purine metabolism and/or uric acid excretion**. The exact cause of the defect usually is unknown.
   a. Hyperuricemia may result from **uric acid overproduction**, **impaired renal clearance of uric acid**, or a combination of these.
   b. Some patients with primary hyperuricemia and gout have a known enzymatic defect, such as hypoxanthine–guanine phosphoribosyltransferase (HGPRT) deficiency or phosphoribosyl-1-pyrophosphate (PRPP) synthetase excess (see Fig. 42-1).
   c. Principally for therapeutic purposes, patients with primary hyperuricemia and gout can be classified as **overproducers** or **underexcretors** of uric acid.
      (1) **Overproducers** (about 10% of patients) synthesize abnormally large amounts of uric acid and excrete excessive amounts—more than 800 to 1000 mg daily on an unrestricted diet or more than 600 mg daily on a purine-restricted diet. They generally have a markedly increased miscible urate pool (greater than 2.5 g).
      (2) **Underexcretors** (about 90% of patients) generally produce normal or near-normal amounts of uric acid but excrete less than 600 mg daily on a purine-restricted diet. They generally have only a slightly increased miscible urate pool.
      (3) Some underexcretors also are overproducers.
2. **Secondary hyperuricemia and gout** develop during the course of another disease or as a result of drug therapy.

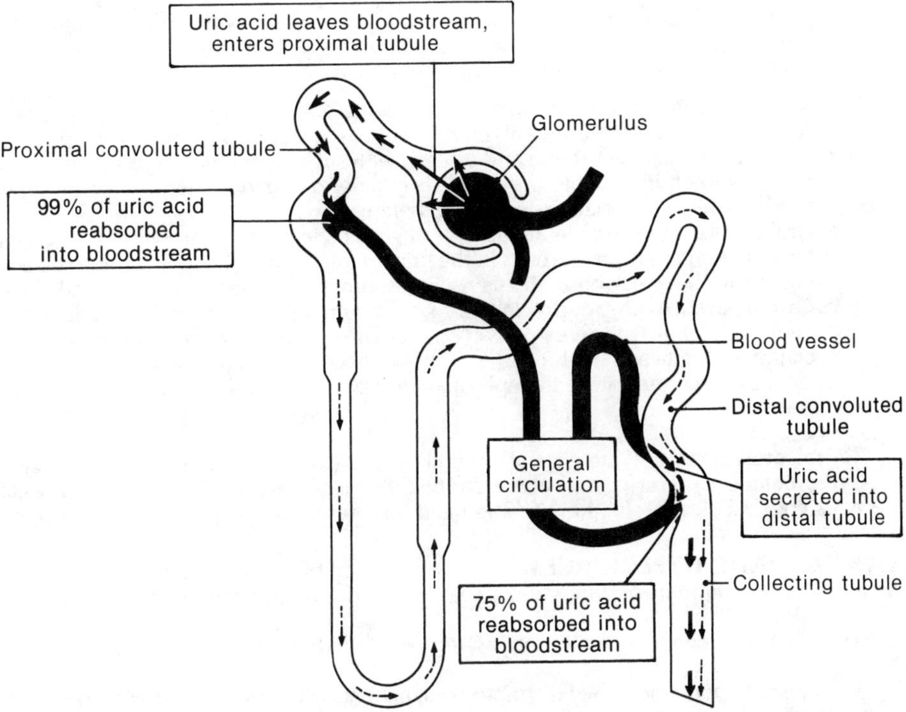

Figure 42-2. Uric acid filtration, reabsorption, and secretion sites. At the glomerulus, uric acid is filtered and enters the proximal tubule. Here, approximately 99% of uric acid is reabsorbed into the bloodstream. At the distal tubule, uric acid is secreted; subsequently, about 75% of the amount secreted is reabsorbed. Therefore, almost all urinary uric acid is excreted at the distal tubule.

a. Hematologic causes of hyperuricemia and gout (associated with increased nucleic acid turnover and breakdown to uric acid)
   (1) Lymphoproliferative disorders
   (2) Myeloproliferative disorders
   (3) Certain hemolytic anemias and hemoglobinopathies

b. Chronic renal failure. In this condition, reduced renal clearance of uric acid can lead to hyperuricemia.

c. Drug-induced
   (1) Aspirin and **other salicylates** inhibit tubular secretion of uric acid when given in low doses (e.g., less than 2 g/day of aspirin). (At high doses, they frequently cause uricosuria.)
   (2) Cytotoxic drugs increase uric acid concentrations by enhancing nucleic acid turnover and excretion.
   (3) Diuretics (except spironolactone) may cause hyperuricemia; most likely, this occurs via volume depletion, which, in turn, increases proximal tubular reabsorption, or via impaired tubular secretion of uric acid.
   (4) Ethambutol and **nicotinic acid** increase uric acid concentrations by competing with urate for tubular secretion sites, thereby decreasing uric acid excretion.
   (5) Heavy alcohol consumption. By forming lactate, which competes with urate for tubular secretion sites, alcohol overuse reduces uric acid excretion.

d. Miscellaneous disorders. Diabetic ketoacidosis, psoriasis, and chronic lead poisoning are examples of conditions that may cause hyperuricemia.

E. Pathophysiology

1. Gouty arthritis develops when **monosodium urate crystals** are deposited in the synovium of involved joints.

2. An **inflammatory response** to monosodium urate crystals leads to an attack of acute gouty arthritis; painful joint swelling is characterized by redness, warmth, and tenderness. A systemic reaction may accompany joint symptoms.

3. If gout progresses untreated, **tophi**, or **tophaceous deposits** (deposits of monosodium urate

crystals), eventually may lead to joint deformity and disability; kidney involvement may lead to renal impairment. However, these developments are uncommon in the general gout population and represent late complications of hyperuricemia.

4. **Renal complications of hyperuricemia and gout** can have serious consequences.
   a. **Acute tubular obstruction.** This complication may develop secondary to uric acid production in the collecting tubules and ureters, with subsequent blockage and renal failure. It is most common in patients with gout secondary to myeloproliferative or lymphoproliferative disorders—especially after chemotherapy.
   b. **Urolithiasis.** Occurring in about 20% of gout patients, this complication is characterized by formation of uric acid stones in the urinary tract. Low urine pH seems to be a contributing factor. The risk of urolithiasis rises as serum and urinary uric acid levels increase.
   c. **Chronic urate nephropathy.** In this complication, urate deposits arise in the renal interstitium. Most clinicians agree, however, that chronic hyperuricemia rarely, if ever, leads to clinically significant nephropathy. The presence of concomitant disease (e.g., diabetes mellitus, hypertension, lead nephropathy) may explain the finding of nephropathy in gout patients.

F. **Clinical presentation.** Four clinical presentations of hyperuricemia and gout may be seen: **Asymptomatic hyperuricemia**, **acute gouty arthritis**, **intercritical gout**, and **chronic tophaceous gout**. Clinical evaluation and the need for intervention depend on the presentation.

II. ASYMPTOMATIC HYPERURICEMIA

II. ASYMPTOMATIC HYPERURICEMIA is characterized by an elevated serum uric acid level but has no signs or symptoms of deposition disease (arthritis, tophi, or urolithiasis).

A. No definitive evidence indicates that asymptomatic hyperuricemia is harmful.

B. Clinicians cannot predict which asymptomatic patients will develop gout symptoms or hyperuricemia-related complications. However, the risk of symptom development and complications increases as the serum uric acid level rises.

C. **Therapy.** Although some asymptomatic patients may receive drug therapy, most do not require treatment. However, any secondary causes of hyperuricemia should be minimized or reversed, if possible.

1. **Drug therapy** to reduce the serum uric acid level is controversial. Some physicians believe that the risk of adverse drug effects and the expense and inconvenience of long-term therapy outweigh the benefits. However, in patients with sustained and marked hyperuricemia, urate-lowering drugs may be given (see section IV C 2).

2. **Supportive interventions** may include maintenance of adequate urine output (to prevent uric acid stone formation), avoidance of high purine foods, and regular medical appointments to monitor the serum uric acid level and check for clinical evidence of deposition disease.

III. ACUTE GOUTY ARTHRITIS

III. ACUTE GOUTY ARTHRITIS. This clinical presentation of gout is characterized by **painful arthritic attacks** of sudden onset.

A. **Pathogenesis.** Monosodium urate crystals form in articular tissues; this process sets off an inflammatory reaction. Trauma, exposure to cold, or another triggering event may be involved in the development of the acute attack.

B. **Signs and symptoms**

1. The **initial attack** comes on abruptly, with severe, progressively worsening arthritic pain, generally involving only one or a few joints.

2. The affected joints typically become hot, swollen, and extremely tender. In his account of his personal experience with gout, seventeenth-century British physician Thomas Sydenham described the pain this way: "Now it is a violent stretching and tearing of the ligaments—now it is a gnawing pain and now a pressure and tightening. So exquisite and lively...is the feeling of the part affected, that it cannot bear the weight of bedclothes nor the jar of a person walking in the room."*

3. The initial attack usually occurs at night or in the early morning as synovial fluid is reabsorbed.

---

*Latham RG (trans): *The Works of Thomas Sydenham, vol. II.* London, Sydenham Society, 1850.

4. The most common site of the initial attack is the first metatarsophalangeal joint; an attack there is known as **podagra**. Other sites that may be affected include the instep, ankle, heel, knee, wrist, elbow, and fingers.

5. The first few untreated attacks typically last 3 to 14 days. Later attacks may affect more joints and take several weeks to resolve.

6. During recovery, as edema subsides, local desquamation and pruritus may occur.

7. **Systemic symptoms** during an acute attack may include fever, chills, and malaise.

C. Diagnostic criteria

1. **Definitive diagnosis** of gouty arthritis can be made by demonstration of monosodium urate crystals in the **synovial fluid** of affected joints. These needle-shaped crystals are termed negatively birefringent when viewed through a polarized light microscope.

2. **Serum analysis** usually reveals an above-normal uric acid level; however, this finding is not specific for acute gout. Other common serum findings include leukocytosis and a moderately elevated erythrocyte sedimentation rate.

3. A **dramatic therapeutic response to colchicine** may be helpful in establishing the diagnosis, but this is not absolute because other causes of acute arthritis may respond as well.

4. Because uric acid crystals may not be found in the affected joints of all acute gout patients, a **probable diagnosis** of acute gouty arthritis can be made using the criteria developed by the American Rheumatism Association. The presence of a minimum of six of the following ten criteria warrants a suggestive diagnosis:
   a. Development of maximum inflammation within 1 day
   b. More than one arthritis attack
   c. Oligoarthritis attack (limited to a few joints)
   d. Painful or swollen first metatarsophalangeal joint
   e. Unilateral attack involving the tarsal joint
   f. Unilateral attack involving the first metatarsophalangeal joint
   g. Redness over the affected joint
   h. Tophus
   i. Asymptomatic swelling in one joint
   j. Hyperuricemia

D. Treatment goals

1. **Relieve pain and inflammation**

2. **Terminate the acute attack**

3. **Restore normal function to the affected joints**

E. Therapy

1. **General therapeutic principles**
   a. The affected joint (or joints) should be immobilized.
   b. Anti-inflammatory drug therapy should begin immediately. For maximal therapeutic effectiveness, these drugs should be kept on hand so that the patient may begin therapy as soon as a subsequent attack begins.
   c. Urate-lowering drugs should not be given until the acute attack is controlled as they may prolong the attack by causing a change in uric acid equilibrium.

2. **Specific drugs.** Any of the following agents may be used:
   a. **Colchicine.** The traditional drug of choice for relieving pain and inflammation and ending the acute attack, colchicine is most effective when initiated 12 to 36 hours after symptoms begin (the period of maximal leukocyte migration). Approximately 75% to 90% of patients respond to the drug when given for an acute attack.
      (1) **Mechanism of action.** Colchicine apparently impairs leukocyte migration to inflamed areas and disrupts urate deposition and the subsequent inflammatory response.
      (2) **Oral regimen**
         (a) During the **initial attack**, 0.5 to 0.6 mg of colchicine is given every hour until:
            (i) A response occurs
            (ii) A total of 6 to 8 mg is administered
            (iii) Intolerable gastrointestinal distress (nausea, vomiting, diarrhea) develops
         (b) Patients typically respond within 12 to 24 hours after therapy begins. Complete relief usually occurs in 1 to 3 days.

(c) During **subsequent attacks**, patients may receive half of the total dose administered for the initial attack, then receive the remaining half as 0.5 mg every hour.

(3) Intravenous regimen

(a) A single dose of 2 to 3 mg is given in 20 to 30 ml of normal saline solution by slow push. If needed, another injection may be given in 6 to 8 hours. Patients should not receive more than 6 mg over a period of 24 hours. Because it causes tissue irritation, colchicine should never be given intramuscularly or subcutaneously.

(b) Intravenous administration may relieve acute gouty arthritis more rapidly than oral administration and helps reduce the risk of gastrointestinal toxicity.

(4) Precautions and monitoring effects

(a) **Gastrointestinal distress** (nausea, vomiting, abdominal cramps, diarrhea) occurs in up to 80% of patients receiving oral colchicine. This dosage form should be avoided in patients with peptic ulcer disease and other gastrointestinal disorders.

(b) **Local extravasation** (causing local pain and necrosis) can occur with administration of intravenous colchicine. This risk can be reduced by use of a secure intravenous line.

(c) **Colchicine therapy** may cause bone marrow depression. This rare effect develops mainly in patients who receive excessive doses or who have underlying renal or hepatic disease. Long-term therapy may result in neurologic, renal, or other toxicity.

b. Nonsteroidal anti-inflammatory drugs (NSAIDs)

(1) These drugs are preferred when treatment is delayed significantly after symptom onset or when the patient cannot tolerate the adverse gastrointestinal effects of colchicine. Some clinicians consider these drugs the agents of choice. Patients typically respond 6 to 24 hours after therapy begins; symptoms usually resolve completely within 3 to 5 days.

(a) **Indomethacin** is given in an initial single oral dose of 75 mg, followed by 50 mg every 6 hours for 2 days, then 50 mg every 8 hours for 1 to 2 days.

(b) **Other NSAIDs**, such as **fenoprofen**, **ibuprofen**, **naproxen**, **sulindac**, and **piroxicam** also have been used successfully in the treatment of acute gout.

(c) **Phenylbutazone** has a well-established efficacy; however, it is now used less frequently because of the development of newer and safer NSAIDs.

(2) Precautions and monitoring effects

(a) **Adverse effects of indomethacin** usually are dose-related. Occurring in 10% to 60% of patients, these effects may warrant drug discontinuation. They primarily include gastrointestinal complaints of nausea and abdominal discomfort and central nervous system effects of headaches and dizziness. Indomethacin should be taken with food or milk to minimize gastric mucosal irritation.

(b) **Adverse effects of phenylbutazone** include sodium and fluid retention; consequently, this drug should be avoided in patients with borderline cardiac reserves or overt congestive heart failure. Gastrointestinal distress (e.g., nausea, abdominal discomfort, and peptic ulceration) also may occur. Rarely, blood dyscrasias (e.g., aplastic anemia, agranulocytosis) develop; they are most common in elderly patients and in those receiving the drug for long periods. To avoid these potential toxicities, phenylbutazone therapy should not exceed 1 week.

F. Adrenocorticotropic hormone (ACTH) and **corticosteroids** are reserved for refractory cases. However, relapse commonly follows drug withdrawal.

IV. INTERCRITICAL GOUT is the symptom-free period after the first attack. This phase may be interrupted by the recurrence of acute attacks.

A. The **onset of subsequent attacks** varies. In most patients, the second attack occurs within 1 year of the first, but in some it may be delayed for 5 to 10 years. A small percentage of patients never experience a second attack. If hyperuricemia is insufficiently treated, subsequent attacks may become progressively longer and more severe and may involve more than one joint.

B. Treatment goals

1. Reduce the frequency and severity of recurrent attacks

2. Minimize urate deposition in body tissues and thus prevent progression to chronic tophaceous gout

C. Therapy

1. Conservative intervention is indicated for patients with infrequent attacks, a serum uricase acid level below 9 mg/dl (measured by the uricase method), no tophi, and no evidence of renal disease or uric acid stones. Such intervention includes the following measures:

a. **Restriction of alcohol consumption** and **dietary purine** (e.g., organ meats, anchovies) helps reduce uric acid concentrations.

b. **High-volume fluid intake** and **increased urinary output** (at least 2 L/day) improve uric acid excretion and minimize renal urate precipitation.

c. **Weight reduction** (in obese patients) sometimes reduces the serum uric acid level slightly.

d. **Colchicine therapy** helps prevent gouty arthritis attacks. This drug may be given in the usual dose of 0.5 to 1.5 mg/day. (However, some patients require as little as 0.5 mg two or three times weekly.) Patients who cannot tolerate colchicine may receive indomethacin instead.

2. **Urate-reducing drug therapy.** The goal of such therapy is to reduce the serum uric acid level below 6 mg/dl. Urate-reducing drugs include **uricosurics**, which increase renal uric acid excretion, and **xanthine oxidase inhibitors**, which reduce uric acid production.

a. **Indications** for urate-reducing therapy include the following:

(1) Frequent gouty arthritis attacks despite conservative intervention

(2) Chronic joint changes with tophi

(3) Uric acid nephrolithiasis

(4) Evidence of renal damage induced by uric acid

(5) A serum uric acid level above 9 mg/dl

b. **Uricosurics** include **probenecid** and **sulfinpyrazone.** They are the preferred agents for underexcretors. Long-term uricosuric therapy reduces the incidence of gouty arthritis attacks, prevents formation of new tophi, and helps resolve existing tophi.

(1) Mechanism of action. Probenecid and sulfinpyrazone block uric acid reabsorption at the proximal convoluted tubule, thereby increasing the rate of uric acid excretion (see Fig. 42-2).

(2) Indications. Uricosurics generally are used to reduce hyperuricemia in patients who excrete less than 600 mg of uric acid per day.

(3) Dosage and administration

(a) Probenecid is given initially in two daily oral doses of 250 mg, then increased to 500 mg twice daily every 1 to 2 weeks until the serum uric acid level drops below 6 mg/dl, to a maximal daily dose of 3 g.

(b) Sulfinpyrazone is given initially in two daily oral doses of 50 mg, then increased by 100 mg weekly, to a maximal daily dose of 800 mg.

(4) Precautions and monitoring effects

(a) Uricosurics are **contraindicated** in patients with urinary tract stones.

(b) These drugs generally are ineffective in patients with creatinine clearances below 25 ml/min.

(c) Aspirin and **other salicylates** antagonize the action of uricosurics.

(d) Uricosuric therapy should not be initiated during an acute gout attack. During the first 6 to 12 months of therapy, these drugs may increase the frequency, severity, and duration of acute attacks (by changing the equilibrium of body urate). Therefore, some clinicians administer prophylactic colchicine concomitantly during the early months of uricosuric therapy.

(e) Patients should maintain a high fluid intake and a urine output (at least 2 L/day) during uricosuric therapy to decrease renal urate precipitation. Alkalinization of the urine to a pH above 6.0 through administration of sodium bicarbonate or Shohl's solution U.S.P. will increase the solubility of uric acid.

(f) Probenecid is well tolerated by most patients, but it occasionally causes adverse effects, such as gastrointestinal distress (especially when given in high doses). It should be administered cautiously to patients with peptic ulcer disease. In rare cases, hypersensitivity reactions will occur.

(g) Sulfinpyrazone causes gastrointestinal distress in 10% to 15% of patients. Hypersensitivity reactions occur rarely. Sulfinpyrazone reduces platelet adhesiveness and may cause blood dyscrasias; periodic blood counts should be done.

c. **Xanthine oxidase inhibitors** include **allopurinol**.

(1) Mechanism of action. Allopurinol and its long-acting metabolite, oxypurinol, block the final steps in uric acid synthesis by inhibiting xanthine oxidase, an enzyme that converts xanthine to uric acid. The drug thus reduces the serum uric acid level while increasing the renal excretion of the more soluble oxypurine precursors; this, in turn, decreases the risk of uric acid stones and nephropathy.

(2) Indications. Allopurinol is the preferred urate-reducing agent for patients in the following categories:

(a) Patients who excrete more than 600 mg of uric acid per day

(b) Patients with recurrent tophaceous deposits or uric acid stones
(c) Patients with renal impairment

(3) **Dosage and administration**. Allopurinol is given initially in a daily dose of 100 to 200 mg (preferably as a single dose), then increased in weekly increments to 300 mg/day. (However, some patients may need 600 to 900 mg/day to control hyperuricemia.) Typically, the uric acid level starts to fall after 1 to 2 days, with a maximal effect for a given dose in 7 to 10 days.

(4) **Precautions and monitoring effects**
(a) Hypersensitivity reactions have been reported.
(b) Minor skin rashes may occur.
(c) Life-threatening toxicity syndrome occurs rarely. This syndrome may include one or all of the following: vasculitis, rash (usually toxic epidermal necrolysis), eosinophilia, hepatic damage, and progressive renal failure.
(d) Allopurinol may induce more frequent acute gout attacks. This risk can be minimized by administration of low doses and concurrent colchicine therapy.
(e) Patients receiving concurrent ampicillin have an increased risk of developing rash.
(f) Patients should maintain a high fluid intake and urine output during allopurinol therapy.

V. CHRONIC TOPHACEOUS GOUT. This rare clinical presentation may develop if hyperuricemia and gout remain untreated for many years.

A. Pathogenesis. Persistent hyperuricemia leads to the development of tophi in the synovia, olecranon bursae, and various periarticular locations. Eventually, articular cartilage may be destroyed, resulting in joint deformities, bony erosions, deposition of tophi within tissues, and renal disease.

B. Clinical evaluation

1. Patients may develop large subcutaneous tophi in the **pinna** of the external ear (the classic site) as well as in other locations.

2. Typically, the urate pool is many times the normal size.

C. Therapy. Allopurinol and probenecid may be given in combination to treat severe cases.

STUDY QUESTIONS

Directions: Each question below contains five suggested answers. Choose the **one best** response to each question.

1. All of the following statements concerning an acute gouty attack are correct EXCEPT

A. the diagnosis of gout is assured by a good therapeutic response to colchicine because no other form of arthritis will respond to this drug
B. to be assured of the diagnosis, monosodium urate crystals must be identified in the synovial fluid of the affected joint
C. attacks frequently occur in the middle of the night
D. an untreated attack may last up to 2 weeks
E. the first attack usually involves only one joint, most frequently the big toe (first metatarsophalangeal joint)

2. A 42-year-old obese black man has been diagnosed as having gout. He has had three acute attacks this year, and his uric acid level is presently 11.5 mg/dl (upper limit of normal is 7 mg/dl). He has no other diseases. Rational treatment of this patient during the interval period between gouty attacks might include any of the following EXCEPT

A. acetaminophen or aspirin 650 mg as needed for joint pain
B. probenecid
C. colchicine
D. allopurinol
E. a decrease in caloric intake

3. A 45-year-old white man is admitted to the hospital with the diagnosis of an acute attack of gout. His serum uric acid is 10.5 mg/dl (normal 3 to 7 mg/dl). Which of the following would be the most effective initial treatment plan?

A. Before treating this patient, immobilize the affected joint and obtain a 24-hour urinary uric acid level to determine which drug, either allopurinol or probenecid, would be the best agent to initiate therapy
B. Begin oral colchicine 0.6 mg every hour until relief is obtained, or gastrointestinal distress occurs, or a maximum of 8 mg has been taken; also begin probenecid 250 mg twice a day concurrently
C. Administer oral indomethacin 75 mg initially, then 50 mg three times a day for 2 to 3 days, then gradually taper the dose over the next few days
D. Administer oral phenylbutazone 200 mg every 6 hours for 3 days, then give 100 mg three times a day for an additional 4 months
E. Give colchicine 0.5 mg intramuscularly followed by 1 mg IV piggyback every 12 hours for 2 weeks

Directions: Each question below contains three suggested answers of which **one or more** is correct. Choose the answer

A if **I only** is correct
B if **III only** is correct
C if **I and II** are correct
D if **II and III** are correct
E if **I, II, and III** are correct

4. Allopurinol is recommended rather than probenecid in the treatment of hyperuricemia in which of the following situations?

I. When the patient has several large tophi on the elbows and knees
II. When the patient has an estimated creatinine clearance of 15 ml/min
III. When the patient has leukemia and there is concern regarding renal precipitation of urate

ANSWERS AND EXPLANATIONS

1. The answer is A. (*III B 1, 3–5, C 1, 3*) Other forms of acute arthritis may respond to colchicine, so that the diagnosis of gout cannot be established unequivocally by a good response to this agent. A definitive diagnosis requires the presence of urate crystals in the affected joint, although the presence of other symptoms or laboratory findings may suggest a probable diagnosis of gout.

2. The answer is A. [*I D 2 c (1); III E 2 a; IV C 1, 2 b (3) (a), (4) (c), c*] Aspirin in doses less than 2 g/day can inhibit uric acid secretion. Weight reduction, allopurinol or probenecid to lower the serum uric acid levels, and prophylactic colchicine are all appropriate interventions in the interval phase to reduce the incidence of acute gouty attacks.

3. The answer is C. [*III E 1 c, 2 a, b (1); IV C 2 b (4) (d)*] The most effective initial plan in treating an acute attack of gout is to administer indomethacin orally, giving 75 mg initially, then 50 mg three times a day for 2 to 3 days, then gradually tapering the dosage over the next few days. Even though joint immobilization is an appropriate initial step, drugs for pain relief should be administered as soon as possible. Uric acid modification therapy (allopurinol or probenecid) should not be initiated until the acute attack is under control. Initiating therapy with probenecid at this point may prolong the acute attack. Phenylbutazone should not be used for longer than 1 week. Cochicine should never be given intramuscularly because it causes tissue irritation.

4. The answer is E (all). [*IV C 2 b (4) (b), c (2)*] In the treatment of hyperuricemia, allopurinol is indicated rather than probenecid when large tophi are present, when the creatinine clearance is less than 25 ml/min (probenecid would be ineffective, but allopurinol dosage would have to be decreased), when the patient is an overproducer of uric acid, and when there is a need to prevent the formation of large amounts of uric acid (e.g., when conditions like leukemia are present).

43
Peptic Ulcer Disease

S. James Matthews

I. GENERAL CONSIDERATIONS

A. Definition. Peptic ulcer disease refers to a group of disorders characterized by circumscribed lesions of the mucosa of the upper gastrointestinal tract (especially the stomach and duodenum). The lesions occur in regions exposed to gastric juices.

B. Manifestations

1. **Duodenal ulcers** almost always develop in the duodenal bulb (the first few centimeters of the duodenum). A few, however, arise between the bulb and the ampulla.

2. **Gastric ulcers** form most commonly in the antrum or at the antral–fundal junction.

3. **Less common forms of peptic ulcer disease**
   a. **Stress ulcers** result from serious trauma or illness, major burns, or ongoing sepsis. The most common site of stress ulcer formation is the proximal portion of the stomach.
   b. **Zollinger-Ellison syndrome** is a severe form of peptic ulcer disease in which intractable ulcers are accompanied by extreme gastric hyperacidity and at least one gastrinoma (a non-beta islet cell tumor of the pancreas or another site).
   c. **Stomal ulcers** (also called marginal ulcers) may arise at the anastomosis or immediately distal to it in the small intestine in patients who have undergone ulcer surgery and have experienced subsequent ulcer recurrence after a symptom-free period.
   d. **Drug-associated ulcers** occur in patients who chronically ingest substances that damage the gastric mucosa, such as nonsteroidal anti-inflammatory drugs (NSAIDs).

C. Incidence. Peptic ulcer disease is the most common disorder of the upper gastrointestinal tract.

1. **Duodenal ulcers** affect roughly 4% to 10% of the United States population; **gastric ulcers** occur in approximately 0.03% to 0.05% of the population.

2. Nearly 80% of peptic ulcers are duodenal; the others are gastric ulcers.

3. Most duodenal ulcers appear in people between ages 20 and 50 years; onset of gastric ulcers usually occurs between ages 45 and 55 years.

4. Duodenal ulcers are twice as common in men as in women; gastric ulcers affect men and women equally.

5. Approximately 10% to 20% of gastric ulcer patients also have a concurrent duodenal ulcer.

D. Description

1. Ulcer size varies. The average duodenal ulcer typically has a diameter of less than 1 cm; most gastric ulcers are somewhat larger (1 to 2.5 cm in diameter).

2. Most ulcers are sharply demarcated and have a round, oval, or elliptical shape.

3. The mucosa surrounding the ulcer typically is inflamed and edematous.

4. Ulcers penetrate the **muscularis propria** and, in some cases, extend into the serosa or even into the pancreas.

5. Fibrous tissue, granulation tissue, and necrotic debris form the ulcer base. During ulcer healing, a scar forms as epithelium from the edges covers the ulcer surface.

6. Nearly all duodenal ulcers are benign; up to 10% of gastric ulcers are malignant.

E. Etiology. The precise cause of peptic ulcer disease has not been defined. However, certain factors are known to increase the risk of developing the disease.

1. Genetic factors

a. Ulcers are at least twice as common in siblings of ulcer patients as in the general population.

b. Blood type. People with blood type O have an above-normal incidence of duodenal ulcers; those with blood type A have a higher incidence of gastric ulcers.

2. Smoking. Smokers have an increased risk of developing peptic ulcer disease. In addition, cigarette smoking delays ulcer healing and increases the risk and rapidity of relapse after the ulcer heals. Nicotine decreases biliary and pancreatic bicarbonate secretion. Smoking also accelerates the emptying of stomach acid into the duodenum.

3. NSAIDs. When ingested chronically, aspirin, indomethacin, and other NSAIDs promote gastric ulcer formation.

a. These drugs may injure the gastric mucosa by allowing back-diffusion of hydrogen ions into the mucosa.

b. NSAIDs also inhibit the synthesis of prostaglandins, substances with a cytoprotective effect on the mucosa.

4. Alcohol. A known mucosal irritant, alcohol causes marked irritation of the gastric mucosa if ingested in large quantities.

5. Coffee. Both regular and decaffeinated coffee contain peptides that stimulate release of gastrin, a hormone that triggers the flow of gastric juice. However, a direct link between coffee and peptic ulcer disease has not been proven.

6. Corticosteroids. According to a recent study, these drugs double the risk (1.8 versus 0.8) of ulcer development. Corticosteroid-induced ulcers have a high incidence of perforation and hemorrhage. To complicate matters, these drugs may mask ulcer symptoms.

7. Associated disorders. Peptic ulcer disease is more common in patients with hyperparathyroidism, emphysema, rheumatoid arthritis, and alcoholic cirrhosis.

8. Advanced age. Degeneration of the pylorus permits bile reflux into the stomach, creating an environment that favors ulcer formation.

9. *Campylobacter pylori*. This bacterial organism has been linked with some cases of duodenal ulcers and gastritis.

10. Psychological factors. Once assigned key rolls in the pathogenesis of peptic ulcer disease, stress and personality type now are viewed as relatively minor influences.

F. Pathophysiology. Ulcers develop when an imbalance exists between factors that protect the gastric mucosa and factors that promote mucosal corrosion.

1. Protective factors

a. Normally, the mucosa secretes a thick mucus that serves as a barrier between luminal acid and epithelial cells. This barrier slows the inward movement of hydrogen ions and allows their neutralization by bicarbonate ions in fluids secreted by the stomach and duodenum.

b. Alkaline and neutral pancreatic biliary juices also help buffer acid entering the duodenum from the stomach.

c. An **intact mucosal barrier** prevents back-diffusion of gastric acids into mucosal cells. It also has the capacity to stimulate local blood flow, which brings nutrients and other substances to the area and removes toxic substances (e.g., hydrogen ions). Mucosal integrity also promotes cell growth and repair after local trauma.

2. Corrosive factors. Peptic ulcer disease reflects the inability of the gastric mucosa to resist corrosion by irritants such as pepsin, hydrochloric acid (HCl), and other gastric secretions.

a. Exposure to gastric acid and pepsin is necessary for ulcer development.

b. Disrupted mucosal barrier integrity allows gastric acids to diffuse from the lumen back into mucosal cells, where they cause injury.

3. Physiologic defects associated with peptic ulcer disease. Researchers have identified various physiologic defects in patients with duodenal and gastric ulcers.

a. Duodenal ulcer patients may have the following defects:

(1) Increased capacity for gastric acid secretion

(a) Some duodenal ulcer patients have up to twice the normal number of parietal cells (which produce HCl).

(b) Nearly 70% of duodenal ulcer patients have elevated serum levels of **pepsinogen I** and a corresponding increase in pepsin-secreting capacity.

(2) Increased parietal cell responsiveness to gastrin
(3) Above-normal postprandial gastrin secretion
(4) Defective inhibition of gastrin release at low pH, possibly leading to failure to suppress postprandial acid secretion
(5) Above-normal rate of gastric emptying, resulting in delivery of a greater acid load to the duodenum

b. Gastric ulcer patients typically exhibit the following characteristics:
(1) Deficient gastric mucosal resistance, direct mucosal injury, or both
(2) Elevated serum gastrin levels (in acid hyposecretors)
(3) Decreased pyloric pressure at rest and in response to acid or fat in the duodenum
(4) Delayed gastric emptying
(5) Increased reflux of bile and other duodenal contents
(6) Subnormal mucosal levels of prostaglandins (these levels normalize once the ulcer heals)

G. Clinical presentation. Signs and symptoms of peptic ulcer disease vary with the patient's age and the location of the lesion. Only about 50% of patients experience classic ulcer symptoms. The remainder are asymptomatic or report vague or atypical symptoms.

1. Pain. Patients typically describe heartburn or a gnawing, burning, aching, or cramp-like pain. Some report abdominal soreness or hunger sensations. It is unclear whether peptic ulcer pain results from chemical stimulation or from spasm.

a. Duodenal ulcer pain usually is restricted to a small, midepigastric area near the xiphoid. Pain may radiate below the costal margins into the back or the right shoulder.

b. Gastric ulcer pain is less localized. It may be referred to the left subcostal region.

c. Pain from a duodenal ulcer frequently awakens the patient between midnight and 2 A.M.; it is almost never present before breakfast. In contrast, gastric ulcer rarely produces nocturnal pain.

d. Food usually relieves duodenal ulcer pain but may cause gastric ulcer pain. This finding may explain why duodenal ulcer patients tend to gain weight, whereas gastric ulcer patients may lose weight. Pain characteristically occurs 90 minutes to 3 hours after meals in duodenal ulcer patients, while pain in gastric ulcer patients is usually present 45 to 60 minutes after a meal.

2. Nausea and vomiting may occur with either ulcer type.

3. Disease course. Both duodenal and gastric ulcers tend to be chronic, with spontaneous remissions and exacerbations. Within a year of the initial symptoms, most patients experience a relapse.

a. In many cases, relapse is seasonal, occurring more often in the spring and autumn.

b. Prophylactic drug therapy usually is not recommended because of the risk of side effects. However, if relapses are frequent or severe, prophylactic drug therapy is instituted.

H. Clinical evaluation

1. Physical findings. Patients with peptic ulcer disease may exhibit superficial and deep epigastric tenderness and voluntary muscle guarding. With duodenal ulcer, patients also may show unilateral spasm over the duodenal bulb. Gastric ulcer patients may have weight loss.

2. Diagnostic test results

a. Blood tests may show hypochromic anemia.

b. Stool tests may detect occult blood if the ulcer is chronic.

c. Gastric secretion tests may reveal hypersecretion of HCl in duodenal ulcer patients and normal or subnormal HCl secretion in gastric ulcer patients.

d. Upper gastrointestinal series (barium x-ray) reveals the ulcer crater in up to 80% of cases. Duodenal bulb deformity suggests a duodenal ulcer.

e. Upper gastrointestinal endoscopy, the most specific test, may be done if barium x-ray yields inconclusive results. This procedure confirms ulcer in at least 95% of cases and may detect ulcers not demonstrable by radiography.

f. Biopsy may be necessary to determine whether a gastric ulcer is malignant.

II. TREATMENT OBJECTIVES

A. Relieve pain and other ulcer symptoms and promote ulcer healing

B. Prevent complications of peptic ulcer disease

C. Maintain adequate nutrition

D. Teach the patient about the disease in order to improve therapeutic compliance

III. THERAPY

A. Drug therapy. Peptic ulcer patients usually are treated with antacids, histamine$_2$ (H_2)-receptor antagonists, or both; other drugs are added as necessary. Drug regimens that suppress nocturnal acid secretion are found to result in the highest duodenal ulcer healing rates. Drug therapy typically provides prompt symptomatic relief and promotes ulcer healing within 4 to 6 weeks.

1. Antacids. These compounds, which neutralize gastric acid, are used to treat ulcer pain and heal the ulcer. Studies show antacids and H_2-receptor antagonists to be equally effective. Antacids are available as **magnesium**, **aluminum**, **calcium**, or **sodium salts**. The most widely used antacids are mixtures of aluminum hydroxide and magnesium hydroxide.

a. Mechanism of action and therapeutic effects. Antacids reduce the concentration and total load of acid in the gastric contents. By increasing gastric pH, they also inhibit pepsin activity. In addition, they strengthen the gastric mucosal barrier.

b. Choice of agent

(1) Nonsystemic antacids (e.g., magnesium or aluminum substances) are preferred to systemic antacids (e.g., sodium bicarbonate) for intensive ulcer therapy because they avoid the risk of alkalosis.

(2) Liquid antacid forms have a greater buffering capacity than tablets. However, tablets are more convenient to carry. With either dosage form, the size and frequency of doses may limit patient compliance.

(3) Antacid mixtures (e.g., aluminum hydroxide with magnesium hydroxide) provide more even, sustained action than single-agent antacids and permit a lower dosage of each compound. In addition, compounds in a mixture may interact so as to negate each other's untoward effects. For instance, the constipating effect of aluminum hydroxide may counter the diarrhea that magnesium hydroxide frequently produces.

(4) Calcium carbonate usually is avoided because it causes acid rebound, may delay pain relief and ulcer healing, and induces constipation. Another potential adverse effect of this compound is hypercalcemia; the risk is increased if calcium carbonate is taken with milk or another alkaline substance. The milk-alkali syndrome (hypercalcemia, alkalosis, azotemia, nephrocalcinosis) may also occur.

c. Administration and dosage

(1) Antacids differ greatly in acid-neutralizing capacity (ANC), defined as the number of milliequivalents (mEq) of a 1 N solution of HCl that can be brought to a pH of 3.5 in 15 minutes. With most duodenal ulcer patients, about 50 mEq/hr of available antacid is needed for ongoing neutralization of gastric contents. Therefore, the required dosage depends on the ANC of the specific antacid.

(2) Buffering action lasts 2 to 3 hours when the antacid is administered 1 hour after a meal. An additional dose taken 3 hours after a meal prolongs buffering for another hour. In contrast, an antacid taken on an empty stomach provides buffering for only 20 to 40 minutes.

(3) Consequently, the typical antacid regimen calls for doses 1 hour and 3 hours after meals and at bedtime.

(4) Dosage

(a) Because the ANC of antacid products varies widely, no standard dosage can be given in terms of milliliters of suspension or number of tablets. However, patients with duodenal ulcers generally require individual dosages of 80 to 160 mEq of ANC (equivalent to 30 to 60 ml of Mylanta or Maalox). Thus, the total daily dosage may be as much as 420 ml of Mylanta or Maalox if the standard seven-times–daily dosing regimen is used. Because of the large doses and the need for frequent administration, compliance with antacid treatment regimens has been low.

(b) Antacid therapy usually continues for 6 to 8 weeks.

d. Precautions and monitoring effects

(1) Calcium carbonate and magnesium-containing antacids should be used cautiously in patients with severe renal disease.

(2) Sodium bicarbonate is contraindicated in patients with hypertension, congestive heart failure, severe renal disease, and edema. It should not be used for ulcer therapy.

(3) All antacids should be used cautiously in elderly patients (especially those with decreased gastrointestinal motility) and renally impaired patients.

(4) Aluminum-containing antacids should be used cautiously in patients who suffer from dehydration or intestinal obstruction.

(5) The combination of calcium carbonate with an alkaline substance (e.g., sodium bicarbonate) and milk may cause the milk-alkali syndrome.

(6) Hypermagnesemia may develop in renally impaired patients using magnesium-containing antacids.
(7) Constipation can occur in patients using calcium carbonate and aluminum-containing antacids.
(8) Diarrhea is a common adverse effect of magnesium-containing antacids. If diarrhea occurs, the patient may alternate the antacid mixture with aluminum hydroxide.
(9) **Significant interactions**. Because antacids alter gastric pH and affect absorption of ingested substances, they have a high potential for drug interactions. To ensure consistent absorption and therapeutic efficacy, orally administered drugs should be given 30 to 60 minutes before antacids.
(a) Antacids bind with **tetracycline**, inhibiting its absorption and reducing its therapeutic efficacy.
(b) Antacids may destroy the coating of **enteric-coated drugs**, leading to premature drug dissolution in the stomach.
(c) Antacids may interfere with the absorption of many drugs, including **cimetidine**, **ranitidine**, **digoxin**, **isoniazid**, **anticholinergics**, **iron products**, and **phenothiazines** [see section III A 2 d (6) (c)].
(d) Antacids may reduce the therapeutic effects of **sucralfate** [see section III A 3 c (2)].

2. H_2-Receptor antagonists. These relatively new drugs may be preferred to other antiulcer agents because of their convenience and lack of effect on gastrointestinal motility.

a. Mechanism of action and therapeutic effects. H_2-receptor antagonists competitively inhibit the action of histamine at parietal cell receptor sites, reducing the volume and hydrogen ion concentration of gastric acid secretions. They accelerate the healing of most ulcers.

b. Choice of agent. Cimetidine, **ranitidine**, or **famotidine** may be administered to treat peptic ulcers or hypersecretory states (e.g., Zollinger-Ellison syndrome). **Nizatidine**, the newest H_2-receptor, may be used to treat and prevent recurrence of duodenal ulcers; its clinical place in therapy has not been thoroughly elucidated.
(1) **Cimetidine**, the first H_2-receptor antagonist approved for clinical use, reduces gastric acid secretion by about 50% (at a total daily dosage of 1000 mg).
(2) **Ranitidine**, a more potent drug, causes a 70% reduction in gastric acid secretion (at a total daily dosage of 300 mg).
(3) **Famotidine** is the most potent H_2-receptor antagonist. After a 40-mg dose, mean nocturnal gastric acid secretion is reduced by 94% for up to 10 hours.

c. Administration and dosage
(1) **Cimetidine** usually is administered orally in a dosage of 300 mg four times daily (with meals and at bedtime) for up to 8 weeks.
(a) Alternatively, duodenal ulcer patients may receive 400 mg twice daily or 800 mg at bedtime. An 800-mg bedtime dose is also effective in treating gastric ulcers.
(b) Hospitalized patients may receive parenteral doses—300 mg diluted to 20 ml, given by intravenous (IV) push over 1 to 2 minutes every 6 hours.
(c) For duodenal ulcer prophylaxis, 400 mg may be given orally at bedtime. (However, in 20% to 40% of patients, the ulcer recurs despite cimetidine prophylaxis.
(2) **Ranitidine** usually is given orally in a dosage of 150 mg twice daily. Duodenal ulcer patients may receive 300 mg at bedtime, alternatively. Therapy continues for up to 8 weeks.
(a) Hospitalized patients may receive ranitidine by IV or intramuscular route (50 mg every 6 to 8 hours).
(b) Prophylactic therapy may be administered to reduce the risk of ulcer recurrence. The approved prophylactic dosage is 150 mg at bedtime.
(3) **Famotidine**, administered to duodenal ulcer patients, is given in an oral dosage of 40 mg at bedtime for acute therapy, for a maximum of 8 weeks. For prophylactic therapy, the dosage is 20 mg at bedtime.
(a) Hospitalized patients may receive an IV injection of 20 mg every 12 hours.
(b) As with cimetidine and ranitidine, the ulcer may recur after drug discontinuation.
(4) **Nizatidine**, for the treatment of duodenal ulcers, is given orally in a dosage of 300 mg once daily at bedtime or 150 mg twice daily for up to 8 weeks. For prophylactic therapy, the dosage is 150 mg at bedtime.

d. Precautions and monitoring effects
(1) Ranitidine must be used cautiously in patients with hepatic impairment. Hepatotoxicity is unusual and occurs most often during IV administration. Cimetidine has also been associated with hepatotoxicity.
(2) Cimetidine may cause such hematologic disorders as thrombocytopenia, agranulocytosis, and aplastic anemia.
(3) All of these agents may cause headache and dizziness. Cimetidine additionally may

lead to confusion, especially in patients over age 60 years or if dosage is not adjusted for patients with decreased kidney or liver function.

(4) Cimetidine has a weak androgenic effect, possibly resulting in male gynecomastia and impotence.

(5) Cimetidine and ranitidine rarely can cause bradycardia, which is reversible on discontinuation of therapy.

(6) **Significant interactions**

(a) Cimetidine binds the cytochrome P-450 system of the liver and thus may interfere with the metabolism of such drugs as **phenytoin**, **theophylline**, **phenobarbital**, **lidocaine**, **warfarin**, **imipramine**, **diazepam**, and **propranolol**.

(b) Cimetidine decreases hepatic blood flow, possibly resulting in reduced clearance of **propranolol** and **lidocaine**.

(c) **Antacids** impair absorption of cimetidine and ranitidine and should be given 1 hour apart from these drugs.

(d) Cimetidine inhibits the excretion of procainamide by competing with the drug for the renal proximal tubular secretion site.

3. **Sucralfate**. This mucosal protectant is a nonabsorbable disaccharide containing sucrose and aluminum.

a. **Mechanism of action and therapeutic effects**. Sucralfate adheres to the base of the ulcer crater, forming a protective barrier against gastric acids and bile salts.

(1) Sucralfate's ulcer-healing efficacy compares favorably to that of the H_2-receptor antagonists.

(2) Duodenal ulcers respond better than gastric ulcers to sucralfate therapy.

b. **Administration and dosage**

(1) An oral agent, sucralfate usually is given in a dosage of 1 g four times daily (1 hour before meals) and at bedtime. Unless radiography or endoscopy documents earlier ulcer healing, therapy continues for 4 to 8 weeks.

(2) Continued sucralfate therapy after remission postpones ulcer relapse more effectively than does cimetidine therapy.

c. **Precautions and monitoring effects**

(1) Constipation is the most common adverse effect of sucralfate.

(2) **Significant interaction**. **Antacids** may reduce mucosal binding of sucralfate, decreasing its therapeutic efficacy. Antacids should be given 30 to 60 minutes apart from sucralfate if used in combination ulcer therapy.

4. **Gastrointestinal anticholinergics** (e.g., belladonna leaf, atropine, propantheline) sometimes are used as adjunctive agents for relief of refractory duodenal ulcer pain. However, these agents have no proven value in ulcer healing.

a. Given in combination with antacids, anticholinergics delay gastric emptying, thereby prolonging antacid retention. They are most effective when taken at night and in large doses.

b. Anticholinergics occasionally are used in patients who do not respond to H_2-receptor antagonists alone.

c. These drugs are contraindicated in patients with gastric ulcers because they prolong gastric emptying. They also are contraindicated in patients with narrow-angle glaucoma and urinary retention.

d. **Adverse effects** of anticholinergics include confusion, dry mouth, blurred vision, urinary retention, and constipation.

5. Certain **prostaglandins** may prove valuable in ulcer therapy. These agents suppress gastric acid secretion and may guard the gastric mucosa against damage from NSAIDs. **Misoprostol** has been approved for use in the prevention of gastric ulcers caused by NSAIDs.

6. **Sedatives** are useful adjuncts in promoting rest for highly anxious ulcer patients.

B. Other therapeutic measures

1. **Modification of diet and social habits**

a. Previously emphasized in ulcer therapy, strict dietary limitations now are considered largely unnecessary.

(1) Bland or milk-based diets formerly were recommended. However, research indicates that these diets do not speed ulcer healing. In fact, most experts now advise ulcer patients to **avoid milk** because recent studies show that milk increases gastric acid secretion. Also, because it leaves the stomach quickly, milk lacks extended buffering action.

(2) Small, frequent meals—also previously recommended—can worsen ulcer pain by causing acid rebound 2 to 4 hours after eating.

b. **Current dietary guidelines** emphasize avoidance of foods and beverages known to exacerbate gastric discomfort or to promote acid secretion. This category typically includes coffee, other caffeinated beverages, and alcohol.

c. **Smoking**. Patients who smoke should be encouraged to quit because smoking markedly slows ulcer healing—even during optimal ulcer therapy.

d. **NSAIDs** should be avoided by ulcer patients.

2. **Surgery**. An ulcer patient who develops complications may require surgery—sometimes on an emergency basis (see section IV). Incapacitating recurrent ulcers also may warrant surgery.

a. **Types of surgical procedures** for ulcer disease include antrectomy and truncal vagotomy (Billroth I procedure), partial gastrectomy and truncal vagotomy (Billroth II procedure), highly selective (proximal gastric) vagotomy, and total gastrectomy (the treatment of choice for Zollinger-Ellison syndrome that is unresponsive to medical management).

b. A **vagotomy** severs a branch of the vagus nerve, thereby decreasing HCl secretion. An **antrectomy**, by removing the antrum, eliminates some acid-secreting mucosa as well as the major source of gastrin.

IV. COMPLICATIONS. Complications of peptic ulcer disease cause approximately 7000 deaths in the United States annually.

A. Hemorrhage. This life-threatening condition develops from widespread gastric mucosal irritation or ulceration with acute bleeding.

1. **Clinical features**. The patient may vomit fresh blood or a coffee-ground–like substance. Other signs include passage of bloody or tarry stools, diaphoresis, and syncope. With major blood loss, manifestations of **hypovolemic shock** may appear: The pulse rate may exceed 110 or systolic blood pressure may drop below 100.

2. **Management**

a. Patient stabilization, bleeding cessation, and measures to prevent further bleeding are crucial.

(1) Airway, breathing, and circulation must be ensured.

(2) IV crystalloids and colloids (e.g., Hetastarch) should be infused as needed.

(3) The patient's electrolyte status must be monitored and any imbalances corrected promptly.

b. **Gastric lavage** may be performed via a nasogastric or orogastric tube; iced saline solution is instilled until the aspirate returns free of blood.

c. Vasoconstrictors, antacids, or H_2-receptor antagonists may be administered. Vasopressin, an agent that causes contraction of gastrointestinal smooth muscle, may be given to constrict vessels and control bleeding.

d. **Emergency surgery** usually is indicated if the patient does not respond to medical management.

B. Perforation. Penetration of a peptic ulcer through the gastric or duodenal wall results in this acute emergency. Perforation most commonly occurs with ulcers located in the anterior duodenal wall.

1. **Clinical features**. Sudden acute upper abdominal pain, rigidity, guarding, rebound tenderness, and absent or diminished bowel sounds are typical manifestations. Several hours after onset, symptoms may abate somewhat; this apparent remission is dangerously misleading because peritonitis and shock may ensue.

2. **Management**. Emergency surgery is almost always necessary.

C. Obstruction. Inflammatory edema, spasm, and scarring may lead to obstruction of the duodenal or gastric outlet. The pylorus and proximal duodenum are the most common obstruction sites.

1. **Clinical features**. Typical patient complaints include postprandial vomiting or bloating, appetite and weight loss, and abdominal distention. Tympany and a succussion splash may be audible on physical examination. Gastric aspiration after an overnight fast typically yields more than 200 ml of food residue or clear fluid contents. (Gastric cancer must be ruled out as the cause of obstruction.)

2. **Management**

a. **Conservative measures** (as in routine ulcer therapy) are indicated in most cases of obstruction.

b. Patients with marked obstruction may require **continuous gastric suction** with careful monitoring of fluid and electrolyte status. A **saline load test** may be performed after 72 hours of continuous suction to test the degree of residual obstruction.

c. If less than 200 ml of gastric contents are aspirated, liquid feedings can begin. **Aspiration** is performed at least daily for the next few days to monitor for retention and to guide dietary modifications as the patient progresses to a full regular diet.

d. Surgery is indicated if medical management fails.

D. Postsurgical complications

1. Dumping syndrome. Affecting about 10% of patients who have undergone partial gastrectomy, this disorder is characterized by rapid gastric emptying.

a. Causes. The mechanism underlying dumping syndrome is poorly defined. However, intestinal exposure to hypertonic chyme may play a key role by triggering rapid shifts of fluid from the plasma to the intestinal lumen.

b. Clinical features. The patient may experience weakness, dizziness, anxiety, tachycardia, flushing, sweating, abdominal cramps, nausea, vomiting, and diarrhea.

(1) Manifestations may develop 15 to 30 minutes after a meal (**early dumping syndrome**) or 90 to 120 minutes after a meal (**late dumping syndrome**).

(2) Reactive hypoglycemia may partly account for some cases of late dumping syndrome.

c. Management. The patient usually is advised to eat six small meals of high protein and fat content and low carbohydrate content. Fluids should be ingested 1 hour before or after a meal but never with a meal. **Anticholinergics** may be given to slow food passage into the intestine.

2. Other postsurgical complications include reflux gastritis, afferent blind loop syndrome, stomal ulceration, diarrhea, malabsorption, early satiety, and iron-deficiency anemia.

STUDY QUESTIONS

Directions: Each question below contains five suggested answers. Choose the **one best** response to each question.

1. Which of the following organisms has been implicated as a possible cause of chronic gastritis and peptic ulcer disease?

A. *Campylobacter jejuni*
B. *Escherichia coli*
C. *Campylobacter pylori*
D. *Calymmatobacterium granulomatis*
E. *Giardia lamblia*

2. All of the following statements concerning antacid therapy used in the treatment of duodenal or gastric ulcers are correct EXCEPT

A. antacids may be used to heal the ulcer but are ineffective in controlling ulcer pain
B. antacids neutralize acid and decrease the activity of pepsin
C. if used alone for ulcer therapy, antacids should be administered 1 hour and 3 hours after meals and at bedtime
D. if diarrhea occurs, the patient may alternate the antacid product with aluminum hydroxide
E. calcium carbonate should be avoided because it causes acid rebound and induces constipation

3. As part of a comprehensive management strategy to treat peptic ulcer disease, patients should be encouraged to do all of the following EXCEPT

A. decrease caffeine ingestion
B. eat only bland foods
C. stop smoking
D. avoid alcohol
E. avoid the use of milk as a treatment modality

4. A gastric ulcer patient requires close follow-up to document complete ulcer healing because

A. perforation into the intestine is common
B. spontaneous healing of the ulcer may occur in 30% to 50% of cases
C. there is the risk of the ulcer being cancerous
D. symptoms tend to be chronic and recur
E. weight loss may be severe in gastric ulcer patients

Directions: Each question below contains three suggested answers of which **one or more** is correct. Choose the answer

A if **I only** is correct
B if **III only** is correct
C if **I and II** are correct
D if **II and III** are correct
E if **I, II, and III** are correct

5. Correct statements concerning cigarette smoking and ulcer disease include which of the following?

I. Smoking delays healing of gastric and duodenal ulcers
II. Nicotine decreases biliary and pancreatic bicarbonate secretion
III. Smoking accelerates the emptying of stomach acid into the duodenum

6. When administered at the same time, antacids can decrease the therapeutic efficacy of which of the following drugs?

I. Sucralfate
II. Ranitidine
III. Cimetidine

Directions: The group of questions below consists of lettered choices followed by several numbered items. For each numbered item select the **one** lettered choice with which it is **most** closely associated. Each lettered choice may be used once, more than once, or not at all.

Questions 7–11

For each effect, select the agent that is most likely associated with it.

A. Sodium bicarbonate
B. Aluminum hydroxide
C. Calcium carbonate
D. Magnesium hydroxide
E. Propantheline

7. May cause diarrhea
8. Cannot be used by patients with heart failure
9. Use with milk and an alkaline substance can cause milk-alkali syndrome
10. May cause dry mouth
11. Can be alternated with an antacid mixture to control diarrhea

ANSWERS AND EXPLANATIONS

1. The answer is C. (*I E 9*) *Campylobacter pylori* commonly is found in patients with peptic ulcer disease and always in association with chronic gastritis. Elimination of the organism has resulted in healing of the gastritis and the duodenal ulcer. More data, however, is needed before a definitive cause-and-effect relationship can be established.

2. The answer is A. (*III A 1*) Antacids have been shown to heal peptic ulcers, and their main use in modern therapy is to control ulcer pain. Antacids should be taken 1 hour and 3 hours after meals because the meal prolongs the acid-buffering effect of the antacid. If diarrhea becomes a problem with antacid use, an aluminum hydroxide product can be alternated with the antacid mixture; this takes advantage of the constipating property of aluminum. Since calcium carbonate causes acid rebound and constipation, its use should be avoided.

3. The answer is B. (*III B 1*) Bland food diets are no longer recommended in the treatment of ulcer disease—research indicates that bland or milk-based diets do not accelerate ulcer healing. Studies show that patients can eat almost anything; however, they should avoid foods that aggravate their ulcer symptoms.

4. The answer is C. (*I D 6*) Five percent to ten percent of gastric ulcers may be due to cancer. The ulcer may respond to therapy; however, failure of the ulcer to decrease satisfactorily in size and to heal with therapy may suggest cancer. Close follow-up is necessary to document complete ulcer healing.

5. The answer is E (all). (*I E 2, III B 1 c*) Clinical studies have shown that smoking increases susceptibility to ulcer disease, impairs spontaneous and drug-induced healing, and increases the risk and rapidity of recurrence of the ulcer. These findings may result in part from nicotine's ability to decrease biliary and pancreatic bicarbonate secretion, thus decreasing the body's ability to neutralize acid in the duodenum. Also, the accelerated emptying of stomach acid into the duodenum may predispose to duodenal ulcer and may decrease healing rates.

6. The answer is E (all). [*III A 1 d (9), 3 c (2)*] The mean peak blood concentration of cimetidine and the area under the 4-hour cimetidine blood concentration curve were both reduced significantly when cimetidine was administered at the same time as an antacid. The absorption of ranitidine is also reduced when it is taken concurrently with an aluminum–magnesium hydroxide antacid mixture. To avoid this interaction, the antacid should be administered 1 hour before or 2 hours after the administration of cimetidine or ranitidine. Antacids may reduce mucosal binding of sucralfate, decreasing its therapeutic efficacy. Antacids should therefore be given 30 to 60 minutes before or after sucralfate.

7–11. The answers are: 7-D, 8-A, 9-C, 10-E, 11-B. [*III A 1 b (3), d (5), 3, 4 d*] Magnesium-containing products tend to cause diarrhea, possibly due to the ability of magnesium to stimulate the secretion of bile acids by the gallbladder. Because of its sodium content, sodium bicarbonate is contraindicated in patients with congestive heart failure, hypertension, severe renal disease, and edema. Sodium bicarbonate is no longer used in peptic ulcer therapy. In addition to causing acid rebound, calcium carbonate, if taken with milk and an alkaline substance for long periods, may cause the milk-alkali syndrome. It also may cause adverse effects such as hypercalcemia, alkalosis, azotemia, and nephrocalcinosis. Propantheline, like other anticholinergic agents, may cause dry mouth, blurred vision, urinary retention, and constipation. These agents are sometimes used as adjuncts to relieve duodenal ulcer pain. They are contraindicated in gastric ulcer because they delay gastric emptying. Aluminum hydroxide is constipating and can be alternated with the patient's current antacid when that antacid product is causing diarrhea.

44
Diabetes Mellitus

Helen L. Figge

I. GENERAL CONSIDERATIONS

A. Definition. Diabetes mellitus (DM) refers to a group of disorders characterized by absent or deficient insulin secretion or peripheral insulin resistance, resulting in hyperglycemia and impaired metabolism.

B. Classification. DM occurs in two major forms.

1. **Type I: Insulin-dependent DM** (IDDM: formerly known as juvenile-onset or ketosis-prone diabetes)
   - **a.** This form is most common in children and in adults up to age 30 years but may occur at any age.
   - **b.** Type I diabetics are predisposed to **ketoacidosis**—accumulation of ketone bodies in body tissues and fluids.
   - **c.** Disease onset is sudden.
   - **d.** Beta cells, insulin-producing cells of the pancreatic islets of Langerhans, are destroyed, causing **absolute insulin deficiency**.
   - **e.** All type I diabetics require insulin replacement therapy.

2. **Type II: Non-insulin-dependent DM** (formerly called adult-onset diabetes; may be insulin requiring)
   - **a.** Most type II diabetics are over age 40 years and obese.
   - **b.** Disease onset typically is gradual.
   - **c.** In most cases, type II DM is characterized by **insensitivity to insulin** in the target tissues, deficient response of pancreatic beta cells to glucose, or both.
   - **d.** Because some insulin is secreted, ketoacidosis is prevented.
   - **e.** Only a minority of type II diabetics require insulin replacement therapy.

C. Incidence. In the United States, DM affects an estimated 1% to 5% of the population. Type I DM accounts for approximately 10% of cases; type II, for about 90% of cases.

D. Etiology. Various factors are thought to contribute to the development of DM.

1. **Type I DM**. Genetic predisposition, environmental factors, and autoimmunity have been proposed.
   - **a.** Certain **genetic markers** in the human leukocyte antigen (HLA) system have been strongly linked with type I DM. In addition, many patients have a family history of the disease; 50% of persons having identical twins with type I DM also are diabetics.
   - **b.** Viruses (e.g., rubella) and toxic chemicals are among the **environmental factors** that researchers believe may affect the pancreas and cause beta cell destruction in persons who are genetically predisposed to DM.
   - **c.** An **autoimmune component** is suggested by the presence of antibodies to islet-cell antigens in most new-onset type I diabetics. An abnormal immune response could cause the body to destroy beta cells because it has misidentified them as foreign.

2. **Type II DM**. Genetic factors and a beta cell or peripheral site defect have been implicated.
   - **a.** Nearly all identical twins of patients with type II DM also have the disease. A high percentage of other type II diabetics have a strong family history of the disease.
   - **b.** A **beta cell defect** is postulated to cause abnormalities in insulin secretion (absent or blunted early secretion phase).
   - **c.** A **peripheral site defect** is postulated to lead to **insulin resistance**—tissue insensitivity to

the action of insulin. This condition may result from a decreased number of insulin receptors or abnormal insulin action at or beyond the receptor. The ability of insulin to bind to cell walls is impaired.

3. **Secondary diabetes** may arise from such conditions as endocrine disorders (e.g., Cushing's syndrome), pregnancy, pancreatic disease, and use of drugs that antagonize insulin (e.g., thiazide diuretics, adrenocorticosteroids).

E. Pathophysiology. In untreated type I and type II DM, the disease follows a typical progression.

1. Without adequate insulin, which transports glucose across cell membranes, glucose transport to most cells diminishes. Also, the conversion of glucose to glycogen diminishes. As a result, glucose is trapped in the bloodstream and **hyperglycemia** occurs. Some glucose also spills into the urine.

2. Hyperglycemia leads to **osmotic diuresis** and subsequent dehydration and electrolyte abnormalities. As diuresis progresses, reductions in cardiac output and blood pressure may occur, leading to circulatory collapse.

3. Without glucose, cells must utilize protein and fat as energy sources.
   a. Fat is broken down into **free fatty acids** and **glycerol**.
   b. In the liver, free fatty acids are further broken down into **ketone bodies**.
   c. Breakdown is so rapid that excessive ketone bodies spill into the bloodstream. (In type II DM, however, the presence of limited amounts of insulin prevents ketonemia.)
   d. Increased amounts of glycerol, another by-product of fat metabolism, worsen hyperglycemia.

F. Clinical evaluation

1. **Physical findings**. Type I DM has an abrupt onset and, in some cases, an acute presentation. With type II DM, symptoms develop gradually; some patients are asymptomatic or have only mild symptoms.
   a. Classic signs and symptoms of untreated DM include polydipsia (excessive thirst), polyuria (excessive urination), polyphagia (excessive hunger), fatigue, weakness, and weight loss. Other common findings are dry, itchy skin; frequent skin and vaginal infections; and visual disturbances.
   b. The type I diabetic may present with signs and symptoms of ketoacidosis (see section IV A 1).
   c. Symptom severity and onset help differentiate type I and type II DM.
   d. Long-standing DM causes typical progressive changes in the retina, kidneys, nervous system, cardiovascular system, and integumentary system. For physical findings reflecting these changes, see section IV B.

2. **Laboratory findings**
   a. The diagnosis of DM is confirmed by a **fasting blood glucose** level of 140 mg/dl or more on at least two occasions.
   b. If the fasting blood glucose level is normal (below 140 mg/dl) but the patient has suggestive signs and symptoms, an **oral glucose tolerance test** (OGTT) will be done.
      (1) Glucose (75 g), dissolved in 300 ml of water, is given after a 12-hour fast.
      (2) A blood glucose level of 200 mg/dl or more at 2 hours and in at least one earlier sample after the glucose dose is administered confirms DM.
   c. A **random blood glucose** level of 200 mg/dl or more also confirms DM.
   d. Reversible factors that promote hyperglycemia (e.g., increased calorie intake, pregnancy, and certain medications) should be ruled out before a diagnosis of DM is established.

II. TREATMENT OBJECTIVES

A. To maintain optimal health, thus permitting a productive life

B. To equalize the supply and demand of insulin to prevent symptomatic hyperglycemia and hypoglycemia

C. To avoid acute disease complications (e.g., ketosis)

D. To prevent or minimize complications of long-standing disease

E. To teach the patient about the disease and ensure therapeutic compliance

III. THERAPY.
Diet, drug therapy, exercise, glucose monitoring, patient education, and self-care are crucial in the management of DM.

A. Diet. All diabetics must eat a well-balanced diet to regulate blood glucose.

1. Type I patients must eat at properly spaced intervals.
2. Type II diabetics—most of whom are obese—should follow a weight-reduction diet (increased weight is associated with more pronounced hyperglycemia). Dietary therapy alone is sufficient to control hyperglycemia in many type II patients.
3. Intake of carbohydrates, proteins, and fats should be regulated, with carbohydrates accounting for 50% to 60% of total caloric intake, proteins accounting for 10% to 15%, and fats accounting for 30% to 35%.
4. Refined and simple sugars should be avoided.
5. High intake of fiber (e.g., bran, beans, fruits, vegetables) seems to improve blood glucose control.
6. Cholesterol intake is limited to less than 300 mg/day.
7. The **food exchange system** increases flexibility in meal planning. This system lists equivalent carbohydrate, protein, and fat values for foods in six basic groups.
8. The **glycemic index**, another meal planning aid, categorizes carbohydrates according to the blood glucose level they produce after ingestion; the lower the level, the lower a given carbohydrate's glycemic index. Although this system may allow diabetics to select carbohydrates more carefully, researchers debate its value because the glycemic index of carbohydrates may change when they are consumed along with proteins or fats.
9. Factors that change the blood glucose level (e.g., stress, exercise) necessitate dietary adjustment. For example, before vigorous exercise, the diabetic should consume 30 to 40 g of a complex carbohydrate, plus protein.

B. Drug therapy. Insulin and sulfonylureas are used in the treatment of DM.

1. **Insulin**
   - **a. Indications**. Insulin replacement therapy is indicated for all type I diabetics and for type II diabetics whose hyperglycemia does not respond to dietary or sulfonylurea therapy.
   - **b. Mechanism of action**. Insulin lowers the blood glucose level by increasing glucose transport across cell membranes, enhancing glucose conversion to glycogen, inhibiting release of free fatty acids from adipose tissue, and inhibiting lipolysis and glycogenolysis.
   - **c. Choice of agent**
     - **(1) Source**. Most commercial insulin is derived from beef and pork; most insulin products contain a mixture of the two. (Pork insulin is less antigenic than beef insulin.) Highly purified monospecies insulin and biosynthetic human insulin (produced by recombinant DNA techniques) are available for patients with insulin allergy or resistance. Use of human insulin in newly diagnosed type I diabetics is preferred because of its reduced antigenicity.
     - **(2) Concentration**. Most insulins come in a concentration of 100 units/ml (U100), dispensed in 10-ml vials.
       - **(a)** Concentrated insulin preparations (U500) are available for patients with insulin resistance.
       - **(b)** Children and adults needing small insulin quantities may use U40 insulin.
     - **(3) Preparations**
       - **(a)** The three major types of insulin differ in onset and duration of action (Table 44-1).
         - **(i) Fast-acting** insulin products include **regular** and **semilente insulin** (insulin zinc suspension).
         - **(ii) Intermediate-acting** insulin products include **lente** and **NPH** (isophane insulin suspension).
         - **(iii) Long-acting** insulin products include **PZI** (protamine zinc insulin) and **ultralente** (extended insulin zinc suspension).
       - **(b) Insulin mixtures**. Some diabetics need a mixture of insulin types (e.g., a rapid-acting insulin to control morning hyperglycemia and an intermediate-acting insulin to control later hyperglycemia).
         - **(i)** Insulin may be mixed by the patient or bought in premixed form (e.g., Mixtard, consisting of 70% NPH insulin and 30% regular insulin).
         - **(ii)** Insulins mixed together should be of the same concentration.
   - **d. Administration and dosage.** Except in special circumstances, insulin is always administered by subcutaneous injection.
     - **(1)** The subcutaneous injection site should be rotated to avoid lipohypertrophy and fibrosis. However, to prevent variations in drug absorption, injections should be given within the same region (e.g., the abdomen).

Table 44-1. Major Characteristics of Insulin Preparations

Preparation	Onset of Action (Hours)	Peak Effect (Hours)	Duration of Action (Hours)
Fast-acting insulins			
Regular	0.25–1	2–6	4–12
Semilente	0.5–1	3–6	8–16
Intermediate-acting insulins			
Lente	1–4	6–16	12–28
NPH*	1.5–4	6–16	12–24
Long-acting insulins			
PZI†	3–8	14–24	24–48
Ultralente	4	18–24	36

*NPH = isophane insulin suspension.

†PZI = protamine zinc insulin.

(2) Patients with acute hyperglycemia or ketoacidosis may require **intravenous** (IV) administration with regular insulin (insulin injection).

(3) **Insulin pump**. This delivery method, which provides tighter glycemic control, is indicated for selected diabetics who need long-term insulin therapy, who have widely fluctuating blood glucose levels, or whose life-styles preclude regular meals. However, there is a risk of developing serious hypoglycemia when using a pump.

(a) The **closed-loop** pump senses and responds to changing blood glucose levels. Through a subcutaneous needle in the thigh or abdominal wall, the pump administers appropriate amounts of insulin continuously. Because it requires blood aspiration, it can be used only in a hospital setting.

(b) The **open-loop** pump does not have a glucose sensor. It infuses insulin in small continuous doses and in large doses that the patient releases when appropriate (e.g., before meals).

e. Precautions and monitoring effects

(1) Improper insulin therapy may induce **hypoglycemia**, especially in patients with unpredictable changes in insulin requirements. Other causes of hypoglycemia include meal skipping, vigorous exercise, and accidental insulin overdose.

(a) Signs and symptoms of insulin hypoglycemia include headache, blurred vision, weakness, diaphoresis, tachycardia, irritability, and confusion.

(b) To reverse insulin hypoglycemia in an **unresponsive patient**, glucose may be injected intravenously or honey or a glucose product (e.g., Glutose) may be inserted into the patient's buccal pouch. In addition, glucagon may be given subcutaneously, intramuscularly, or intravenously at a dose of 0.5 to 1 unit (0.5 to 1 mg).

(c) A **conscious patient** may be given a food or a beverage containing a simple, fast-acting carbohydrate (e.g., candy, fruit juice) to raise the blood glucose level.

(2) Local or systemic insulin allergy may occur, particularly after the first dose. Manifestations include allergic urticaria, anaphylaxis, and angioedema.

(3) **Lipoatrophy** (subcutaneous fat loss triggered by an immune reaction) may occur at the injection site. (Purer insulin forms have reduced the incidence of this adverse reaction.)

(4) **Lipohypertrophy** and fibrosis may develop in patients who do not rotate injection sites.

(5) **Insulin resistance** is defined as the need for more than 200 U/day of insulin (in the absence of ketoacidosis). This condition may result from obesity, infection, glucocorticoid excess, or a high concentration of circulating IgG anti-insulin antibodies.

(a) Nearly all patients receiving insulin develop such antibodies; however, in cases of insulin resistance, serum insulin-binding capacity usually exceeds 30 U/L.

(b) The condition may resolve spontaneously. In some cases, though, it necessitates a switch to a less antigenic insulin (e.g., to pork or human insulin), use of multiple injections of regular insulin rather than an intermediate-acting product, or prednisone therapy (60 mg/day) to suppress the immune response.

(6) Too much insulin can cause the **Somogyi effect** (insulin rebound syndrome). In this syndrome, nocturnal hypoglycemia stimulates a surge of counterregulatory hormones, triggering morning hyperglycemia.

(7) Various factors may change a diabetic's insulin requirements.

(a) Infection, weight gain, puberty, inactivity, hyperthyroidism, and Cushing's disease tend to **increase** insulin needs.
(b) Renal failure, adrenal insufficiency, malabsorption, hypopituitarism, weight loss, and increased exercise tend to **reduce** insulin needs.

(8) Regular glucose self-monitoring is needed to evaluate changing insulin requirements and therapeutic efficacy (see sections III D and E).

(9) PZI and regular insulin must not be mixed together in the same syringe.

(10) **Significant interactions**
(a) A decreased response to insulin may occur when **corticosteroids, nicotinic acid,** or **thiazide diuretics** are administered concomitantly.
(b) Hypoglycemic effects may increase, leading to prolonged hypoglycemia, with concomitant use of insulin and **monoamine oxidase (MAO) inhibitors**, **beta blockers**, **salicylates**, **oxytetracycline**, **fenfluramine**, **alcohol**, **sulfonylureas**, **or pentamidine**.

2. **Sulfonylureas** (oral hypoglycemics) are used to control hyperglycemia in selected diabetics.

a. **Indications**. These drugs help reduce blood glucose levels in type II DM that does not respond to diet alone. Because the action of sulfonylureas seems to depend on functioning beta cells, these drugs are not useful in type I diabetics.

b. **Mechanism of action**. As an **acute** action, sulfonylureas stimulate beta cell tissue to secrete insulin. In the **long-term**, these drugs appear to reduce cellular insulin resistance.

c. **Choice of agent**. First-generation sulfonylureas include **acetohexamide**, **chlorpropamide**, **tolbutamide**, and **tolazamide**. Second-generation agents, considerably more potent, include **glipizide** and **glyburide**. The most clinically significant difference among sulfonylureas is **duration of action** (Table 44-2).

(1) **Tolbutamide**, with the shortest duration, is administered mainly to elderly type II diabetics for whom hypoglycemia is a more serious complication.

(2) **Acetohexamide**, **tolazamide**, **glipizide**, and **glyburide** have intermediate durations. (The duration of acetohexamide is prolonged in renal disease.)

(3) **Chlorpropamide** has the longest duration and poses a risk to patients with renal or hepatic impairment. It also causes more severe and frequent side effects (including hypoglycemia and hyponatremia) than the other sulfonylureas.

d. **Administration and dosage** (see Table 44-2)

e. **Precautions and monitoring effects**

(1) Sulfonylureas are contraindicated in patients without functioning beta cells, children, pregnant and lactating women, and patients with allergy to sulfa agents. They also are contraindicated during stressful conditions that increase the risk of hyper- or hypoglycemia.

(2) These agents should not be used in patients with severe renal or hepatic impairment.

(3) Sulfonylurea therapy has been associated with a possible increased risk of cardiovascular mortality and morbidity.

(4) Hypoglycemia and alcohol intolerance may occur during sulfonylurea therapy. Alcohol intolerance is less common with second-generation agents.

(5) Sulfonylureas should not be discontinued without a physician's approval.

(6) Untoward reactions to sulfonylureas include gastrointestinal disturbances (e.g., nausea, gastric discomfort, vomiting, constipation), tachycardia, headache, skin rash, and hematologic problems (e.g., agranulocytosis, pancytopenia, hemolytic anemia).

(7) Sulfonylureas pose a risk of cholestatic jaundice.

Table 44-2. Dosages and Other Characteristics of Sulfonylureas

Agent	Usual Daily Dosage (mg)	Number of Daily Doses	Duration of Action (Hours)	Metabolism Site
First-generation agents				
Acetohexamide	250–1500	1–2	12–18	Liver, kidney
Chlorpropamide	100–500	1	60	Kidney
Tolazamide	100–1000	1–2	12–14	Liver
Tolbutamide	500–3000	2–3	6–12	Liver
Second-generation agents				
Glipizide	2.5–40	1–2	24	Liver, kidney
Glyburide	1.25–20	1–2	24	Liver, kidney

(8) Sulfonylurea therapy has a relatively **high failure rate** (25% to 40%).
(a) In **primary therapeutic failure**, the agent fails to control hyperglycemia within the first 4 weeks after initiation.
(b) In **secondary therapeutic failure**, the drug controls hyperglycemia initially but fails to maintain control. Approximately 5% to 30% of initial responders experience secondary therapeutic failure.

(9) **Significant interactions**
(a) Prolonged hypoglycemia and masking of hypoglycemia symptoms may occur with concomitant use of **beta blockers** and **clonidine.**
(b) **Alcohol, salicylates, nonsteroidal anti-inflammatory drugs, methyldopa, chloramphenicol, warfarin, MAO inhibitors, probenicid**, and **ranitidine** may intensify the hypoglycemic effects of sulfonylureas.
(c) A decreased hypoglycemic response may occur with concomitant use of **corticosteroids, aminophylline, bleomycin, thiazide diuretics, ethacrynic acid, levodopa, rifampin, phenytoin**, and **oral contraceptives.**

C. Exercise. A carefully planned and religiously followed exercise program enhances glucose uptake by cells, thereby reducing the blood glucose level.

1. **Aerobic exercise** (e.g., swimming, walking, running) has a desirable hypoglycemic effect because it uses glucose as fuel; aerobic exercise also promotes cardiovascular health.

2. **Anaerobic exercise** (e.g., weight-lifting) should be avoided by diabetics because it induces stress that leads to increased blood glucose levels. Also, anaerobic exercise may cause deleterious cardiovascular effects (e.g., increased blood pressure).

D. Glucose monitoring. Frequent measurement of the blood glucose level is a key aspect of DM therapy. It helps determine therapeutic efficacy, guide and refine any adjustments to drug therapy, and, when performed by the patient at home, permits better understanding of the glycemic effects of specific foods.

1. **Urine glucose testing**
a. Various testing kits are available.
(1) Tests using the **copper sulfate reduction method** (e.g., Clinitest tablets) yield the most accurate results. This method is indicated for type I diabetics.
(a) This test method reveals glycosuria.
(b) The presence of urine sugars other than glucose may cause a false-positive result.
(c) Use of such drugs as levodopa, probenicid, penicillins, isoniazid, barbiturates, and salicylates may cause false-positive results. Use of cephalosporins may complicate interpretation of test results.
(2) The **glucose oxidase method** reveals reactions between urine glucose and oxidase. Tests using this method (e.g., Chemstrip uG, Diastix, Tes-Tape) consist of reagent strips or paper tape.
(a) The test is performed by quickly dipping the strip or tape in and out of the urine, then holding it in the air to read it.
(b) Use of salicylates, levodopa, vitamin C, and Pyridium (phenazopyridine) may alter test results.
(c) This test method tends to underestimate high urine glucose concentrations.
b. To ensure uniform interpretation, all urine glucose test results should be read in **mg% sugar** rather than in plus marks.
c. Urine glucose tests are less accurate than blood glucose tests and do not always reflect blood glucose levels. Also, they do not detect hypoglycemia.

2. **Blood glucose testing**. This type of testing is indicated for patients who require tight glycemic control to avoid hypoglycemia.
a. Some patients (especially type I diabetics) need to measure their blood glucose level several times daily—typically before or after meals.
b. Blood glucose tests are more reliable than urine glucose tests.
c. Various test methods and products are available.
(1) **Reagent strips** (e.g., Chemstrip bG, Dextrostix, Visidex II) are visual tests in which a blood droplet is applied to the test strip.
(2) **Glucose meters** (e.g., Glucometer II, Accu-Chek bG), more precise than reagent strips, give a numerical blood glucose value.
(3) The **hemoglobin A_{1c} test**, also known as the glycohemoglobin or glycosylated hemoglobin test) shows long-term glycemic control and serves as an index of therapeutic efficacy or compliance.

(a) A hemoglobin variant produced by glycosylation of hemoglobin A, hemoglobin A_{1c} is more abundant in diabetics than nondiabetics.
(b) The hemoglobin A_{1c} level reflects the average blood glucose level over the preceding 120 days. (The glycosylation rate remains constant over the 120-day life span of red blood cells.)
(c) A hemoglobin A_{1c} level of 7.5% or lower indicates good glycemic control; a level of 9.0% or higher reflects poor control.

E. Patient education and self-care. Patient education about the disease and patient participation in medical care are crucial aspects of DM management.

1. **Patient education** improves understanding of the disease, thereby promoting compliance with dietary, drug, and exercise regimens and glucose self-monitoring. Patients also must be taught how to prevent, recognize, and treat hypoglycemia and hyperglycemia.
2. Appropriate **self-care measures** are necessary to avoid the potentially dire consequences of trauma and skin abrasions resulting from disease complications such as neuropathy and peripheral vascular compromise.
   a. The patient must inspect the skin daily for abrasions, pain, or swelling and see a physician promptly for treatment. Injuries should be covered immediately with sterile gauze.
   b. Even minor trauma, especially to the legs and feet, should be avoided.
   c. Daily foot cleansing should be performed using only soap and water (with a thermometer to check water temperature if the patient has neuropathy-induced sensation loss). Skin should be dried gently and vegetable oil applied.
   d. Corns and calluses should be removed by a podiatrist.
   e. Only properly fitting, low-heeled shoes should be worn.

F. Pancreas and islet cell transplantation. These experimental procedures may be performed to treat some cases of DM.

G. Disease management in pregnancy. Approximately 2% to 3% of pregnant women with no history of DM develop diabetes or impaired glucose tolerance—presumably from the increased insulin requirements of pregnancy.

1. DM in pregnancy carries an increased risk of neonatal morbidity.
2. Tight glycemic control is especially important during pregnancy to avoid neonatal complications. Continuous insulin infusion (via an insulin pump) or multiple insulin injections may be required.
3. Sulfonylureas are contraindicated in pregnant women.
4. Weight reduction is not recommended because this could compromise fetal development.
5. Some experts advise termination of pregnancy by induced labor or cesarean section at 37 to 38 weeks gestation.
6. Glucose tolerance usually normalizes within a few weeks after delivery.

IV. COMPLICATIONS

A. Acute complications. Life-threatening complications of DM include diabetic ketoacidosis and hyperglycemic hyperosmolar nonketotic coma. Hypoglycemia, another acute complication, usually stems from drug therapy [see section III B 1 e (1)].

1. **Diabetic ketoacidosis (DKA).** Affecting only type I diabetics, this disorder typically arises after a short period (hours or days) of deteriorating glycemic control.
   a. **Precipitating causes** include stress, infection, exercise, excessive alcohol consumption, improper insulin therapy, and dietary noncompliance—conditions that lead to an absence or deficiency of insulin.
   b. DKA is often the presenting disorder in children with previously undiagnosed type I DM.
   c. **Hyperglycemia** and **ketonemia** trigger osmotic diuresis, electrolyte loss, hypovolemia, and metabolic acidosis.
   d. **Physical findings** include Kussmaul's respirations, acetone breath odor, dehydration, dry skin, poor skin turgor, reduced level of consciousness (ranging from confusion to coma), and abdominal pain. Without treatment, death ensues.
   e. **Laboratory findings** include elevated levels of blood glucose and ketone bodies (e.g., acetone, acetoacetate), low arterial pH and carbon dioxide partial pressure (PCO_2) values, and

abnormal serum electrolyte values.

f. **Therapy** involves fluid, insulin, and electrolyte replacement.

2. **Hyperglycemic hyperosmolar nonketotic coma (HHNC)**, which occurs in type II diabetics, has a higher mortality rate than DKA.
   a. **Precipitating factors** include various illnesses and conditions that increase insulin requirements [e.g., severe burns, gastrointestinal bleeding, central nervous system (CNS) injury, acute myocardial infarction].
      (1) Use of certain drugs (e.g., steroids, glucagon, thiazide diuretics, cimetidine, and propranolol) also can trigger HHNC.
      (2) Such medical procedures as IV hyperalimentation and peritoneal dialysis increase the risk for HHNC.
   b. **Physical findings** include polyuria, polydipsia, dehydration, hypotension, rapid respirations, abdominal discomfort, nausea, vomiting, tachycardia, palpitations, focal neurologic signs, and reduced level of consciousness.
   c. **Laboratory findings** include an extremely elevated blood glucose level (800 to 1000 mg/dl) and a serum osmolarity of 280 mOsm/kg or more.
   d. **Therapy** involves fluid, insulin, and electrolyte replacement.

B. Chronic complications. DM is associated with a high risk for a number of chronic illnesses.

1. **Cardiovascular disease**
   a. **Atherosclerosis** and **peripheral vascular disease** are more severe and more common in diabetics than in nondiabetics; also, disease onset typically is earlier.
   b. **Microvascular changes**, characterized by **thickening of the capillary basement membrane**, may lead to retinopathy and skin changes.
   c. Diabetics have a higher incidence of **hypertension** than nondiabetics.

2. **Ocular complications**
   a. **Premature cataracts** are most common in diabetics with severe chronic hyperglycemia.
   b. **Diabetic retinopathy**, a consequence of microvascular changes, affects approximately 50% of diabetics within 10 years of disease onset.
      (1) This syndrome is the leading cause of new blindness in the United States.
      (2) **Retinal microaneurysm**, the earliest sign of retinopathy, may progress to **punctate hemorrhage**, **exudation**, and **proliferative retinopathy**.
      (3) Retinal detachment, secondary glaucoma, and vision loss may ensue.

3. **Diabetic nephropathy**, another manifestation of microvascular pathology, ultimately may lead to renal insufficiency or failure.
   a. Diabetic nephropathy is characterized by **proteinuria**, **microalbuminuria**, **glomerular lesions**, and **renal arteriosclerosis**.
   b. Diabetics account for approximately 25% of patients with end-stage renal failure.

4. **Diabetic neuropathies** typically involve both the autonomic and peripheral nervous systems.
   a. Gastric atony, incontinence, diarrhea, and impotence reflect autonomic involvement.
   b. Peripheral neuropathy may give rise to impaired perception of pain and temperature (particularly in the lower extremities).
   c. **Ischemia** may cause skeletal muscle atrophy and motor abnormalities.

5. **Skin and mucous membrane complications** stem from vascular changes and neuropathy.
   a. Diabetics have an increased risk for infection, such as *Candida* infections of the skin and vagina. Erythema commonly develops beneath the breasts and between fingers; eruptive xanthomas occur most often in long-standing, poorly controlled DM.
   b. **Atrophic lesions** (round painless lesions) and **diabetic dermopathy** (reddish-brown papular spots) are common, especially on the lower extremities.
   c. An ulcerating necrotic lesion called **necrobiosis lipoidica diabeticorum** may develop on the anterior leg surface or the dorsum of the ankle.
   d. Injury, infection, neuropathy, vascular disease, or ischemia may lead to **gangrene**, which is 20 times more common in diabetics than nondiabetics.

STUDY QUESTIONS

Directions: Each question below contains five suggested answers. Choose the **one best** response to each question.

1. Current criteria used in the diagnosis of diabetes mellitus include all of the following symptoms EXCEPT

A. fasting hyperglycemia
B. polyuria
C. polydypsia
D. weight gain
E. weight loss

2. The most useful glucose test employed in monitoring diabetes mellitus therapy is

A. urine monitoring
B. blood monitoring
C. renal function monitoring
D. cardiovascular monitoring
E. vascular monitoring

3. Which of the following statements concerning insulin replacement therapy is most likely true?

A. Most commercial insulin products vary little with respect to time, course, and duration of hypoglycemic activity
B. Regular insulins cannot be mixed with NPH (isophane insulin suspension)
C. Regular insulin cannot be given intravenously
D. Cutting down on carbohydrate consumption is a necessity for all diabetic patients
E. Insulin therapy does not have to be monitored closely

4. A mass of adipose tissue that develops at the injection site is usually due to the patient's neglect in rotating the insulin injection site. This is known as

A. lipoatrophy
B. hypertrophic degenerative adiposity
C. lipohypertrophy
D. atrophic skin lesion
E. dermatitis

5. Sulfonylureas are a primary mode of therapy in the treatment of

A. insulin-dependent (type I) diabetes mellitus patients
B. diabetic patients experiencing severe hepatic or renal dysfunction
C. diabetic pregnant women
D. patients with diabetic ketoacidosis
E. non-insulin–dependent (type II) diabetes mellitus patients

6. Patients taking chlorpropamide should avoid products containing

A. acetaminophen
B. ethanol
C. vitamin A
D. penicillins
E. milk products

7. Which of the following is the standard recommended dose of glyburide?

A. 0.5 to 2 mg per day
B. 1.25 to 20 mg per day
C. 50 to 100 mg per day
D. 200 mg per day
E. 200 to 1000 mg per day

ANSWERS AND EXPLANATIONS

1. The answer is D. (*I E, F 1* a) Frequent urination (polyuria), thirst (polydypsia), and weight loss are all common signs of diabetes. When these symptoms are present, it is necessary to have a fasting blood glucose level drawn to determine a diabetic state. A fasting blood glucose level of greater than or equal to 140 mg/dl on more than one occasion is diagnostic of a diabetic state.

2. The answer is B. (*III D 1, 2*) Blood glucose monitoring is the most useful form of monitoring glucose levels. Urine monitoring provides only gross estimates of the current status and cannot rule out hypoglycemia. Renal function and cardiovascular and vascular functions provide evidence of long-standing disease and are not useful for monitoring daily progress.

3. The answer is D. [*III A, B 1* c *(3) (a)*] Many commercial insulin preparations vary with respect to duration of activity and time for peak plasma level. Regular insulin can be mixed with NPH (isophane insulin suspension) and can be given intravenously. All insulin therapies should be monitored closely and on a daily basis. Careful regulation of carbohydrate intake is very important for all diabetic patients—carbohydrate consumption plays a major role in the balance of glucose metabolism and antagonizes the effects of insulin therapy.

4. The answer is C. [*III B 1* e *(4)*] Lipohypertrophy consists of masses of adipose tissue that develop at the injection site, usually in patients who do not rotate the injection sites properly. The masses gradually disappear if injection in these sites is avoided.

5. The answer is E. (*III B 2* a) Sulfonylureas should not be used as primary therapy in insulin-dependent (type I) diabetes mellitus patients, in those who have severe hepatic or renal dysfunction, or in those patients who are pregnant. Diabetic ketoacidosis should never be treated with sulfonylureas. This condition must be treated with insulin, fluids, and electrolyte replacement.

6. The answer is B. [*III B 2* c *(3),* e *(4), (9) (b)*] Acute injestion of ethanol (alcohol) by patients who are taking any antidiabetic agent carries the risk of severe hypoglycemia especially due to the potential hypoglycemic effects of ethanol, (especially if consumed in the fasting state).

7. The answer is B. (*III B 2* c; *Table 44-2*) The standard recommended dose of glyburide is 1.25 to 20 mg per day. Doses greater than 20 mg are not recommended by the manufacturer. Patients may be started on a low dose (e.g., 1.25 mg per day) and titrated up to an effective oral dose, as clinically indicated.

45
Thyroid Disease

John E. Janosik

I. PHYSIOLOGY

A. Thyroid hormone regulation

1. The thyroid gland synthesizes, stores, and secretes hormones that are important to growth and development and the metabolic rate. These hormones are **thyroxine (T_4)** and **triiodothyronine (T_3)**.
2. The thyroid gland also secretes **calcitonin**, which reduces blood calcium ion concentration.
3. Thyroid hormone secretion and transport are controlled by **thyroid-stimulating hormone (thyrotropin; TSH)**. TSH is released by the anterior pituitary gland, which is triggered by **thyrotropin-releasing hormone (TRH)**, secreted from the hypothalamus.
4. The process produces increased blood levels of thyroid hormone (circulating free T_4 and free T_3), which in turn signals the pituitary to stop releasing TSH (acting as **negative feedback**).
5. Conversely, low blood levels of free hormone trigger pituitary release of TSH, which stimulates the thyroid gland to secrete T_4 and T_3 until free hormone levels return to normal. At this point, the pituitary gland ceases to release TSH, which completes the feedback loop (Fig. 45-1).
6. This homeostatic mechanism attempts to maintain the level of circulating thyroid hormone within a very narrow range.

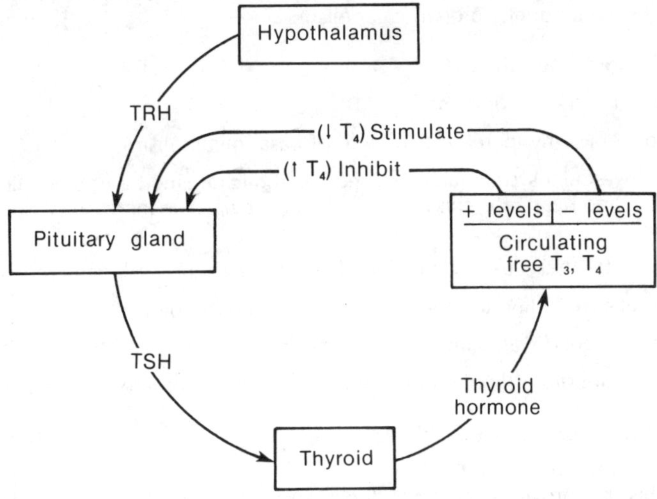

Figure 45-1. Thyroid hormone regulation loop. This carefully balanced hormone regulation system uses both positive (stimulating) and negative (inhibiting) feedback to maintain homeostasis. Disruption of any of these elements can produce serious consequences, such as myxedema crisis (underavailability of thyroid hormone) or thyroid storm (overabundance of thyroid hormone). *TRH* = thyroid-releasing hormone; *TSH* = thyroid-stimulating hormone; T_4 = thyroxine; T_3 = triiodothyronine.

B. Biosynthesis (Fig. 45-2)

1. Essential to synthesis of thyroid hormones is dietary iodine, reduced to **inorganic iodide**, which the thyroid actively extracts from the plasma (through iodide trapping, also known as the **iodide pump**). Some of this iodide is stored within the colloid; some diffuses into the lumen of thyroid follicles.
2. Iodide is oxidized by peroxidase and bound to tyrosyl residues within the thyroglobulin molecule in a process called **organification**.
3. The synthesis begins with iodide binding to tyrosine, forming **monoiodotyrosine (MIT)**.
4. MIT then binds another iodide to form **diiodotyrosine (DIT)**.
5. Then, slowly, a coupling reaction binds MIT and DIT, producing **T_3**, **reverse triiodothyronine (rT_3)**, and **T_4**.

C. Hormone transport

1. After TSH stimulation of the thyroid gland, T_3 and T_4 are cleaved from thyroglobulin and released into the circulation.
2. Once in the circulation, thyroid hormone is transported bound to several plasma proteins. This helps to protect the hormone from premature metabolism and excretion, prolongs its half-life in the circulation, and allows it to reach its site of action.
3. The majority of thyroid hormone is transported by **thyroxine-binding globulin (TBG)**. Prealbumin and albumin also serve as carriers.

D. Hormone metabolism

1. Peripheral conversion of T_4 to T_3 takes place in the pituitary gland, liver, and kidneys and accounts for about 80% of T_3 generation.
2. Deiodination accounts for the majority of hormone degradation. The major steps in this process are shown in Figure 45-3.
3. Deiodinated hormones are excreted in feces and urine.
4. Minor nondeiodination pathways of metabolism include conjugation with sulfate and glucuronide, deamination, and decarboxylation.

E. Hormone function. Although the effects of thyroid hormones are known, the basic mechanisms producing these effects elude precise definition. Among the likely basic premises is that they seem to activate the messenger RNA transcription process and can promote protein synthesis or (in excessive amounts) protein catabolism.

F. Thyroid hormones affect:

1. Growth and development
2. Calorigenics (by increasing the rate of basal metabolism)
3. Cardiovascular system (an increased metabolic rate increases blood flow and, in turn, cardiac output and heart rate; this may be related in part to an increased tissue sensitivity to catecholamines)
4. The central nervous system (CNS) [increasing or diminishing cerebration]
5. Musculature (a fine tremor characterizes hyperthyroidism)
6. Sleep (fatigued wakefulness with hyperthyroidism or somnolence with hypothyroidism)
7. Lipid metabolism (lipid mobilization and degradation are stimulated)

G. Thyroid function studies (Table 45-1)

1. **Serum total thyroxine (TT_4)**
   a. This test provides the most direct reflection of thyroid function through indicating hormone availability to tissues. Total (free and bound) T_4 is determined by radioimmunoassay, which is sensitive and rapid.
   b. Changes in thyroid-globulin concentration, especially TBG (which increases during pregnancy), alter the total concentration of T_4 and may produce a misleading high or low test result.
   c. However, these changes in TBG do not affect the concentration of free T_4. Therefore, to

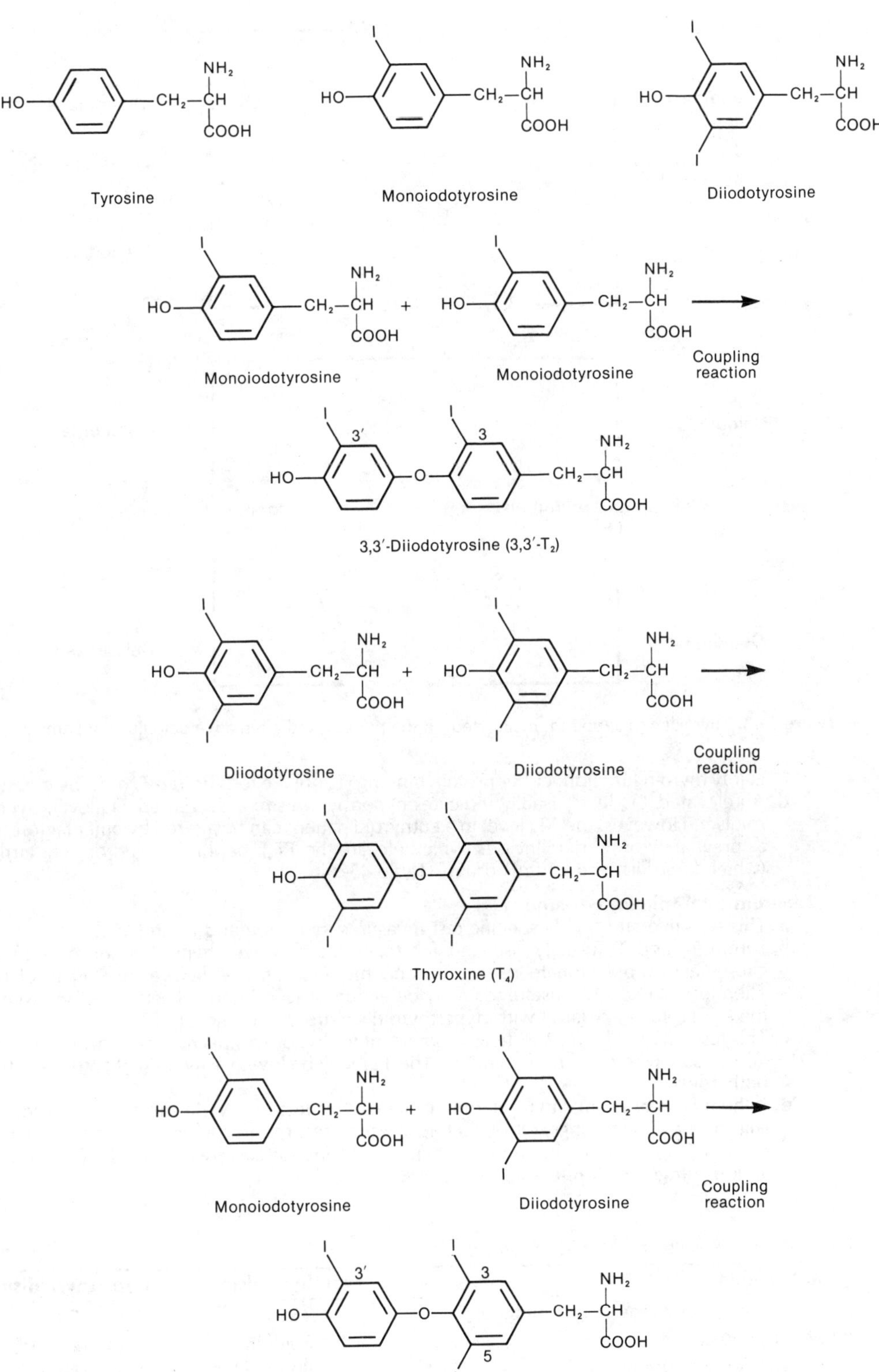

Figure 45-2. Biosynthesis of thyroid hormones. The major products are thyroxine (T_4) and triiodothyronine (T_3). These are formed in the follicle cells of the thyroid gland by iodination of tyrosine residues. Monoiodo- and diiodotyrosine residues are formed first. These then react to form T_3 and T_4.

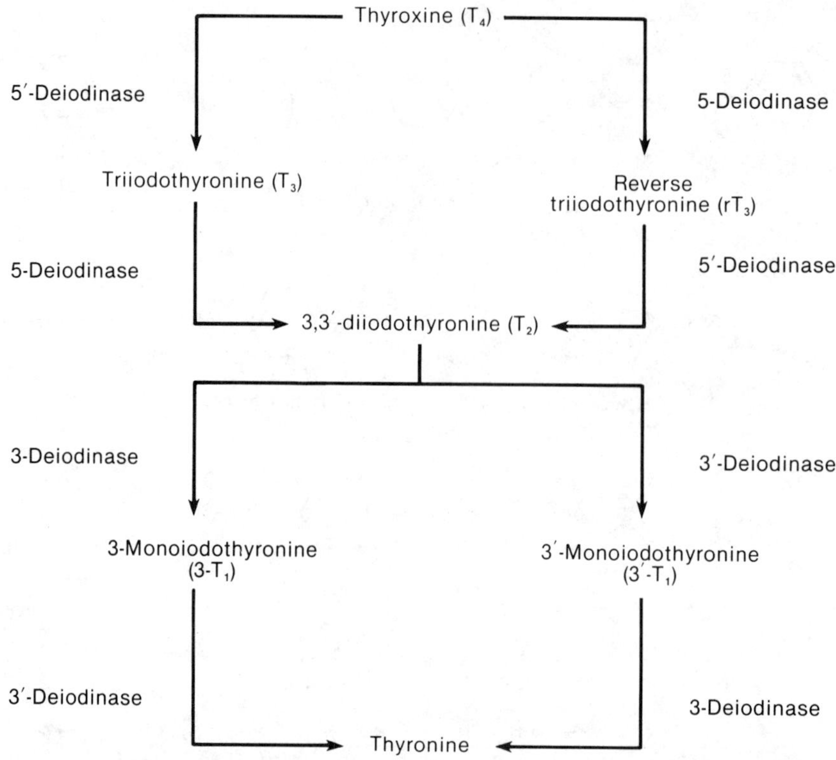

Figure 45-3. Thyroxine metabolism: major steps in the primary and alternative deiodination pathways.

clarify thyroid function, either protein binding (T_3 uptake test) or free T_4 must be measured.

d. An elevated TT_4 level usually indicates hyperthyroidism; a decreased TT_4 level, hypothyroidism. However, the TT_4 level in a euthyroid patient can be altered by other factors, such as pregnancy or febrile illnesses (which elevate the TT_4), nephrotic syndrome or cirrhosis (which lower it), and various drugs. (Table 45-2).

2. Serum total triiodothyronine (TT_3)

a. This sensitive and highly specific test measures total (free and bound) T_3.

b. Serum T_3 and T_4 usually rise and fall together; however, hyperthyroidism commonly causes a disproportionate rise in T_3, and the TT_3 can rise before the TT_4 level does. Therefore, TT_3 can be useful for early detection or to rule out hyperthyroidism. Many of the symptoms associated with hyperthyroidism are due to elevated TT_3.

c. This test may not be diagnostically significant for hypothyroidism, in which TT_3 levels may fall but stay within the normal range. The TT_3 may be low in only 50% of patients with hypothyroidism.

d. If there is an abnormality in binding proteins, this test may yield the same misleading results as the TT_4 readings. Other factors affecting test results include pregnancy (which increases TT_3 levels), malnutrition or hepatic or renal disease (which lower TT_3 levels), or various drugs (see Table 45-2).

Table 45-1. Test Results in Thyroid Disorders

Thyroid Function Test	Hypothyroidism	Hyperthyroidism
Serum resin triiodothyronine (RT_3U) uptake	↓ (< 35%)	↑ (> 45%)
Serum total thryoxine (TT_4)	↓ (< 5 μg/dl)	↑ (> 12 μg/dl)
Serum total triiodothyronine (TT_3)	↓ (< 80 ng/dl)	↑ (> 180 ng/dl)
Free thyroxine index (FTI)	↓ (< 5.5)	↑ (< 10.5)
Serum thyrotropin (TSH)	↑ (> 6 μU/ml)	↓ (< 0.5 μU/ml)

↑ = increased levels.
↓ = decreased levels.

Table 45-2. Effects of Drugs on Thyroid Function Tests

Drug	Serum T_4	Resin T_3 Uptake	Free Thyroxine Index (FTI)	Serum T_3	Serum TSH	Comment
p-Aminosalicylic acid (PAS)	↓	(nd)	↓	(nd)	↑*	Antithyroid effect, rarely, with long-term use
Aminoglutethimide (*Cytadren*)	↓	(nd)	(nd)	(nd)	↑	
Anabolic steroids and androgens	↓	↑	0	↓*	(nd)	Decreased serum TBG
Antithyroid drugs: propylthiouracil or methimazole (*Tapazole*)	↓	↓	↓	↓	0 or ↑	TSH may increase if patient becomes hypothyroid
Asparaginase (*Elspar*)	↓	↑	(nd)	↓*	↑*	Decreased serum TBG
Barbiturates	↓[a]	(nd)	↓	(nd)	(nd)	Stimulates T_4 metabolism
Contraceptives, oral	↑	↓	0	↑	0	TBG usually increased
Corticosteroids	0 or ↓	0 or ↑	0 or ↓	↓	↓	Usual doses decrease TBG; high doses may increase TBG
Danazol (*Danocrine*)	↓	↑	0[b]	↓	0 or ↓	Decreased serum TBG
Estrogens	↑	↓	0	↑	0	Increased serum TBG
Ethionamide (*Trecator*)	↓	(nd)	↓*	(nd)	↑*	Antithyroid effect
Fluorouracil (*Adrucil*; others)	↑	↓	(nd)	↑	0	Patients clinically euthyroid; TBG increased
Heparin, intravenous	↑[c]	0 or ↑	↑*	0	(nd)	FTI is increased with some measures
Hypoglycemics (sulfonylureas)	0[d]	0[d]	0[d]	(nd)	(nd)	
Iodides, inorganic	0	0	0	(nd)	(nd)	
Iodides, organic	0	0	0	(nd)	(nd)	
Levodopa and levodopa–carbidopa (*Sinemet*)	0	0	0	0	↓[e]	
Levothyroxine (*Levothroid*; others)	↑ (s)[f,g]	↑ or 0 or ↓[f,g]	0 or ↑[f,g]	↑ or 0[f,g]	↑ or 0[f]	
Liothyronine (*Cytomel*; others)	↓[f]	0 or ↓[f]	↓[f]	↑ or ↓[f,g]	0[f]	
Liotrix (*Euthroid; Thyrolar*)	0[f] or ↓ (s)	0[f]	0[f]	0[f,g]	0[f]	
Lithium carbonate (*Eskalith*; others)	0 or ↓	0 or ↓	0 or ↓	0 or ↓	0 or ↑	

Continued on next page

Table 45-2. Continued

Drug	Serum T_4	Resin T_3 Uptake	Free Thyroxine Index (FTI)	Serum T_3	Serum TSH	Comment
Methadone (*Dolophine*)	↑ (s)	↓	0	↑	0	Increased serum TBG
Mitotane (*Lysodren*)	↓	0	0*	(nd)	(nd)	
Nitroprusside (*Nipride*)	↓	(nd)	(nd)	(nd)	(nd)	Clinical hypothyroidism
Oxyphenbutazone (*Oxalid; Tandearil*) and phenylbutazone (*Azolid; Butazolidin*)	0 or ↓	↑	↓	(nd)	↑*	May compete with T_4 for TBG binding. Rarely, overt hypothyroidism and goiter may occur
Perphenazine (*Trilafon*)	↑	↓	↓	↑	0*	
Phenytoin (*Dilantin*; others)	↓	0 or ↑ (s)	0 or ↓ (s)	↓	0	Stimulates T_4 metabolism and may compete with T_4 for TBG binding
Propranolol (*Inderal*)	0 or ↑[h]	0[i]	(nd)	↓[j]	0	
Resorcinol (excessive topical use)	↓	↓	↓	↓	↑	
Salicylates (large doses)	↓	↑ (s)	↓*	↓	0*	Compete with T_4 for TBG binding

↑ = increased; ↓ = decreased; 0 = no effect; (s) = slight effect; (nd) = no data (Adapted from *The Medical Letter* 23:31, 1981).
TBG = thyroxine binding globulin.
* Effect deduced rather than based on reported clinical evidence.

a. Patients requiring thyroid replacement therapy have decreased serum thyroxine when barbiturates are given.
b. Free thyroxine index may increase slightly, but usually remains in the normal range.
c. T_4 assay by competitive protein binding is spuriously increased, but T_4-RIA is probably not affected. Free thyroxine measured by dialysis may be increased.
d. May occasionally decrease serum T_4 and increase resin T_3 uptake.
e. Slight decrease in euthyroid patients; but in long-standing hypothyroid patients, levodopa considerably decreases the elevated TSH.
f. In a patient on adequate doses for thyroid replacement.
g. Increased T_4, FTI, and T_3 tend to return to normal after several months of therapy with levothyroxine. After liothyronine, T_3 may be elevated 2 hours after a dose and depressed 24 hours after a dose.
h. Increased T_4 levels are reported in one study, but not in others.
i. With short-term propranolol in hyperthyroid patients.
j. In euthyroid subjects, the decreased serum T_3 returns to normal with continued propranolol therapy.

3. **Resin triiodothyronine uptake (RT_3U)**
   a. This test clarifies whether abnormal T_4 levels are due to a thyroid disorder or to abnormalities in the binding proteins, because it evaluates the binding capacity of TBG.
   b. If an abnormal amount (high or low) of thyroid hormone is present in the blood, the RT_3U results **change in the same direction** as the altered level—elevated in hyperthyroidism; decreased in hypothyroidism.
   c. However, if abnormalities in binding proteins underlie the abnormal levels of TT_4, TT_3, or both, the RT_3U results **change in the opposite direction**—decreasing as TBG increases; increasing as TBG decreases.
   d. Various drugs can cause spurious changes in the RT_3U (see Table 45-2).

4. **Serum thyrotropin (TSH)**
   a. This test is the most sensitive test for detecting the hypothyroid state because the hypothalamic–pituitary axis compensates very quickly for even slight decreases in circulating free hormone by releasing more TSH. The TSH levels may be elevated even before low circulating levels of TT_4 are detectable by diagnostic testing.
   b. Serum TSH is not a reliable test for hyperthyroidism (in which TSH is suppressed) because low levels and low-normal levels of TSH may be indistinguishable with the current technology.
   c. Effects of drugs on the serum TSH are shown in Table 45-2.

5. **Free thyroxine index (FTI)**
   a. This is not a separate test but rather an estimation of the free T_4 level through a mathematical interpretation of the relationship between RT_3U and serum T_4 levels:

$$\text{FTI} = \frac{TT_4 \times RT_3U}{\text{mean serum } RT_3U}$$

   b. FTI values are elevated in hyperthyroidism or when the TBG is low; decreased in hypothyroidism or when the TBG is elevated.
   c. Effects of drugs on the FTI are shown in Table 45-2.

II. HYPOTHYROIDISM

A. Definition. The inability of the thyroid gland to supply sufficient thyroid hormone results in varying degrees of hypothyroidism, from mild, clinically insignificant forms to the life-threatening extreme, myxedema coma.

B. Classification

1. **Primary hypothyroidism** is due to:
   a. Gland destruction or dysfunction caused by disease or medical therapies (e.g., radiation, surgical procedures)
   b. Failure of the gland to develop or congenital incompetence (i.e., **cretinism**)

2. **Secondary hypothroidism** is due to a pituitary disorder that inhibits TSH secretion. The thyroid gland is normal but lacks appropriate stimulation by TSH.

3. **Tertiary hypothyroidism** refers to a condition in which the pituitary–thyroid axis is intact, but the hypothalamus lacks the ability to secrete TRH to stimulate the pituitary.

C. Causes

1. **Hashimoto's thyroiditis,** which is a chronic lymphocytic thyroiditis that is considered to be an autoimmune disorder

2. **Treatment of hyperthyroidism**, such as radioactive iodine therapy, subtotal thyroidectomy, or administration of antithyroid agents

3. **Surgical excision**

4. **Goiter** (enlargement of the thyroid gland)
   a. **Endemic goiter** results from inadequate intake of dietary iodine. This is common in regions with iodine-depleted soil and in areas of endemic malnutrition.
   b. **Sporadic goiter** can follow ingestion of certain drugs or foods containing **progoitrin** (L-5-vinyl-2-thio-oxazolidone), which is inactive and converted by hydrolysis to goitrin. Goitrins inhibit oxidation of iodine to iodide and prevent iodide from binding to thyroglobulin, thereby decreasing thyroid hormone production. Progoitrin has been isolated in cabbage, kale, peanuts, brussels sprouts, mustard, rutabaga, kohlrabi, spinach, cauliflower, and horseradish. **Goitrogenic drugs** include propylthiouracil, iodides, phenylbutazone, cobalt, and lithium.

c. **Less common causes** include acute (usually traumatic) and subacute thyroiditis, nodules, nodular goiter, and thyroid cancer.

D. Signs and symptoms

1. Early clinical features tend to be somewhat vague: lethargy, fatigue, forgetfulness, sensitivity to cold, unexplained weight gain, and constipation.

2. Progressively, the characteristic features of myxedema emerge: dry, flaky, inelastic skin; coarse hair; slowed speech and thought; hoarseness; puffy face, hands, and feet; eyelid droop; hearing loss; menorrhagia; decreased libido; slow return of deep tendon reflexes (especially in the Achilles tendon). If untreated, myxedema coma will develop.

E. Laboratory findings (see Table 45-1)

F. Treatment goal is replacement therapy using oral agents (Table 45-3).

G. Therapeutic agents

1. **Desiccated thyroid**
   a. Once the agent of choice, desiccated thyroid has fallen out of favor since standardized synthetic levothyroxine preparations have become available.
   b. **Dessicated thyroid preparations** are not considered bioequivalent; they have evidenced varying amounts of active substances. Although they met established USP criteria for iodine content, variation in activity was noted. The content assay, while specific for iodine, was unable to specify the ratio of T_3 to T_4, and this ratio varies with animal source. Porcine gland preparations have a higher T_3 to T_4 ratio than those from ovine or bovine sources.

2. **Fixed ratio (liotrix) preparations.** In an effort to standardize the T_3: T_4 ratio, substances that mimic glandular content were developed. However, the T_3 component proved unnecessary (because T_4 is metabolized to T_3) and even disadvantageous (because of T_3-induced adverse effects; e.g., tremor, headache, palpitations, diarrhea).

3. **Levothyroxine**
   a. Predictable results and lack of T_3-induced side effects have made levothyroxine the agent of choice.
   b. The two major brands of levothyroxine preparations (Levothroid and Synthroid) have been compared for bioequivalency and were shown to be equivalent in patients with hypothyroidism.
   c. The usual adult maintenance dose is 100 to 200 μg/day.

H. Precautions and monitoring effects

1. Adult patients with a history of cardiac disease and elderly patients should begin therapy with lower doses (e.g., 25 μg/day of levothyroxine). After 2 to 4 weeks, the dose should be increased gradually to an individually adjusted maintenance dose (usually less than 100 μg daily).

2. Patients should be observed on initiation of therapy for possible **cardiac complications**, such as angina, palpitations, or arrhythmias.

3. **Serum thyroid levels** should be monitored, particularly T_4, TSH, and RT_3U levels, as well as the FTI. Tests should be carried out on a monthly basis until a maintenance dose is determined. Thereafter, one or two tests per year are adequate.

4. Levothyroxine administration, especially long-term therapy, can induce **thyrotoxicosis**; T_4 levels can rise even though the dosage remains unchanged.

I. Myxedema coma is a life-threatening complication with a high mortality rate.

1. It is most common in elderly patients with preexisting, although usually undiagnosed, hypothyroidism.

2. **Precipitating factors** include alcohol, sedative, or narcotic use; overuse of antithyroid agents; abrupt discontinuation of thyroid hormone therapy; infection; exposure to cold temperatures; and iatrogenic insult due to radiation therapy or thyroid surgery.

3. The patient usually declines from profound lethargy to coma, hypothermia, and a significant decrease in respiratory rate, potentially leading to respiratory failure as the crisis progresses. Hypometabolism produces a fluid and electrolyte imbalance that leads to fluid retention and hyponatremia. Cardiac effects include decreased heart rate and contractility, decreasing cardiac output.

Table 45-3. Thyroid Replacement Preparations

Preparation	Trade Names	Advantage	Disadvantage	Comments	Source
Desiccated thyroid	Thyroid USP Enseals Thyroid Strong Armour Thyroid Thyrar	Low cost	Some preparations have unpredictable results Inconsistent T_3:T_4 ratio T_3 increases adverse effects	Contains T_3 Some brands are standardized by iodine content*	Porcine, bovine, or ovine thyroid glands
Thyroglobulin	Proloid	Low cost	Unpredictable results T_3 increases adverse effects	Contains T_3	Porcine thyroid gland
Liothyronine	Cytomel	Predictable results Useful for myxedema crisis	Lacks T_4	Usually reserved for myxedema crisis	Synthetic
Liotrix	Euthroid Thyrolar	Standardized formulation	T_3 increases adverse effects Expensive	Fixed T_3:T_4 ratio of 1:4 Metabolism of T_4 to T_3 renders T_3 component unnecessary	Synthetic
Levothyroxine	Levothyroid Synthroid	Predictable results IV preparation available	Expensive	Agent of choice Does not contain T_3 All preparations are not interchangeable	Synthetic

T_3 = triiodothyronine.
T_4 = thyroxine.
*Iodine content, as well as T_3:T_4 ratio, varies with species.

4. **Treatment** consists of rapid restoration of T_3 and T_4 levels to normal.
   a. A loading dose of levothyroxine 400 to 500 μg is given as an intravenous bolus. Liothyronine, 25 μg, is then given orally every 6 hours.
   b. Treatment is continued until improvement is noted. Afterwards, liothyronine is discontinued and levothyroxine is changed to the oral preparation. A maintenance dose is then determined (see section II H).

III. HYPERTHYROIDISM

A. Definition. Hyperthyroidism is the overabundance of thyroid hormone. **Thyrotoxicosis** is the general term applied to overactivity of the thyroid gland.

B. Graves' disease (diffuse toxic goiter)

1. The most common form of hyperthyroidism, Graves' disease occurs primarily, but not exclusively, in young women.
2. The basis of this disease is an **autoimmune disorder** in which antibodies bind to and activate TSH receptors, resulting in the overproduction of thyroid hormone.
   a. These antibodies are termed long-acting thyroid stimulators (LATS) because their duration of action extends beyond that of TSH. As TSH is only mimicked, not overabundant, neither testing for TSH nor attempts to influence it are productive.
   b. Antibody titers are often elevated in patients with Graves' disease.
3. **Signs and symptoms** characteristic of Graves' disease include:
   a. Diffusely enlarged nontender goiter
   b. Nervousness, irritability, anxiety, insomnia
   c. Heat intolerance and profuse sweating
   d. Weight loss despite increased appetite
   e. Tremor, muscle weakness
   f. Palpitations and tachycardia
   g. Exophthalmos, stare, and lid lag (slow upper lid closing)
   h. Diarrhea
   i. Thrill or bruit over the thyroid
   j. Periorbital edema

C. Plummer's disease (toxic nodular goiter)

1. This **form of thyrotoxicosis** is less common than Graves' disease. Its underlying cause remains unknown, but its incidence is highest in patients over 50 years of age, and it usually arises from a long-standing nontoxic goiter.
2. The thyrotoxicosis is a result of one or more adenomatous nodules autonomously secreting excessive thyroid hormone, which suppresses the rest of the gland. Scanning confirms the diagnosis if it indicates that activity and iodine uptake are confined to the nodular mass unless TSH is introduced.
3. The **signs and symptoms** are essentially the same as for Graves' disease except that one or more nodular masses are found, rather than diffuse glandular enlargement, and ophthalmopathy is usually absent. Cardiac abnormalities (congestive heart failure, tachyarrhythmias) are commonly seen with Plummer's disease.

D. Less common forms of hyperthyroidism

1. **Jodbasedow phenomenon** is an overproduction of thyroid hormone following a sudden, large increase in iodine ingestion—through either a sudden reversal of an iodine-deficient diet or the introduction of iodide or iodine in contrast agents or drugs, such as the antiarrhythmic agent amiodarone.
2. **Factitious hyperthyroidism** occurs with abusive ingestion of thyroid replacement agents, usually in a misguided effort to lose weight. Diagnosis is aided by the absence of glandular swelling and of exophthalmos and the lack of autoimmune activity found in Graves' disease.

E. Laboratory findings (see Table 45-1).

F. Treatment goal. Symptomatic relief is provided until definitive treatment can be effected.

G. Therapeutic agents

1. **Beta adrenergic blocking agents—propranolol**

a. Propranolol helps to reduce some of the peripheral manifestations (e.g., tachycardia, sweating, severe tremor, and nervousness) of hyperthyroidism.
b. In addition to providing symptomatic relief, propranolol inhibits the peripheral conversion of T_4 to T_3.

2. Antithyroid agents—propylthiouracil (PTU) and methimazole

a. **Action.** These agents may help attain remission through direct interference with thyroid hormone synthesis. Both agents inhibit iodide oxidation and iodotyrosyl coupling. In addition, PTU (but not methimazole) diminishes peripheral deiodination of T_4 to T_3.

b. **Therapeutic uses** of these drugs include:
(1) **Definitive treatment** in which remission is achieved
(2) **Adjunctive therapy**, with radioactive iodine until the radiation takes effect
(3) **Preoperative preparation**, to establish and maintain a euthyroid state until definitive surgery can be performed

c. **Dosages**
(1) **Propylthiouracil**
(a) For adults, the initial dose is 300 to 450 mg/day in three divided doses (i.e., 100 to 150 mg every 8 hours). Adult patients with severe disease may require as much as 600 to 1200 mg/day initially.
(b) The initial dose is continued for about 2 months; then a maintenance dose of 100 to 150 mg/day is given, as a single dose or divided into two doses.
(c) Maintenance therapy is continued for approximately 1 year, then gradually discontinued over 1 to 2 months while the patient is monitored for signs of recurrent hyperthyroidism. The patient may remain in remission for several years. A recurrent episode of hyperthyroidism is most likely to occur within 3 to 6 months of drug discontinuation.
(d) If hyperthyroidism recurs after drug therapy is stopped, the agent should be restarted and alternative therapy should be considered (e.g., thyroid gland ablation or removal).
(2) **Methimazole**
(a) The initial dose range is 5 to 60 mg/day, in three divided doses, depending on disease severity. After 2 months of therapy, a maintenance dose of 5 to 30 mg/day is initiated.
(b) Maintenance therapy is continued for approximately 1 year, at which time the drug is gradually discontinued, usually over 1 to 2 months.

d. **Precautions and monitoring effects**
(1) Serum thyroid levels and the FTI should be monitored for a return to normal.
(2) Goiter size should decrease with reduced hormone output.
(3) The incidence of **adverse effects** is less than 1% with PTU and less than 3% with methimazole. The adverse effects are similar for the two agents.
(a) The most bothersome are dermatologic reactions (e.g., rash, urticaria, pruritus, hair loss, skin pigmentation). Others include headache, drowsiness, paresthesia, nausea, vomiting, vertigo, neuritis, loss of taste, arthralgia, and myalgia.
(b) Severe adverse effects—agranulocytosis, granulocytopenia, thrombocytopenia, drug fever, hepatitis, and hypoprothrombinemia—occur less frequently. Patients receiving methimazole who are over 40 years old and are receiving doses above 40 mg/day are at increased risk of developing agranulocytosis. Patients receiving PTU who are over 40 years old are at increased risk of developing agranulocytosis, but no dose association has been established.

3. Radioactive iodine (RAI)

a. **Action.** The thyroid gland picks up the radioactive element ^{131}I as it would regular iodine. The radioactivity subsequently destroys some of the cells that would otherwise concentrate iodine and produce T_4, thus decreasing thyroid hormone production.

b. **Advantages**
(1) **High cure rate**—almost 100% for patients with Graves' disease and only slightly less for patients with Plummer's disease
(2) **Avoids surgical risks**—such as adverse reaction to anesthetics, hypoparathyroidism, nerve palsy, bleeding, and hoarseness
(3) **Less expensive**—avoids costs of hospitalization

c. **Disadvantages**
(1) Risk of delayed **hypothyroidism**
(2) Slight, though undocumented, risk of **genetic damage**
(3) **Multiple doses**, which may be required, delaying therapeutic efficacy for a long period (many months or a year)

d. **Dosage.** A dose of 80 to 100 microcuries of ^{131}I per estimated gram of thyroid gland is recommended. Some protocols use lower dosages, but these may be less effective, requiring retreatment. When the dose is higher, there is a potential risk that hypothyroidism will develop.

e. Precautions and monitoring effects

(1) Radioiodine therapy is generally reserved for patients past the childbearing years because effects on future offspring are not known.

(2) Response to ^{131}I is hard to gauge, and patients must be monitored early for recurrence of hyperthyroidism, and later for hypothyroidism, which may develop even 20 years or more after therapy.

4. Subtotal thyroidectomy. Partial removal of the thyroid gland may be indicated if drug therapy fails or radioactive iodine is undesirable. This is a difficult procedure, but the success rate is high and the cure rapid. Risks include those mentioned in [section III G 3 b (2)], precipitating thyroid storm, and permanent postoperative hypothyroidism. The risk of inducing thyroid storm can be minimized by obtaining a euthyroid state through use of antithyroid agents or propranolol (see section III G 1).

H. Complications

1. Hypothyroidism may occur iatrogenically or, it has been proposed, as a natural sequel to Graves' disease.

2. Thyroid storm (thyrotoxic crisis) is a sudden exacerbation of hyperthyroidism caused by rapid release (leakage) of thyroid hormone. It is invariably fatal if not treated rapidly. In this crisis, unchecked hypermetabolism leads ultimately to dehydration, shock, and death.

a. Precipitating factors include thyroid trauma or surgery, radioiodine therapy, infection, and sudden discontinuation of antithyroid therapy.

b. It is **characterized** by a TT_4 level of 25 to 30 μg/dl, rapidly rising fever, tachycardia disproportionate to the fever, and unexplained, pronounced restlessness and tremor.

c. Treatment

(1) PTU, in doses of 150 to 250 mg orally every 6 hours, is the preferred agent, since PTU blocks peripheral deiodination of T_4 to T_3, while methimazole does not. However, if necessary, methimazole, 15 mg orally every 6 hours, can be used instead.

(2) Propranolol, in doses of 20 to 200 mg orally every 6 hours or 1 to 3 mg intravenously every 4 to 6 hours, should be administered unless contraindicated (e.g., because the patient has congestive heart failure).

(3) Potassium iodide, in doses of 50 to 100 mg every 12 hours, is given (after PTU) to minimize intrathyroidal iodine uptake.

(4) Other supportive therapy includes rehydration, cooling, antibiotics, rest, and sedation.

STUDY QUESTIONS

Directions: Each question below contains five suggested answers. Choose the **one best** response to each question.

1. What is the correct formula to use for calculating the free thyroxine index?

A. $T_4 \times RT_3U$/mean serum RT_3U
B. $T_4 \times T_3$/mean serum RT_3U
C. $T_3 \times RT_3U$/mean serum RT_3U
D. $T_4 \times RT_3U \times$ mean serum RT_3U
E. $T_3 \times RT_3U \times$ mean serum RT_3U

2. What precursor is required for thyroxine biosynthesis?

A. Triiodothyronine
B. Threonine
C. Tyrosine
D. Thyrotropin
E. Iodine

3. All of the following conditions are causes of hyperthyroidism EXCEPT

A. Graves' disease
B. Hashimoto's thyroiditis
C. toxic multinodular goiter
D. triiodothyronine toxicosis
E. Plummer's disease

4. Which of the following preparations is used to attain remission of thyrotoxicosis?

A. Propranolol
B. Liotrix
C. Levothyroxine
D. Propylthiouracil
E. Desiccated thyroid

5. The thyroid gland normally secretes which of the following substances into the serum?

A. Thyrotropin-releasing hormone
B. Thyrotropin
C. Diiodothyronine
D. Thyroglobulin
E. Thyroxine

6. The most sensitive test for the diagnosis of hypothyroidism is a serum

A. triiodothyronine resin uptake
B. total thyroxine
C. total triiodothyronine
D. thyrotropin
E. iodine

7. All of the following conditions are causes of hypothyroidism EXCEPT

A. thyroidectomy
B. surgical excision
C. Hashimoto's thyroiditis
D. goitrin-induced iodine deficiency
E. Graves' disease

8. All of the following are common tests to monitor patients receiving replacement therapy for hypothyroidism EXCEPT

A. thyrotropin stimulation test
B. serum thyrotropin
C. free thyroxine index
D. triiodothyronine resin uptake
E. total thyroxine

9. Which of the following pairs of preparations has been most studied for bioequivalency?

A. Euthroid — Thyrolar
B. Thyroglobulin — Proloid
C. Levothroid — Synthroid
D. Cytomel — Synthroid
E. Desiccated thyroid — Armour Thyroid

10. The inhibition of pituitary thyrotropin secretion is controlled by which of the following?

A. Free thyroxine
B. Thyroid-releasing hormone
C. Free thyroxine index
D. Reverse triiodothyronine
E. Total thyroxine

ANSWERS AND EXPLANATIONS

1. The answer is A. (*I G 5*) The free thyroxine index (FTI) is a mathematical interpretation of the relationship between the resin triiodothyronine uptake (RT_3U) and serum thyroxine (T_4) levels, compared to the mean population value for RT_3U. The FTI is calculated using reported values for total thyroxine (TT_4) and RT_3U. The normal FTI value in euthyroid patients is 5.5 to 12.

2. The answer is C. (*I B*) Biosynthesis of thyroid hormones begins with iodide binding to tyrosine, which forms monoiodotyrosine (MIT). Monoiodotyrosine binds another iodide atom to form diiodotyrosine (DIT). Once MIT and DIT are formed, a coupling reaction occurs, which produces triiodothyronine (T_3), thyroxine (T_4), reverse triiodothyronine (rT_3), and other byproducts.

3. The answer is B. (*II C 1; III B–D*) Hashimoto's thyroiditis (chronic lymphocytic thyroiditis) is a cause of hypothyroidism. The incidence of Hashimoto's thyroiditis is 1% to 2%, and it increases with age. It is more common in females than in males and in whites than in blacks. There may be a familial tendency. Patients with Hashimoto's thyroiditis have elevated titers of antibodies to thyroglobulin: A titer of greater than 1:32 is seen in over 85% of patients. Two variants of Hashimoto's thyroiditis have been described: gland fibrosis and idiopathic thyroid atrophy, which is most likely an extension of Hashimoto's thyroiditis.

4. The answer is D. (*III G 2*) In hyperthyroid patients, remission of thyrotoxicosis is achieved with propylthiouracil (PTU) by two mechanisms: (1) interference of iodination of the tyrosyl residues, ultimately reducing production of thyroxine; (2) inhibition of peripheral conversion of thyroxine to triiodothyronine. Propranolol is commonly used as an adjunct to PTU for symptomatic management of hyperthyroidism.

5. The answer is E. (*I A 1*) The major compounds secreted by the thyroid gland, after its stimulation by thyrotropin, are triiodothyronine (T_3) and thyroxine (T_4). Once released from the thyroid, T_3 and T_4 are transported by plasma proteins, namely thyroxine-binding globulin, thyroxine-binding prealbumin, and albumin.

6. The answer is D. (*I G 4 a*) Thyrotropin is normally secreted from the anterior pituitary gland and stimulates the thyroid gland to secrete thyroxine (T_3) and triiodothyronine (T_4). The serum T_4 concentration feeds back to the pituitary and controls TSH secretion. Any defect in the feedback mechanism causes TSH fluctuations.

7. The answer is E. (*II C; III B 1*) Graves' disease (diffuse toxic goiter) is the most common form of hyperthyroidism. It occurs most often in women in the third and fourth decades of life. There is a genetic and familial predisposition. The etiology is linked to an autoimmune reaction between immunoglobulin G (IgG) and the thyroid.

8. The answer is A. (*II H 3*) The thyrotropin (TSH) stimulation test measures thyroid tissue response to exogenous TSH. It is not commonly used to monitor thyroid replacement therapy. It may be useful in the initial diagnosis of hypothyroidism.

9. The answer is C. (*II G 3 b*) Many brands of levothyroxine are currently available. Both generic and trade-name preparations have been studied, with an emphasis on Levothroid and Synthroid. The importance of bioequivalency becomes apparent when patients have received different brands of levothyroxine and have exhibited changes in therapeutic response to equivalent replacement doses.

10. The answer is A. (*I A 4*) An increase in the blood level of thyroid hormone [circulating free thyroxine (T_4) and free triiodothyronine (T_3)] signals the pituitary to stop releasing thyroid-stimulating hormone (thyrotropin; TSH). The free fraction of thyroxine is available to bind at the pituitary receptors.

46
Renal Failure

Susan A. Krikorian

I. ACUTE RENAL FAILURE

A. Definition. Acute renal failure (ARF) is the sudden, potentially reversible interruption of kidney function, resulting in retention of nitrogenous waste products in body fluids.

B. Classification and etiology. ARF is classified according to its cause.

1. **Prerenal ARF** stems from impaired renal perfusion, which may result from:
   a. **Reduced arterial blood volume** (e.g., from hemorrhage or from vomiting, diarrhea, or other gastrointestinal fluid loss)
   b. **Urinary losses** from excessive diuresis
   c. **Decreased cardiac output** (e.g., from congestive heart failure or pericardial tamponade)
   d. **Renal vascular obstruction** (e.g., from renal artery stenosis)

2. **Intrarenal ARF** (also called **intrinsic** or **parenchymal ARF**) reflects structural kidney damage brought on by any of the following conditions:
   a. **Acute tubular necrosis (ATN)**, the leading cause of ARF. ATN may:
      (1) **Stem from exposure to nephrotoxic agents** (e.g., aminoglycosides, anesthetics, pesticides, organic solvents, heavy metals, radiopaque contrast materials)
      (2) **Stem from ischemic injury** (e.g., from surgery, circulatory collapse, severe hypotension)
      (3) **Be pigment-associated** (e.g., hemolysis, **myoglobinuria**)
   b. **Acute glomerulonephritis**
   c. **Tubular obstruction**, as from hemolytic reactions or uric acid crystals
   d. **Acute inflammation** (e.g., acute tubulointerstitial nephritis, papillary necrosis)
   e. **Renal vasculitis**
   f. **Radiation nephritis**

3. **Postrenal ARF** results from obstruction of the urinary flow anywhere along the urinary tract. Causes include:
   a. **Ureteral obstruction**, as from calculi, uric acid crystals, or thrombi
   b. **Tubular obstruction**, as from uric acid or oxalate crystal accumulation
   c. **Bladder obstruction**, as from calculi, thrombi, tumors, or infection
   d. **Urethral obstruction**, as from strictures, tumors, or prostatic hypertrophy
   e. **Extrinsic obstruction**, as from hematoma, inflammatory bowel disease, or accidental surgical ligation

C. Pathophysiology. ARF progresses in three phases.

1. **Oliguric phase**
   a. Urine output sometimes drops markedly—to 500 ml/day or less (**oliguria**). In some cases, urine output falls below 100 ml/day (**anuria**). However, recently it has been shown that up to 59% of patients are nonoliguric.
   b. Nitrogenous waste products accumulate in the blood.
      (1) **Azotemia** reflects urea accumulation.
      (2) Serum creatinine, sulfate, phosphate, and organic acid levels also climb rapidly.
   c. The serum sodium concentration falls below normal, from intracellular fluid shifting and dilution.
   d. Unless dietary potassium is restricted or body potassium is removed, **hyperkalemia** can occur. Without treatment, this condition may lead to neuromuscular depression and paralysis, impaired cardiac conduction, arrhythmias, respiratory muscle paralysis, cardiac arrest, and ultimately death.

2. **Diuretic phase**
   a. This phase begins when urine output rises above 500 ml/day (typically, after a few days to 6 weeks of oliguria).
   b. Usually, urine output rises in increments of several milliliters to 300 to 500 ml/day, then increases more rapidly.
   c. Azotemia and associated laboratory findings may persist until urine output reaches 1000 to 2000 ml/day.
   d. Diuresis may reflect removal of excess extracellular fluid that accumulated during the oliguric phase. The diuresis is caused by a gradual recovery of renal function or may be due to a tubular concentrating defect. Osmotic diuresis may occur as well.
   e. The diuretic phase carries a high risk of fluid and electrolyte abnormalities, gastrointestinal bleeding, infection, and respiratory failure.

3. **Recovery phase**. During this period, renal function gradually returns to normal. However, residual impairment may decrease renal reserve.

D. Clinical evaluation

1. **Physical findings**. Initially, ARF causes azotemia and, in most cases, oliguria. Later, electrolyte abnormalities and other severe systemic effects occur.
   a. **Urine output** typically is low—from 20 to 500 ml/day.
   b. Signs and symptoms of **hyperkalemia** (a result of reduced potassium excretion by impaired kidneys) include:
      (1) Neuromuscular depression (paresthesias, muscle weakness, and paralysis)
      (2) Diarrhea, abdominal distention
      (3) Irritability and anxiety
      (4) Slow or irregular pulse
      (5) Electrocardiographic changes, with potential cardiac arrest
   c. **Uremia**, caused by excessive nitrogenous waste retention, may lead to nausea, vomiting, diarrhea, edema, confusion, fatigue, convulsions, neuromuscular irritability, and coma.
   d. **Metabolic acidosis**, most common when ARF is complicated by infection or reduced cardiac output, is evidenced by:
      (1) Deterioration of mental status (mental obtudation, coma, lethargy)
      (2) Depressed cardiac contractility and decreased vascular resistance, leading to hypotension, pulmonary edema, and ventricular fibrillation.
      (3) Nausea and vomiting
      (4) Muscle weakness and irritability
      (5) Respiratory abnormalities (e.g., hyperventilation, Kussmaul's respirations)
   e. **Hyperphosphatemia** may arise from decreased phosphate excretion (the kidneys are the main regulators of serum phosphate).
      (1) The principal effect of serum phosphate elevation is the formation of insoluble calcium phosphate complexes.
      (2) The signs and symptoms relate to resultant hypocalcemia and metastatic soft tissue calcification.
      (3) Manifestations of hyperphosphatemia include the following:
         (a) Neuromuscular irritability, tetany
         (b) Hypotension
         (c) Soft-tissue calcification (reflecting hypocalcemia, which typically accompanies hyperphosphatemia)
   f. **Hypocalcemia** resulting from hyperphosphatemia, may cause:
      (1) Neuromuscular abnormalities (e.g., paresthesias, muscle cramps and spasms; tetany and seizures with severe hypocalcemia)
      (2) Mental status changes (e.g., confusion; changes in mood, intellect, and memory)
      (3) Hyperactive deep tendon reflexes, Trousseau's and Chvostek's signs
      (4) Abdominal cramps
      (5) Stridor, dyspnea
      (6) Hypotension
   g. **Hyponatremia** results from dilution and intracellular fluid shifts during the diuretic phase of ARF. Physical findings include:
      (1) Lethargy, weakness, seizures, cognitive impairment, possible reduction in level of consciousness
      (2) Gait disturbances, muscle twitching
   h. **Intravascular volume depletion**, suggesting **prerenal failure**, may cause:
      (1) Flat jugular venous pulses (when the patient lies supine)
      (2) Orthostatic changes in blood pressure and pulse
      (3) Poor skin turgor, dry mucous membranes

i. Other findings that suggest **prerenal failure** include:
  (1) An abdominal bruit, possibly indicating renal artery stenosis
  (2) Pulsus paradoxus, suggesting pericardial tamponade
  (3) Increased jugular venous pressure, pulmonary rales, and a third heart sound (signaling congestive heart failure)
j. Postrenal failure caused by obstructed urinary flow may manifest itself in:
  (1) A suprapubic or flank mass
  (2) Bladder distention
  (3) Costovertebral angle tenderness
  (4) Prostate enlargement

2. Diagnostic test results
a. Urinalysis, crucial in the evaluation of kidney function, includes an examination of sediment; identification of proteins, glucose, ketones, blood, and nitrites; and measurement of urinary pH and urine specific gravity (concentration) or osmolality (dilution).
  (1) Urinary sediment examination
    (a) With prerenal or postrenal ARF, hyaline casts, red blood cells, and white blood cells may appear.
    (b) With intrarenal ARF, urinalysis usually shows tubular cells, tubular epithelial cell casts, and many brown pigmented granular casts.
    (c) Waxy casts reflect advanced renal failure.
  (2) The presence of **blood** (hematuria) or **proteins** (proteinuria) indicates renal dysfunction.
  (3) Urine specific gravity ranges from 1.010 to 1.016 in ARF.
  (4) Urine osmolality typically rises in prerenal ARF, decreases in ATN (a cause of intrarenal ARF).
b. Measurement of **urine sodium** and **creatinine** levels can help classify ARF.
  (1) In prerenal ARF, the urine creatinine level increases and the urine sodium level decreases.
  (2) In intrarenal ARF resulting from ATN, the urine creatinine level drops and the urine sodium level rises.
c. The **creatinine clearance test**, an index of the **glomerular filtration rate (GFR)**, allows estimation of the number of functioning nephrons; decreased creatinine clearance indicates renal dysfunction.
d. Blood studies provide an index of renal excretory function and body chemistry status. Findings typical of ARF include:
  (1) Increased blood urea nitrogen (BUN) level
  (2) Increased serum creatinine level
  (3) Possible increase in hemoglobin and hematocrit values
  (4) Abnormal serum electrolyte values
    (a) Serum potassium level above 5 mEq/L, reflecting hyperkalemia
    (b) Serum phosphate level above 2.6 mEq/L (4.8 mg/dl), indicating hyperphosphatemia
    (c) Serum calcium level below 4 mEq/L (8.5 mg/dl), reflecting hypocalcemia. However, the serum calcium level must be correlated with the serum albumin level. Each rise or fall of 1 g/dl of serum albumin beyond its normal range is responsible for an increase or decrease in serum calcium of approximately 0.8 mg/dl. Consequently, a below-normal serum albumin level may result in a deceptively low calcium level.
    (d) Serum sodium level below 135 mEq/L, reflecting hyponatremia
  (5) Abnormal arterial blood gas values [pH below 7.35, bicarbonate concentration (HCO_3^-) below 22], reflecting metabolic acidosis
e. The **renal failure index** (the ratio of the urine sodium concentration to the urine-to-serum creatinine ratio) helps determine the etiology of ARF. Typically, this index is less than 1 in prerenal ARF or acute glomerulonephritis (a cause of intrarenal ARF); it is greater than 2 in postrenal ARF and in other intrarenal causes of ARF.
f. Electrocardiography (ECG) may show evidence of hyperkalemia—tall, peaked T waves; widening QRS complexes; prolonged P-R interval, then decreased amplitude and disappearance of P waves; and, ultimately, ventricular fibrillation and cardiac arrest.
g. Radiographic findings
  (1) Ultrasound may detect upper urinary tract obstruction.
  (2) Kidney-ureter-bladder radiography may reveal:
    (a) Urinary tract calculi
    (b) Enlarged kidneys (suggesting ATN)
    (c) Asymmetrical kidneys, suggesting unilateral renal artery disease, ureteral obstruction, or chronic pyelonephritis

(3) **Radionuclide scans** may reveal:
(a) Bilateral differences in renal perfusion, suggesting serious renal disease
(b) Bilateral differences in dye excretion, suggesting parenchymal disease or obstruction as the cause of ARF
(c) Diffuse, slow, dense radionuclide uptake, suggesting ATN
(d) Patchy or absent radionuclide uptake, possibly indicating severe, acute glomerulonephritis

(4) **Computed tomography scans** may provide better visualization of an obstruction.

h. **Renal biopsy** may be performed in selected patients when other test results are inconclusive.

E. Treatment objectives

1. **Correct any reversible causes of ARF**, thus preventing or minimizing further renal damage or complications
   a. Nephrotoxic drugs should be discontinued; gastric lavage may be performed or an antidote administered to treat ingestion of other nephrotoxic compounds.
   b. Infection should be treated.
   c. Obstructions should be removed.

2. **Correct and maintain proper fluid and electrolyte balance**, thereby reducing the renal work load and permitting tissue recovery

3. **Treat body chemistry alterations** (e.g., hyperkalemia, metabolic acidosis)

4. **Improve urine output**

5. **Treat systemic manifestations of ARF**

F. Therapy

1. **Conservative management** alone may suffice in uncomplicated ARF.
   a. **Fluid management**
      (1) Fluid intake should be restricted to match fluid losses—both sensible losses (via urine, stool, and tube drainage) and insensible losses (via the skin and respiratory tract).
      (2) Volume overload must be avoided or corrected to prevent or minimize the risk of hypertension and congestive heart failure.
      (3) The patient should be weighed daily to help determine fluid volume status.
   b. **Dietary measures**
      (1) Because catabolism usually accompanies renal failure, the patient should receive a high-calorie, low-protein diet. Such a diet helps to:
         (a) Reduce the renal work load by decreasing the production of end products of protein metabolism that the kidneys cannot excrete
         (b) Prevent ketoacidosis
         (c) Alleviate manifestations of uremia (e.g., nausea, vomiting, confusion, fatigue)
      (2) If edema or hypertension is present, sodium intake should be restricted.
      (3) In many cases, potassium intake must be limited.

2. **Management of body chemistry alterations**
   a. **Treatment of hyperkalemia**
      (1) **Dialysis** may be used to treat acute, life-threatening hyperkalemia. See section II F 6 for a discussion of this procedure.
      (2) **Calcium gluconate**
         (a) **Mechanism of action and therapeutic effects**. Calcium gluconate replaces and maintains body calcium, thereby counteracting the cardiotoxicity caused by acute hyperkalemia.
         (b) **Onset of action** is a few minutes.
         (c) **Administration and dosage**. When used to reverse hyperkalemia-induced cardiotoxicity, calcium gluconate is given intravenously, as 10 to 20 ml of a 10% solution (0.45 mEq Ca^{2+}/ml). (Doses of up to 50 ml of a 10% solution are safe when given slowly.) The initial dose may be followed by another 50 ml of a 10% solution placed in a larger fluid volume (e.g., dextrose injection) and administered more slowly.
         (d) **Precautions and monitoring effects**
            (i) Calcium gluconate is contraindicated in patients with ventricular fibrillation or renal calculi.
            (ii) The infusion rate should not exceed 0.5 ml/min. Patients should remain recumbent for about 15 minutes after infusion.
            (iii) The ECG should be monitored during calcium gluconate therapy.

(iv) Calcium gluconate should not be mixed with solutions containing sodium bicarbonate because this can lead to precipitation.
(v) Adverse effects include tingling sensations and renal calculus formation.

(e) **Significant interaction**. Calcium gluconate may cause increased digitalis toxicity when administered concurrently with **digitalis preparations**.

(3) Sodium bicarbonate. This drug may be given as an emergency measure for severe hyperkalemia or metabolic acidosis.

(a) **Mechanism of action and therapeutic effects**. Sodium bicarbonate restores bicarbonate that the renal tubules cannot reabsorb from the glomerular filtrate, thereby increasing arterial pH. This results in the shifting of potassium into cells and a reduction in the serum potassium concentration.

(b) **Onset of action** is 15 to 30 minutes.

(c) **Administration and dosage**

(i) Sodium bicarbonate is given intravenously.
(ii) The dosage is calculated as follows:

$$[50\% \text{ of body weight (in kg)}] \times (\text{desired arterial } HCO_3^- - \text{actual } HCO_3^-)$$

(iii) Usually, the dose is infused over 4 to 8 hours or less.

(d) **Precautions and monitoring effects**

(i) To avoid sodium and fluid overload, this drug must be given cautiously. Half of the patient's bicarbonate deficit is replaced over the first 12 hours of therapy.
(ii) Sodium bicarbonate solution may precipitate calcium salts and should not be mixed in the same infusion fluid.
(iii) Arterial blood gas values and serum electrolyte levels should be monitored closely during sodium bicarbonate therapy.

(4) Regular insulin with 50% dextrose

(a) **Mechanism of action and therapeutic effect**. This drug combination deposits potassium with glycogen into the liver, thereby reducing the serum potassium concentration.

(b) **Onset of action** is 15 to 30 minutes.

(c) **Administration and dosage**. Regular insulin with 50% dextrose is administered intravenously as 100 ml of 50% dextrose containing 10 U of regular insulin. It is given over 30 minutes.

(d) **Precautions and monitoring effects**

(i) The serum glucose level should be monitored during therapy.
(ii) The patient should be assessed closely for signs and symptoms of fluid overload.

(5) Sodium polystyrene sulfonate (SPS)

(a) **Mechanism of action**. SPS is a potassium-removing resin that exchanges sodium ions for potassium ions in the intestine (1 g of SPS is exchanged for every 0.5 to 1 mEq/L of potassium). The resin is then distributed throughout the intestines and excreted in the feces.

(b) **Therapeutic effect**. Administered as an adjunctive treatment for hyperkalemia, SPS reduces potassium levels in the serum and other body fluids.

(c) **Onset of action** when SPS is administered orally is 2 hours; it is 1 hour when administered via retention enema.

(d) **Administration and dosage**

(i) SPS usually is given orally (or, rarely, through a nasogastric tube). The typical dosage is 15 to 30 g in a suspension of 70% sorbitol, given every 4 to 6 hours.
(ii) When oral or nasogastric administration is not possible (as when nausea, vomiting, or paralytic ileus is present), SPS may be given by **retention enema**. The usual dosage is 30 to 50 g in 100 ml of sorbitol as a warm emulsion, inserted deep into the sigmoid colon every 6 hours. Insertion may be done via a rubber tube that is taped in place or via a Foley catheter with a balloon inflated distal to the anal sphincter.

(e) **Precautions and monitoring effects**

(i) The patient's electrolyte levels should be monitored closely during SPS therapy.
(ii) SPS therapy usually continues until the serum potassium level drops to 4 to 5 mEq/L.
(iii) The patient should be assessed regularly for signs of potassium depletion (e.g., irritability, confusion, cardiac arrhythmias, ECG changes, muscle weakness).
(iv) Sodium overload may occur during SPS therapy.
(v) For oral administration, the resin should be mixed only with water or sorbitol, never with orange juice (which has a high potassium content); for rectal administration, it should be mixed only with water and sorbitol, never with mineral oil.

(vi) Adverse effects of SPS include constipation, fecal impaction (with rectal administration), nausea, vomiting, and diarrhea.

(vii) SPS should not be used as the sole agent in the treatment of severe hyperkalemia; other agents should be used in conjunction with this drug.

(f) **Significant interaction. Magnesium hydroxide** and other nonabsorbable cation-donating laxatives and antacids may decrease the effectiveness of potassium exchange by SPS and may cause systemic alkalosis.

b. **Treatment of metabolic acidosis. Sodium bicarbonate** may be given if the arterial pH is below 7.35. See section I F 2 a (3) for a discussion of this drug.

c. **Treatment of hyperphosphatemia**

(1) **Dialysis** may be used to treat acute, life-threatening hyperphosphatemia accompanied by acute hypocalcemia (see section II F 6).

(2) **Aluminum hydroxide** (an aluminum-containing antacid)

(a) **Mechanism of action and therapeutic effect**. Aluminum hydroxide binds excess phosphate in the intestine, thereby reducing the serum phosphate concentration.

(b) **Onset of action** is 6 to 12 hours.

(c) **Administration and dosage**. Aluminum hydroxide is administered orally, in tablet or suspension form. For the treatment of hyperphosphatemia, the dosage ranges from 0.5 to 2 g (tablets) or from 15 to 30 ml (suspension), given three or four times daily with meals.

(d) **Precautions and monitoring effects**

(i) Aluminum hydroxide may cause constipation and anorexia.

(ii) Serum phosphate levels should be monitored because the drug can cause phosphate depletion.

(iii) Aluminum hydroxide can cause calcium resorption and bone demineralization.

(e) Calcium carbonate may be given instead of aluminum hydroxide to treat hyperphosphatemia.

d. **Treatment of hypocalcemia**. Immediate treatment is necessary if the patient has severe hypocalcemia, as evidenced by tetany.

(1) **Calcium gluconate**. [See section I F 2 a (2) for a discussion of this drug in the treatment of hyperkalemia.]

(a) **Mechanism of action and therapeutic effect**. This drug replaces and maintains body calcium, raising the serum calcium level immediately.

(b) **Administration and dosage**. When used to reverse hypocalcemia, calcium gluconate is administered intravenously in a dosage of 1 to 2 g over a period of 10 minutes, followed by a slow infusion (over 6 to 8 hours) of an additional 1 g.

(c) **Precautions and monitoring effects** and **significant interaction**. See section I F 2 a (2) (c) and (d).

(2) **Oral calcium salts**. Calcium carbonate, chlorate, gluconate, lactate, or levulinate may be given by mouth when oral intake is permitted or if the patient has relatively mild hypocalcemia symptoms. The usual adult dose is 41 to 62 g/day, given in three or four divided doses.

e. **Treatment of hyponatremia**

(1) Moderate or asymptomatic hyponatremia may warrant only fluid restriction.

(2) **Sodium chloride**. This drug may be given for severe or symptomatic hyponatremia (a serum sodium level below 120 mEq/L).

(a) **Mechanism of action and therapeutic effect**. Sodium chloride replaces and maintains sodium and chloride concentrations, thereby increasing extracellular tonicity.

(b) **Administration and dosage**

(i) A 3% or 5% solution of sodium chloride is given by slow intravenous (IV) infusion. The amount of solution needed is calculated from the following equation:

(Normal serum sodium level − actual serum sodium level) × total body water

(ii) Typically, 400 ml are given.

(c) **Precautions and monitoring effects**

(i) This treatment is controversial and must be used with extreme caution.

(ii) Sodium chloride must be given very slowly to avoid circulatory overload, pulmonary edema, or central pontine myelinolysis.

(iii) Serum electrolyte levels must be monitored frequently during therapy.

(iv) Excessive infusion may cause hypernatremia and other serious electrolyte abnormalities and may worsen existing acidosis.

3. **Management of systemic manifestations**

a. **Treatment of fluid overload and edema**. As water and sodium accumulate in extracellular fluid during ARF, fluid overload and edema may occur. **Diuretics** and **dopamine** may be given to reduce fluid volume excess and edema and to convert oliguric ARF to nonoliguric ARF. Treatment should be initiated as soon as possible after oliguria begins. Mannitol (an osmotic diuretic) or a loop diuretic may be used; thiazide diuretics are avoided in renal failure because they are ineffective when creatinine clearance is less than 25 ml/min and may worsen the patient's clinical status.

(1) **Step 1. Loop (high-ceiling) diuretics**. These agents include **bumetanide**, **furosemide**, and **ethacrynic acid**. Loop diuretics are more potent and faster-acting than thiazide diuretics.

(a) **Mechanism of action and therapeutic effects**. Loop diuretics inhibit sodium and chloride reabsorption at the loop of Henle, promoting water excretion and thus helping to relieve oliguria and edema.

(b) **Onset of action** for an oral dose is 1 hour; it is several minutes for an IV dose. Duration of action for an oral dose is 6 to 8 hours; it is 2 to 3 hours for an IV dose.

(c) **Administration and dosage**

(i) **Furosemide**, the most commonly used loop diuretic, usually is administered intravenously in patients with ARF to hasten the therapeutic effect. The dose, based on desired urine output, is titrated to the patient's needs; the usual initial dose is 1 to 1.5 mg/kg. If the first dose does not produce a urine output of 10 to 15 ml within 20 to 30 minutes, a double dose is administered; if the desired response still does not occur, a triple dose is administered 20 to 30 minutes after this.

(ii) **Bumetanide** may be given to patients who are unresponsive or allergic to furosemide. The usual dose, administered intravenously or intramuscularly in the treatment of ARF, is 0.5 to 1 mg/day (however, some patients may require up to 20 mg/day). A second or third dose may be given at intervals of 2 to 3 hours. When bumetanide is given orally, the dose is 0.5 to 2 mg/day, repeated up to two times, if necessary, at intervals of 2 to 3 hours.

(iii) **Ethacrynic acid** is less commonly used to treat ARF because ototoxicity (sometimes irreversible) is associated with its use. It may be given intravenously (slowly over several minutes) in a dose of 50 to 100 mg. The usual oral dose is 50 to 200 mg/day; some patients may require up to 200 mg twice daily.

(d) **Precautions and monitoring effects**

(i) Loop diuretics must be used cautiously because they may cause orthostatic hypotension, fluid and electrolyte abnormalities (e.g., volume depletion and dehydration, hypocalcemia, hypokalemia, hypochloremia, hyponatremia, hypomagnesemia), and ototoxicity (transient deafness, especially with rapid IV injection). Furosemide and ethacrynic acid may cause agranulocytosis.

(ii) Gastrointestinal reactions include abdominal pain and discomfort, diarrhea
(iii) (with furosemide and ethacrynic acid), and nausea (with bumetanide).
Blood pressure and pulse rate should be assessed during diuretic therapy.
(iv) Serum electrolyte levels should be monitored frequently and the patient as-
(v) sessed regularly for signs and symptoms of electrolyte abnormalities.
Blood glucose levels should be monitored in diabetic patients receiving loop di-
(vi) uretics because these agents may cause hyperglycemia and impaired glucose tolerance.
Patients who are allergic to sulfonamides may be hypersensitive to bumetanide
(vii) and furosemide.

(e) **Significant interactions**

(i) **Aminoglycoside antibiotics** may potentiate ototoxicity when administered with any loop diuretic.

(ii) **Indomethacin** may hamper the diuretic response to furosemide and bumetanide; **probenecid** may hamper the diuretic response to bumetanide.

(iii) Ethacrynic acid may potentiate the anticoagulant effects of **warfarin**.

(iv) **Clofibrate** may magnify the effects of furosemide.

(v) Sweating and flushing may occur when **chloral hydrate** is administered to patients receiving IV furosemide.

(2) **Step 2. Mannitol**, an osmotic diuretic, is a nonreabsorbable polysaccharide.

(a) **Mechanism of action and therapeutic effect**. Mannitol increases the osmotic pressure of the glomerular filtrate; fluid from interstitial spaces is then drawn into blood vessels, expanding plasma volume and maintaining or increasing the urine flow. (This drug may be given to **prevent ARF in high-risk patients**, such as those undergoing surgery or suffering from severe trauma or hemolytic transfusion reactions.)

(b) **Onset of action** is 15 to 30 minutes. Duration of action is 3 to 4 hours.

(c) **Administration and dosage**. Mannitol is available in solutions ranging from 5% to 25%. For the treatment of oliguric ARF or the prevention of ARF, the usual initial dose is 12.5 to 25 g, administered intravenously; the maximum daily dose is 100 g, administered intravenously.The exact concentration of the solution is determined by the patient's fluid requirements.

(d) Precautions and monitoring effects

(i) Mannitol is contraindicated in patients with anuria, pulmonary edema or congestion, severe dehydration, and intracranial hemorrhage (except during craniotomy).

(ii) This drug may cause or worsen pulmonary edema and circulatory overload. If signs and symptoms of these problems develop, the infusion should be stopped.

(iii) Other adverse effects of mannitol include fluid and electrolyte abnormalities, water intoxication, headache, confusion, blurred vision, thirst, nausea, and vomiting.

(iv) Vital signs, urine output, daily weights, cardiopulmonary status, and serum and urine sodium and potassium levels should be monitored during mannitol therapy.

(v) Mannitol solutions with undissolved crystals should not be given.

(3) Dopamine. This vasopressor, an immediate metabolic precursor of epinephrine and norepinephrine, is a potent sympathomimetic agent.

(a) Mechanism of action and therapeutic effect. Given at low doses, dopamine stimulates dopaminergic receptors, located mainly in splanchnic blood vessels; this results in vessel dilation, which leads, in turn, to enhanced renal blood flow and urine output. Dopamine may be used to prevent as well as treat ARF.

(b) Administration and dosage. Dopamine is given intravenously in doses of 1 to 5 μg/kg/min. The dose is titrated to the desired response.

(c) Precautions and monitoring effects

(i) Dopamine may cause hypotension, tachycardia, arrhythmias, palpitations, anginal pain, ECG abnormalities (e.g., widening QRS complexes), and vasoconstriction. These signs and symptoms may warrant slowing of the infusion rate.

(ii) Adverse gastrointestinal effects include nausea and vomiting.

(iii) Extravasation may result in necrosis and tissue sloughing.

(iv) Dopamine must be used cautiously in patients receiving monoamine oxidase (MAO) inhibitors.

(v) During the infusion, the patient's blood pressure, pulse, cardiac function, urine output, and extremity temperature and color should be assessed.

(d) Significant interactions

(i) Phenytoin may cause reduced blood pressure.

(ii) Ergot alkaloids can lead to dangerously elevated blood pressure.

b. Treatment of other systemic manifestations. ARF typically causes hematologic, gastrointestinal, and skin disturbances. See section II F 6 for a discussion of the management of these problems.

4. Dialysis. Hemodialysis or peritoneal dialysis may be necessary in ARF patients who develop anuria; acute fluid overload; severe hyperkalemia, metabolic acidosis, or hyperphosphatemia; GFR below 5 ml/min; BUN level above 100 mg/dl; or serum creatinine level above 10 mg/dl. For a discussion of dialysis, see section II F 8.

II. CHRONIC RENAL FAILURE

A. Definition. Chronic renal failure (CRF) is the progressive, irreversible deterioration of renal function. Usually resulting from long-standing disease, it sometimes derives from ARF that does not respond to treatment.

Table 46-1. Drugs with Significant Renal Elimination*

Allopurinol	Methotrexate
Aminoglycosides	N-aceytlprocainamide
Atenolol	Nadolol
Cephalosporins	Penicillin
Cisplatin	Phenobarbital
Digoxin	Sulfonamides
Ethambutol	Vancomycin
Lithium carbonate	

*In patients with renal impairment, these drugs will accumulate and may cause toxic effects. The dosage should be decreased or dosing intervals reduced; in some cases, both these measures should be taken. Serum drug concentrations should be monitored, especially if the drug has a narrow therapeutic index.

B. Classification and pathophysiology

1. CRF typically progresses through four stages and may be classified according to its stage:
   a. **Mild CRF**, characterized by slightly decreased renal reserve (GFR of 50 to 70 ml/min)
   b. **Moderate CRF**, characterized by a further decrease in renal reserve (GFR of 10 to 50 ml/min, causing renal insufficiency). Despite some loss of renal function, homeostasis is preserved.
   c. **Severe CRF**, characterized by manifest renal failure (GFR of 5 to 10 ml/min). At this stage, slight azotemia occurs.
   d. **End-stage renal disease**, characterized by uremia (GFR below 5 ml/min). Fluid and electrolyte imbalances develop, azotemia worsens, and systemic manifestations appear.

2. As CRF progresses through these stages, **nephron destruction** worsens, leading to deterioration in the kidneys' filtration, reabsorption, and endocrine functions.

3. Renal function typically does not diminish until about 75% of kidney tissue is damaged. Eventually, the kidneys become shrunken, fibrotic masses.

C. Etiology. Major causes of CRF in adults include:

1. Chronic glomerular disease (approximately 50% to 60% of cases)
2. Chronic interstitial nephritis
3. Hereditary renal disease
4. Long-standing vascular disease (e.g., renal artery stenosis)
5. Systemic hypertension
6. Long-standing obstructive uropathy (e.g., renal calculi)
7. Chronic exposure to nephrotoxic agents
8. Chronic endocrine disease (e.g., diabetic neuropathy)

D. Clinical evaluation

1. **Physical findings**. Signs and symptoms, which vary widely, usually do not appear until renal insufficiency (moderate CRF) progresses to renal failure (severe CRF).
   a. **Metabolic** abnormalities include hyponatremia, later becoming sodium overload; hyperkalemia; fluid overload; and metabolic acidosis. See section I D 1 b, d, g, and h for specific findings associated with metabolic abnormalities.
   b. **Neurologic** manifestations range from short attention span, apathy, and listlessness to confusion, clouded sensorium, convulsions, and coma. **Neuromuscular** findings include peripheral neuropathy (pain, itching, and a burning sensation in the feet and legs) progressing to paresthesia and motor nerve dysfunction.
   c. **Cardiovascular** problems include hypertension, arrhythmias, pericarditis, and peripheral edema.
   d. **Gastrointestinal** manifestations include nausea, vomiting, constipation, stomatitis, and unpleasant taste. Ulcers, pancreatitis, and uremic colitis sometime develop.
   e. **Respiratory** problems include dyspnea (if congestive heart failure is present), Kussmaul's respirations (a sign of acidosis), increased susceptibility to infection, pulmonary edema, pleuritic pain, and uremic pleuritis.
   f. **Integumentary** findings typically include pale, yellowish, dry, scaly skin; severe itching; uremic frost; ecchymoses; purpura; and brittle nails and hair.
   g. **Musculoskeletal** changes range from muscle and bone pain to pathologic fractures and calcifications in the brain, heart, eyes, joints, and vessels.
   h. Hematologic disturbances include anemia. The signs and symptoms of anemia arise from lack of erythropoietin and reduced life span of red blood cells and include:
      (1) Pallor of the skin, nail beds, palms, conjunctivae, and buccal mucosa
      (2) Abnormal bruising or ecchymoses
      (3) Dyspnea, angina pectoris
      (4) Extreme fatigue

2. **Diagnostic test results**
   a. **Creatinine clearance** may range from 0 to 70 ml/min, reflecting renal impairment.
   b. **Blood tests** typically show:
      (1) Elevated BUN and serum creatinine levels
      (2) Reduced arterial pH and HCO_3^- concentration
      (3) Reduced serum calcium level

(4) Increased serum potassium and phosphate levels
(5) Possible reduction in the serum sodium level
(6) Normochromic, normocytic anemia; hematocrit 20% to 30%

c. **Urinalysis** may reveal glycosuria, proteinuria, erythrocytes, leukocytes, and casts. Specific gravity is fixed at 1.010.

d. **Radiographic findings**. Kidney–ureter–bladder radiography, IV pyelography, renal scan, renal arteriography, and nephrotomography may be performed. Typically, these tests reveal small kidneys (less than 8 cm in length).

E. Treatment objectives

1. Improve patient comfort and prolong life

2. Treat systemic manifestations of CRF

3. Correct body chemistry abnormalities

F. Therapy

1. **Conservative management**—dietary measures and fluid restriction—help relieve some symptoms of CRF and may increase patient comfort and prolong life until dialysis or renal transplantation is required or available. See section I F 1 a and b for a discussion of these measures.

2. **Treatment of edema and chronic heart failure**. **Digitalis preparations** and **diuretics** may be given to manage edema and chronic heart failure and to increase urine output.

a. **Digitalis preparations**. Also known as cardiotonic glycosides, these agents include **digitalis leaf**, **deslanoside**, **digoxin**, **digitoxin**, and **gitalin**. See Chapter 34 for a discussion of these drugs.

b. **Diuretics**. An osmotic diuretic (mannitol), a loop diuretic, or a thiazide-like diuretic may be given.

(1) **Osmotic and loop diuretics**. See section I F 3 a (1) and (2) for information on the use of these drugs in renal failure.

(2) **Thiazide-like diuretics**. **Metolazone** is the most commonly used diuretic in CRF.

(a) **Mechanism of action and therapeutic effect**. Metolazone reduces the body's fluid and sodium volume by increasing sodium reabsorption in the ascending limb of the loop of Henle, thereby increasing urinary excretion of fluid and sodium.

(b) **Administration and dosage**. This drug is given orally in doses of 5 to 20 mg/day; the dose is titrated to the patient's needs. Furosemide and metolazone act synergistically. Combination use is common.

(c) **Precautions and monitoring effects**

(i) Metolazone should not be given to patients with hypersensitivity to sulfonamide derivatives, including thiazides.
(ii) To avoid nocturia, the daily dose should be given in the morning.
(iii) This drug may cause hematologic reactions, such as agranulocytosis, aplastic anemia, and thrombocytopenia.
(iv) Fluid volume depletion, hypokalemia, hyperuricemia, hyperglycemia, and impaired glucose tolerance may occur during metolazone therapy.
(v) This drug may cause hypersensitivity reactions, such as vasculitis and pneumonitis.

(d) **Significant interactions**

(i) **Diazoxide** may potentiate the antihypertensive, hyperglycemic, and hyperuricemic effects of metolazone.
(ii) **Colestipol** and **cholestyramine** decrease the absorption of metolazone.

3. **Treatment of hypertension**. **Antihypertensive agents** may be needed if blood pressure becomes dangerously high as a result of edema and the high renin levels occurring in CRF. Antihypertensive therapy should be initiated in the lowest effective dose and titrated according to patient needs.

a. **Angiotensin-converting enzyme (ACE) inhibitors** (e.g., captopril, enalapril, lisinopril) are widely used to treat CRF because they help preserve renal function and typically cause fewer adverse effects than other antihypertensive agents. See Chapter 33 for a discussion of ACE inhibitors.

b. **β-adrenergic blockers** (e.g., propranolol, atenolol) reduce blood pressure through various mechanisms. For a discussion of these agents, see Chapter 33.

c. **Other antihypertensive agents** are sometimes used in the treatment of CRF, including **α-adrenergic stimulants** (e.g., clonidine, methyldopa) and **vasodilators** (e.g., prazosin, hydralazine). See Chapter 33, for information on these drugs.

4. **Treatment of hyperphosphatemia** involves administration of a **phosphate binder** (e.g., aluminum hydroxide or calcium carbonate) [see section I F 2 c].

5. Treatment of hypocalcemia

a. Oral calcium salts [see section I F 2 d (2)]

b. Vitamin D

(1) Mechanism of action and therapeutic effect. Vitamin D promotes intestinal calcium and phosphate absorption and utilization and thus increases the serum calcium concentration.

(2) Choice of agent. For the treatment of hypocalcemia in ARF and other renal disorders, **calcitriol** (vitamin D_2, the active form of vitamin D) is the preferred vitamin D supplement because of its greater efficacy and relatively short duration of action. Other single-entity preparations include dihydrotachysterol (obtained by vitamin D_2 reduction); ergocalciferol (pure vitamin D_2); and calcifediol (the product of the initial step in vitamin D_3 activation).

(3) Administration and dosage. Calcitriol is given orally; the dose is titrated to the patient's needs (0.5 to 1 μg/day may be effective).

(4) Precautions and monitoring effects

(a) Vitamin D administration may be dangerous in patients with renal failure and must be used with extreme caution.

(b) Vitamin D toxicity may cause a wide range of signs and symptoms, including headache, dizziness, ataxia, convulsions, psychosis, soft-tissue calcification, conjunctivitis, photophobia, tinnitus, nausea, diarrhea, pruritus, and muscle and bone pain.

(c) Vitamin D has a narrow therapeutic index, necessitating frequent measurement of BUN and serum and urine calcium and potassium levels.

(d) Because hyperphosphatemia generally accompanies hypocalcemia in renal failure, dietary phosphate should be restricted and binding agents should be given during vitamin D therapy to prevent calcification and deterioration in renal function. See section I F 2 c (2) for information on aluminum hydroxide, a binding agent.

6. Treatment of other systemic manifestations of CRF

a. Treatment of **anemia** includes administration of **iron** and **folate supplements** (e.g., ferrous sulfate, folic acid).

(1) Severe anemia may warrant infusion of **fresh frozen packed cells** or **washed packed cells**.

(2) To increase red blood cell production, **androgens** may be given.

b. Treatment of **gastrointestinal disturbances**

(1) Antiemetics help control nausea and vomiting.

(2) Cimetidine may be given to relieve gastric irritation.

(3) Dioctyl sodium succinate or **methylcellulose** may be used to prevent constipation.

(4) Enemas may be given to remove blood from the gastrointestinal tract.

c. Treatment of skin problems. An **antipruritic agent** (e.g., diphenhydramine) may be used to alleviate itching.

7. Management of body chemistry abnormalities. See section I F 2.

8. Dialysis. When CRF progresses to end-stage renal disease and no longer responds to conservative measures, long-term dialysis or renal transplantation is necessary to prolong life.

a. Hemodialysis is the preferred dialysis method for patients with a reduced peritoneal membrane, hypercatabolism, or acute hyperkalemia.

(1) This technique involves shunting of the patient's blood through a dialysis membrane-containing unit for diffusion, osmosis, and ultrafiltration. The blood is then returned to the patient's circulation.

(2) Vascular access may be obtained via an arteriovenous fistula or an external shunt.

(3) The procedure takes only 3 to 8 hours; most patients need only two or three treatments each week. With proper training, patients can perform hemodialysis at home.

(4) The patient receives **heparin** during hemodialysis to prevent clotting.

(5) Various complications may arise, including hemorrhage, hepatitis, anemia, septicemia, cardiovascular problems, air embolism, rapid shifts in fluid and electrolyte balance, itching, nausea, vomiting, headache, seizures, aluminum osteodystrophy.

b. Peritoneal dialysis is the preferred dialysis method for patients with bleeding disorders and cardiovascular disease.

(1) The peritoneum is used as a semipermeable membrane. A plastic catheter inserted into the peritoneum provides access for the dialysate, which draws excess fluids, wastes, and electrolytes accross the peritoneal membrane periodically by osmosis and diffusion.

(2) Peritoneal dialysis can be carried out in three different modes.

(a) Intermittent peritoneal dialysis is an automatic cycling mode lasting 8 to 10 hours, performed three times each week. This mode allows nighttime treatment and is appropriate for working patients.

(b) Continuous ambulatory peritoneal dialysis is performed daily for 24 hr/day with four exchanges daily. The patient can remain active during the treatment.

(c) **Continuous cyclic peritoneal dialysis** may be used if the other two modes fail to improve creatinine clearance. Dialysis takes place at night; the last exchange is retained in the peritoneal cavity during the day, then drained that evening.

(3) The **advantages** of peritoneal dialysis include lack of serious complications, retention of normal fluid and electrolyte balance, simplicity, reduced cost, patient independence, and reduced need or no need for heparin administration.

(4) **Complications** of peritoneal dialysis include hyperglycemia, constipation, and inflammation or infection at the catheter site. Also, this method carries a high risk of peritonitis.

9. **Renal transplantation**. This surgical procedure allows some patients with end-stage CRF to live normal and—in many cases—longer lives.

a. **Histocompatibility** must be tested beforehand to minimize the risk of transplant rejection and failure. Human leukocyte antigen (HLA) type, mixed lymphocyte reactivity, and blood group types are determined to assess histocompatibility.

b. Renal transplant material may be obtained from a living donor or a cadaver.

c. Three types of **graft rejection** can occur.

(1) **Hyperacute** (immediate) **rejection** results in graft loss within minutes to hours after transplantation.

(a) Acute urine flow cessation and bluish or mottled kidney discoloration are intraoperative signs of hyperacute rejection.

(b) Postoperative manifestations include kidney enlargement, fever, anuria, local pain, sodium retention, and hypertension.

(c) Treatment for hyperacute rejection is immediate nephrectomy.

(2) **Acute rejection** may occur 4 to 60 days after transplantation.

(a) Findings may include fever, oliguria, and graft enlargement (however, in some cases, only subtle signs, such as abnormal laboratory test results, occur).

(b) Initial treatment is **steroid administration**; if the condition does not respond to steroids, nephrectomy is necessary.

(3) **Chronic rejection** occurs later than 60 days after transplantation.

(a) Signs and symptoms include low-grade fever, increased proteinuria, azotemia, hypertension, oliguria, weight gain, and edema.

(b) Treatment may include **alkylating agents**, **cyclosporine**, **antilymphocyte globulin**, and **corticosteroids**. In some cases, nephrectomy is necessary.

d. **Complications** of renal transplantation include:

(1) Infection, diabetes, hepatitis, and leukopenia, resulting from immunosuppressive therapy

(2) Hypertension, resulting from various causes

(3) Cancer (e.g., lymphoma, cutaneous malignancies, head and neck cancer, leukemia, and colon cancer)

(4) Pancreatitis and mental and emotional disorders (e.g., suicidal tendencies, severe depression), brought on by steroid therapy

STUDY QUESTIONS

Directions: Each question below contains five suggested answers. Choose the **one best** response to each question.

1. Treatment for metabolic acidosis associated with acute renal failure (ARF) should begin when total serum carbon dioxide is less than 15 mEq/L and blood pH is less than 7.35. Which of the following agents should be administered in this situation?

 A. Calcium supplements
 B. Furosemide
 C. Atenolol
 D. Sodium bicarbonate
 E. Mannitol

2. The drug of choice in the treatment of hyperkalemia-induced arrhythmias is

 A. calcium gluconate
 B. calcium carbonate
 C. sodium bicarbonate
 D. digoxin
 E. sodium polysterene sulfonate

3. Which of the following diuretics is the drug of choice for the management of oliguric acute renal failure (ARF) with urine output less than 20 ml/hr?

 A. Bumetanide
 B. Furosemide
 C. Hydrochlorothiazide
 D. Metolazone
 E. Mannitol

4. All of the following diuretics will produce diuresis when the creatinine clearance is less than 25 ml/min EXCEPT

 A. hydrochlorothiazide
 B. metolazone
 C. mannitol
 D. bumetanide
 E. furosemide

5. Which of the following drugs is given in combination with low-dose continuous dopamine infusion to produce a brisk diuresis in acute renal failure (ARF)?

 A. Hydrochlorothiazide
 B. Metolazone
 C. Sodium bicarbonate
 D. Furosemide
 E. Mannitol

6. Certain agents are thought to be kidney-protective and have a low incidence of side effects. Which of the following drugs is preferred in treating hypertension in patients with chronic renal failure (CRF)?

 A. Vasodilators
 B. α-Adrenergic stimulants
 C. β-Blockers
 D. Angiotensin converting enzyme (ACE) inhibitors
 E. Enzymatic buffers

ANSWERS AND EXPLANATIONS

1. The answer is D. [*I F 2 a (3), b*] Sodium bicarbonate administered intravenously is the treatment of choice for metabolic acidosis. The agent replaces bicarbonate stores and leads to an increase in both total serum carbon dioxide and blood pH values.

2. The answer is A. [*I F 2 a (2)*] Calcium gluconate administered intravenously is the drug of choice in the treatment of hyperkalemia-induced arrhythmias, with an average adult dose of 1 g. Onset of action is usually within a few minutes. Calcium gluconate antagonizes the effect of high serum potassium levels on cardiac conduction.

3. The answer is B. (*I F 3 a*) Furosemide, which is a loop diuretic usually administered intravenously, is the diuretic drug of choice in the management of oliguric acute renal failure (ARF). The loop diuretics act in the medullary and cortical ascending limbs of the loop of Henle. The agents inhibit sodium and chloride reabsorption. They also produce renal vasodilatation, resulting in an increase in renal blood flow. The onset of diuretic action of furosemide administered intravenously is quick (within minutes), and duration of action lasts 2 to 3 hours.

Bumetanide, another loop diuretic, offers no advantage over furosemide except in those patients refractory to the diuretic action of furosemide. Some patients refractory to furosemide may respond to bumetanide. Hydrochlorothiazide does not produce diuresis when creatinine clearance is less than 25 ml/min. Mannitol is an osmotic diuretic and may be used in selected patients who are refractory to the loop diuretics. Metolazone, a thiazide diuretic, is sometimes used in combination with furosemide for its added diuretic action.

4. The answer is A. (*I F 3 a*) Hydrochlorothiazide is a thiazide diuretic. Generally, thiazide diuretics do not produce diuresis when creatinine clearance is less than 25 ml/min. The thiazide diuretics inhibit sodium and chloride reabsorption in the kidney tubules but also inherently decrease renal blood flow. Although metolazone has the same pharmacologic action as the thiazide diuretics, it does not substantially decrease renal blood flow and may produce diuresis when creatinine clearance reaches 25 ml/min or below.

5. The answer is D. [*I F 3 a (1), (3)*] Dopamine given intravenously at a continuous low-dose rate of between 1 and 5 μg/kg/min is primarily dopaminergic. Low-dose continous dopamine infusion may be used alone or with furosemide in patients refractory to furosemide or mannitol alone.

6. The answer is D. (*II F 3 a*) Angiotensin-converting enzyme (ACE) inhibitors (e.g., captopril, enalapril, lisinopril) are widely used to treat hypertension in CRF patients. They are thought to help preserve renal function and typically cause fewer adverse effects than other antihypertensive agents.

47
Cancer Chemotherapy

Robert J. Cersosimo

I. GENERAL CONSIDERATIONS

A. Definition. Cancer is a new tissue growth (neoplasm) in which undifferentiated cells proliferate uncontrollably.

B. Classification. The major histologic categories of cancerous tumors are:

1. **Carcinomas**, originating in epithelial tissue
2. **Sarcomas**, originating primarily in connective tissues
3. **Leukemias** and **lymphomas**, originating in the blood and lymphatic systems, respectively

C. Incidence

1. Cancer is the second leading cause of death in the United States.
2. Each year, nearly 1 million new cancer cases are diagnosed and roughly 500,000 Americans die of cancer.
   a. In adult males, the most common cancers are lung, prostate, and colorectal cancer.
   b. In adult females, the leading cancers are breast, colorectal, and lung cancer.
   c. Among American children, cancer is second to accidents as the most common cause of death.
      (1) Each year, approximately 6000 new cancer cases are reported and 1700 cancer deaths occur in children.
      (2) The most common cancers in children under age 15 are acute leukemia, brain and other central nervous system (CNS) tumors, and lymphomas.

D. Etiology. The cause of cancer remains largely unknown. However, various factors have been implicated.

1. **Carcinogens**. Asbestos, radiation, cigarettes, and certain hormones are proven cancer-causing agents.
2. **Viruses**. Various forms of cancer have been associated with specific viruses. For example, there is evidence of a relationship between the Epstein-Barr virus, which causes infectious mononucleosis, and nasopharyngeal cancer and Burkitt's lymphoma.
3. **Genetics**. Wilms' tumor may have a familial inheritance pattern.
4. **Immune deficiency**. An inhibited immune response (e.g., from aging, stress, or severe systemic infection) may promote cancer by preventing the body from recognizing and destroying cancer cells.
5. **Diet**. A diet that is high in fats and proteins and low in fiber may promote certain cancers.

E. Cell cycle. All cells—normal and cancerous—pass through various life-cycle phases.

1. **G_0 phase**. During this resting phase, the cell is not preparing for cell division. Cells remain in this phase for variable periods.
2. **G_1 phase**. The cell prepares for synthesis of deoxyribonucleic acid (DNA).
3. **S phase**. DNA synthesis takes place.
4. **G_2 phase**. The cell prepares for division.

5. **M (mitosis) phase**. Cell division takes place, resulting in the creation of two daughter cells from each cell.

F. Cancer cell and tumor characteristics

1. **Genetic change**. Chromosomal research suggests that cancer reflects a genetic change at the cellular level.

2. **Uncontrolled proliferation**. Unlike normal cells, cancer cells do not respond to various signals that regulate cell, tissue, and organ growth. Consequently, they proliferate at an uncontrollable rate.

3. **Invasiveness**. Cancer cells tend to invade and destroy surrounding tissues.

4. **Metastasis**. A cancerous tumor may shed cells into the bloodstream and lymphatic vessels. From here, the cells disperse to distant sites in which secondary tumors develop. Local extension (e.g., tumor spread into a body cavity) also represents metastasis.

5. **Growth fraction and Gompertzian growth**
   a. The **growth fraction** of a tumor indicates the percentage of its cells undergoing DNA synthesis and division at any given time.
   b. Tumor growth reflects the **Gompertzian growth** pattern.
      (1) Young tumors grow rapidly.
      (2) As tumors enlarge with age, their growth rate decreases or reaches a plateau.
   c. Thus, young tumors typically have a higher growth fraction than older tumors. Generally, large, slow-growing tumors have low growth fractions.
   d. Because anticancer drugs are more effective against dividing than nondividing cells, these drugs are more successful against young tumors, which have a higher percentage of dividing cells.

6. **Tumor doubling time**. Reflecting the time needed for a tumor to double in size, doubling time varies from one tumor type to another. However, tumors of the same type share similar doubling times. For example:
   a. Burkitt's lymphoma doubles in approximately 24 hours.
   b. Small-cell lung cancer doubles in roughly 30 days.
   c. Colorectal cancer takes more than 600 days to double.

G. Clinical evaluation. Diagnostic tests for cancer include those that identify the primary tumor site, locate any secondary foci, and help stage and grade the tumor.

1. X-rays, isotope scans, computed tomography (CT) scans, and magnetic resonance imaging (MRI) are used to identify the tumor site and stage the disease.

2. **Biopsy** allows histologic analysis of tumor tissue.

3. **Tumor marker substances** may suggest which form of cancer is present, help detect disease spread, and when measured during therapy, permit evaluation of therapeutic efficacy and tumor recurrence.
   a. Levels of **carcinoembryonic antigen** (CEA) may be elevated when cancer of the lung, breast, pancreas, or colon is present. However, a number of nonmalignant conditions may also cause elevated CEA levels (e.g., alcoholic liver disease, pancreatitis, heavy cigarette smoking, ulcerative colitis, a recent blood transfusion.)
   b. Levels of **alpha-fetoprotein (AFP)** may be increased in cancer of the testis, pancreas, or stomach. AFP levels may also be elevated in noncancerous conditions (e.g., viral hepatitis).

4. **Disease staging** helps guide anticancer therapy.
   a. Each malignacy has its own specific staging system. For example, Hodgkin's disease is classified as stages I to IV; prostate cancer, as stages A to D.
   b. The **TNM system** is an attempt to standardize cancer staging. The letters T, N, and M refer to **t**umor size, lymph **n**ode involvement, and the presence or absence of **m**etastases. Subscript numbers appended to the T and the N give an idea of the tumor size and the extent of nodal involvement, while a plus sign or minus sign (or a zero) appended to the M indicates whether metastases are present or absent.

5. **Tumor grading** determines the degree of cancer cell differentiation, helps gauge the tumor's growth rate, and identifies the tumor on the basis of corresponding normal cells.

II. TREATMENT OBJECTIVES

A. Induce tumor regression or cure

B. Prevent metastasis

C. Improve the quality of life by reducing pain and other disease symptoms

III. THERAPY*

A. Cancer chemotherapy

1. General considerations

a. Therapeutic effects. Anticancer drugs destroy cancer cells by interfering with cell growth and division.

(1) **Cell-cycle–specific** agents destroy cells only during a specific phase of the cell cycle. Generally, such drugs are most effective for tumors with a high growth fraction.

(2) **Cell-cycle–nonspecific** agents can destroy cancer cells during several or all cell cycle phases. These drugs are most useful for tumors with a low growth fraction.

(3) Cancer chemotherapy is most successful in early disease stages, when fewer cancer cells are present and the patient can better tolerate the toxic effects of chemotherapy.

b. Therapeutic goal. The aim of chemotherapy is **total cell kill**.

(1) Anticancer drugs kill a **fixed percentage** rather than a fixed number of cancer cells. Surviving cancer cells may cause a relapse.

(2) Consequently, to achieve a cure, chemotherapy must destroy all cancer cells.

(3) Total cell kill is more likely to occur when several anticancer drugs are given together, as in combination chemotherapy (see section III A I e).

c. Drug classification. Cancer chemotherapeutic agents generally are classified according to their chemical structure, mechanism of action, or source. The major drug groups are **alkylating agents**, **antimetabolites**, **natural products**, **hormonal agents**, and **miscellaneous drugs**.

d. Choice of agent(s) is based mainly on tumor characteristics, such as the tumor site, stage, histologic origin, and expected susceptibility to specific agents (as indicated by clinical experience or research).

e. Combination chemotherapy. Now used more commonly than single-agent therapy, combination chemotherapy usually involves three or more agents.

(1) Combination regimens may have a dramatically higher response rate than single-agent therapy.

(2) Drugs given in combination generally should have different mechanisms of action, should act during different cell cycle phases, should have known activity as single agents, and should be associated with different adverse effects.

(a) Cell-cycle–specific drugs may be given in combination with cell-cycle–nonspecific agents.

(b) Examples of combination regimens include:

(i) **MOPP**: Mechlorethamine, Oncovin (vincristine), procarbazine, and prednisone (therapeutic for Hodgkin's disease)

(ii) **FAM**: Fluorouracil, Adriamycin (doxorubicin), and mitomycin (therapeutic for various gastrointestinal carcinomas)

f. Dosing frequency. To allow normal cells to recover between doses, most chemotherapeutic drugs are administered in short courses interrupted by rest periods.

g. Administration route. Most agents are given systemically via oral or intravenous (IV) administration. However, in some cases, they are given regionally or locally (e.g., via intraperitoneal, intra-arterial, or intrathecal administration).

h. Therapeutic response

(1) **Criteria**. During therapy, the following parameters are monitored to evaluate therapeutic efficacy.

(a) **Tumor response**. X-rays, ultrasound, radionuclide scans, CT scans, or MRI may be used to determine **tumor response**.

(i) **Complete response** indicates no evidence of the tumor.

(ii) **Partial response** generally means that there has been at least a 50% reduction in the product of two perpendicular diameters in one or more measurable lesions, and that this shrinkage has lasted for at least 1 month, with no new tumors elsewhere.

(iii) **Minimal response** usually indicates tumor shrinkage of less than 50%.

(iv) **No response** (also called **stable disease**) means that the tumor has neither shrunk nor grown.

***Note:** The therapeutic indications cited in this chapter are FDA-approved uses for the drugs mentioned. Many cancer chemotherapeutic agents have also been used in various other forms of cancer on an investigational basis.

(v) **Progression** indicates tumor growth despite therapy.

(vi) **Cure** usually refers to a complete response that has been maintained without therapy for at least 5 years (or, in the case of breast cancer and certain other tumors, 10 years).

(b) **Organ function**. Normalization of any organs previously affected by the tumor suggests a positive therapeutic response.

(c) **Marker substances**. A significant reduction in levels of such marker substances as CEA, AFP, and prostatic acid phosphatase indicates tumor shrinkage.

(d) **Performance status**. The patient's ability to perform self-care and normal daily activities serves as an index of the palliative value of chemotherapy. The Karnofsky scale is commonly used to evaluate performance status (Table 47-1).

(2) **Resistance to therapy**. Various factors can lead to a poor therapeutic response.

(a) **Low growth fraction**. Tumors with a low percentage of rapidly dividing cells are less sensitive to chemotherapy.

(b) **Inadequate drug penetration**. As a tumor expands, it may outgrow its blood and nutrient supply, reducing the amount of drug that reaches the tumor.

(c) **De novo (natural) resistance**. In any large cell population, some cells possess natural resistance to a given chemotherapeutic agent. Old, large tumors typically contain greater numbers of resistant cells than do young, small tumors—especially after exposure to chemotherapy.

(d) **Metastases**. As a tumor grows, the risk of metastasis rises. Metastatic tumors increase the body's total tumor burden, decreasing the odds for destruction of all cancer cells via chemotherapy.

(e) **Pharmacologic sanctuaries**. Cancer cells in the CNS usually do not respond to systemic chemotherapy because most chemotherapeutic agents cannot penetrate the blood–brain barrier.

(f) **Patient intolerance**. The severe side effects of chemotherapy may necessitate early drug discontinuation before all cancer cells have been eliminated.

2. Alkylating agents

a. The first chemotherapy drugs in use, these agents were developed from nitrogen mustard or its derivatives. This category includes the following subgroups:

(1) **Nitrogen mustards**—chlorambucil, cyclophosphamide, ifosfamide, mechlorethamine, melphalan, and uracil mustard

(2) **Alkyl sulfonates**—busulfan

Table 47-1. The Karnofsky Performance Scale

Patient's General Condition	Performance Status (%)	Description
Can perform normal activities; no special care needed	100	Normal activity; no complaints or evidence of disease
	90	Normal activity; minor signs/symptoms of disease
	80	Normal activity with effort; some signs/symptoms of disease
Able to live at home but unable to work; performs self-care with some assistance	70	Can perform self-care but cannot carry on normal activity or active work
	60	Requires occasional help but can perform most self-care activities
	50	Requires considerable help with self-care; needs frequent medical care
Cannot perform self-care; requires institutional care or its equivalent	40	Disabled; requires special care and assistance
	30	Severely disabled; hospitalization indicated
	20	Very ill; hospitalization and active support necessary
	10	Moribund; rapidly progressing fatal disease process
	0	Deceased

(3) **Nitrosoureas**—carmustine, lomustine, and streptozocin
(4) **Triazenes**—dacarbazine
(5) **Ethylenimines**—thiotepa

b. Mechanism of action. Alkylating agents affix an alkyl group to cellular DNA, causing cross-linking of DNA strands that triggers cell death. Cell-cycle–nonspecific, these agents kill nondividing as well as dividing cells.

(1) **Chlorambucil** is indicated for chronic lymphocytic leukemia, Hodgkin's disease, and non-Hodgkin's lymphomas.
(2) **Cyclophosphamide** is given to treat a wide range of cancers, including lymphomas, leukemias, cancer of the breast and ovary, neuroblastoma, and retinoblastoma. In addition, it is sometimes used as an immunosuppressant to minimize organ transplant rejection.
(3) **Mechlorethamine (nitrogen mustard)** is given for lymphomas. In the treatment of other cancers (e.g., breast and ovarian cancer), it has largely been replaced by other alkylating agents.
(4) **Melphalan** is used primarily in the treatment of multiple myeloma. It is also indicated for epithelial ovarian carcinoma.
(5) **Uracil mustard** is indicated for lymphomas, chronic lymphocytic and myelocytic leukemia, and mycosis fungoides.
(6) **Busulfan** is indicated for chronic myelocytic leukemia.
(7) **Carmustine (BCNU)** is used to treat lymphomas, multiple myeloma, and cancer of the brain.
(8) **Lomustine (CCNU)** is used for cancer of the brain and Hodgkin's disease.
(9) **Streptozocin** is given to treat metastatic pancreatic islet cell carcinoma.
(10) **Dacarbazine (DTIC)** is indicated for metastatic malignant melanoma and Hodgkin's disease.
(11) **Thiotepa** is indicated for the treatment of superficial bladder tumors. It is also used for palliative treatment of tumors of the breast and ovary. It is occasionally administered by intracavitary instillation to treat pleural, pericardial, or peritoneal effusions.
(12) **Ifosfamide**, the newest alkylating agent, is indicated for testicular germ cell tumors.

3. Antimetabolites

a. The first drugs developed specifically against tumors, antimetabolites have a narrower spectrum than other chemotherapeutic agents. They are most effective during the S phase of the cell cycle. This drug category includes the following subgroups:

(1) **Folic acid analogues**—methotrexate
(2) **Purine analogues**—mercaptopurine and thioguanine
(3) **Pyrimidine analogues**—cytarabine, floxuridine, and fluorouracil

b. Mechanism of action

(1) **Methotrexate** competitively inhibits dihydrofolate reductase, preventing folic acid reduction to tetrahydrofolate.
(2) **Mercaptopurine** and **thioguanine** are converted by hypoxanthine-guanine phosphoribosyl transferase to their corresponding nucleotides, which inhibit purine synthesis.
(3) **Cytarabine**, **floxuridine**, and **fluorouracil** are activated to their corresponding nucleotides, which inhibit DNA synthesis.

c. Indications

(1) **Methotrexate** is used to treat acute lymphoblastic and meningeal leukemia; non-Hodgkin's lymphoma; choriocarcinoma; lymphosarcoma; mycosis fungoides; and cancer of the breast, testis, head and neck, and lung. In addition, it is administered for such noncancerous conditions as psoriasis.
(2) **Mercaptopurine (6-mercaptopurine)** is indicated for the treatment of acute lymphocytic leukemia and acute and chronic myeloblastic leukemia.
(3) **Thioguanine (6-thioguanine)** is indicated for acute myelocytic leukemia.
(4) **Cytarabine** is indicated for acute leukemia—especially acute myelocytic leukemia in adults.
(5) **Floxuridine** is indicated for gastrointestinal adenocarcinoma metastatic to the liver.
(6) **Fluorouracil** is administered for cancer of the breast, colon and rectum, pancreas, and stomach.

4. Natural products

a. This category of naturally occurring substances includes the following subgroups:

(1) **Vinca alkaloids**—vinblastine and vincristine
(2) **Epipodophyllotoxins**—etoposide
(3) **Antibiotics**—bleomycin, dactinomycin, daunorubicin, doxorubicin, mitomycin, mitoxantrone, and plicamycin
(4) **Enzymes**—asparaginase

b. Mechanism of action

(1) **Vinblastine** and **vincristine** are M-phase specific, blocking cell division by interfering with mitosis.

(2) **Etoposide** blocks cells at the S–G_2 interface; in high doses, it causes G_2 arrest.

(3) **Bleomycin** inhibits DNA synthesis and causes chain scission and fragmentation of DNA. It is most effective during phases G_1 and G_2.

(4) **Dactinomycin**, **daunorubicin**, and **doxorubicin** intercalate with DNA, distorting DNA-dependent ribonucleic acid (RNA) synthesis and DNA synthesis.

(5) **Mitomycin** alkylates DNA, inhibiting DNA synthesis and leading to a cell growth imbalance that causes cell death.

(6) **Mitoxantrone** is thought to interact with the enzyme topoisomerase II, which is needed for supercoiling of the DNA helix.

(7) **Plicamycin** complexes with DNA, inhibiting RNA synthesis.

(8) **Asparaginase** depletes asparagine, an amino acid necessary for growth of certain cancer cells.

c. Indications

(1) **Vinblastine** is given for the treatment of metastatic testicular tumors, lymphomas, Kaposi's sarcoma, breast cancer, choriocarcinoma, and mycosis fungoides.

(2) **Vincristine** is indicated for lymphomas, leukemias (especially acute leukemias in children), neuroblastoma, Wilms' tumor, and rhabdomyosarcoma.

(3) **Etoposide (VP-16)** is indicated for testicular cancer and small-cell lung cancer.

(4) **Bleomycin** is indicated for lymphomas and cancer of the testis, head and neck, cervix, and skin.

(5) **Dactinomycin (actinomycin D)** is used primarily for Wilms' tumor, sarcomas, and methotrexate-resistant choriocarcinomas.

(6) **Daunorubicin** is therapeutic for acute myelocytic leukemia and acute lymphocytic leukemia.

(7) **Doxorubicin** is indicated for cancer of the breast, ovary, lung, bladder, stomach, and thyroid; osteogenic and soft tissue sarcomas; Hodgkin's disease; non-Hodgkin's lymphomas; Wilms' tumor; neuroblastoma; and acute leukemia.

(8) **Mitomycin** is given in the treatment of cancer of the pancreas.

(9) **Mitoxantrone** is currently used for management of acute nonlymphocytic leukemia.

(10) **Plicamycin (mithramycin)** is given for testicular cancer. It also has value in such conditions as hypercalcemia and hypercalciuria (especially when associated with cancer involving the bone).

(11) **Asparaginase (L-asparaginase)** is used almost exclusively in combination with other drugs to treat acute lymphocytic leukemia.

5. Hormonal agents

a. These drugs alter the hormonal environment of certain hormone-dependent tumors, interrupting the neoplastic process. Hormonal agents are classified in the following subgroups:

(1) **Adrenocorticosteroids** (e.g., prednisone, dexamethasone)

(2) **Progestins** (e.g., medroxyprogesterone, megestrol)

(3) **Androgens** (e.g., fluoxymesterone, testosterone, dromostanolone)

(4) **Estrogens** (e.g., estradiol, diethylstilbestrol)

(5) **Antiestrogens** (e.g., tamoxifen)

(6) **Gonadotropin-releasing hormone analogues** (e.g., leuprolide)

b. Mechanism of action. Hormonal agents have various mechanisms. Those relating to chemotherapeutic actions are discussed below. For details on the general mechanisms of these drugs, see Chapter 13.

(1) **Adrenocorticosteroids** attach to corticosteroid-binding proteins in leukemic cells. They also cause lympholysis, suppress mitosis, and inhibit cellular protein synthesis.

(2) **Progestins** bind to specific progesterone receptors and promote maturation and maintenance of normal endothelial tissue. Their activity in other tumors is unknown.

(3) **Androgen** activity is uncertain. Androgens may inhibit estrogen receptors or reduce estrogen formation from adrenal products.

(4) **Estrogens** bind to receptor proteins, leading to increased RNA and protein synthesis and stimulation of DNA synthesis. In prostate cancer, estrogens inhibit the release of luteinizing hormone-releasing factor (LHRF), thereby reducing luteinizing hormone (LH) levels; this ultimately leads to a decline in testicular androgen production.

(5) **Antiestrogens** bind to estrogen receptors, possibly in a way that leads to severely impaired growth of estrogen-dependent tumors.

(6) **Gonadotropin-releasing hormone analogues** initially stimulate, then suppress, the secretion of follicle-stimulating hormone and luteinizing hormone; testosterone inhibition results.

c. **Indications**
   (1) **Adrenocorticosteroids** are given adjunctively in the treatment of leukemia, lymphomas, breast cancer, and multiple myeloma.
   (2) **Progestins** are useful against breast and endometrial cancer.
   (3) **Androgens** are indicated for advanced post-menopausal breast cancer.
   (4) **Estrogens** are given for cancerous breast tumors containing estrogen receptors and for prostatic cancer.
   (5) **Antiestrogens** are used to treat advanced postmenopausal and premenopausal breast cancer. They are most effective against tumors containing estrogen receptors.
   (6) **Gonadotropin-releasing hormone analogues** are indicated for advanced prostate cancer.

6. **Miscellaneous agents**. This category includes **cisplatin**, **hydroxyurea**, **interferon alfa-2a** and **alfa-2b**, **mitotane**, and **procarbazine**.
   a. **Mechanism of action**
   (1) **Cisplatin** cross-links DNA strands and binds to cytoplasmic and nuclear proteins, resulting in cell death. It is cell-cycle–nonspecific.
   (2) **Hydroxyurea** inhibits ribonucleoside diphosphate reductase, thus interfering with DNA synthesis.
   (3) **Interferon alfa-2a** and **alfa-2b** bind to specific membrane receptors on the cell surface, triggering a series of immunologic responses leading to suppression of viral replication and cell proliferation.
   (4) **Mitotane** selectively attacks adrenocortical cells and rapidly reduces adrenocorticosteroid levels.
   (5) **Procarbazine** is metabolized to active agents, which may damage DNA and inhibit RNA, DNA, and protein synthesis.
   b. **Indications**
   (1) **Cisplatin** (*cis*-platinum) is used in the treatment of cancer of the testis, ovary, and bladder.
   (2) **Hydroxyurea** is indicated primarily for acute and chronic granulocytic leukemia, metastatic malignant melanoma, cancer of the head and neck, and ovarian carcinoma.
   (3) **Interferon alfa-2a** and **alfa-2b** are used in the treatment of hairy-cell leukemia and Kaposi's sarcoma.
   (4) **Mitotane** is therapeutic for inoperable adrenocortical cancer.
   (5) **Procarbazine** is given primarily to treat Hodgkin's disease.

7. **Precautions and monitoring effects**. Drugs used in cancer chemotherapy have a very narrow therapeutic index—the dosage needed to achieve a therapeutic response usually proves toxic to the body's rapidly proliferating cells (e.g., bone marrow, gastrointestinal tract mucosa, hair follicles, and fetal tissue). However, with early detection of drug toxicity, drug dosages can be modified or the drug regimen altered to minimize toxic effects.
   a. **Contraindications to chemotherapy**
   (1) **Infection**. Because chemotherapeutic agents are immunosuppressive, they generally are withheld until infection has been eliminated.
   (2) **Poor hematologic status**. Chemotherapy can severely depress bone marrow function. Consequently, it usually is reserved for patients with adequate leukocyte, platelet, and erythrocyte levels.
   b. **Indications for cautious use**
   (1) **Impaired renal or hepatic function**. Severe drug toxicity may result from inadequate drug metabolism or excretion—a common consequence of hepatic or renal impairment.
   (2) **Poor nutritional status**. Malnutrition predisposes the chemotherapy patient to severe toxicity.
   c. **Common toxic drug effects**
   (1) **Myelosuppression** (bone marrow suppression) is the most common dose-limiting toxic effect, occurring with nearly every chemotherapeutic drug. Unless drug dosages are chosen carefully, bleeding and infection can result.
   (a) With most drugs, the **nadir** (point of maximum myelosuppression) generally occurs about 10 to 14 days after drug administration.
   (b) **Recovery** (return of normal bone marrow function) usually takes place 18 to 21 days after drug administration.
   (c) Leukocytes and platelets—both with short life spans—are the most commonly affected blood cells. Erythrocytes are less commonly suppressed because of their much longer life span.
   (i) Dosages of most chemotherapeutic drugs should be reduced when the white blood cell (WBC) count drops below 4000 cells/mm^3. Chemotherapeutic drugs

are withheld when the WBC count falls below 2500 cells/mm³ or the platelet count drops below 80,000 cells/mm³.

(ii) Usually, chemotherapy can resume when the WBC count rises above 4000 cells/mm³ and the platelet count exceeds 120,000 cells/mm³.

(d) **Delayed myelosuppression**. With such drugs as carmustine, lomustine, and mitomycin, maximum myelosuppression typically occurs around the fourth or fifth week after therapy begins. For this reason, these drugs usually are given at 6-week intervals to allow bone marrow recovery.

(e) **Nonsuppressive agents**. Because bleomycin, vincristine, and asparaginase rarely cause significant myelosuppression at commonly administered doses, these agents are considered nonsuppressive.

(2) **Adverse gastrointestinal effects**

(a) **Nausea and vomiting**, common with many chemotherapeutic drugs, result from stimulation of the brain's chemoreceptor trigger zone. See Table 47-2 for a comparison of the emetic potential of various agents.

(i) Onset of nausea and vomiting usually occurs within 3 to 4 hours after drug administration; in many cases, symptoms subside in less than 24 hours. A few drugs (e.g., cisplatin) may cause prolonged distress.

(ii) Severe nausea and vomiting may reduce patient tolerance of chemotherapy.

(iii) Antiemetic therapy—initiated before chemotherapeutic drugs are administered—can minimize or prevent nausea and vomiting.

(b) **Stomatitis** and **mucositis**, most common with the antimetabolites and antibiotics, reflect damage to the oral mucosa.

(i) Symptoms may range from mild inflammation to ulcerations of the mouth.

(ii) Mouth ulcers may warrant drug discontinuation until the ulcers heal. When therapy resumes, dosages may need to be reduced.

(iii) Treatment is symptomatic (e.g., local anesthetics); generally, lesions heal within 7 to 10 days.

(c) **Diarrhea** reflects irritation of the bowel mucosa resulting from death of gastrointestinal tract cells. This adverse effect is most likely to occur with the antimetabolites (especially methotrexte).

(3) **Alopecia** (hair loss) stems from damage to hair follicles.

(a) Chemotherapeutic drugs may cause loss of some or all hair—eyelashes, eyebrows, and axillary hair as well as scalp hair.

(b) Hair loss typically begins 1 to 2 weeks after chemotherapy begins and progresses as therapy continues.

(c) The degree of alopecia varies with the drug administered. Some drugs cause only hair thinning; others, total baldness. Doxorubicin is associated with a high incidence of alopecia; other agents only occasionally cause significant hair loss.

(d) Usually, alopecia is reversible, with hair regrowth beginning about 8 weeks after chemotherapy ends. Sometimes, hair begins to regrow during chemotherapy. Regrowth may be a different color or texture than the original hair.

(4) **Local tissue damage**. Spillage or extravasation (escape of medication from the vein into neighboring tissue) can seriously damage tissue. Significant damage is most likely to occur with extravasation of such agents as doxorubicin, daunorubicin, dactinomycin, plicamycin, mitomycin, and mechlorethamine.

(a) **Signs and symptoms** of extravasation include pain, itching, burning, stinging, inflammation, swelling, and temperature changes. Within a few weeks, necrosis, sloughing, or ulceration may occur, accompanied by severe pain.

Table 47-2. Relative Incidence of Nausea and Vomiting Associated with Major Chemotherapeutic Agents

Very High (90% or More)	High (60%–90%)	Moderate (30%–60%)	Low (10%–30%)	Very Low (<10%)
Cisplatin	Carmustine	Asparaginase	Bleomycin	Busulfan
Dacarbazine	Cyclophosphamide	Daunorubicin	Cytarabine	Chlorambucil
Mechlorethamine	Dactinomycin	Doxorubicin	Etoposide	Thioguanine
Streptozocin	Ifosfamide	Fluorouracil	Hydroxyurea	Vincristine
	Lomustine	Mitomycin	Melphalan	
	Plicamycin	Mitoxantrone	Mercaptopurine	
	Procarbazine		Methotrexate	
			Tamoxifen	
			Thiotepa	
			Vinblastine	

(b) **Causes** of extravasation include improper injection technique, inappropriate equipment or injection site, accidental needle or catheter movement, and fragile veins.

(c) To **prevent** extravasation, the following measures should be taken.
  (i) A clean venipuncture should be performed.
  (ii) The needle should be taped securely; proper needle placement should be verified.
  (iii) During drug administration, the injection site should be observed frequently for infiltration and erythema.

(d) **Management** of extravasation includes the following measures.
  (i) The infusion should be stopped and the needle left in place. An empty syringe may be fitted onto the needle to try to aspirate the drug out of the area.
  (ii) A corticosteroid may be instilled to reduce local inflammation.
  (iii) To treat extravasation of **doxorubicin**, some experts recommend injection of sodium bicarbonate through the needle to reduce cell metabolism and thus minimize damage. However, this step is controversial because sodium bicarbonate itself may cause tissue damage.
  (iv) Ice may be applied after the IV line is removed. Heat is often recommended after extravasation of a **vinca alkaloid**.
  (v) Severe extravasation causing an extensive lesion may necessitate skin grafting via plastic surgery.

(e) Because some chemotherapeutic agents may be mutagenic, carcinogenic, or teratogenic, health care personnel who prepare and administer chemotherapy should learn and follow **safe handling guidelines**.
  (i) Every pharmacy that prepares chemotherapeutic dosage forms should establish safe handling guidelines and thoroughly train personnel to follow them.
  (ii) The American Society of Hospital Pharmacists and the Occupational Safety and Health Administration are among several organizations that have established guidelines for the storage, preparation, administration, and disposal of chemotherapeutic agents. Specific guidelines used in hospitals and other institutions may vary.

d. Drug-specific toxicities

(1) Doxorubicin, daunorubicin, and mitoxantrone: **Cardiotoxicity**. These agents may lead to early or chronic cardiac effects.
  (a) Early effects include electrocardiographic (ECG) changes (e.g., sinus tachycardia, flattened T waves, ST-segment depression) and arrhythmias.
  (b) Chronic cardiotoxicity, manifested by cardiomyopathy, is dose-related and cumulative.
    (i) The **maximum cumulative lifetime** dose of doxorubicin and daunorubicin should be limited to 550 mg/m^2 of the body surface area. The maximum cumulative dose of mitoxantrone is 140 mg/m^2 of body surface area.
    (ii) Risk factors for cardiomyopathy include advanced age (over 70), prior radiation therapy that included the heart in the radiation port, preexisting heart disease, and concurrent or prior administration of another drug with cardiotoxic potential. The presence of any of these risk factors calls for discontinuation of doxorubicin or daunorubicin therapy after a cumulative lifetime dose of 400 mg/m^2 of the body surface area. Mitoxantrone should be discontinued before the cumulative dose of 140 mg/m^2 is reached.

(2) Vinca alkaloids: **Neurotoxicity**. Administration of vincristine and, to a lesser extent, vinblastine may lead to toxic neurologic effects.
  (a) **Peripheral neuropathy**, an early sign of neurotoxicity, frequently is manifested by tingling in the extremities.
  (b) Other signs and symptoms of neurotoxicity include loss of deep tendon reflexes, paresthesias, muscle weakness and cramps, constipation, urinary retention, ataxia, and cranial nerve palsies.
  (c) Neurotoxicity may warrant drug discontinuation.
  (d) To minimize the risk of neurotoxicity, vincristine should not be given in doses exceeding 2 mg.

(3) Cisplatin: **Renal toxicity**. This drug may cause dose-related renal tubular impairment.
  (a) Renal damage is cumulative; with high doses or repeated therapeutic courses, the damage may be irreversible, resulting in kidney failure.
  (b) The risk of renal toxicity can be minimized by initiating good hydration before chemotherapy and maintaining it for at least 24 to 48 hours afterward.
  (c) A diuretic (e.g., mannitol) may be given before and during cisplatin administration to reduce the risk of renal toxicity.

(4) **Cyclophosphamide: Bladder toxicity**. Hemorrhagic cystitis arises in up to 10% of patients receiving this drug.

(a) Toxicity presumably stems from bladder irritation caused by reactive drug metabolites.

(b) Signs and symptoms of hemorrhagic cystitis include dysuria, urinary frequency, hematuria, and pubic or lower abdominal pain. These problems usually call for temporary drug discontinuation.

(c) A high fluid intake during and for 48 hours after cyclophosphamide administration may help prevent bladder toxicity.

(5) **Bleomycin: Pulmonary toxicity**

(a) Signs and symptoms of drug-induced pulmonary toxicity include fine rales, cough, dyspnea, fever, and pulmonary infiltrates.

(b) Deterioration of pulmonary function may result in life-threatening pulmonary fibrosis (seen in approximately 1% of patients).

(c) Risk factors for pulmonary toxicity include advanced age (over 70), preexisting pulmonary disease, and a cumulative lifetime bleomycin dose exceeding 400 mg.

B. Other treatments. For cancers that initially manifest as localized tumors causing localized symptoms, **surgery** or **radiation therapy** may be indicated as the initial treatment.

1. **Surgery** may have both diagnostic and therapeutic value.

   a. **Biopsy** of surgically removed tissue permits histologic analysis and pathologic staging.

   b. Tumor removal may be curative, palliative, reconstructive, or rehabilitative.

2. **Radiation therapy** involves use of ionizing radiation to reduce the rate of cancer cell mitosis, to impair DNA synthesis, and for other actions aimed at cancer control.

   a. This treatment is used to control or arrest the development of various forms of cancer.

   b. In patients with certain inoperable cancers, radiation provides palliative treatment of symptoms.

3. **Combined modality therapy**

   a. **Surgery and radiation therapy** may be combined to increase the survival odds, avoid radical surgery, and preserve anatomical function.

   (1) **Preoperative radiation** can reduce a large tumor to an operable size as well as reduce the risk of perioperative disease spread.

   (2) **Postoperative radiation** can help prevent the proliferation or metastasis of residual cancer cells.

   b. **Systemic chemotherapy may be used after surgery, radiation therapy, or both.** This approach is especially suitable for the treatment of localized tumors that are likely to metastasize at an early stage and for which effective chemotherapy is available.

   (1) When administered after surgery, chemotherapy aims to eradicate microscopic residual cancer cell clusters along the tumor margins and helps prevent metastatic spread.

   (2) Recent studies show prolonged survival when adjuvant chemotherapy is administered to women who have undergone previous surgery for breast cancer.

STUDY QUESTIONS

Directions: Each question below contains five suggested answers. Choose the **one best** response to each question.

1. The growth of a malignant tumor is characterized by all of the following EXCEPT

A. genetic change passed on to each new cell
B. uncontrolled proliferation of the cancer cells
C. metastasis to other areas of the body
D. a constant continuously rapid rate of cell multiplication
E. invasiveness into neighboring tissue

2. A general effect of all cancer chemotherapy agents is

A. higher response rate to combination therapy
B. activity limited to tumor cells
C. cell-cycle–nonspecificity
D. dose-limiting myelosuppression
E. activity directed primarily against frequently replicating cells

3. All of the following are criteria for combination therapy with antineoplastic agents EXCEPT

A. they should employ different mechanisms of action
B. they should be physically compatible in the same intravenous solution
C. they should have non-overlapping side effects
D. they should have known activity as single agents
E. they should be administered at optimal doses and administration schedules

4. The most frequent dose-limiting adverse effect associated with cancer chemotherapy is

A. alopecia
B. mucositis
C. nausea and vomiting
D. myelosuppression
E. renal dysfunction

5. The nadir of white blood cell and platelet counts after administration of most cancer chemotherapeutic agents generally occurs

A. 3 to 5 days after treatment
B. 6 to 8 days after treatment
C. 10 to 14 days after treatment
D. 21 to 24 days after treatment
E. 28 to 35 days after treatment

6. Of the cancer chemotherapy agents listed, nausea and vomiting are most commonly associated with

A. cisplatin
B. vincristine
C. thioguanine
D. chlorambucil
E. busulfan

7. Cardiotoxicity is often associated with doxorubicin administration. Assuming no risk factors are present, at what cumulative dose should doxorubicin be discontinued?

A. 400 mg
B. 450 mg/m^2
C. 500 mg
D. 550 mg/m^2
E. 650 mg

8. To help prevent an episode of hemorrhagic cystitis during chemotherapy with cyclophosphamide, a patient should

A. abstain from alcoholic beverages for 48 hours
B. receive a corticosteroid for 48 hours
C. follow a low-salt diet beginning before chemotherapy
D. avoid aspirin or aspirin-containing products
E. drink plenty of water during and at least 48 hours after therapy

9. Which of the following agents is associated with delayed myelosuppression?

A. Methotrexate
B. Mitomycin
C. Mercaptopurine
D. Mechlorethamine
E. Megestrol acetate

10. The maximum cumulative lifetime dose of bleomycin is 400 mg because the drug is toxic to the

A. lungs
B. kidneys
C. liver
D. heart
E. pancreas

ANSWERS AND EXPLANATIONS

1. The answer is D. (*I F 1–5*) The growth of a malignant tumor is characterized by genetic change, uncontrolled proliferation, metastasis, and invasiveness. Tumor growth follows a Gompertzian growth pattern; that is, an initially rapid rate of growth followed by a plateau phase, not a continuously rapid growth.

2. The answer is E. (*III A 1*) A general effect of all cancer chemotherapy agents is activity directed primarily against frequently replicating cells. Some anticancer drugs are cell-cycle–specific, while others are cell-cycle–nonspecific. The activity of cancer chemotherapy agents is not limited to tumor cells, unfortunately: These agents also harm normal cells. While most chemotherapeutic agents produce myelosuppression, there are a few that are considered to be non-myelosuppressive.

3. The answer is B. [*III A 1 e (2)*] Combination therapy drugs should ideally have different mechanisms of action, have different side effects, have known activity as single agents, and should be administered at optimal doses and administration schedules. The only answer that is not a criterion for combination therapy is that they should be physically compatible in the same intravenous solution. This is not necessary for drugs to be effective in combination.

4. The answer is D. [*III A 7 c (1)*] The most frequent dose-limiting side effect associated with cancer chemotherapy is myelosuppression. With few exceptions, almost every antineoplastic agent will cause bone marrow suppression. Although alopecia and nausea and vomiting are common adverse effects, their incidence and severity varies with the agent employed. Mucositis is common with some agents but may not occur with others. Only a few chemotherapeutic agents are associated with significant renal dysfunction.

5. The answer is C. [*III A 7 c (1) (a)*] The point of maximum bone marrow suppression, characterized by the nadir of the white blood cell and platelet counts, generally occurs 10 to 14 days after administration of cancer chemotherapy. Although the levels of these cells may begin to decline earlier, the suppression is maximal as stated above. Cell counts generally recover around day 21. Only a few drugs are associated with delayed marrow suppression, which would produce maximum suppression at 4 to 5 weeks.

6. The answer is A. [*III A 7 c (2) (a); Table 47-2*] The frequency of nausea and vomiting associated with cancer chemotherapeutic agents is presented in Table 47-2. From the table it can be seen that the incidence of gastric distress is quite variable, ranging from less than 10% for busulfan, chlorambucil, thioguanine, and vincristine, to 90% or more for cisplatin.

7. The answer is D. [*III A 7 d (1) (b) (i)*] The chronic cardiotoxicity associated with doxorubicin requires that the maximum cumulative lifetime dose be limited to 550 mg/m^2 of the body surface area. Risk factors include advanced age (over 70 years of age), prior radiation therapy that included the heart in the radiation port, preexisting heart disease, and prior or concurrent administration of another drug with cardiotoxic potential.

8. The answer is E. [*III A 7 d (4) (c)*] Hemorrhagic cystitis may occur during chemotherapy with cyclophosphamide. Prevention is best accomplished with the consumption of plenty of water during and at least 48 hours after therapy. Abstention from alcohol, corticosteroid administration, a low-salt diet, or avoidance of aspirin—or aspirin-containing compounds—will not prevent or minimize the damage.

9. The answer is B. [*III A 7 c (1) (d)*] Delayed marrow suppression is unusual with cancer chemotherapy, but it does occur with a few drugs, notably mitomycin and the nitrosoureas (carmustine, lomustine, streptozocin). Bone marrow suppression most commonly occurs within the first 2 weeks after administration of chemotherapy, reaching a maximum in 10 to 14 days; this would be the case with methotrexate, mercaptopurine, and mechlorethamine. Megetrol, a hormonal agent, is not marrow-suppressive.

10. The answer is A. [*III A 7 d (5)*] Because bleomycin is potentially harmful to the lungs, the maximum cumulative lifetime dose of this drug is 400 mg. Bleomycin is not generally associated with damage to the liver, heart, or pancreas. Although this agent is primarily eliminated from the body through the kidneys, it is not a renal toxin.

Appendix A: Prescription Dispensing Information

Prescriptions

PARTS OF A PRESCRIPTION

A prescription is an order for medication issued by a physician, dentist, veterinarian, or other properly licensed medical practitioner (prescriber) to be filled by a pharmacist and used by the patient. Medication orders are similar to prescriptions but are intended for patients in an institutional setting.

A prescription generally contains the following information:

1. Name, address, and age of the patient
2. Date on which the prescription was written
3. Superscription symbol, or ℞, meaning "take thou" or "recipe"
4. Inscription, the name and amount of medication prescribed
5. Subscription, the dispensing and compounding instructions to the pharmacist
6. Signa or Sig, the directions to the patient
7. Signature of the prescriber
8. Name, address, and telephone number of the prescriber
9. Drug Enforcement Agency (DEA) registry number for controlled substances
10. Refill information

The following is an example of a prescription for a common generic drug:

Noel Legraphs, M.D.
3917 Wellspring Lane
Boston, MA 02115

(617) 123-4567 Date: 2/05/89

Name: John Smith Age: 28
Address: Brookline, MA 02146

℞

Penicillin VK 250 mg

Disp. tabs #40

Sig: One tablet q.i.d. for 10 days

______________ M.D.

Refills 1 DEA #

The following is an example of a prescription that requires extemporaneous compounding:

Noel Legraphs, M.D.
3917 Wellspring Lane
Boston, MA 02115

(617) 123-4567 Date: 2/05/89

Name: John Smith Age: 28
Address: Brookline, MA 02146

℞

Codeine phosphate 0.24 g
Ammonium chloride 7.2 g
Phenergan expectorant
qs ad 120.0 ml

M. et ft syrup

Sig: One tsp q 4 to 6 hr prn cough

______________ M.D.

Refills 0 DEA #

THE PRESCRIPTION LABEL

The prescription label should provide accurate and specific information to the patient for identification and use of the medication so that proper compliance by the patient may be attained. A prescription label usually contains the following information:

1. Pharmacy name and address
2. Prescription number
3. Date on which the prescription was dispensed
4. Name of the physician
5. Name of the patient
6. Directions for use of the medication
7. Name of the medication, including potency and quantity. A compounded prescription containing more than two ingredients generally does not have all the ingredients labeled.
8. Initials of the pharmacist
9. Expiration date or beyond-use date of the medication
10. Appropriate auxiliary or strip labels, as needed
11. For generic medication, the manufacturer's name or abbreviation

Additional information may be included on the label according to local state law.

```
LEGRAPHS                102 MAIN ST.
                        EVERYWHERE, PA
711942870               03/22/89
JOHN SMITH              H.B. JONES, M.D.

TAKE 1 TABLET 4 TIMES A DAY FOR
10 DAYS
                        0040TB REFILLS 0
PENICILLIN  VK  250MG TABL
UNITE POTENCY EXP 03/90

FINISH ALL THIS MEDICATION
TAKE ON EMPTY STOMACH
```

AUXILIARY LABELS

Auxiliary, or strip, labels should attract the patient's attention and should contain special additional information regarding the use of and the precautions and/or storage conditions for the medication. Generally, auxiliary labels should use positive statements, such as "For the ear," as opposed to negative statements, such as "Not to be swallowed." If appropriate, auxiliary labels in Spanish or other language may be helpful for the patient.

An auxiliary label for suspensions and emulsions might read "Shake well"; for heat-sensitive materials such as insulin, "Keep in refrigerator"; for topical ointments and creams, "For external use only." A positive statement indicates exactly where the product is to be instilled or applied, e.g., "For the ear." Warnings concerning alcohol consumption, exposure to sunlight, and possible discoloration of urine or feces may also appear on labels.

Appendix B: Common Prescription Drugs

Generic Drugs

Generic Name	Brand Name	Company	Category
Acetaminophen/codeine*	Tylenol/Codeine	McNeil	Non-opioid/opioid analgesic
Acyclovir	Zovirax	Burroughs Wellcome	Antiviral
Albuterol*	Ventolin Aerosol	Allen & Hanbury (Glaxo)	Beta-2 adrenergic bronchodilator
	Proventil Aerosol	Schering	Beta-2 adrenergic bronchodilator
Allopurinol	Zyloprim	Burroughs Wellcome	Xanthine oxidase inhibitor (reduces uric acid)
Alprazolam	Xanax	Upjohn	Benzodiazepine, anti-anxiety
Amiloride HCl/hydrochlorothiazide	Moduretic	Merck Sharp & Dohme	Diuretic/antihypertensive
Amitriptyline hydrochloride*	Elavil	Merck Sharp & Dohme	Tricylic antidepressant
Amoxicillin*	Trimox	Squibb	Penicillin antibiotic
	Polymox	Bristol	Penicillin antibiotic
	Amoxil	Beecham	Penicillin antibiotic
	Wymox	Wyeth-Ayerst	Penicillin antibiotic
Amoxicillin/clavulanate potassium	Augmentin	Beecham	Penicillin antibiotic/beta lactamase inhibitor
Ampicillin*	Totacillin	Beecham	Penicillin antibiotic
	Amcill	Warner Chilcott	Penicillin antibiotic
	Omnipen	Wyeth-Ayerst	Penicillin antibiotic
Atenolol	Tenormin	ICI Pharma	Beta adrenergic blocker
Atenolol/chlorthalidone	Tenoretic	ICI Pharma	Beta adrenergic blocker/diuretic
Azatadine maleate/pseudoephedrine sulfate	Trinalin	Schering	Antihistamine/decongestant
Betaxolol hydrochloride	Betoptic	Alcon	Cardioselective beta-1 adrenergic receptor blocking agent (ophthalmic)
Bumetanide	Bumex	Roche	Loop diuretic
Buspirone hydrochoride	BuSpar	Mead Johnson	Anxiolytic
Butalbital/acetaminophen/caffeine	Fioricet	Sandoz	Sedative/analgesic
Butalbital/aspirin/caffeine*	Fiorinal	Sandoz	Sedative/analgesic
Butalbital/aspirin/caffeine/codeine	Fiorinal/Codeine	Sandoz	Sedative/analgesic
Captopril	Capoten	Squibb	Angiotensin converting enzyme (ACE) inhibitor/antihypertensive
Carbamazepine*	Tegretol	Geigy	Anticonvulsant
Carbidopa/levodopa	Sinemet	Merck Sharp & Dohme	Aromatic amino acid decarboxylase inhibitor/antihypertensive
Cefaclor	Ceclor	Lilly	Cephalosporin antibiotic
Cefadroxil monohydrate	Duricef	Mead Johnson	Cephalosporin antibiotic
Cefuroxime axetil	Ceftin	Allen & Hanbury (Glaxo)	Cephalosporin antibiotic
Cephalexin	Keftab	Dista	Cephalosporin antibiotic
Cephalexin*	Keflex	Dista	Cephalosporin antibiotic

*Generic product available.

Continued on next page

Generic Drugs—*Continued*

Generic Name	Brand Name	Company	Category
Chlorpheniramine maleate d-pseudoephedrine HCl	Deconamine	Berlex	Antihistamine/decongestant
Chlorpropamide*	Diabinese	Pfizer	Oral hypoglycemic
Chlorthalidone*	Hygroton	Rorer	Diuretic/antihypertensive
Chlorzoxazone	Parafon Forte DSC	McNeil	Skeletal muscle relaxant
Cimetidine	Tagamet	Smith Kline & French	Histamine H_2 receptor antagonist
Clemastine fumarate/phenylpropanolamine hydrochloride	Tavist-D	Sandoz	Antihistamine/nasal decongestant
Clindamycin phosphate	Cleocin T	Upjohn	Antibiotic (topical)
Clonidine hydrochloride	Catapres	Boehringer Ingelheim	Antihypertensive
Clorazepate dipotassium*	Tranxene	Abbott	Benzodiazepine
Clotrimazole	Lotrimin	Schering	Antifungal
	Gyne-Lotrimin	Schering	Antifungal
Clotrimazole/betamethasone	Lotrisone	Schering	Antifungal/corticosteroid topical cream
Codeine phosphate/iodinated glycerol*	Tussi-Organidin	Wallace	Antitussive/mucolytic expectorant
Codeine phosphate/iodinated glycerol/dextromethorphan*	Tussi-Organidin DM	Wallace	Antitussive/mucolytic expectorant
Conjugated estrogens	Premarin Oral	Wyeth-Ayerst	Estrogenic agent
Cromolyn sodium*	Intal	Fisons	Mast cell stabilizer/antiallergy
	Nasalcrom	Fisons	Mast cell stabilizer/antiallergic nasal solution
Crystalline warfarin sodium	Coumadin Oral	Du Pont	Oral anticoagulant
Cyclobenzaprine hydrochloride	Flexeril	Merck Sharp & Dohme	Muscle relaxant
Desipramine hydrochloride*	Norpramin	Merrell Dow	Tricyclic antidepressant
Desoximetasone	Topicort	Hoechst-Roussel	Corticosteroid (topical)
Diazepam*	Valium	Roche	Benzodiazepine
Dicyclomine hydrochloride*	Bentyl	Lakeside	Antispasmodic-irritable bowel syndrome
Diflunisal	Dolobid	Merck Sharp & Dohme	Nonsteroidal anti-inflammatory agent (NSAID)
Digoxin*	Lanoxin	Burroughs Wellcome	Cardiac glycoside
Diltiazem hydrochloride*	Cardizem	Marion	Calcium ion influx inhibitor
Diphenoxylate HCl/atropine sulfate*	Lomotil	Searle	Antispasmodic/anticholinergic (antidiarrheal combination)
Dipivefrin hydrochloride (dipvalyl epinephrine)	Propine	Allergan	Antiglaucoma
Dipyridamole*	Persantine	Boehringer Ingelheim	Coronary vasodilator
Doxepin hydrochloride*	Sinequan	Roerig	Psychotropic/antianxiety
Enalapril maleate	Vasotec	Merck Sharp & Dohme	Angiotensin converting enzyme (ACE) inhibitor/antihypertensive
Erythromycin ethylsuccinate*	E.E.S	Abbott	Macrolide antibiotic
	Erythrocin	Abbott	Macrolide antibiotic
Erythromycin ethylsuccinate/sulfisoxazole acetyl*	Pediazole	Ross	Antibiotic combination (otitis media)

Erythromycin stearate*	Erythrocin stearate	Abbott	Macrolide antibiotic
Erythromycin*	PCE	Abbott	Macrolide antibiotic (enteric coated particles)
	Ery-Tab	Abbott	Macrolide antibiotic delayed release (enteric coated tablet)
	E-Mycin	Upjohn	Macrolide antibiotic (enteric coated)
	ERYC	Parke-Davis	Macrolide antibiotic (delayed release)
	E-Mycin 333	Upjohn	Macrolide antibiotic
Extended phenytoin sodium	Dilantin Sodium	Parke-Davis	Antiepileptic
Fenoprofen calcium*	Nalfon	Dista	Nonsteroidal anti-inflammatory agent (NSAID)
Flunisolide	Nasalide	Syntex	Topical anti-inflammatory steroid (nasal solution)
Fluocinonide*	Lidex	Syntex	Corticosteroid topical cream
Fluoxetine hydrochloride	Prozac	Dista	Antidepressant
Flurazepam hydrochloride*	Dalmane	Roche	Benzodiazepine
Furosemide*	Lasix Oral	Hoechst-Roussel	Diuretic
Gemfibrozil	Lopid	Parke-Davis	Lipid regulating agent
Glipizide	Glucotrol	Roerig	Oral hypoglycemic
Glyburide	DiaBeta	Hoechst-Roussel	Oral hypoglycemic
Glyburide	Micronase	Upjohn	Oral hypoglycemic
Haloperidol*	Haldol	McNeil	Major tranquilizer/psychotropic
Hydrochlorothiazide*	HydroDIURIL	Merck Sharp & Dohme	Diuretic/antihypertensive
Hydrocodone bitartrate*	Vicodin	Knoll	Opioid analgesic
Hydrocodone polistirex/phenyltoloxamine polistirex	Tussionex	Pennwalt	Narcotic antitussive/antihistamine (Pennkinetic extended release suspension)
Hydrocortisone combination suppository*	Anusol-HC	Parke-Davis	Hydrocortisone combination hemorrhoidal rectal suppository
Hydroxyzine hydrochloride*	Atarax	Roerig	Antianxiety/antihistamine
Ibuprofen*	Motrin	Upjohn	Nonsteroidal anti-inflammatory agent (NSAID)
	Rufen	Boots-Flint	Nonsteroidal anti-inflammatory agent (NSAID)
Indapamide	Lozol	Rorer	Antihypertensive/diuretic
Indomethacin*	Indocin SR	Merck Sharp & Dohme	Nonsteroidal anti-inflammatory agent (NSAID), sustained release
Indomethacin*	Indocin	Merck Sharp & Dohme	Nonsteroidal anti-inflammatory agent (NSAID)
Ipratropium bromide	Atrovent	Boehringer Ingelheim	Anticholinergic bronchodilator
Isophane	Iletin I NPH	Lilly	Insulin (beef-pork)
Isophane NPH insulin	Humulin N	Lilly	Insulin (human)
Isosorbide dinitrate*	Isordil	Wyeth-Ayerst	Coronary vasodilator
Ketoconazole	Nizoral	Janssen	Antifungal
Labetalol hydrochloride	Normodyne	Key	Adrenergic blocker/antihypertensive
Levonorgestrel/ethinyl estradiol	Triphasil-28	Wyeth-Ayerst	Combination oral contraceptive
Levothyroxine sodium*	Synthroid	Boots-Flint	Thyroid hormone
Loperamide hydrochloride	Immodium	Janssen	Antidiarrheal
Lorazepam*	Ativan	Wyeth-Ayerst	Benzodiazepine

*Generic product available.

Continued on next page

Generic Drugs—*Continued*

Generic Name	Brand Name	Company	Category
Meclizine hydrochloride*	Antivert	Roerig	Antihistamine
Medroxyprogesterone Acetate*	Provera	Upjohn	Progestational agent
Metaproterenol sulfate*	Alupent Aerosol	Boehringer Ingelheim	Beta adrenergic bronchodilator
	Alupent Syrup	Boehringer Ingelheim	Beta adrenergic bronchodilator
Methyldopate hydrochloride*	Aldomet	Merck Sharp & Dohme	Antihypertensive
Methyldopa/hydrochlorothiazide*	Aldoril	Merck Sharp & Dohme	Antihypertensive/diuretic
Methylphenidate hydrochloride*	Ritalin	CIBA	Mild central nervous system stimulant
Methylprednisolone*	Medrol Oral	Upjohn	Glucocorticoid
Metoclopramide hydrochloride*	Reglan	Robins	Upper GI (gastrointestinal) tract motility stimulator
Metoprolol tartrate	Lopressor	Geigy	Beta adrenergic blocker
Miconazole nitrate	Monistat Dual-Pak	Ortho	Antifungal vaginal suppository and cream with applicator
	Monistat-7	Ortho	Antifungal vaginal suppository
Minocycline hydrochloride	Minocin	Lederle	Tetracycline antibiotic
Multivitamin and fluoride supplement	Poly-Vi-Flor	Mead Johnson	Multivitamin and fluoride supplement drops
Multivitamin/multimineral combination	Stuartnatal 1 + 1	Stuart	Multivitamin/multimineral pre- or postnatal supplement
Nadolol	Corgard	Princeton	Beta adrenergic blocker
Naproxen	Naprosyn	Syntex	Nonsteroidal anti-inflammatory agent (NSAID)
Naproxen sodium	Anaprox	Syntex	Nonsteroidal anti-inflammatory agent (NSAID/analgesic)
Nicotine polacrilex	Nicorette	Lakeside	Nicotine gum
Nifedipine*	Procardia	Pfizer	Calcium ion channel blocker
Nitrofurantoin macrocrystals	Macrodantin	Norwich Eaton	Antibacterial
Nitroglycerin*	Nitrostat	Parke-Davis	Coronary vasodilator/anti-anginal agent
	Nitro-Bid	Marion	Coronary vasodilator
	Transderm-Nitro	CIBA	Coronary vasodilator/anti-anginal agent
	Nitro-Dur II	Key	Coronary vasodilator (transdermal)
Norethindrone/ethinyl estradiol*	Ortho-Novum 7/7/7-28	Ortho	Combination oral contraceptive
	Ortho-Novum 1/35-21	Ortho	Combination oral contraceptive
	Ortho-Novum 1/35-28	Ortho	Combination oral contraceptive
	Ortho-Novum 7/7/7-21	Ortho	Combination oral contraceptive
	Ovcon	Mead Johnson	Combination oral contraceptive
	Tri-Norinyl	Syntex	Combination oral contraceptive
Norethindrone/mestranol*	Ortho-Novum 1/50-28	Ortho	Combination oral contraceptive
	Ortho-Novum 1/50-21	Ortho	Combination oral contraceptive
Norgestrel/ethinyl estradiol*	Lo/Ovral-28	Wyeth-Ayerst	Combination oral contraceptive
	Lo/Ovral-21	Wyeth-Ayerst	Combination oral contraceptive
Nortriptyline hydrochloride	Pamelor	Sandoz	Antidepressant
Oxazepam*	Serax	Wyeth-Ayerst	Benzodiazepine
Oxycodone/acetaminophen*	Tylox	McNeil	Opioid/non-opioid analgesic
	Percocet-5	Du Pont	Opioid/non-opioid analgesic
Oxycodone/aspirin*	Percodan	Du Pont	Opioid/non-opioid analgesic

Penicillin VK (potassium)*	Veetids	Squibb	Penicillin antibiotic
	V-Cillin K	Lilly	Penicillin antibiotic
	Pen-Vee K	Wyeth-Ayerst	Penicillin antibiotic
	LEDERCILLIN VK	Lederle	Penicillin antibiotic
	Beepen-VK	Beecham	Penicillin antibiotic
	Betapen-VK	Bristol	Penicillin antibiotic
Pentazocine HCl/naloxone HCl	Talwin-Nx	Winthrop	Strong analgesic/narcotic antagonist
Pentoxifylline	Trental	Hoechst-Roussel	Improves blood flow in chronic occlusive artery disease
Perphenazine/amitriptyline*	Triavil	Merck Sharp & Dohme	Antipsychotic/antidepressant
Phenobarbital*	Phenobarbital	Lilly	Barbiturate
Phenobarbital/belladonna alkaloids*	Donnatal	Robins	Barbiturate/belladonna alkaloids (hydroscyamine sulfate; atropine sulfate; scopolamine hydrobromide anticholinergic)
Phenylephrine/chlorpheniramine tannates	Rynatan	Wallace	Nasal decongestant/antihistamine combination
Phenylpropanolamine hydrochloride combination	Naldecon	Bristol	Nasal decongestant/antihistamine combination (phenylpropanolamine HCl/phenylephrine HCl/phenyltoloxamine)
Phenylpropanolamine hydrochloride /guaifenesin*	Entex LA	Norwich Eaton	Decongestant/expectorant (long acting)
Piroxicam	Feldene	Pfizer	Nonsteroidal anti-inflammatory agent (NSAID)
Polymyxin B/neomycin/hydrocortisone*	Cortisporin Otic	Burroughs Wellcome	Antibiotic/corticosteroid combination
Potassium chloride*	Slow-K	CIBA	Potassium supplement
	Klotrix	Mead Johnson	Potassium supplement
	Micro-K 10	Robins	Potassium supplement
	K-Tab	Abbott	Potassium supplement
	Micro-K	Robins	Potassium supplement
Prazepam	Centrax	Parke-Davis	Benzodiazepine
Prazosin hydrochloride	Minipress	Pfizer	Antihypertensive
Prednisone*	Deltasone	Upjohn	Corticosteroid
	Orasone	Reid-Rowell	Corticosteroid
Prednisone acetate/sodium sulfacetamide	Bleph-10	Allergan	Corticosteroid/antibiotic (ophthalmic)
Prochlorperazine*	Compazine	Smith Kline & French	Phenothiazine antinauseant
Promethazine HCl/codeine phosphate*	Phenergan/codeine	Wyeth-Ayerst	Phenothiazine antihistamine/opioid analgesic-antitussive
Promethazine hydrochloride*	Phenergan	Wyeth-Ayerst	Phenothiazine/antihistamine
Propoxyphene napsylate/acetaminophen*	Darvocet-N-100	Lilly	Analgesic
Propranolol hydrochloride	Inderal LA	Wyeth-Ayerst	Beta adrenergic blocker
Propranolol hydrochloride*	Inderal	Wyeth-Ayerst	Beta adrenergic blocker
Ranitidine hydrochloride	Zantac	Glaxo	Histamine H_2 receptor antagonist
Sucralfate	Carafate	Marion	Anti-ulcer
Sulindac	Clinoril	Merck Sharp & Dohme	Nonsteroidal anti-inflammatory agent (NSAID)
Temazepam*	Restoril	Sandoz	Benzodiazepine

*Generic product available.

Continued on next page

Generic Drugs—*Continued*

Generic Name	Brand Name	Company	Category
Terbutaline sulfate	Brethine	Geigy	Beta adrenergic bronchodilator
Terfenadine	Seldane	Merrell Dow	Antihistamine
Tetracycline hydrochloride*	Sumycin	Squibb	Tetracycline antibiotic
	Achromycin V	Lederle	Tetracycline antibiotic
Theophylline anhydrous*	Theo-Dur	Key	Bronchodilator
	Slo-bid	Rorer	Bronchodilator (timed release)
Thiothixene hydrochloride*	Navane	Roerig	Psychotropic
Thioridazine hydrochloride*	Mellaril	Sandoz	Phenothiazine psychotropic
Timolal maleate	Timoptic	Merck Sharp & Dohme	Intraocular pressure lowering agent in glaucoma treatment
Tobramycin	Tobrex	Alcon	Aminoglycoside antibiotic (ophthalmic)
Tolmetin sodium	Tolectin DS	McNeil	Nonsteroidal anti-inflammatory agent (NSAID)
Trazodone hydrochloride*	Desyrel	Mead Johnson	Antidepressant
Tretinoin	Retin-A Acne	Ortho	Retinoic acid (vitamin A) topical
Triamterene/hydrochlorothiazide	Maxzide	Lederle	Diuretic/antihypertensive
Triamterene/hydrochlorothiazide*	Dyazide	Smith Kline & French	Diuretic/antihypertensive
Triazolam	Halcion	Upjohn	Triazolbenzodiazepine, hypnotic
Trimethoprim/sulfamethoxazole*	Bactrim DS	Roche	Antifolate/antibacterial (double strength)
	Septra DS	Burroughs Wellcome	Antifolate/antibacterial (double strength)
	Septra	Burroughs Wellcome	Antifolate/antibacterial
Verapamil hydrochloride	Calan SR	Searle	Slow channel calcium blocker (sustained release)
Verapamil hydrochloride*	Calan	Searle	Slow channel calcium blocker

*Generic product available.

Brand Drugs

Brand Name	Generic Name	Company	Category
Achromycin V	Tetracycline hydrochloride*	Lederle	Tetracycline antibiotic
Aldomet	Methyldopate hydrochloride*	Merck Sharp & Dohme	Antihypertensive
Aldoril	Methyldopa/hydrochlorothiazide	Merck Sharp & Dohme	Antihypertensive/diuretic
Alupent Aerosol	Metaproterenol sulfate*	Boehringer Ingelheim	Beta adrenergic bronchodilator
Alupent Syrup	Metaproterenol sulfate*	Boehringer Ingelheim	Beta adrenergic bronchodilator
Amcill	Ampicillin*	Warner Chilcott	Penicillin antibiotic
Amoxil	Amoxicillin*	Beecham	Penicillin antibiotic
Anaprox	Naproxen sodium	Syntex	Nonsteroidal anti-inflammatory agent (NSAID)/analgesic
Antivert	Meclizine hydrochloride*	Roerig	Antihistamine
Anusol-HC	Hydrocortisone combination suppository	Parke-Davis	Hydrocortisone combination hemorrhoidal rectal suppository
Atarax	Hydroxyzine hydrochloride*	Roerig	Antianxiety/antihistamine
Ativan	Lorazepam	Wyeth-Ayerst	Benzodiazepine
Atrovent	Ipratropium bromide	Boehringer Ingelheim	Anticholinergic bronchodilator
Augmentin	Amoxicillin/clavulanate potassium	Beecham	Penicillin antibiotic/beta lactamase inhibitor
Bactrim DS	Trimethoprim/sulfamethoxazole	Roche	Antifolate/antibacterial (double strength)
Beepen-VK	Penicillin VK (potassium)*	Beecham	Penicillin antibiotic
Bentyl	Dicyclomine hydrochloride	Lakeside	Antispasmodic-irritable bowel syndrome
Betapen-VK	Penicillin VK (potassium)*	Bristol	Penicillin antibiotic
Betoptic	Betaxolol hydrochloride	Alcon	Cardioselective beta-1 adrenergic receptor blocking agent (ophthalmic)
Bleph-10	Prednisone acetate/sodium sulfacetamide	Allergan	Corticosteroid/antibiotic (ophthalmic)
Brethine	Terbutaline sulfate	Geigy	Beta adrenergic bronchodilator
Bumex	Bumetanide	Roche	Loop diuretic
BuSpar	Buspirone hydrochloride	Mead Johnson	Anxiolytic
Calan	Verapamil hydrochloride*	Searle	Slow channel calcium blocker
Calan SR	Verapamil hydrochloride	Searle	Slow channel calcium blocker (sustained release)
Capoten	Captopril	Squibb	Angiotensin converting enzyme (ACE) inhibitor/ antihypertensive
Carafate	Sucralfate	Marion	Anti-ulcer
Cardizem	Diltiazem hydrochloride	Marion	Calcium ion influx inhibitor
Catapres	Clonidine hydrochloride	Boehringer Ingelheim	Antihypertensive
Ceclor	Cefaclor	Lilly	Cephalosporin antibiotic
Ceftin	Cefuroxime axetil	Allen & Hanbury (Glaxo)	Cephalosporin antibiotic
Centrax	Prazepam	Parke-Davis	Benzodiazepine

*Generic product available.

Continued on next page

Brand Drugs—*Continued*

Brand Name	Generic Name	Company	Category
Cleocin T	Clindamycin phosphate	Upjohn	Antibiotic (topical)
Clinoril	Sulindac	Merck Sharp & Dohme	Nonsteroidal anti-inflammatory agent (NSAID)
Compazine	Prochlorperazine	Smith Kline & French	Phenothiazine antinauseant
Corgard	Nadolol	Princeton	Beta adrenergic blocker
Cortisporin Otic	Polymyxin B/neomycin/hydrocortisone	Burroughs Wellcome	Antibiotic/corticosteroid combination
Coumadin Oral	Crystalline Warfarin Sodium	Du Pont	Oral anticoagulant
Dalmane	Flurazepam hydrochloride	Roche	Benzodiazepine
Darvocet-N-100	Propoxyphene napsylate/acetaminophen	Lilly	Analgesic
Deconamine	Chlorpheniramine maleate/ d-pseudoephedrine HCl	Berlex	Antihistamine/decongestant
Deltasone	Prednisone*	Upjohn	Corticosteroid
Desyrel	Trazodone hydrochloride	Mead Johnson	Antidepressant
DiaBeta	Glyburide	Hoechst-Roussel	Oral hypoglycemic
Diabinese	Chlorpropamide	Pfizer	Oral hypoglycemic
Dilantin Sodium	Extended phenytoin sodium	Parke-Davis	Antiepileptic
Dolobid	Diflunisal	Merck Sharp & Dohme	Nonsteroidal anti-inflammatory agent (NSAID)
Donnatal	Phenobarbital/belladonna alkaloids	Robins	Barbiturate/belladonna alkaloids (hydroscyamine sulfate; atropine sulfate; scopolamine hydrobromide anticholinergic)
Duricef	Cefadroxil monohydrate	Mead Johnson	Cephalosporin antibiotic
Dyazide	Triamterene/hydrochlorothiazide*	Smith Kline & French	Diuretic/antihypertensive
Elavil	Amitriptyline hydrochloride*	Merck Sharp & Dohme	Tricyclic antidepressant
Entex LA	Phenylpropanolamine HCl/guaifenesin	Norwich Eaton	Decongestant/expectorant (long acting)
ERYC	Erythromycin*	Parke-Davis	Macrolide antibiotic (delayed release)
Erythrocin	Erythromycin ethylsuccinate*	Abbott	Macrolide antibiotic
Erythrocin stearate	Erythromycin stearate*	Abbott	Macrolide antibiotic
Ery-Tab	Erythromycin*	Abbott	Macrolide antibiotic delayed release (enteric coated tablet)
E-Mycin	Erythromycin*	Upjohn	Macrolide antibiotic (enteric coated)
E-Mycin 333	Erythromycin*	Upjohn	Macrolide antibiotic
E.E.S.	Erythromycin ethylsuccinate*	Abbott	Macrolide antibiotic
Feldene	Piroxicam	Pfizer	Nonsteroidal anti-inflammatory agent (NSAID)
Fioricet	Butalbital/acetaminophen/caffeine	Sandoz	Sedative/analgesic
Fiorinal	Butalbital/aspirin/caffeine	Sandoz	Sedative/analgesic
Fiorinal/Codeine	Butalbital/aspirin/caffeine/codeine	Sandoz	Sedative/analgesic
Flexeril	Cyclobenzaprine hydrochloride	Merck Sharp & Dohme	Muscle relaxant
Glucotrol	Glipizide	Roerig	Oral hypoglycemic
Gyne-Lotrimin	Clotrimazole*	Schering	Antifungal
Halcion	Triazolam	Upjohn	Triazolbenzodiazepine, hypnotic
Haldol	Haloperidol	McNeil	Major tranquilizer/psychotropic
Humulin N	Isophane NPH insulin	Lilly	Insulin (human)
HydroDIURIL	Hydrochlorothiazide*	Merck Sharp & Dohme	Diuretic/antihypertensive

Hygroton	Chlorthalidone*	Rorer	Diuretic/antihypertensive
Iletin I NPH	Isophane	Lilly	Insulin (beef-pork)
Immodium	Loperamide hydrochloride	Janssen	Antidiarrheal
Inderal	Propranolol hydrochloride*	Wyeth-Ayerst	Beta adrenergic blocker
Inderal LA	Propranolol hydrochloride	Wyeth-Ayerst	Beta adrenergic blocker
Indocin	Indomethacin*	Merck Sharp & Dohme	Nonsteroidal anti-inflammatory agent (NSAID)
Indocin SR	Indomethacin	Merck Sharp & Dohme	Nonsteroidal anti-inflammatory agent (NSAID), sustained release
Intal	Cromolyn sodium	Fisons	Mast cell stabilizer/antiallergy
Isordil	Isorbide dinitrate*	Wyeth-Ayerst	Coronary vasodilator
Keflex	Cephalexin*	Dista	Cephalosporin antibiotic
Keftab	Cephalexin	Dista	Cephalosporin antibiotic
Klotrix	Potassium chloride*	Mead Johnson	Potassium supplement
K-Tab	Potassium chloride*	Abbott	Potassium supplement
Lanoxin	Digoxin*	Burroughs Wellcome	Cardiac glycoside
Lasix Oral	Furosemide*	Hoechst-Roussel	Diuretic
LEDERCILLIN VK	Penicillin VK (potassium)*	Lederle	Penicillin antibiotic
Lidex	Fluocinonide	Syntex	Corticosteroid topical cream
Lomotil	Diphenoxylate HCl/atropine sulfate	Searle	Antispasmodic/anticholinergic (antidiarrheal combination)
Lopid	Gemfibrozil	Parke-Davis	Lipid regulating agent
Lopressor	Metoprolol tartrate	Geigy	Beta adrenergic blocker
Lotrimin	Clotrimazole	Schering	Antifungal
Lotrisone	Clotrimazole/betamethasone	Schering	Antifungal/corticosteroid topical cream
Lozol	Indapamide	Rorer	Antihypertensive/diuretic
Lo/Ovral-21	Norgestrel/ethinyl estradiol*	Wyeth-Ayerst	Combination oral contraceptive
Lo/Ovral-28	Norgestrel/ethinyl estradiol*	Wyeth-Ayerst	Combination oral contraceptive
Macrodantin	Nitrofurantoin macrocrystals	Norwich Eaton	Antibacterial
Maxzide	Triamterene/hydrochlorothiazide	Lederle	Diuretic/antihypertensive
Medrol Oral	Methylprednisolone	Upjohn	Glucocorticoid
Mellaril	Thioridazine hydrochloride*	Sandoz	Phenothiazine psychotropic
Micronase	Glyburide	Upjohn	Oral hypoglycemic
Micro-K	Potassium chloride*	Robins	Potassium supplement
Micro-K 10	Potassium chloride*	Robins	Potassium supplement
Minipress	Prazosin hydrochloride	Pfizer	Antihypertensive
Minocin	Minocycline hydrochloride	Lederle	Tetracycline antibiotic
Moduretic	Amiloride HCl/hydrochlorothiazide	Merck Sharp & Dohme	Diuretic/antihypertensive
Monistat Dual-Pak	Miconazole nitrate	Ortho	Antifungal vaginal suppository and cream with applicator
Monistat-7	Miconazole nitrate	Ortho	Antifungal vaginal suppository
Motrin	Ibuprofen*	Upjohn	Nonsteroidal anti-inflammatory agent (NSAID)
Naldecon	Phenylpropanolamine HCl combination	Bristol	Nasal decongestant/antihistamine combination (phenylpropanolamine HCl/phenylephrine HCl/phenyltoloxamine citrate/chlorpheniramine maleate)

*Generic product available.

Continued on next page

Brand Drugs—*Continued*

Brand Name	Generic Name	Company	Category
Nalfon	Fenoprofen calcium	Dista	Nonsteroidal anti-inflammatory agent (NSAID)
Naprosyn	Naproxen	Syntex	Nonsteroidal anti-inflammatory agent (NSAID)
Nasalcrom	Cromolyn sodium*	Fisons	Mast cell stabilizer/antiallergic nasal solution
Nasalide	Flunisolide	Syntex	Topical anti-inflammatory steroid (nasal solution)
Navane	Thiothixene hydrochloride	Roerig	Psychotropic
Nicorette	Nicotine polacrilex	Lakeside	Nicotine gum
Nitrostat	Nitroglycerin	Parke-Davis	Coronary vasodilator/anti-anginal agent
Nitro-Bid	Nitroglycerin	Marion	Coronary vasodilator
Nitro-Dur II	Nitroglycerin	Key	Coronary vasodilator (transdermal)
Nizoral	Ketoconazole	Janssen	Antifungal
Normodyne	Labetalol hydrochloride	Key	Adrenergic blocker/antihypertensive
Norpramin	Desipramine hydrochloride*	Merrell Dow	Tricyclic antidepressant
Omnipen	Ampicillin*	Wyeth-Ayerst	Penicillin antibiotic
Orasone	Prednisone*	Reid-Rowell	Corticosteroid
Ortho-Novum 1/35-21	Norethindrone/ethinyl estradiol*	Ortho	Combination oral contraceptive
Ortho-Novum 1/35-28	Norethindrone/ethinyl estradiol*	Ortho	Combination oral contraceptive
Ortho-Novum 1/50-21	Norethindrone/mestranol*	Ortho	Combination oral contraceptive
Ortho-Novum 1/50-28	Norethindrone/mestranol*	Ortho	Combination oral contraceptive
Ortho-Novum 7/7/7-21	Norethindrone/ethinyl estradiol*	Ortho	Combination oral contraceptive
Ortho-Novum 7/7/7-28	Norethindrone/ethinyl estradiol*	Ortho	Combination oral contraceptive
Ovcon	Norethindrone/ethinyl estradiol*	Mead Johnson	Combination oral contraceptive
Pamelor	Nortriptyline hydrochloride	Sandoz	Antidepressant
Parafon Forte DSC	Chlorzoxazone	McNeil	Skeletal muscle relaxant
PCE	Erythromycin*	Abbott	Macrolide antibiotic (enteric coated particles)
Pediazole	Erythromycin ethylsuccinate/ sulfisoxazole acetyl	Ross	Antibiotic combination (otitis media)
Pen-Vee K	Penicillin VK (potassium)*	Wyeth-Ayerst	Penicillin antibiotic
Percocet-5	Oxycodone/acetaminophen*	Du Pont	Opioid/non-opioid analgesic
Percodan	Oxycodone/aspirin*	Du Pont	Opioid/non-opioid analgesic
Persantine	Dipyridamole*	Boehringer Ingelheim	Coronary vasodilator
Phenergan	Promethazine hydrochloride	Wyeth-Ayerst	Phenothiazine/antihistamine
Phenergan/codeine	Promethazine HCl/codeine phosphate	Wyeth-Ayerst	Phenothiazine antihistamine/opioid analgesic-antitussive
Phenobarbital	Phenobarbital*	Lilly	Barbiturate
Polymox	Amoxicillin*	Bristol	Penicillin antibiotic
Poly-Vi-Flor	Multivitamin and fluoride supplement	Mead Johnson	Multivitamin and fluoride supplement drops
Premarin Oral	Conjugated estrogens	Wyeth-Ayerst	Estrogenic agent
Procardia	Nifedipine	Pfizer	Calcium ion channel blocker
Propine	Dipivefrin HCl (dipvalyl epinephrine)	Allergan	Antiglaucoma
Proventil Aerosol	Albuterol	Schering	Beta-2 adrenergic bronchodilator
Provera	Medroxyprogesterone Acetate	Upjohn	Progestational agent
Prozac	Fluoxetine hydrochloride	Dista	Antidepressant

Reglan	Metoclopramide hydrochloride*	Robins	Upper GI (gastrointestinal) tract motility stimulator
Restoril	Temazepam	Sandoz	Benzodiazepine
Retin-A Acne	Tretinoin	Ortho	Retinoic acid (vitamin A) topical
Ritalin	Methylphenidate hydrochloride	CIBA	Mild central nervous system stimulant
Rufen	Ibuprofen*	Boots-Flint	Nonsteroidal anti-inflammatory agent (NSAID)
Rynatan	Phenylephrine/chlorpheniramine/ pyrilamine tannates	Wallace	Nasal decongestant/antihistamine combination
Seldane	Terfenadine	Merrell Dow	Antihistamine
Septra	Trimethoprim/sulfamethoxazole*	Burroughs Wellcome	Antifolate/antibacterial
Septra DS	Trimethoprim/sulfamethoxazole	Burroughs Wellcome	Antifolate/antibacterial (double strength)
Serax	Oxazepam	Wyeth-Ayerst	Benzodiazepine
Sinemet	Carbidopa/levodopa	Merck Sharp & Dohme	Aromatic amino acid decarboxylase inhibitor/ antihypertensive
Sinequan	Doxepin hydrochloride	Roerig	Psychotropic/antianxiety
Slow-K	Potassium chloride*	CIBA	Potassium supplement
Slo-bid	Theophylline anhydrous*	Rorer	Bronchodilator (timed released)
Stuartnatal 1 + 1	Multivitamin/multimineral combination	Stuart	Multivitamin/multimineral pre- or postnatal supplement
Sumycin	Tetracycline hydrochloride*	Squibb	Tetracycline antibiotic
Synthroid	Levothyroxine sodium +	Boots-Flint	Thyroid hormone
Tagamet	Cimetidine	Smith Kline & French	Histamine H_2 receptor antagonist
Talwin Nx	Pentazocine HCl/naloxone HCl	Winthrop	Strong analgesic/narcotic antagonist
Tavist-D	Clemastine fumarate/ phenylpropanolamine HCl	Sandoz	Antihistamine/nasal decongestant
Tegretol	Carbamazepine	Geigy	Anticonvulsant
Tenoretic	Atenolol/chlorthalidone	ICI Pharma	Beta adrenergic blocker/diuretic
Tenormin	Atenolol	ICI Pharma	Beta adrenergic blocker
Theo-Dur	Theophylline anhydrous*	Key	Bronchodilator
Timoptic	Timolal maleate	Merck Sharp & Dohme	Intraocular pressure lowering agent in glaucoma treatment
Tobrex	Tobramycin	Alcon	Aminoglycoside antibiotic (ophthalmic)
Tolectin DS	Tolmetin sodium	McNeil	Nonsteroidal anti-inflammatory agent (NSAID)
Topicort	Desoximetasone	Hoechst-Roussel	Corticosteroid (topical)
Totacillin	Ampicillin*	Beecham	Penicillin antibiotic
Transderm-Nitro	Nitroglycerin	CIBA	Coronary vasodilator/anti-anginal agent
Tranxene	Clorazepate dipotassium	Abbott	Benzodiazepine
Trental	Pentoxifylline	Hoechst-Roussel	Improves blood flow in chronic occlusive artery disease
Triavil	Perphenazine/amitriptyline	Merck Sharp & Dohme	Antipsychotic/antidepressant
Trimox	Amoxicillin*	Squibb	Penicillin antibiotic
Trinalin	Azatadine maleate/pseudoephedrine sulfate	Schering	Antihistamine/decongestant
Triphasil-28	Levonorgestrel/ethinyl estradiol	Wyeth-Ayerst	Combination oral contraceptive
Tri-Norinyl	Norethindrone/ethinyl estradiol*	Syntex	Combination oral contraceptive
Tussionex	Hydrocodone polistirex/ phenyltoxamine polistirex	Pennwalt	Narcotic antitussive/antihistamine (Pennkinetic extended release suspension)

*Generic product available.

Continued on next page

Brand Drugs—*Continued*

Generic Name	Brand Name	Company	Category
Tussi-Organidin	Codeine phosphate/iodinated glycerol	Wallace	Antitussive/mucolytic expectorant
Tussi-Organidin DM	Codeine phosphate/iodinated glycerol /dextromethorphan	Wallace	Antitussive/mucolytic expectorant
Tylenol/Codeine	Acetaminophen/codeine*	McNeil	Non-opioid/opioid analgesic
Tylox	Oxycodone/acetaminophen	McNeil	Opioid/non-opioid analgesic
Valium	Diazepam*	Roche	Benzodiazepine
Vasotec	Enalapril maleate	Merck Sharp & Dohme	Angiotensin converting enzyme (ACE) inhibitor/ antihypertensive
Veetids	Penicillin VK (potassium)*	Squibb	Penicillin antibiotic
Ventolin Aerosol	Albuterol	Allen & Hanbury (Glaxo)	Beta-2 adrenergic bronchodilator
Vicodin	Hydrocodone bitartrate	Knoll	Opioid analgesic
V-Cillin K	Penicillin VK (potassium)*	Lilly	Penicillin antibiotic
Wymox	Amoxicillin*	Wyeth-Ayerst	Penicillin antibiotic
Xanax	Alprazolam	Upjohn	Benzodiazepine, anti-anxiety
Zantac	Ranitidine hydrochloride	Glaxo	Histamine H_2 receptor antagonist
Zovirax	Acyclovir	Burroughs Wellcome	Antiviral
Zyloprim	Allopurinol	Burroughs Wellcome	Xanthine oxidase inhibitor (reduces uric acid)

*Generic product available.

Common Abbreviations

There is considerable variation in the use of capitalization, italicization, and punctuation in abbreviations. The forms of abbreviation in this list are those most often encountered by pharmacists.

Abbreviation	Meaning
A, aa., or $\overline{aa}$	of each
a.c.	before meals
ad	to, up to
a.d.	right ear
ad lib.	at pleasure, freely
a.m.	morning
amp.	ampule
ante	before
aq.	water
a.s.	left ear
a.u.	each ear, both ears
b.i.d.	twice a day
BP	British Pharmacopoeia
BSA	body surface area
c. or $\bar{c}$	with
cap. or caps.	capsule
cp	chest pain
D.A.W.	dispense as written
cc or cc.	cubic centimeter
comp.	compound, compounded
dil.	dilute
D.C., dc, or disc.	discontinue
disp.	dispense
div.	divide, to be divided
dl or dL	deciliter
d.t.d.	give of such doses
DW	distilled water
D_5W	dextrose 5% in water
elix.	elixir
e.m.p.	as directed
et	and
ex aq.	in water
fl or fld	fluid
fl oz	fluid ounce
ft.	make
g or Gm	gram
gal.	gallon
GI	gastrointestinal
gr or gr.	grain
gtt or gtt.	drop, drops
H	hypodermic
h. or hr.	hour
h.s.	at bedtime
IM	intramuscular
inj.	injection
IV	intravenous
IVP	intravenous push
IVPB	intravenous piggy back
K	potassium
l or L	liter
lb.	pound
M	mix
m^2 or M^2	square meter
mcg, mcg., or μg	microgram
mEq	milliequivalent
mg or mg.	milligram
ml. or mL	milliliter
μl or μL	microliter
♍	minim
N&V	nausea and vomiting
Na	Sodium
N.F.	National Formulary
No.	number
noct.	night, in the night
non rep.	do not repeat
NPO	nothing by mouth
N.S., NS, or N/S	normal saline
½ NS	half strength normal saline
O	pint
o.d.	right eye, every day
o.l.	left eye
o.s.	left eye
OTC	over the counter
o.u.	each eye, both eyes
o_2	both eyes
oz.	ounce
p.c.	after meals
PDR	Physicians Desk Reference
p.m.	afternoon; evening
p.o.	by mouth
pr	for the rectum
prn or p.r.n.	as needed
pt.	pint
pulv.	powder
pv	for vaginal use
q.	every
q.d.	every day
q.h.	every hour

q. 4 hr.	every four hours
q.i.d.	four times a day
q.o.d.	every other day
q.s.	a sufficient quantity
q.s. ad	a sufficient quantity to make
R	rectal
R.L. or R/L	Ringer's lactate
℞	prescription
s. or s̄	without
Sig.	write on label
sol.	solution
S.O.B.	shortness of breath
s.o.s.	if there is need (once only)
ss. or $\overline{ss}$	one half
stat.	immediately
subc, subq, or s.c.	subcutaneously
sup. or supp	suppository
susp.	suspension
syr.	syrup
tab.	tablet
tal.	such, such a one
tal. dos.	such doses
tbsp. or T	tablespoonful
t.i.d.	three times a day
tr. or tinct.	tincture
tsp. or t.	teaspoonful
U or u.	unit
u.d. or ut dict.	as directed
ung.	ointment
U.S.P. or USP	United States Pharmacopoeia
w/v	weight/volume

Drug Product Abbreviations and Dosage Forms

Drug Product	Example	Company	Description/Comment
Caplet	Advil Caplet	Whitehall	Ibuprofen in a capsule-shaped compressed tablet (caplet)
Chronotab	Disophrol Chronotab	Schering	Dexbrompheniramine maleate/pseudoephedrine sulfate controlled release tablet
CR	Norspace CR	Searle Pharmaceuticals	Disopyramide phosphate (controlled release) capsule
Depo	Depo-Medrol	Upjohn	Sterile methylprednisolone acetate suspension
Dispertabs	PCE	Abbott	Erythromycin enteric coated particles in a tablet
Dospan	Tenuate Dospan	Lakeside (Merrell Dow)	Diethylproprion hydrochloride controlled release tablet
DS	Septra DS	Burroughs Wellcome	Trimethoprim/Sulfamethoxazole (Double Strength)
Enduret	Preludin Enduret	Boehringer-Ingelheim	Phenmetrazine hydrochloride prolonged action tablets
Extencaps	Micro-K Extencaps	A.H. Robins	Microencapsulated potassium chloride controlled release capsule
Extentab	Dimetane Extentabs	A.H. Robins	Brompheniramine maleate extended (controlled) release tablets
Filmtab	Erythrocin Stearate Filmtab	Abbott Pharmaceuticals	Erythromycin stearate film coated compressed tablet
Forte	Thiosulfil Forte	Ayerst Laboratories	Higher dose (0.5 g) sulfamethizole (Forte = stronger)
Gradumet	Desoxyn Gradumet	Abbott Pharmaceuticals	Methamphetamine hydrochloride sustained release tablet
Gyrocap	Slo-Bid Gyrocaps	Rorer	Theophylline anhydrous controlled release capsule
Infatab	Dilantin Infatabs	Parke-Davis	Phenytoin tablets, USP
Kapseals	Dilantin Kapseals	Parke-Davis	Extended phenytoin sodium capsule (Kapseal = sealed hard gelatin capsule)
LA	Inderal LA	Ayerst Laboratories	Propranalol hydrochloride (long acting) capsule
Oros	Acutrim	CIBA Geigy	Phenylpropanolamine HCl controlled release osmotic tablet
Pennkinetic	Tussionex	Pennwalt	Hydrocodone polistirex/chlorpheniramine polistirex extended release ion exchange suspension
Perles	Tessalon Perles	Du Pont	Benzonatate in a soft gelatin capsule (Perle)
Plateau Caps	Nitro-Bid Plateau Caps	Marion	Nitroglycerin controlled release capsules
Progestasert	Progestasert	Alza	Intrauterine progesterone contraceptive system
Pulvule	Darvon Compound	Eli Lilly	Propoxyphene hydrochloride/aspirin/caffeine capsule (Pulvule)
Repetabs	Polaramine Repetabs	Schering	Dexchlorpheniramine maleate repeat action tablets

Continued on next page

Drug Product	Example	Company	Description/Comment
RTU	Flagyl I.V. RTU	Searle Pharmaceuticals	Metronidazole injection ready-to-use (RTU)
SA	Sudafed SA	Burroughs Wellcome	Pseudoephedrine hydrochloride sustained release (sustained action) tablet
Sequels	Ferro-Sequels	Lederle Laboratories	Ferrous (iron) fumarate sustained release capsule
Spansule	Dexedrine Spansule	Smith Kline & French	Dextroamphetamine sulfate controlled release capsule
Spinhaler	Intal Inhaler	Fisons	Cromolyn sodium inhalation aerosol for delivery of powder from capsule
Sprinkle	Theo-Dur Sprinkle	Key Pharmaceuticals	Microencapsulated theophylline granules contained in capsule which may be swallowed whole or sprinkled on food
SR	Elixophyllin SR	Berlex Laboratories	(Sustained release) theophylline
Tabloid	Empirin Aspirin tablets	Burroughs Wellcome	Compressed tablet (Tabloid) containing 325 mg aspirin
Tembids	Isordil Tembids Capsules	Wyeth-Ayerst	Isosorbide dinitrate controlled release capsule
Tempules	Nicobid Tempules	Rorer	Niacin timed release capsule
Ten-tab	Tepanil Ten-tab	3M Riker Laboratories	Diethylproprion hydrochloride sustained release tablets
Timesule	Isoclor Timesule	Fisons	Chlorpheniramine maleate/pseudoephedrine sulfate controlled release capsule
Tubex	Closed injection system	Wyeth-Ayerst	Injection system for delivering premeasured doses of medication
-Dur	Theo-Dur	Key Pharmaceuticals	Theophylline anhydrous sustained release

Metrology

METRIC, APOTHECARY, AND AVOIRDUPOIS SYSTEMS

Metric system

1. Basic units

Mass = g or gram
Length = m or meter
Volume = L or liter
1 cc (cubic centimeter) of water is approximately equal to 1 mL and weighs 1 g.

2. Prefixes

kilo-	10^3 or 1000 times the basic unit
hekto-	10^2 or 100 times the basic unit
deka-	10 or 10 times the basic unit
deci-	10^{-1} or 0.1 times the basic unit
centi-	10^{-2} or 0.01 times the basic unit
milli-	10^{-3} or 0.001 times the basic unit
micro-	10^{-6} or one-millionth of the basic unit
nano-	10^{-9} or one-billionth of the basic unit
pico-	10^{-12} or one-trillionth of the basic unit

Examples of these prefixes include milligram (mg), which equals one-thousandth of a gram and deciliter (dL), which equals 100 mL or 0.1 L.

Apothecary system

1. Volume (fluids or liquid)

60 minims (♍) = 1 fluidrachm or fluidram (fʒ) or (ʒ)
8 fluidrachms (480 minims) = 1 fluid ounce (f℥ or ℥)
16 fluidounces = 1 pint (pt or 0)
2 pints (32 fluidounces) = 1 quart (qt)
4 quarts (8 pints) = 1 gallon (gal or C)

2. Mass (weight)

20 grains (gr) = 1 scruple (℈)
3 scruples (60 grains) = 1 drachm or dram (ʒ)
8 drachms (480 grains) = 1 ounce (℥)
12 ounces (5760 grains) = 1 pound (lb)

Avoirdupois system

1. Volume

1 fluidrachm = 60 min.
1 fluid ounce = 8 fl. dr.
= 480 min.
1 pint = 16 fl. oz.
= 7680 min.
1 quart = 2 pt.
= 32 fl. oz.
1 gallon = 4 qt.
= 128 fl. oz.

2. Mass (weight)

The *grain* is common to both the apothecary and avoirdupois systems.

437.5 grains (gr) = 1 ounce (oz)

16 ounces (7000 grains) = 1 pound (lb)

CONVERSION

Exact equivalents

Exact equivalents are used for the conversion of specific quantities in pharmaceutical formulas and prescription compounding.

1. Length

1 meter (m) = 39.37 in.

1 inch (in) = 2.54 cm.

2. Volume

1 mL = 16.23 minims (♏)

1 ♏ = 0.06 mL

1 f ʒ = 3.69 mL

1 f ℥ = 29.57 mL

1 pt = 473 mL

1 gal (U.S.) = 3785 mL

3. Mass

1 g = 15.432 gr

1 kg = 2.20 lb (avoir.)

1 gr = 0.065 g or 65 mg

1 oz (avoir.) = 28.35 g

1 ℥ (apoth.) = 31.1 g

1 lb (avoir.) = 454 g

1 lb (apoth.) = 373.2 g

4. Other equivalents

1 oz (avoir.) = 437.5 gr

1 ℥ (apoth.) = 480 gr

1 gal (U.S.) = 128 fl ℥

1 fl ℥ (water) = 455 gr

1 gr (apoth.) = 1 gr (avoir)

Approximate equivalents

Approximate equivalents may be used by physicians in prescribing the dose quantities using the metric and apothecary systems of weights and measures, respectively.

Household units are often used to inform the patient of the size of the dose. In view of the almost universal practice of employing the *teaspoon* ordinarily available in the household for the administration of medicine, the teaspoon may be regarded to represent 5 mL. When accurate measurement of a liquid dose is required, the USP recommends that a calibrated oral syringe or dropper is used.

1 fluid dram = 1 teaspoonful
= 5 mL

4 fluidounces = 120 mL

8 fluidounces = 1 cup
= 240 mL

1 grain = 65 mg

1 Kg = 2.2 pounds (lbs)

Temperature Conversion

Centigrade (Celsius) to Fahrenheit: (°C × 9/5) + 32 = °F
Fahrenheit to Centigrade (Celsius): (°F − 32) × 5/9 = °C

MILLIEQUIVALENTS PER LITER (mEq/L)

$$\text{mEq/L} = \frac{\text{weight of salt (g)} \times \text{valence of ion} \times 1000}{\text{molecular weight of salt}}$$

$$\text{weight of salt} = \frac{\text{mEq/L} \times \text{molecular weight of salt}}{\text{valence of ion} \times 1000}$$

Drugs That Should Not Be Crushed

Pharmacists may encounter patients who, for one reason or another, cannot swallow tablets or capsules. When an alternative liquid formulation is not available, pulverizing the solid dosage form before administration may serve as a quick, safe solution to the problem.

But not all pharmaceutical products may be crushed before administration. Controlled-release formulations can deliver dangerous immediate doses of their active ingredients if the integrity of the delivery system is destroyed. And enteric-coated products must remain intact in order to prevent their dissolution in the stomach.

Listed below are controlled-release and enteric-coated products that should not be crushed or chewed.

In general, capsules containing sustained-release or enteric-coated particles may not be opened and their contents administered on a spoonful of soft food. Instruct patients not to chew the particles, though. (Patients should, in fact, be discouraged from chewing any medication unless it is specifically formulated for that purpose.)

This list should not be considered all-inclusive. Generic and alternate brands of some products may exist. Tablets intended for sublingual or buccal administration (not included in this list) should also be administered only as intended, in an intact form.

Actifed 12-Hour capsules	Burroughs Wellcome	cr
Acutrim tablets	CIBA	cr
Adipost capsules	Ascher	cr
Aerolate SR	Fleming	cr
Aerolate JR	Fleming	cr
Aerolate III	Fleming	cr
Afrinol Repetab tablets	Schering	cr
Aller-Chlor capsules	Rugby	cr
Allerest 12-Hour capsules	Pharmacraft	cr
AL-R capsules	Saron	cr
Ammonium Chloride Enseals tablets	Lilly	ec
APF Arthritis Pain Formula tablets	Whitehall	ec
Artane Sequels	Lederle	cr
Arthritis Bayer Timed Release Aspirin	Glenbrook	cr
ASA Enseals	Lilly	ec
Atrohist Sprinkle tablets	Adams	cr
Atrohist L.A. tablets	Adams	cr

Avazyme tablets	Wallace	ec
Azulfidine EN-tab tablets	Pharmacia	ec
Belladenal-S tablets	Sandoz	cr
Bellergal-S tablets	Sandoz	cr
Bisacodyl tablets	various	ec
Bontril Slow-Release capsules	Carnrick	cr
Bromfed capsules	Muro	cr
Bromfed-PD capsules	Muro	cr
Bromphen tablets	Schein	cr
Bromphen TD tablets	Schein	cr
Bromphen Compound TD tablets	Schein	cr
Bronkodyl S-R capsules	Winthrop-Breon	cr
Carter's Little Pills	Carter	ec
Cerespan capsules	USV	cr
Chexit tablets	Dorsey	cr
Choledyl tablets	Parke-Davis	ec
Choledyl SA tablets	Parke-Davis	cr
Chlor-Trimeton Repetabs tablets	Schering	cr
Chlor-Trimeton Decongestant Repetabs	Schering	cr
Chymoral tablets	Armour	ec
Combid Spansule capsules	SK&F	cr
Comhist LA capsules	Norwich Eaton	cr
Compazine Spansule capsules	SK&F	cr
Congess SR capsules	Fleming	cr
Congess JR capsules	Fleming	cr
Constant-T tablets	Geigy	cr
Contac capsules	Menley & James	cr
Contac caplets	Menley & James	cr
Control capsules	Thompson	cr
Cosprin tablets	Glenbrook	ec
Cotazym-S capsules	Organon	ec
Cystospaz-M capsules	Webcon	cr
Dallergy-Jr capsules	Laser	cr
Deconamine SR capsules	Berlex	cr
Deconsal LA tablets	Adams	cr
Deconsal Sprinkle capsules	Adams	cr
Dehist capsules	Forest	cr
Demazin Repetabs tablets	Schering	cr
Depakote tablets	Abbott	ec
Desoxyn Gradumet tablets	Abbott	cr
Dexatrim capsules	Thompson	cr
Dexedrine Spansule capsules	SK&F	cr
Diamox Sequel capsules	Lederle	cr
Diethylstilbestrol Enseal tablets	Lilly	ec
Dilatrate-SR capsules	Reed & Carnrick	cr
Dimetane Extentab tablets	Robins	cr
Dimetapp Extentab tablets	Robins	cr
Disobrom tablets	Geneva	cr
Disophrol Chronotab tablets	Schering	cr
Donnatal Extentab tablets	Robins	cr

Donnazyme tablets	Robins	cr
Double-Sal tablets	Vale	ec
Dristan 12-Hour capsules	Whitehall	cr
Drixoral tablets	Schering	cr
Drize capsules	Ascher	cr
Dulcolax tablets	Boehringer Ingelheim	ec
Duotrate capsules	JMI	cr
Duraphyl tablets	Forest	cr
Duraquin tablets	Parke-Davis	cr
Easprin tablets	Parke-Davis	ec
Ecotrin tablets	Menley & James	ec
Ecotrin Duentric capsules	Menley & James	ec
Ecotrin Maximum Strength Duentric	Menley & James	ec
Ectasule Minus III capsules	Fleming	cr
Ectasule Minus Jr. capsules	Fleming	cr
Ectasule Minus Sr. capsules	Fleming	cr
Elixophyllin SR capsules	Berlex	cr
E-Mycin tablets	Upjohn	ec
Encaprin capsules	Norwich Eaton	ec
Encaprin Maximum Strength capsules	Norwich Eaton	ec
Entex-LA tablets	Norwich Eaton	cr
Entozyme tablets	Robins	cr
ERYC capsules	Parke-Davis	ec
Ery-Tab tablets	Abbott	ec
Eskalith-CR tablets	SK&F	cr
Extendryl JR capsules	Fleming	cr
Extendryl SR capsules	Fleming	cr
Feco-T tablets	Blaine	cr
Fedahist Gyrocaps capsules	Rorer	cr
Feosol capsules	Menley & James	ec
Fergon capsules	Winthrop-Breon	ec
Ferralyn Lanacap capsules	Lannett	cr
Fero-Grad-500 tablets	Abbott	cr
Fero-Gradumet tablets	Abbott	cr
Ferro-Sequel capsules	Lederle	cr
Ferrous Sulfate Enseal tablets	Lilly	ec
Festal II tablets	Hoechst	ec
Genabid capsules	Goldine	cr
Guaifed capsules	Muro	cr
Hispril Spansule capsules	SK&F	cr
Histabid capsules	Glaxo	cr
Histatapp-TD tablets	Upsher-Smith	cr
Histaspan-D capsules	USV	cr
Histaspan-Plus capsules	USV	cr
Humibid LA tablets	Adams	cr
Iberet-500 tablets	Abbott	cr
Iberet-Folic-500 tablets	Abbott	cr
Ilotycin tablets	Dista	ec
Inderal LA capsules	Ayerst	cr
Inderide LA capsules	Ayerst	cr
Indocin-SR capsules	MSD	cr

Iso-Bid capsules	Geriatric	cr
Isochron tablets	Forest	cr
Isoclor Timesule capsules	Fisons	cr
Isordil Tembid capsules	Wyeth	cr
Isordil Tembid tablets	Wyeth	cr
Kaon-Cl tablets	Adria	cr
Kaon-CL-10 tablets	Adria	cr
K-Dur tablets	Key	cr
K-Tab tablets	Abbott	cr
Kloraspan tablets	Wesley	cr
Klor-Con 8/Klor-Con 10 tablets	Upsher-Smith	cr
Klotrix tablets	Mead Johnson	cr
LaBID tablets	Norwich Eaton	cr
Levsinex Timecap capsules	Rorer	cr
Levsinex with Pb Timecap capsules	Rorer	cr
Lithobid tablets	CIBA	cr
Mandalets tablets	Quality Gen.	ec
Mandameth tablets	Major	ec
Measurin tablets	Winthrop-Breon	cr
Meprospan capsules	Wallace	cr
Mestinon Timespan tablets	Roche	cr
Micro-K Extencap capsules	Robins	cr
Mol-Iron Chronosule capsules	Schering	cr
MS Contin tablets	Purdue Frederick	cr
Naldecon tablets	Bristol	cr
Niac capsules	Forest	cr
Nico-400 Plateau Cap capsules	Marion	cr
Nicobid Tempule capsules	USV	cr
Nitro-Bid Plateau Cap capsules	Marion	cr
Nitroglyn capsules	Key	cr
Nitrospan capsules	USV	cr
Nitrostat-SR capsules	Parke-Davis	cr
Nolamine tablets	Carnrick	cr
Norflex tablets	Riker	cr
Norpace-CR capsules	Searle	cr
Novafed capsules	Merrell Dow	cr
Novafed-A capsules	Merrell Dow	cr
Novahistine LP tablets	Lakeside	cr
Ornade Spansule capsules	SK&F	cr
P-200 tablets	Boots	cr
Pabalate tablets	Robins	ec
Pabalate-SF tablets	Robins	ec
Pancrease capsules	McNeil	ec
Pancreatin Enseals Triple Strength tablets	Lilly	ec
Pavabid Plateau Cap capsules	Marion	cr
PBR/12 capsules	Scott-Alison	cr
PBZ-SR tablets	Geigy	cr
PCE tablets	Abbott	cr
Pentol SA tablets and capsules	Major	cr

Peritrate-SA tablets	Parke-Davis	cr
Phenetron Compound tablets	Lannett	ec
Phyllocontin tablets	Purdue Frederick	cr
Polaramine Repetab tablets	Schering	cr
Poly-Histine-DX capsules	Bock	cr
Potassium Chloride Enseal tablets	Lilly	ec
Potassium Iodide Enseal tablets	Lilly	ec
Prelu-2 capsules	Boehringer Ingelheim	cr
Preludin Enduret tablets	Boehringer Ingelheim	cr
Procan-SR tablets	Parke-Davis	cr
Prolamine Maximum Strength Capsules	Thompson	cr
Promine-SR tablets	Major	cr
Pronestyl-SR tablets	Squibb	cr
Purebrom Compound TD tablets	Purepac	cr
Quibron Bidcaps capsules	Mead Johnson	cr
Quibron-T/SR tablets	Mead Johnson	cr
Quinaglute Dura-Tab tablets	Berlex	cr
Quinatime tablets	Bolar	cr
Quinidex Extentab tablets	Robins	cr
Releserp-5 capsules	Scott-Alison	cr
Respbid tablets	Boehringer Ingelheim	cr
Ritalin-SR tablets	CIBA	cr
Robimycin Robitab tablets	Robins	ec
Rondec-TR tablets	Ross	cr
Roxanol-SR tablets	Roxane	cr
Ru-Tuss tablets	Boots	cr
Ru-Tuss II capsules	Boots	cr
Singlet tablets	Lakeside	cr
Slo-bid Gyrocaps capsules	Rorer	cr
Slo-Phyllin Gyrocaps capsules	Rorer	cr
Slow-Fe tablets	CIBA	cr
Slow-K tablets	CIBA	cr
Sodium Chloride Enseal tablets	Lilly	ec
Sodium Salicylate Enseal tablets	Lilly	ec
Somophyllin-CRT capsules	Fisons	cr
Sorbitrate-SA tablets	Stuart	cr
Span-FF capsules	MetroMed	cr
Span Niacin tablets	Scrip	cr
Sudafed 12 Hour capsules	Burroughs Wellcome	cr
Sustaire tablets	Pfipharmecs	cr
Tamine SR tablets	Geneva	cr
Tavist-D tablets	Sandoz	cr
Tedral-SA tablets	Parke-Davis	cr
Teldrin Spansule capsules	Menley & James	cr
Temaril Spansule capsules	SK&F	cr
Ten-K tablets	Geigy	cr

Tenuate Dospan tablets	Lakeside	cr
Tepanil Ten-tab tablets	Riker	cr
Theo-24 capsules	Searle	cr
Theobid Duracap capsules	Glaxo	cr
Theobid Jr Duracap capsules	Glaxo	cr
Theochron tablets	Forest	cr
Theoclear-LA capsules	Central	cr
Theo-Dur tablets	Key	cr
Theo-Dur Sprinkle capsules	Key	cr
Theolair-SR tablets	Riker	cr
Theophyl-SR capsules	McNeil	cr
Theospan-SR capsules	Laser	cr
Theo-Time capsules	Major	cr
Theovent capsules	Schering	cr
Thorazine Spansule capsules	SK&F	cr
Thyroid Enseal tablets	Lilly	ec
Tranxene-SD tablets	Abbott	cr
Trental tablets	Hoechst	cr
Triaminic-12 tablets	Dorsey	cr
Triaminic TR tablets	Dorsey	cr
Triaminic Juvulet tablets	Dorsey	cr
Trilafon Repetab tablets	Schering	cr
Trinalin Repetabs tablets	Schering	cr
Tussagesic tablets	Dorsey	cr
Tuss-Ornade Spansule capsules	SK&F	cr
Uniphyl tablets	Purdue Frederick	cr
Uracel 5 tablets	Vortech	ec
Valrelease capsules	Roche	cr
Verin tablets	Verex	cr
Zorprin tablets	Boots	cr

Controlled release = cr; enteric coated = ec.

Appendix C: Pharmacy Schools and Organizations

Colleges and Schools of Pharmacy

UNITED STATES

Although all schools listed have accredited first professional degree programs, not all PharmD programs have been accredited by the American Council on Pharmaceutical Education. The accreditation status of programs can be obtained by contacting the ACPE, 311 West Superior, Chicago, Illinois 60610, (312) 664-3575.

Alabama

School of Pharmacy
Auburn University
Alabama 36849-5501
205/844-4740

School of Pharmacy
Samford University
800 Lakeshore Drive
Birmingham, Alabama 35229
205/870-2820

Arizona

College of Pharmacy
The University of Arizona
Tucson, Arizona 85721
602/626-1427

Arkansas

College of Pharmacy
University of Arkansas for Medical Sciences
4301 West Markham - Slot 522
Little Rock, Arkansas 72205-7122
501/686-5557

California

School of Pharmacy
University of California S-926
San Francisco, California 94143-0446
415/476-1225

School of Pharmacy
University of the Pacific
3601 Pacific Avenue
Stockton, California 95211
209/946-2561

School of Pharmacy
University of Southern California
1985 Zonal Avenue
Los Angeles, California 90033-1086
213/224-7501

Colorado

School of Pharmacy
University of Colorado
Box 297
Boulder, Colorado 80309-0297
303/492-6278

Connecticut

School of Pharmacy
The University of Connecticut
Box U-92
372 Fairfield Road
Storrs, Connecticut 06269-2092
203/486-2129

District of Columbia

College of Pharmacy and Pharmacal Sciences
Howard University
2300 4th Street, N.W.
Washington, DC 20059
202/636-6530

Florida

College of Pharmacy and Pharmaceutical Sciences
Florida Agricultural and Mechanical University
P.O. Box 367
Tallahassee, Florida 32307
904/599-3578

Southeastern College of Pharmaceutical Sciences
1750 N.E. 168th Street
N. Miami Beach, Florida 33162-3097
305/949-4000

College of Pharmacy
University of Florida
Box J-484
Health Science Center
Gainesville, Florida 32610
904/392-9713

Georgia

Southern School of Pharmacy
Mercer University
345 Boulevard, N.E.
Atlanta, Georgia 30312
404/653-8800

College of Pharmacy
The University of Georgia
Athens, Georgia 30602
404/542-1911

Idaho

College of Pharmacy
Idaho State University
Pocatello, Idaho 83209-0009
208/236-2175

Illinois

College of Pharmacy
University of Illinois at Chicago
833 South Wood St., Box 6998
M/C 874
Chicago, Illinois 60680-6998
312/996-7240

Indiana

College of Pharmacy
Butler University
46th & Sunset Avenue
Indianapolis, Indiana 46208
317/283-9322

School of Pharmacy and Pharmacal Sciences
Purdue University
West Lafayette, Indiana 47907-0708
317/494-1357

Iowa

College of Pharmacy
Drake University
28th & Forest
Des Moines, Iowa 50311
515/271-2172

College of Pharmacy
The University of Iowa
Iowa City, Iowa 52242
319/335-8794

Kansas

School of Pharmacy
University of Kansas
2056 Malott
Lawrence, Kansas 66045-2500
913/864-3591

Kentucky

College of Pharmacy
University of Kentucky
Rose Street - Pharmacy Building
Lexington, Kentucky 40536-0082
606/257-2738

Louisiana

School of Pharmacy
Northeast Louisiana University
700 University Avenue
Monroe, Louisiana 71209-0470
318/342-2180

College of Pharmacy
Xavier University of Louisiana
7325 Palmetto Street
New Orleans, Louisiana 70125
504/483-7424

Maryland

School of Pharmacy
University of Maryland
20 North Pine Street
Baltimore, Maryland
21201-1180
301/328-7650

Massachusetts

Massachusetts College of
Pharmacy and Allied Health
Sciences
179 Longwood Avenue
Boston, Massachusetts 02115
617/732-2800

College of Pharmacy and Allied
Health Professions
Northeastern University
360 Huntington Avenue
Boston, Massachusetts 02115
617/437-3321

Michigan

School of Pharmacy
Ferris State University
901 South State Street
Big Rapids, Michigan 49307
616/592-2254

College of Pharmacy
The University of Michigan
Ann Arbor, Michigan
48109-1065
313/764-7312

College of Pharmacy and Allied
Health Professions
Wayne State University
105 Shapero Hall
Detroit, Michigan 48202-3489
313/577-1574

Minnesota

College of Pharmacy
University of Minnesota
5-130 Health Sciences Unit F
308 Harvard Street, S.E.
Minneapolis, Minnesota
55455-0343
612/624-1900

Mississippi

School of Pharmacy
The University of Mississippi
University, Mississippi
38677-9814
601/232-7265

Missouri

St. Louis College of Pharmacy
4588 Parkview Place
St. Louis, Missouri 63110-1088
314/367-8700

School of Pharmacy
University of Missouri - Kansas
City
5005 Rockhill Road
Kansas City, Missouri 64110
816/276-1607

Montana

School of Pharmacy and Allied
Health Sciences
University of Montana
Missoula, Montana 59812
406/243-4621

Nebraska

School of Pharmacy and Allied
Health Professions
Creighton University
California at 24th Street
Omaha, Nebraska 68178
402/280-2950

College of Pharmacy
University of Nebraska
42nd & Dewey Avenue
Omaha, Nebraska 68105-1065
402/559-4333

New Jersey

College of Pharmacy
Rutgers University
The State University of New
Jersey
Post Office Box 789
Piscataway, New Jersey
08855-0789
201/932-2666

New Mexico

College of Pharmacy
University of New Mexico
Albuquerque, New Mexico
87131
505/277-2461

New York

Arnold & Marie Schwartz
College of Pharmacy and
Health Sciences
Long Island University
75 DeKalb Ave. at University
Plaza
Brooklyn, New York 11201
718/403-1060

College of Pharmacy and Allied
Health Professions
St. John's University
Grand Central and Utopia
Parkways
Jamaica, New York 11439
718/990-6161

School of Pharmacy
State University of New York at
Buffalo
C126 Cooke-Hochstetter
Complex
Buffalo, New York 14260
716/636-2823

Albany College of Pharmacy
Union University
106 New Scotland
Albany, New York 12208
518/445-7211

North Carolina

School of Pharmacy
Campbell University
Post Office Box 1090
Buies Creek, North Carolina 27506
919/893-4111

School of Pharmacy
University of North Carolina
Beard Hall #7360
Chapel Hill, North Carolina 27599-7360
919/966-1121

North Dakota

College of Pharmacy
North Dakota State University
Fargo, North Dakota 58105
701/237-7456

Ohio

College of Pharmacy
Ohio Northern University
Ada, Ohio 45810
419/772-2275

College of Pharmacy
The Ohio State University
500 West 12th Avenue
Columbus, Ohio 43210-1291
614/292-2266

College of Pharmacy
University of Cincinnati-Medical Center
Mail Location #4
Cincinnati, Ohio 45267
513/558-3784

College of Pharmacy
The University of Toledo
2801 West Bancroft Street
Toledo, Ohio 43606
419/537-2019

Oklahoma

School of Pharmacy
Southwestern Oklahoma State University
100 Campus Drive
Weatherford, Oklahoma 73096
405/774-3105

College of Pharmacy
University of Oklahoma
P.O. Box 26901
Oklahoma City, Oklahoma 73190-5040
405/271-6484

Oregon

College of Pharmacy
Oregon State University
Corvallis, Oregon 97331-3507
503/737-3424

Pennsylvania

School of Pharmacy
Duquesne University
Pittsburgh, Pennsylvania 15282
412/434-6380

School of Pharmacy
Philadelphia College of Pharmacy and Science
Woodland Avenue at 43rd Street
Philadelphia, Pennsylvania 19104
215/596-8800

School of Pharmacy
Temple University
3307 North Broad Street
Philadelphia, Pennsylvania 19140
215/221-4990

School of Pharmacy
University of Pittsburgh
1103 Salk Hall
Pittsburgh, Pennsylvania 15261
412/648-8579

Puerto Rico

College of Pharmacy
University of Puerto Rico
GPO Box 5067
San Juan, Puerto Rico 00936-5067
809/758-2525 (ext) 5400

Rhode Island

College of Pharmacy
University of Rhode Island
Kingston, Rhode Island 02881-0809
401/792-2761

South Carolina

College of Pharmacy
Medical University of South Carolina
171 Ashley Avenue
Charleston, South Carolina 29425-2301
803/792-3115

College of Pharmacy
University of South Carolina
Columbia, South Carolina 29208
803/777-4151

South Dakota

College of Pharmacy
South Dakota State University
Box 2202C
Brookings, South Dakota 57007-0197
605/688-6197

Tennessee

College of Pharmacy
University of Tennessee
874 Union Avenue
Memphis, Tennessee 38163
901/528-6036

Texas

College of Pharmacy and Health Sciences
Texas Southern University
3100 Cleburne
Houston, Texas 77004
713/527-7164

College of Pharmacy
University of Houston
4800 Calhoun
Houston, Texas 77204-5511
713/749-4106

College of Pharmacy
University of Texas at Austin
Austin, Texas 78712-1074
512/471-1737

Utah

College of Pharmacy
University of Utah
Salt Lake City, Utah 84112
801/581-6731

Virginia

School of Pharmacy
Virginia Commonwealth University
MCV Campus – Box 581
410 North 12th Street
Richmond, Virginia 23298-0581
804/786-7346

Washington

School of Pharmacy
University of Washington
T-341 Health Science Center, SC-69
Seattle, Washington 98195
206/543-2030

College of Pharmacy
Washington State University
Pullman, Washington 99164-6510
509/335-8664

West Virginia

School of Pharmacy
West Virginia University Health Sciences Center
Morgantown, West Virginia 26506
304/293-5101

Wisconsin

School of Pharmacy
University of Wisconsin-Madison
425 North Charter Street
Madison, Wisconsin 53706
608/262-1416

Wyoming

School of Pharmacy
University of Wyoming
P.O. Box 3375
Laramie, Wyoming 82071-3375
307/766-6120

Canada

Faculty of Pharmacy and Pharmaceutical Sciences
The University of Alberta
Edmonton, Alberta
T6G 2N8 Canada

Faculty of Pharmaceutical Sciences
University of British Columbia
2146 East Mall
Vancouver, B.C.
V6T 1W5

College of Pharmacy
Dalhousie University
5968 College Street
Halifax, Nova Scotia
B3H 3J5 Canada

Ecole De Pharmacie
University Laval
Quebec (Quebec)
G1K 7P4 Canada

The Faculty of Pharmacy
The University of Manitoba
Winnipeg, Manitoba
R3T 2N2 Canada

Memorial University of Newfoundland
Health Science Complex
St. John's, Newfoundland
A1B 3B6 Canada

Faculty of Pharmacy
University of Montreal
C.P. 6128 Succursale A
Montreal, Quebec
H3C 3J7 Canada

College of Pharmacy
University of Saskatchewan
Saskatoon, Saskatchewan
S7N 0W0 Canada

Faculty of Pharmacy
University of Toronto
Toronto, Ontario
M5S 1A1 Canada

Philippines

University of the Philippines
Padre Faura, Manila
Philippines

Malaysia

School of Pharmaceutical Sciences
University Sains Malaysia
Minden, Penang 11800
Malaysia 011-04-888333

Reprinted with permission from the American Association of Colleges of Pharmacy: Colleges and Schools of Pharmacy. *Amer J Pharm Educ* 52:497–498, 1988.

Pharmacy Acronyms and Abbreviations

The following are most commonly used acronyms and abbreviations in pharmacy and licensure:

AACP American Association of Colleges of Pharmacy
ACA American College of Apothecaries
ACPE American Council of Pharmaceutical Education
AFPE American Foundation on Pharmaceutical Education

AIHP	American Institute of the History of Pharmacy
APhA	American Pharmaceutical Association
ASCP	American Society of Consultant Pharmacists
ASHP	American Society of Hospital Pharmacists
ASP	American Society of Pharmacognosy
ASPL	American Society of Pharmacy Law
CLEAR	The National Clearinghouse on Licensure, Enforcement & Regulation
CPSC	Consumer Product Safety Commission
DEA	Drug Enforcement Administration
DWA	Drug Wholesalers Association, Inc.
FDA	Food & Drug Administration
FAHRB	Federation of Association of Health Regulatory Boards
HHS	Department of Health and Human Services
NACDS	National Association of Chain Drug Stores
NAPM	National Association of Pharmaceutical Manufacturers
NARD	National Association of Retail Druggists
NDTC	National Drug Trade Conference
NPC	National Pharmaceutical Council
NCPIE	National Council on Patient Information and Education
NCPDP	National Council on Third Party Prescription Drug Programs
NABP	National Association of Boards of Pharmacy
NABPF	National Association of Boards of Pharmacy Foundation
NABPLEX	National Association of Boards of Pharmacy Licensure Examination
PA	The Proprietary Association
PMA	Pharmaceutical Manufacturers Association
USP	United States Pharmacopeial Convention, Inc.

The following are abbreviations used internally by NABP:

ACT	American College Testing
ACE	Advisory Committee on Examinations
BVC	Bureau of Voluntary Compliance
CBL	Committee on Constitution and Bylaws
CCE	Committee on Continuing Education
CIP	Committee on Institutional Pharmacy
CIT	Committee on Internship Training
CLL	Committee on Law Enforcement/Legislation
EC	Executive Committee
FDLE	Federal Drug Law Examination
FPGEC	Foreign Pharmacy Graduate Examination Commission
FPGEC-SC	Foreign Pharmacy Graduate Examination Commission Steering Committee
FPGEE	Foreign Pharmacy Graduate Equivalency Examination
NRC	NABPLEX Review Committee
NSC	NABPLEX Steering Committee
UTD	Uniform Testing Date

Pharmacy Organizations

American Association of Colleges of Pharmacy
1426 Prince Street
Alexandria, VA 22314
(703) 739-2330

American College of Apothecaries
University of Tennessee
847 Union Avenue
Memphis, TN 38163
(901) 528-6037

American College of Clinical Pharmacy
3101 Broadway, Suite 350
Kansas City, MO 64111
(816) 531-2177

American Foundation for Pharmaceutical Education
618 Somerset Street
P.O. Box 7126
North Plainfield, NJ 07060
(201) 561-8077

American Institute of the History of Pharmacy
c/o Pharmacy Building
University of Wisconsin
Madison, WI 53706
(608) 262-5378

American Pharmaceutical Association
2215 Constitution Avenue NW
Washington, DC 20037
(202) 628-4410

American Society of Consultant Pharmacists
2300 Ninth Street S., Suite 515
Arlington, VA 22204
(703) 920-8492

American Society of Hospital Pharmacists
4630 Montgomery Avenue
Bethesda, MD 20814
(301) 657-3000

American Society of Pharmacognosy
University of Rhode Island
College of Pharmacy
Kingston, RI 02881
(401) 792-2752

American Society for Pharmacy Law
College of Pharmacy
Washington State University
Pullman, WA 99164-6510
(509) 335-4776

Association of Pharmacy Technicians
10123 Alliance Road, Suite 130
P.O. Box 42696
Cincinnati, OH 45242
(513) 793-3555

Drug Chemical and Allied Trades Assn., Inc.
42-40 Bell Blvd., Suite 604
Bayside, NY 11361-2890
(718) 229-8891

Food and Drug Law Institute
1000 Vermont Avenue NW, Suite 1200
Washington, DC 20005
(202) 371-1420

Generic Pharmaceutical Industry Association
200 Madison Ave., Suite 2404
New York, NY 10016
(212) 683-1881

Metropolitan Pharmaceutical Secretaries Association
P.O. Box 8194
St. Louis, MO 63156
(314) 531-6929

National Association of Boards of Pharmacy
O'Hare Corporate Center
1300 Higgins Road, Suite 103
Park Ridge, IL 60068
(312) 698-6227

National Association of Chain Drug Stores
413 N. Lee Street
P.O. Box 1417-D49
Alexandria, VA 22313
(703) 549-3001

NARD
205 Daingerfield Road
Alexandria, VA 22314
(703) 683-8200

National Association of Pharmaceutical Manufacturers
747 Third Avenue
New York, NY 10017
(212) 838-3720

National Catholic Pharmacists Guild of U.S.
1012 Surrey Hills Drive
St. Louis, MO 63117
(314) 645-0085

National Council of State Pharmaceutical Assn. Executives
156 East Market Street, Suite, 900
Indianapolis, IN 46204
(317) 634-4968

National Council on Patient Information and Education
16251 1st Street NW, Suite 1010
Washington, DC 20006
(202) 466-6711

National Institutes of Health
Building 10, Room 1S-257
Bethesda, MD 20205
(301) 496-4363

National Pharmaceutical Association
College of Pharmacy, Box 934
Howard University
Washington, DC 20059
(202) 636-6544/6530

National Pharmaceutical Council
1894 Preston White Drive
Reston, VA 22091
(703) 620-6390

National Pharmaceutical Foundation
P.O. Box 5439, Takoma Park Station
Washington, DC 20912
(202) 829-5008

National Wholesale Druggists Association
P.O. Box 238
Alexandria, VA 22313
(703) 684-6400

Parenteral Drug Association, Inc.
Avenue of the Arts Building
1346 Chestnut Street, Suite 1407
Philadelphia, PA 19107
(215) 735-9752

Pharmaceutical Manufacturers Association
1100 15th Street NW
Washington, DC 20005
(202) 835-3400

The Proprietary Association
1150 Connecticut Avenue NW, Suite 1200
Washington, DC 20036
(202) 429-9260

State Pharmaceutical Editorial Association
222 W. Adams Street, Suite 400
Chicago, IL 60610
(312) 236-1135

U.S. Adopted Names (USAN)
American Medical Association
535 N. Dearborn Street
Chicago, IL 60610
(312) 645-4904

U.S. Navy
Defense Medical Standardization Board
Fort Detrick
Frederick, MD 21701-5013
(301) 663-7387

U.S. Pharmacopeial Convention, Inc.
12601 Twinbrook Parkway
Rockville, MD 20852
(301) 881-0666

U.S. Public Health Service
CA2, 5600 Fishers Lane
Parklawn Building, Room 9-05
Rockville, MD 20857
(301) 443-1993

Veterans Administration
810 Vermont Avenue NW
Washington, DC 20420
(202) 233-3277

Directors and Addresses for State Pharmacy Associations

Alabama	F. Howard Gray Jr., 340 Dexter Ave., Montgomery 36104 (205) 262-0027
Alaska	William F. Davine, 13121 Biscayne Circle, Anchorage 99516 (907) 345-0644
Arizona	Warren Ellison, 2202 N. Seventh St., Phoenix 85006 (602) 258-8121
Arkansas	Norman F. Canterbury, 417 S. Victory, Little Rock 72201 (501) 372-5250
California	Robert C. Johnson, 1112 I St., Suite 300, Sacramento 95814 (916) 444-7811
Colorado	S. Thomas Gray, 770 Grant St., #244, Denver 80203 (303) 861-0328
Connecticut	Daniel C. Leone, 943 Silas Deane Hwy., Wethersfield 06109 (203) 563-4619
Delaware	Christine Bailey, 707 Philadelphia Pike, Wilmington 19809 (302) 762-6019
D.C.	Vasant G. Telang, 6400 Georgia Ave., N.W., Suite 6, Washington 20012 (202) 829-1515
Florida	James B. Powers, 610 N. Adams St., Tallahassee 32301 (904) 222-2400
Georgia	Larry L. Braden, R. Ph., P.O. Box 95527, Atlanta 30347 (404) 231-5074
Hawaii	Gene McBride, P.O. Box 1198, Honolulu 96807 (808) 547-4745
Idaho	JoAn Condie, 1365 N. Orchard, Room 103, Boise 83706 (208) 376-2273
Illinois	Alan Granat, 222 W. Adams St., Suite 400, Chicago 60606 (312) 236-1135

Indiana	David A. Clark, 156 E. Market St., Suite 900, Indianapolis 46204 (317) 634-4968
Iowa	Thomas R. Temple, 8515 Douglas, Suite 24, Des Moines 50322 (515) 270-0713
Kansas	Kenneth W. Schafermeyer, 1308 W. 10th St., Topeka 66604 (913) 232-0439
Kentucky	George Jones, 1228 U.S. Hwy, 127 S., Frankfort 40602 (502) 227-2303
Louisiana	Linda M. Foreman, 2337 St. Claude Ave., New Orleans 70117 (504) 949-7545
Maine	Stanley Stewart, P.O. Box 817, Bangor 04401 (207) 989-3133
Maryland	David A. Banta, 650 W. Lombard St., Baltimore 21201 (301) 727-0746
Massachusetts	Jeffrey J. Burgoyne, P.O. Box 160, 13 Ray Ave., Burlington 01803 (617) 272-7879
Michigan	Larry D. Wagenknecht, 815 N. Washington Ave., Lansing 48906 (517) 484-1466
Minnesota	William E. Bond, 2221 University Ave., S.E., Suite 326, Minneapolis 55414 (612) 378-1414
Mississippi	Phylliss M. Moret, R.Ph., 401 E. Capitol St., Suite 504, Jackson 39201 (601) 944-0416
Missouri	Greg Wood, 410 Madison Ave., Jefferson City 65101 (314) 636-7522
Montana	Robert H. Likewise, P.O. Box 4718, Helena 59604 (406) 449-3843
Nebraska	Tom R. Dolan, R.Ph., 600 S. 12th, Lower Level, Lincoln 68508 (402) 475-4274
Nevada	Kathleen Boyce, 3660 Baker Ln., Reno 89509 (702) 826-3981
New Hampshire	Maurice E. Goulet, 194 N. Main St., Concord 03301 (603) 225-2231
New Jersey	Alvin N. Geser, 118 W. State St., Trenton 08608 (609) 394-5596
New Mexico	Jack E. Hilligoss, 4800 Zuni, S.E., Albuquerque 87108 (505) 265-8720
New York	Elizabeth Lasky, Pine West Plaza IV, Washington Ave. Ext., Albany 12205 (518) 869-6595
North Carolina	A. H. Mebane III, P.O. Box 151, Chapel Hill 27514 (919) 967-2237; (800) 852-7343
North Dakota	Bruce Stoelting, Box 350, Richardton 58652 (701) 225-8650
Ohio	Philip W. Cramer, 395 E. Broad St., Suite 320, Columbus 43215 (614) 221-2391
Oklahoma	John D. Donner, Box 18731, 45 N.E. 52nd St., Oklahoma City 73154 (405) 528-3338
Oregon	Chuck Gress, 1460 State St., Salem 97301 (503) 585-4887
Pennsylvania	Carmen A. DiCello, R.Ph., 508 N. Third St., Harrisburg 17101-1199 (717) 234-6151
Puerto Rico	Elizabeth Silva Rivera, G.P.O. Box 206, San Juan 00936 (809) 753-7157
Rhode Island	Denis B. Barton, 500 Prospect St ., Pawtucket 02860 (401) 725-4141
South Carolina	Robert H. Burnside Jr., 1405 Calhoun St., Columbia 29201 (803) 254-1065
South Dakota	Galen Jordre, Box 518 Pierre 57501 (605) 224-2338
Tennessee	Tom C. Sharp Jr., 226 Capitol Blvd., Suite 705, Nashville 37219 (615) 256-3023
Texas	Luther R. Parker, P.O. Box 14709, Austin 78761 (512) 836-8350
Utah	C. Neil Jensen, 1062 E. 21st St. S., Suite 212, Salt Lake City 84106 (801) 484-9141
Vermont	Philip J. O'Neill, P.O. Box 926, Bennington 05201 (802) 442-5943
Virginia	Paul Galanti, 3119 W. Clay St., Richmond 23230 (804) 355-7941
Washington	Raymond A. Olson, 1420 Maple Ave., S.W., Suite 101, Renton 98055-3196 (206) 228-7171
West Virginia	Richard D. Stevens, 4004 MacCorkle Ave., S.E., Suite 4, Charleston 25304 (304) 925-7204
Wisconsin	Robert E. Henry, 202 Price Pl., Madison 53705 (608) 238-5515
Wyoming	Richard R. Abood, 1115 E. Custer, Laramie 82070 (307) 766-6126

Directors and Addresses for State Boards of Pharmacy

State	Director and Address
Alabama	James W. McLane, 1 Perimeter Park South, Suite 425 S., Birmingham 35243 (205) 967-0130
Alaska	Margaret D. Soden, R.Ph., 3222 Anella Ave., Fairbanks 99709 (907) 479-6793
Arizona	L. A. Lloyd, 5060 N. 19th Ave., Suite 101, Phoenix 85015 (602) 255-5125
Arkansas	Lester Hosto, P.D., P.O. Box 55356, Little Rock 72225 (501) 661-2833
California	Lorie Rice, 1020 N St., Room 448, Sacramento 95814-5784 (916) 445-5014
Colorado	David L. Simmons, 1525 Sherman St., Room 128, Denver 80203 (303) 866-2526
Connecticut	Edward C. Liska, State Office Building, Room G-1A, Hartford 06106 (203) 566-4832 or 3917
Delaware	Martin Golden, Robbins Building, 802 Silver Lake Blvd., Silver Lake Plaza, Dover 19901 (302) 736-4798
D.C.	Carlyle McAdams, 614 H St., N.W., Room 923, Washington 20001 (202) 727-7468
Florida	C. Rod Presnell, 130 N. Monroe St., Suite 170, Tallahassee 32399-0750 (904) 488-7546
Georgia	James M. Jordan, 166 Pryor St., S.W., Atlanta 30303 (404) 656-3912
Hawaii	Jerold Sakoda, P.O. Box 3469, Honolulu 96801 (808) 548-3086
Idaho	L. R. Hansen, 650 W. State St., Room 102-B, Boise 83720 (208) 334-2356
Illinois	Gary L. Clayton, 320 W. Washington St., Springfield 62786 (217) 782-0458
Indiana	William Keown, 1 American Sq., Suite 1020, Box 82067, Indianapolis 46282-0004 (317) 232-2960
Iowa	Norman C. Johnson, 1209 East Ct., Executive Hills West, Des Moines 50319 (515) 281-5944
Kansas	Tom Hitchcock, 900 Jackson, Room 513, Topeka 66612-1220 (913) 296-4056
Kentucky	Richard L. Ross, 1228 U.S. 127 S., Frankfort 40601 (502) 564-3833
Louisiana	Howard B. Bolton, 5615 Corporate Blvd., Suite 8E, Baton Rouge 70808 (504) 925-6496
Maine	Richard O. Campbell, 1 Northwood Rd., Lewiston 04240 (207) 783-9769
Maryland	Roslyn Scheer, 201 W. Preston St., Baltimore 21201 (301) 225-5910
Massachusetts	Harold R. Partamian, 100 Cambridge St., 15th Floor, Boston 02202 (617) 727-9955
Michigan	Cathy Seyka, P.O. Box 30018, 611 W. Ottawa St., Lansing 48909 (517) 373-0620
Minnesota	David E. Holmstrom, 2700 University Ave., W., #107, St. Paul 55114-1079 (612) 642-0541
Mississippi	H. W. Holleman, 2310 Hwy. 80, W., Suite 1165, Jackson 39204 (601) 354-6750
Missouri	Kevin E. Kinkade, P.O. Box 625, Jefferson City 65102 (314) 751-2334
Montana	Warren R. Amole Jr., 510 First Ave. N., Suite 100, Great Falls 59401 (406) 761-5131 or 444-5436
Nebraska	Leland C. Lucke, P.O. Box 95007, 301 Centennial Mall S., Lincoln 68509 (402) 471-2115
Nevada	David Boston, 1201 Terminal Way, Suite 212, Reno 89502 (702) 322-0691
New Hampshire	Paul G. Boisseau, Health & Human Services Building, Hazen Dr., Concord 03301 (603) 271-2350
New Jersey	Robert J. Terranova, 1100 Raymond Blvd., Suite 325, Newark 07102 (201) 648-2433
New Mexico	Charles A. Pineau, 4125 Carlisle, N.E., Albuquerque 87107 (505) 841-6311

New York	Cultural Education Center, Room, 3035 Albany 12230 (518) 474-3848
North Carolina	David R. Work, P.O. Box H, 602H Jones Ferry Rd., Carrboro 27510 (919) 942-4454
North Dakota	William J. Grosz, P.O. Box 1354, Bismarck 58502 (701) 258-1535
Ohio	Franklin Z. Wickham, 65 Front St., Room 504, Columbus 43266-0320 (614) 466-4143
Oklahoma	Joe Schwemin, 4545 N. Lincoln, Suite 112, Oklahoma City 73105 (405) 521-3815
Oregon	Ruth Vandever, 1400 S.W. Fifth Ave., State Office Building, Room 904A, P.O. Box 231, Portland 97207 (503) 229-5849
Pennsylvania	Maurice Mervis, Box 2649, Harrisburg 17105 (717) 783-7157
Puerto Rico	Irza Torres Aguiar, P.O. Box 9342, 800 Robert J. Todd Ave. Ext. 222, Santurce 00908 (809) 725-8161
Rhode Island	Felix A. Lima, 304 Cannon Building, 75 Davis St., Providence 02908 (401) 277-2837
South Carolina	C. Douglas Chavous, P.O. Box 11927, Columbia 29211 (803) 734-1010
South Dakota	Galen Jordre, Box 518 Pierre 57501 (605) 224-2338
Tennessee	J. Floyd Ferrel! Jr., 1808 West End Building, 10th Floor Nashville, 37219-5322 (615) 741-2718
Texas	Fred S. Brinkley, Jr., 8505 Cross Park Dr., Suite 110, Austin 78754 (512) 832-0661
Utah	David E. Robinson, 160 East 300 S., P.O. Box 45802, Salt Lake City 84145 (801) 530-6634
Vermont	James F. Milne, Pavilion Office Building, Montpelier 05602 (802) 828-2372
Virginia	J. B. Carson, 1601 Rolling Hills Dr., Richmond 23229 (804) 662-9911
Washington	Donald H. Williams, 319 E. Seventh Ave., WEA Building, FF-21, Olympia 98504 (206) 753-6834
West Virginia	C. Herbert Traubert, 150 Rockdale Rd., Follansbee 26037 (304) 527-1270
Wisconsin	Robert Ward, P.O. Box 8935, 1400 E. Washington Ave., Madison 53708 (608) 266-8794
Wyoming	Marilynn H. Mitchell, 1720 S. Poplar St., Suite 5, Casper 82601 (307) 234-0294

Appendix D: Licensure Requirements

A State-by-State Rundown of Requirements

All states require candidates for licensure to have graduated from an accredited college of pharmacy and to be of good moral character. All states, except California, use the National Association of Boards of Pharmacy Licensure Examination (NABPLEX®). Virtually every state allows students to retake the exam in case of failure. (A few states also require students to take the Federal Drug Law Exam or a practical exam. Contact the appropriate state board about additional examinations.) Some states require full citizenship, and many states require a candidate to be at least 18 years of age.

Most states will grant a license on the basis of the candidate having been licensed in another state. Individual state boards can be contacted for special requirements and fees. There are two states that do not reciprocate licensure—Florida and California.

	Internship Requirements			
State	**Total Hours**	**Postgrad Hours**	**Continuing Education Requirements for Licensure**	**Industry Intern Credit**
Alabama	1,500	400	15 hours a year	No
Alaska	1,500	160	15 hours a year	No
Arizona	1,500	None	30 hours in two years	500 hours
Arkansas	2,000	1,000	6 hours a year	May be allowed
California	1,500	1,000*	30 hours in two years	Yes
Colorado	1,800	200	No	No
Connecticut	1,500	None	Proposed	May be allowed
Delaware	1,500	None	30 hours in two years	500 hours
District of Columbia	1,500/1,000	None	Proposed	No
Florida	2,080 (varies)	None	15 hours a year	No
Georgia	1,500	None	30 hours in two years	No
Hawaii	2,000	None	No	Yes
Idaho	1,500	None	15 hours a year	One-half credit
Illinois	400	None	30 hours in two years	No
Indiana	1,040	520	30 hours in two years	No
Iowa	1,500	None	30 hours in two years	May be allowed
Kansas	1,500	None	15 hours a year	May be allowed
Kentucky	1,500	None	15 hours a year	400 hours
Louisiana	1,500/1 year	500	15 hours a year	No
Maine	1,500	None	15 hours a year	May be allowed
Maryland	1,560	None	Proposed	Yes
Massachusetts	1,500	None	30 hours in two years	Up to 400 hours
Michigan	1,000	None	30 hours in two years	Up to 400 hours
Minnesota	1,500	None	30 hours in two years	May be allowed
Mississippi	1,500	None	20 hours in two years	300 hours
Missouri	1,500	None	10 hours a year	200 hours
Montana	1,500	None	15 hours a year	May be allowed
Nebraska	1,500	None	30 hours in two years	May be allowed
Nevada	1,500	None	30 hours in two years	No
New Hampshire	1,500	None	15 hours a year	May be allowed
New Jersey	1,000	Varies	30 hours in two years	No
New Mexico	1 year	None	15 hours a year	Yes
New York	6 months	None	No	No
North Carolina	1,500	None	10 hours a year	Up to 500 hours

Continued on next page

State	Internship Requirements: Total Hours	Internship Requirements: Postgrad Hours	Continuing Education Requirements for Licensure	Industry Intern Credit
North Dakota	1,500	None	30 hours in two years	400 hours
Ohio	1,500	None	45 hours in three years	300 hours
Oklahoma	2,000	None	15 hours a year	Yes
Oregon	1,500	400	15 hours a year	No
Pennsylvania	1,500	None	30 hours in two years‡	300 hours
Puerto Rico	1,000	None	35 hours in three years	300 hours
Rhode Island	1,500	None	15 hours a year	One-half credit
South Carolina	1,500	None	Proposed	1,000 hours max.
South Dakota	1,500	None	12 hours a year	400 hours
Tennessee	1,500	None	15 hours a year	Up to 500 hours
Texas	1,500	None	No	May be allowed
Utah	1,500	None	No	May be allowed
Vermont	1,500	None	Proposed	Up to 750 hours
Virginia	6 months	None	No	Yes
Washington	1,500	None	15 hours a year	300 hours
West Virginia	1,500	None	Proposed	520 hours
Wisconsin	2,000	1,000	No	500 hours
Wyoming	1,500	None	6 hours a year	500 hours

Appendix E: General References

Pharmaceutics

Ansel, HC: *Introduction to Pharmaceutical Dosage Forms*, 4th ed, Lea & Febiger, Philadelphia, 1985

Gennaro, AR: *Remington's Pharmaceutical Sciences*, 17th ed, Mack Publishing, Easton, Pa., 1985

Gibaldi, M: *Biopharmaceutics and Clinical Pharmacokinetics*, 3rd ed, Lea & Febiger, Philadelphia, 1984

Lachman, L.; Lieberman, HH; Kanig, JL: *The Theory and Practice of Industrial Pharmacy*, 3rd ed, Lea & Febiger, Philadelphia, 1986

Martin, A; Swarbrick, J; Cammarata, A: *Physical Pharmacy*, 3rd ed, Lea & Febiger, Philadelphia, 1983

Notari, RE: *Biopharmaceutics and Clinical Pharmacokinetics. An Introduction*, 4th ed, Marcel Dekker, Inc., New York, 1987

Rowland, M; Tozer, TN: *Clinical Pharmacokinetics. Concepts and Applications*, 2nd ed, Lea & Febiger, Philadelphia, 1989

Shargel, L; Yu, ABC: *Applied Biopharmaceutics and Pharmacokinetics*, 2nd ed, Appleton-Century-Crofts, Norwalk, Conn., 1985

Stoklosa, MJ; Ansel, AC: *Pharmaceutical Calculations*, 8th ed, Lea & Febiger, Philadelphia, 1986

The United States Pharmacopeia XXI, United States Pharmacopeial Convention, Inc., Rockville, Md., 1985

Medicinal Chemistry and Pharmacology

Albert, A: *Selective Toxicity*, 7th ed, Chapman and Hall, New York, 1985

Csaky, TZ; Barnes, BA: *Cutting's Handbook of Pharmacology*, 7th ed, Appleton-Century-Crofts, Norwalk, Conn., 1984

Doull, J; Klaassen, CD; Amdur, MO: *Casarett and Doull's Toxicology. The Basic Science of Poisons*, 2nd ed, MacMillan Publishing, New York, 1980

Foye, WO: *Principles of Medicinal Chemistry*, 3rd ed, Lea & Febiger, Philadelphia, 1989

Gibson, GG; Skett, P: *Introduction to Drug Metabolism*, Chapman and Hall, New York, 1986

Gilman, AG; Goodman, LS; Rall, TW; Murad, F: *Goodman and Gilman's The Pharmacologic Basis of Therapeutics*, Macmillan Publishing, New York, 1985

Jacob, LS: *Pharmacology*, 2nd ed, Harwal Publishing, Media, Pa., 1987

Lemke, TL: *Review of Organic Functional Groups: Introduction to Medicinal Organic Chemistry*, 2nd ed, Lea & Febiger, Philadelphia, 1988

Nogrady, T: *Medicinal Chemistry*, Oxford University Press, New York, 1988

Professional Pharmacy Practice

AMA Drug Evaluations, American Medical Association, WB Saunders, Philadelphia, 1986

Facts and Comparisons, Facts and Comparisons, Inc., JB Lippincott, St. Louis (published annually)

Handbook of Nonprescription Drugs, 8th ed, American Pharmaceutical Association, Washington, 1986

Hansten, PD; Horn, JR: *Drug Interactions*, 6th ed, Lea & Febiger, Philadelphia, 1989

Hassan, WE, Jr: *Hospital Pharmacy*, 5th ed, Lea & Febiger, Philadelphia, 1986

McElvoy, GK: *Drug Information*, American Society of Hospital Pharmacists, Bethesda, Md., 1989

Pharmacy Law Digest, Facts and Comparisons, Inc., JB Lippincott, St. Louis, 1988

Physicians' Desk Reference, Medical Economics, Oradell, N.J. (published annually)

Turco, S; King, RE: *Sterile Dosage Forms*, 3rd ed, Lea & Febiger, Philadelphia, 1987

United States Pharmacopeia Dispensing Information (three volumes), United States Pharmacopeial Convention, Rockville, Md., 1989

Clinical Pharmacy

Benet, LZ; Massoud, N; Gambertoglio, JG: *Pharmacokinetic Basis for Drug Treatment*, Raven Press, New York, 1984

Braunwald, E; Isselbacher, KJ; Petersdorf, RG; Martin, JB; Fauci, AS: *Harrison's Principles of Internal Medicine*, 11th ed, McGraw-Hill, New York, 1987

DiPiro, JT; Talbert, RL; Hayes, PE; Yee, PE; Posey, LM: *Pharmacotherapy. A Pathophysiologic Approach*, Elsevier, New York, 1988

Dorland's Illustrated Medical Dictionary, 27th ed, WB Saunders, Philadelphia, 1988

Evans, WE; Schentag JJ; Jusko, WJ: *Applied Pharmacokinetics. Principles of Therapeutic Drug Monitoring*, 2nd ed, Applied Therapeutics, Spokane, Wash., 1986

Haddad, LM; Winchester, JF: *Clinical Management of Poisoning and Drug Overdose*, WB Saunders, Philadelphia, 1983

Harvey, AM; Johns, RJ; McKusick, VA; Owen, AH, Jr; Ross, RS: *Principles and Practice of Medicine*, 21st ed, Appleton-Century-Crofts, Norwalk, Conn., 1984

Herfindal, ET; Hirschman, JL: *Clinical Pharmacy and Therapeutics*, 3rd ed, Williams & Wilkins, Baltimore, 1984

Knoben, JE; Anderson, PO: *Handbook of Clinical Drug Data*, 6th ed, Drug Intelligence Publications, Hamilton, Ill., 1988

Krupp, MA; Schroeder, SA; Tierney, LM, Jr: *Current Medical Diagnosis and Treatment*, Appleton-Lange, Norwalk, Conn., 1987

Orlando, MJ; Saltman, RJ: *Manual of Medical Therapeutics*, 25th ed, Little, Brown, Boston, 1986

Shirkey, HC: *Pediatric Therapy*, 5th ed, CV Mosby, St. Louis, 1975

Stedman's Medical Dictionary, 23rd ed, Williams & Wilkins, Baltimore, 1976

Wallach, J: *Interpretation of Diagnostic Tests*, Little, Brown, Boston, 1986

Young, LY; Koda-Kimble, MA: *Applied Therapeutics: The Clinical Use of Drugs*, 4th ed, Applied Therapeutics, Vancouver, Wash., 1988

Index

Page numbers in *italics* denote illustrations; those followed by (T) denote tables; those followed by Q denote questions; and those followed by E denote explanations.

A

C

D

E

I

P

Q

R

S

U

V

W

X

Z

Young's Rule

Child's Dose: = $\frac{\text{Age (yr)}}{\text{Age (yr)} + 12}$ x Adult dose

Clark's Rule

Child's Dose: $\frac{\text{Childs wt (lb)}}{150}$ x Adult dose

Lean Body mass

LBm = 110 lb + 5 lbs for every inch over 5feet

for males ↗

for females ↘

LBm = 100 lbs + 5 lbs for every inch over 5feet.

vol 70w/v

one fluid ounce of H_2O = 455 grains

one ounce (apoth) = 480 grains